ARTHROSCOPIC SURGERY

principles & practice

ARTHROSCOPIC SURGERY
principles & practice

Lanny L. Johnson, M.D.

Clinical Professor of Surgery
Michigan State University
College of Human Medicine
East Lansing, Michigan

VOLUMES ONE AND TWO

THIRD EDITION

with **3,196** illustrations, including **1,958** in full color

The C. V. Mosby Company

ST. LOUIS • TORONTO • PRINCETON   1986

MOSBY

A TRADITION OF PUBLISHING EXCELLENCE

Acquisition editor: Eugenia A. Klein
Developmental editor: Kathryn H. Falk
Manuscript editor: Timothy O'Brien
Book design: Kay M. Kramer
Cover design: John Rokusek
Production: Jeanne A. Gulledge

THIRD EDITION

The C.V. Mosby Company
11830 Westline Industrial Drive, St. Louis, Missouri 63146

Library of Congress Cataloging-in-Publication Data

Johnson, Lanny L., 1933-
  Arthroscopic surgery.

  Rev. ed. of: Diagnostic and surgical arthroscopy.
2nd ed. 1981.
  Includes bibliographies and index.
  1. Joints—Surgery. 2. Arthroscopy. I. Johnson,
Lanny L., 1933-   . Diagnostic and surgical
arthroscopy. II. Title. [DNLM: 1. Arthroscopy.
2. Joint Diseases. 3. Knee Joint—surgery. WE 870 J67c]
RD680.J65   1986   617'.472   85-31997
ISBN 0-8016-2591-2 (set)

C/W/W 9 8 7 6 5 4 3 2

i trust the book honors
my mother and father

JANET LUCE JOHNSON

and

WILLARD L. JOHNSON

1908-1982

Preface
to the third edition

This textbook was written for students by a student. In assembling this text, I have learned a great deal; I trust the reader will also.

My main motive has been to satisfy my curiosity. In the absence of our own observations or experiments, we are restricted to what someone else has said. Let's look for ourselves. I have not ignored what I have learned in the past, but I will not be bound by it. As a result, some material was, is, and will be controversial. It is not my desire to prove I am right, but to know what is right and to do it. To accomplish this purpose, observations must be subject to whether they are scientific or unscientific, believable or unbelievable, but especially true or untrue.

If there is error, I hope both you and I recognize it. It is my intent to be honest. Please forgive where the text is not perfect; it could not be, because the author isn't.

Arthroscopy is in its infancy. I believe that the present state of the art is a reflection of what will become standard operating procedure. The instruments, implants, and approaches may vary, but basic anatomical and pathological principles will be similar.

This textbook is not and should not be considered authoritative, as it represents only my experience. Limitations of time and space create deletions from literature. The necessity of concluding a manuscript for publication may explain the absence of certain topics to future readers. It seems the task of writing a book on arthroscopic surgery is like describing an atomic bomb explosion just before full development of mushroom cloud. If the publication date is delayed, then some of the excitement and unknown effects (fallout) of arthroscopy would be history.

The first text was entitled *The Comprehensive Arthroscopic Examination of the Knee*. That is all that could be said in 1977. The second edition, in 1981, was called *Diagnostic and Surgical Arthroscopy: The Knee and Other Joints*. Now, with arthroscopic procedures well integrated into orthopedics, this edition is titled *Arthroscopic Surgery: Principles and Practice*. With such rapid growth the next edition may well be called *Endoscopy in Orthopaedics*.

I have attempted to record principles that were anatomically sound, pathologically reasonable, and technically possible. Much of the emphasis is on biological rather than bionic solutions to the disease process. The inclusion of patient and practice management principles reflects arthroscopy's central position in orthopedic care. There is some intentional repetition, with cross-references to fuller discussions in other chapters. This was necessary because I anticipate this text will be used as a topical reference, and rarely read cover to cover.

I trust this text will benefit the serious surgeon and answer some questions for the curious. It should be a launching pad for understanding and ideas for both author and reader.

Finally I hope the information is helpful, the photos and drawings illustrative, and the reading a pleasant experience.

P.T.L.

Lanny L. Johnson

Preface
to second edition

When *Comprehensive Arthroscopic Examination of the Knee* was published in 1977, clinical trials were underway with the Intra-articular Shaver. Since then my practice has rapidly become that of an arthroscopic surgeon. I enjoy general orthopedics and still consider myself an orthropedic surgeon, yet the excitement and advancements in the field of arthroscopy cannot be ignored. I believe it will become a major discipline within orthopedic surgery.

I am concerned about the role of arthroscopic surgery in the care of patients. Arthroscopic surgery should not replace sound clinical judgment. It will not solve all knee problems. Proficiency in these techniques should not allow one to ignore or avoid treating ligamentous instability. Arthroscopy is not the only means to successful clinical results. Every effort has been made in this text to illustrate the role of arthroscopy in clinical management and care of a patient.

In preparation for this edition it was necessary to reread the first edition. It was apparent to me that my dogmatism would have to be tempered with the phrase "at the present time." The developments in arthroscopic surgery have been happening so fast that personal communication is required to keep pace. Even so, every effort has been made, including some last-minute revisions, to have this text reflect the state of the art at publication time. As my experience and knowledge increased, prejudices were broken. Methods and concepts are changing.

Knowledge of the knee joint is essential for a successful diagnostic arthroscopy. Basic arthroscopic skills must be mastered before progressing to even the simplest arthroscopic surgical manipulation. The comprehensive arthroscopic setup and surgical techniques should follow the development of these other skills.

Arthroscopic surgery was, and still is, technically difficult; but it is not impossible. It is not the summation of many tricks that leads to success, but rather sound surgical principles. These principles are just being applied in a different discipline from what we have been accustomed to, that is, endoscopic techniques and microsurgical instrumentation, as well as television monitoring. The careful integration of established surgical principles such as exposure, asepsis, hemostasis, and gentleness to this new medium will yield clinical success. This text is dedicated to the demonstration of a rationale for this method of treatment, an exploration of technical details, and encouragement. Arthroscopic surgery is a means of treatment that produces less morbidity and results equal to, if not better than, previously established methods.

Arthroscopic surgical techniques are best learned by observation of a surgeon experienced in these methods. Repeat visits are recommended after personal experience has been gained. The surgeon should not enter into this adventure halfway. Purchase of all the necessary equipment is essential for success. Perhaps most important is an abundance of patience. The yields in knowledge and understanding make one forget the toil of plowing, planting, and harvesting.

This text is not intended to be a "consumer's report." The instruments shown are those which were available and most fitting at the time the techniques were being developed. There are many good arthroscopes and instruments that are not mentioned in this book. It was not economical to purchase duplicates of each tool from various companies. Therefore no attempt has been made to evaluate or make comparisons of companies producing various products. The equipment demonstrated has produced satisfactory results in my experience.

This text is truly a composition. The term "we" clearly reflects the team effort so essential in arthroscopic surgery. The acknowledgments identify the many contributors. Many of the concepts and maneuvers outlined might seem simple and obvious to you; they did to us also after we had thought of them.

I have come to understand that what I called training and experience was often just prejudicial thinking. The arthroscopic surgical experience has convinced me of that, and I hope this text will challenge you and some of your previous concepts.

Again, P.T.L.

Lanny L. Johnson

Preface
to first edition

Arthroscopy is a dynamic, colorful, and exciting experience for the physician. It is best appreciated by performing the procedure. A one-on-one method of teaching is ideal, but because of time and logistics, it is just not possible. The second-best method of experiencing arthroscopy or learning the technique is by movie photography or television.

In this book, an attempt has been made to duplicate the experience of arthroscopy by logos, photographic selection, diagrams, and design. The color illustrations were carefully chosen to be representative rather than comprehensive.

This book is written for the physician who desires the practical details necessary to successfully accomplish a complete inspection of the knee joint. A description of technical details is necessarily labored. The role of the assistant is included to help the inexperienced arthroscopist.

The physician who perseveres will be rewarded with increased knowledge from arthroscopy. The patient will benefit in better diagnostic judgments and therapeutic designs.

I acknowledge and am exceedingly grateful to my assistant, Mrs. Ruth L. Becker, LPN, who has contributed many of the details of this technique. Her contribution has been recognized by the many visiting physicians as being the most essential ingredient in my ability to perform arthroscopy so easily. I agree.

I appreciate the encouragement I received from Dr. David Shneider, who has been able to completely duplicate this technique with great facility and finesse. Using these methods, he has made observations that have added to my understanding.

Gloria Aveiro typed manuscript and revisions at times undoubtedly inconvenient for her; for this I am grateful. For most of the black-and-white photographs, I thank Tom A. Cannel.

Most of all I appreciate Mary Ann, my wife, and our daughters, Charlotte Ann and Autumn Lynn, who have been faithful in many adventures, including this book.

P.T.L.

Lanny L. Johnson

Acknowledgments

Thank you, Mary Ann, for being my wife (and remaining so during the writing of this book). To Charlotte and Autumn, my daughters, who accepted quality time instead of quantity and now will have both.

Ruth Becker, L.P.N., my assistant for many years, has been loyal and thought the best of me and has not taken into account any wrong suffered through it all.

I acknowledge my colleagues, both supporters and detractors. The supporters provided comfort and encouragement, the detractors incentive. Without both, complacency could have set in, course corrections ignored, and completeness neglected.

I appreciated the tutorage of Eugene Bricker, Fred C. Reynolds, the late H. Relton McCarroll, the late Arthur H. Stein, Jr., and Joseph A. Boyes for influencing the surgeon in me. I have often borrowed on their example and instruction during this arthroscopic adventure.

My professional associates have given much of their time, ideas and support. Thanks to Michael D. Austin, James M. Bullock, David A. Detrisac, Floyd G. Goodman, David Shneider, and John A. Jerome.

The staff of the arthroscopy suite at Ingham Medical Center have patiently labored through many changes and rechanges, locally known as progress. They are:

Cynthia Everett, R.N., C.N.O.R., Judith Penrod, R.N., and Joan Dufresne, R.N.

Jean Fox, S.T., Julie Murray, C.S.T., and Susan Harris, L.P.N. Unit secretary, Sally Lopez. Orderly, Thomas Krycinski. Recovery room nurse, Helen Reck, R.N. ASC outpatient nurses, Betty Lockwood, R.N., and Carole Fairman, R.N.

The physicians and staff of Ingham Medical Center's pathology department were responsible for providing histopathological material. Their willingness to cut, recut, stain, and restain specimens is appreciated. They are B. Newton, M.D., E. Elsenety, M.D., M. Fatteh, M.D., M. Jimenez, Sue Rinckey, Gain Kelly, Sally Walker, Doug Porter, Mary Bryhan, Amy Fickies, Carol Crampton, Mary Ann Rogers, and Tricia Fraas.

A thank-you is not enough for the patience given and accommodations made by anesthesiologists Bert Bez, Suk Chang, Y. Chi, Darryl Smith, Dennis Wyatt, and Wayne Hanish.

Because technology was such a great part of arthroscopic development, it could not have happened without many friends from industry. Leonard Bonnell and I were side by side in developing motorized instrumentation. Doug Sjostrom provided prototypes that did what I hoped. Robert Brissette engineered the arthroplasty system, bringing a new demension to reconstructive procedures in arthroscopy.

More recently Gordon Robinson, Dan Bauman, and Paul Dean have brought my computerized medical record to reality.

Thanks to Dean Z. Look for managing recent developments in the arthroscopic environment and instruments and devices for reconstructive procedures in the knee and shoulder.

The actual production of this text was more difficult for me than learning arthroscopic surgery was. Eugenia Klein, Kathy Falk, Tim O'Brien, and Jeanne Gulledge and the other people at C.V. Mosby probably could have learned arthroscopy with a similar effort. They made this text possible.

At my end, Karen Lindstromberg got me started with the manuscript. Mary Jo Slingerland was Mosby's velvet-covered iron-fist enforcer, walking me through the rereading and the other details that were not my favorite activities.

Thanks to Richard Fritzler for illustrations we all can appreciate. (You should know that I restricted his artistic ability in favor of simplicity.)

As you can see, I am just the author of this book that had many, many contributors.

P.T.L.

Lanny L. Johnson

Contents

Contents

Contents

Contents

Development

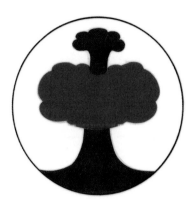

The use of the arthroscope has dramatically changed the practice of orthopedic surgery. Present techniques evolved from the contributions of many pioneers of arthroscopy. In 1931, Takagi used a 3.5 mm diameter endoscope in a joint distended with fluid to perform what was probably the first arthroscopic procedure.[50] That same year, Burman published data dealing primarily with arthroscopy of the knee and other joints in cadavers[7,8] (Fig. 1-1). Watanabe developed some basic principles for arthroscopy of the knee as well as an arthroscope that bears his name.[50] His techniques were brought to North America in 1968 by Dr. Robert W. Jackson of Toronto.[25]

Casscells published a book on diagnostic arthroscopy of the knee in 1971.[11] At about the same time, O'Connor had the vision to move beyond diagnostic into operative arthroscopy.[41,42]

Enormous technological advances in arthroscopy occurred during the 1970s. The bulk of arthroscopic history can be found in contemporary literature. Eikelaar,[15] Fraider,[19] Joyce and Jackson,[32] and Orbon and Poehling[43] have presented excellent comprehensive historical reviews of arthroscopy. I have made no attempt to duplicate their efforts; this book concerns itself with more recent developments.

The clinical value of arthroscopy was questioned even into the mid-1970s. At this time, American orthopedic surgeons could be divided into three categories: those who looked and saw something—the "look-see" group; those who looked and did not see anything—the "look-no-see" group; and those who did not choose to look—the "no-look" group. The "look-see" group was very enthusiastic and was identified by various and sundry labels by others. The "look-no-see"

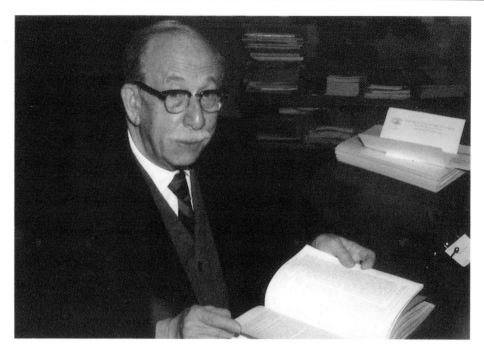

FIG. 1-1. Dr. Michael Burman, 1901-1975. His vision for arthroscopy was demonstrated by cadaver experiments in 1931. (Courtesy Sierge Parisian.)

TABLE 1-1. Percentages of survey respondents performing arthroscopy

	Diagnostic	Knee	Operative	Other joints
1978*		50%		6%
1981	50%		75%	5%
1983	75%		98%	26%

*No designation of diagnostic or operative was available in 1978.

group became discouraged. The "no-look" group determined that arthroscopy was a fad, and these people often professed that they could make a better diagnosis clinically. Of course, the arthroscopic revolution followed.

In the early 1970s, it was easy to know personally every surgeon in the United States who performed arthroscopy. Now, a little more than 10 years later, it might be possible to know every surgeon who does not. The results of the 1978 membership questionnaire of the American Academy of Orthopaedic Surgeons showed that 50% of the respondents used arthroscopy. A similar survey in 1981 showed that 75% used arthroscopic techniques, and by 1983, arthroscopy was used by 98%. Table 1-1 summarizes the responses of orthopedic surgeons to the various questionnaires. The future for arthroscopic surgical technique in the United States appears to be even greater; the results of a survey I undertook in 1982 indicated that 98% of residents in orthopedics planned to include arthroscopic surgery in their orthopedic practices.[31]

INSTRUMENTATION
Arthroscopes

The Watanabe No. 21 arthroscope had a large diameter and a light bulb attached to the end. It was a bulky instrument. There was risk of injurious heat and fracture of the light bulb.

Subsequently, endoscopes using conventional lens systems were introduced. These were rapidly replaced by the Hopkins design rod-lens systems.

In 1970 the first miniature self-focusing arthroscope was developed through the joint efforts of the Nippon Sheet Glass Company and the Department of Orthopedic Surgery in Tokoyo Teishin Hospital. The scope, 1.7 mm in diameter, was used through a cannula having an outside diameter of 2 mm and provided a 37-degree field of view in saline. It was introduced in North America in 1972 by Mr. Leonard Bonnell. To my knowledge it was first used for arthroscopy by Drs. Clement Sledge and J. Drennan Lowell at the Robert Brigham Hospital in Boston.

After viewing their technique, Mr. Harold Neumann assessed the uses and the requirements for such a small-diameter endoscope. The original Watanabe No. 24 arthroscope was redesigned in four ways. The diameter of the arthroscope was increased from 1.7 to 2.2 mm, which improved the illumination by a factor of four and resulted in more rugged assembly. The design was changed to allow for an adaptable light guide to improve handling and ease of sterilization. The eyepiece, which required manual focusing, was changed to a fixed focal length to eliminate confusion and contamination during the procedure. A long, lightweight handle was designed for manipulation of the arthroscope and positioning of the ocular at a distance from the surgeon's hand; in this way the physician's head and eye were away from the sterile field, and his or her sterile gloved hand was protected from potential contamination.

The three-piece instrument, the Needlescope, was available for the market in the fall of 1972 (Fig. 1-2). It had an inclined view of approximately 15 degrees and a field of view of 47 degrees in saline. It was rejected by many arthroscopists because of its fragility, low illumination, and reduced optical clarity as compared with existing larger-diameter endoscopes of different construction.

By June 1976 a third model of the Needlescope was available. It had an enhanced optical design, including a better lens to increase its field of view in saline to 70 degrees while retaining the 15-degree inclined view. Another modification improved the light illumination capacity by at least two f-stops. Now there was a small-diameter endoscope with an angle of vision comparable to a larger endoscope and the optical clarity of larger arthroscopes. The use of television enhanced the brightness electronically.

Recently interest in arthroscopy of smaller joints, not only diagnostic but operative, has revived interest in small-diameter arthroscopes. I now use a Storz small-diameter rod-lens scope. It has excellent optics for both direct and television viewing (see Fig. 4-2).

Originally the small diameter of the Needlescope made it an excellent alternative to the Watanabe scope in the knee joint. The small diameter allowed punc-

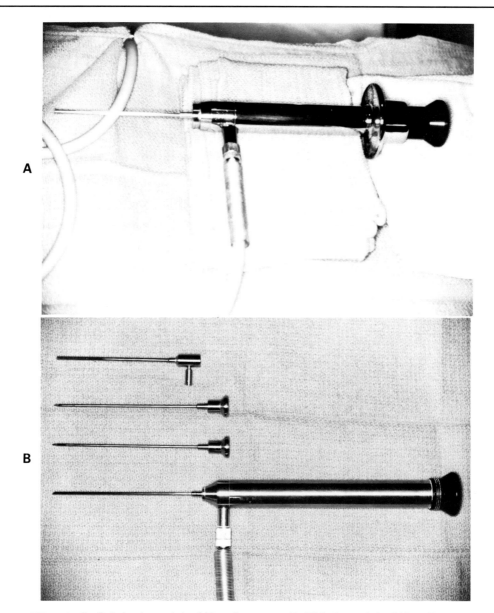

FIG. 1-2. A, Original model of Needlescope. **B,** Third model of Needlescope.

ture wounds small enough for local anesthesia, which was especially important when the arthroscopic procedure preceded an arthrotomy. As routine arthroscopic surgical procedures developed in the late 1970s, a 30-degree inclined view rod-lens endoscope became the instrument of choice (see Fig. 4-2). It had a field of view of 80 degrees in air. It provided optical clarity, greater light-carrying capacity, and better illumination for image transmission on television. In 1985 Storz introduced the 120-degree field of view, 4 mm arthroscope. The wider view is of benefit for photography and nondynamic viewing of large areas of the joint. The 90-degree angle or inclined-view scope is of benefit for orientation and visualization of patellar tracking or extended viewing in the shoulder joint to see over the anterior glenoid from the posterior portal. These arthroscopes are only used in conjunction with the 4 mm, 30-degree inclined view of Hopkins rod-lens design.

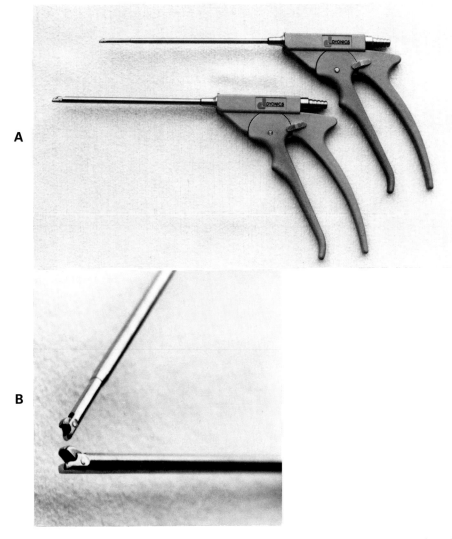

FIG. 1-3. A, The Dyonics vacuum suction punch represents recent developments in hand instrumentation. **B,** Close-up view of the tips.

Hand instrumentation

The original hand instrumentation for arthroscopy was borrowed from other disciplines; the neurosurgical Dandy probe, the gynecological basket resection forceps, and microsurgical knife blades. From this beginning, modifications were made to adapt the instruments to the arthroscopic environment (see Chapter 4).

Presently hand instruments designed specifically for arthroscopic surgery are available. The probes now go through cannula systems. The cutting shapes of the basket forceps are more conforming, effective, and durable. Various configurations available range from 0 to 90 degrees of angulation. The most recent advancement is the suction punch developed by the Dyonics Corporation in conjunction with Dr. Terry Whipple (Fig. 1-3).

The microsurgical knife blades originally used have been replaced with

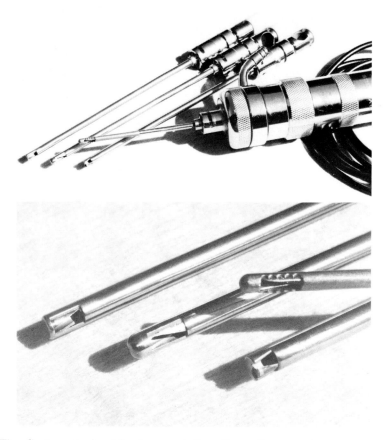

FIG. 1-4. The first motorized instrumentation for arthroscopic surgery was introduced by Dyonics, Inc., in 1978.

blades that have less potential for breakage. The configurations of the knives are designed to conform to the condylar shape. Retrograde blades are available for various specific tasks of cutting meniscus or retinaculum.

Hand instrumentation for arthroscopy has expanded from instruments for resection to instruments for repair. Several manufacturers have introduced meniscus suturing systems. A stapling system for knee and shoulder ligaments has also been developed.

Motorized instrumentation

In 1976 the first motorized instrumentation for arthroscopic surgery was developed by me in collaboration with engineer Leonard Bonnell. Our purpose was to develop a powered cutter for arthroscopic surgical meniscectomy. Because it seemed technically impossible at the time to expose the meniscus, we chose the spacious patellofemoral area and chondromalacia as the pathological model. Using a heart-lung machine for flow measurements, we demonstrated the ability to debride and remove intraarticular tissue through a motorized rotating-cutting device with suction. The device was called the Intra-articular Shaver System and was marketed by Dyonics. The development of various resection shapes followed, including the cutter, the whisker, and the trimmer, as well as the original bullet-shaped shaver (Fig. 1-4). This greatly facilitated arthroscopic techniques including meniscectomy and chondroplasty.

In 1979 I, in conjunction with Mr. Robert Brissette, developed the Abrasion Arthroplasty System including its abrader and synovial resectors (see Fig. 4-47). This allowed further opportunities for arthroscopic surgery in cases of synovial disease and degenerative arthritis. Later, the same instruments played an integral role in the development of arthroscopic reconstructive procedures. These systems have been integrated with a new electric motor, electronically keyed drain cases, and power supply. It is now called the Dyonics Arthroscopic Surgical System (see Fig. 4-44).

ARTHROSCOPIC TECHNIQUES
Diagnostic arthroscopy

Originally arthroscopic procedures were performed with the patient under general anesthesia. These procedures were done with the Watanabe No. 21 endoscope, which required an incision of approximately 1 cm and a rather elaborate irrigation system through the endoscope. This was a single-portal technique, which allowed only limited visualization of the anterior or superior chambers. McGinty and O'Connor subsequently adapted the rod-lens arthroscope to the classic Watanabe technique.

The instrumentation for arthroscopic surgical procedures was not well developed in 1972. Therefore it seemed that, although the prospect of viewing the anterior chambers of the knee joint was attractive, the length of the procedure, the size of the incision including suture closure, and the use of a general anesthetic detracted from the clinical practical application of arthroscopy. In fact, it seemed at that time to me and to others that it was difficult to make a strong argument for arthroscopic inspection when the knee joint, especially its anterior chambers, could be better visualized by an arthrotomy with less time and effort than by arthroscopy. Unfortunately, the same reasoning continued into the late 1970s, with many prominent surgeons indicating that the clinical examination was better than any possible arthroscopic evaluation. By 1984 this argument had passed.

I was not attracted to the Watanabe technique because of the objections previously mentioned. Instead my attention was directed to the Needlescope and the possibility of performing diagnostic arthroscopy using local anesthesia. On October 30, 1972 I performed arthroscopy using the Needlescope with the patient under local anesthesia and with tourniquet control. This procedure was performed on an athlete who had reinjured his knee after conventional knee surgery. The joint was examined and a loose body identified; this was subsequently removed by arthrotomy. The intraarticular structures were visualized, the joint was cleansed, and a diagnosis of postsurgical degenerative arthritis with nonradiopaque loose bodies was confirmed.

I was excited about the ease with which this examination was accomplished and the observations I had made. My enthusiasm was not shared by others. In fact, the endoscope manufacturer doubted the success of the procedure on the basis of letters received from established arthroscopists. Although there were limitations in technique and interpretation of the arthroscopic image, I was encouraged enough to offer this procedure to other patients with knee problems. In the following month I performed ten arthroscopies. This experience increased my confidence and ability to visualize the interior compartment of the joint by arthroscopy with local anesthetic. Subsequently, I learned that Bircher reported arthroscopic examinations using a local anesthetic.[6] Also, Clayton had used the Watanabe No. 21 arthroscope with a local anesthetic in the suprapatellar pouch in patients with rheumatoid arthritis in the 1960s.[12]

It was impossible to see the entire meniscus from the anterior portal, even with a small scope. This necessitated inspection of the posterior compartments transcutaneously to see the posteromedial and posterolateral areas of the meniscus. I reported on my experiences with my first 100 cases of diagnostic arthroscopy of the knee at the International Congress at Rotterdam, the Netherlands, in 1973.[29] Most of the cases were performed with the patient under local anesthesia.

In 1975 I reported my first 400 diagnostic arthroscopic cases performed with a local anesthetic at the annual meeting of the American Academy of Orthopaedic Surgeons. The routine arthroscopy included multiple punctures: posteromedial, posterolateral, and suprapatellar. The patients were not given preoperative medication or any intraarticular anesthetic agent. The technique was developed to such a state that the multiple arthroscopic punctures were little different from multiple needle aspiration sites. Visualization was comprehensive. The short operative time was the result of abundant case experience. A detailed analysis of these cases was included in the first edition of this text.

Anesthesia

Subsequently McGinty and Mapza reported a method of outpatient local anesthesia in 1978.[38] They used not only lidocaine in the skin but also bupivacaine (Marcaine) intraarticularly for long-lasting anesthetic effect. This allowed them to perform arthroscopies of up to 1 hour in duration. There are now a number of reports in the literature concerning the use of local anesthesics and arthroscopy. Most arthroscopic procedures are performed with general anesthesia and integrate the diagnostic and operative procedures.

Other joints

In 1977 Dr. David Shneider and I showed an exhibit on arthroscopy of the shoulder, elbow, and ankle at the American Academy of Orthopaedic Surgeons meeting in Las Vegas. It attracted very little attention. Since that time the use of diagnostic arthroscopy of other joints has increased, so that approximately 26% of surgeons were performing that type of procedure by September, 1983 (see Table 1-1).

Operative arthroscopy

The first arthroscopic meniscectomies were reported in 1925 by Dr. Philip H. Kreuscher in the Illinois Medical Journal.[34] The author proposed this as a reasonable method and advised total meniscectomy. Watanabe reported his first arthroscopic meniscectomy in 1962.

Dr. Richard O'Connor introduced operative arthroscopy to the United States. His procedure involved resecting meniscal tissue with the use of instrumentation borrowed from other disciplines, primarily the basket forceps. He developed an operating arthroscope. This instrument combined an arthroscope with adjacent channels for instrument delivery, and it permitted visualization of the lesion and placement of instruments in front of the arthroscope.

Dr. Robert W. Metcalf's superb technical skills, audiovisual demonstrations, case experience, and seminar presentation advanced arthroscopic surgery. He introduced the concepts of probing and triangulation. These techniques compensated for the two-dimensional imagery of endoscopic viewing. Triangulation also provided a means of learning coordination of two instruments within the joint. These techniques facilitated the introduction of hand surgical instrumentation. Metcalf emphasized atraumatic technique and preservation of meniscal tissue. The controversy of partial versus total meniscal resection was settled by the arthroscopic observations of McGinty and Metcalf.

After it was established that partial meniscectomy was preferable to total, attention was shifted to repair. Both Hughston and DeHaven reported on open surgical meniscal repair, and the possibility of arthroscopic meniscal healing was introduced. In the second edition of this textbook, I reported arthroscopic observations of meniscal vascularity that supported Scapenelli's injection studies. Arnoczky and Warren repeated the injection studies, with emphasis on the human meniscus.

Several surgeons have demonstrated various arthroscopic techniques of performing meniscal repair.[11a,23a] Arnoczky and Warren have reported on dog meniscal repair, including vascular injection studies and the concept of vascular access channels.[3] Recently they demonstrated meniscal grafting in dogs using cryopreserved allografts. I have recently performed both pedicle-based rotational and free meniscal autografts in humans (see Chapter 11).

Metcalf's observations of the benefits of arthroscopically monitored lateral release were supported by McGinty for patellar subluxation and dislocation.

Dr. Ronald Yamamoto reported on the concept of medial retinacular repair for acute patellar dislocation. Dr. Michael D. Austin, one of my associates, introduced arthroscopic patellar realignment with medial imbrication. In this surgery the patella is repositioned (see Chapter 10).

Arthroscopically delivered implants have been introduced for repair of ligaments (see Chapters 12 and 15).

Arthroscopic surgical techniques have been expanded to the treatment of intraarticular fractures of the femoral and tibial condyles.[26a]

Since 1982 I have been treating selected cases of anterior cruciate ligament injuries by arthroscopic methods. Experimental artificial cruciate ligament replacements are being performed by arthroscopically monitored procedures.

Arthroscopic management of degenerative joint disease has included partial- and full-thickness debridement and even resection of osteophytes. Arthroscopic debridement may be combined with high tibial osteotomy. Osteochondritic lesions are also amenable to reconstitution by arthroscopic means (see Chapter 9).

Arthroscopic synovectomy is used in both rheumatoid and degenerative joint disease (see Chapter 13).

Like diagnostic arthroscopy, operative arthroscopy has been extended to joints other than the knee. Debridement procedures have been performed on most synovial joints. Andrews et al. (1984) have adapted arthroscopic techniques to treat the shoulders of throwing athletes. The shoulder joint is the focus of most of the attention at present. Gross, Wiley, and I have devised arthroscopic procedures to repair the Bankart lesion of recurrent dislocation of the shoulder (see Chapter 15). Furthermore both Wiley and I have seen the benefits of arthroscopic debridement in rotator cuff disease, even with tears. I have extended the treatment to arthroscopic subacromial bursectomy, acromionectomy, and coracoacromial ligament sectioning in anterior impingement syndromes. Rotator cuff repairs have been performed by Caspari, Hergenroder, and me using a miniature staple.[9,24a] Arthroscopic ankle fusion has been successfully performed at Ingham Medical Center.[47]

OTHER ENERGY SOURCES FOR ARTHROSCOPIC SURGERY

In 1981, in response to a problem hemoarthrosis following lateral release surgery, Dr. James M. Fox popularized the use of electrocautery cutting and electrocoagulation in patellar lateral retinacular release. This technique requires special instrumentation and knowledge of electroconductivity. It is performed in a medium of CO_2 or sterile water. Fox has demonstrated, as have others, that this decreases the incidence of postoperative hemarthrosis. Hemostasis may be improved by electrocautery and most specifically electrocoagulation.

There are some potential disadvantages. First there is the possibility of the rare electrical current accident. The possibility of severe postoperative pain caused by water extravasation must also be managed. The operative procedure is slower than knife blade cutting, and the equipment is expensive for a single-use procedure.

Ewing has further investigated the possibility of expanding the use of electrosurgery within arthroscopy.[17] He has devised various cutting tips that allow meniscal resection, and he is encouraged by his early results. The potential for articular cartilage injury does exist because the electrosurgical energy is neither unidirectional nor polarized, but rather a multidirectional dispersion of energy.

Whipple et al. have done some excellent basic laboratory work in the use of laser for arthroscopic meniscectomy[52] (Fig. 1-5). They showed that the CO_2 laser could resect meniscal tissue in laboratory animals. The problems include removal of smoke and debris, inaccurate beam direction, and the drying effect of the CO_2 medium on tissues. The debris or char was cleansed from the joint within approximately 4 weeks. The remaining tissue, adjacent to the meniscus cut, demonstrated good healing. Drying in the CO_2 air medium was not a problem if the operative procedure was short. Presently these researchers are developing a laser-competent arthroscope in anticipation of future human investigation.

At the same time, Drs. James B. Smith and Thomas Nancst have carried out arthroscopic laser surgical procedures on patients. They circumvented injury to the adjacent tissue by cutting close to the tip of the probe, where temperatures did not reach 50° Centigrade. A temperature at which protein coagulates was reached less than 1 mm from the tip of the probe. They believe that the meniscus is a poor heat conductor and therefore that injury to the adjacent tissues is unlikely. In fact, they point out that the injury of approximately 75 μm would be produced by a conventional scapel incision. This depth of cutting is supported by Whipple et al.[51,52].

Their initial clinical trials were done in CO_2 medium, and various inflows and suction apparatus were used to keep smoke and debris off the laser lens. The intraarticular pressure was at 80 mm Hg. A red light from a helium-neon

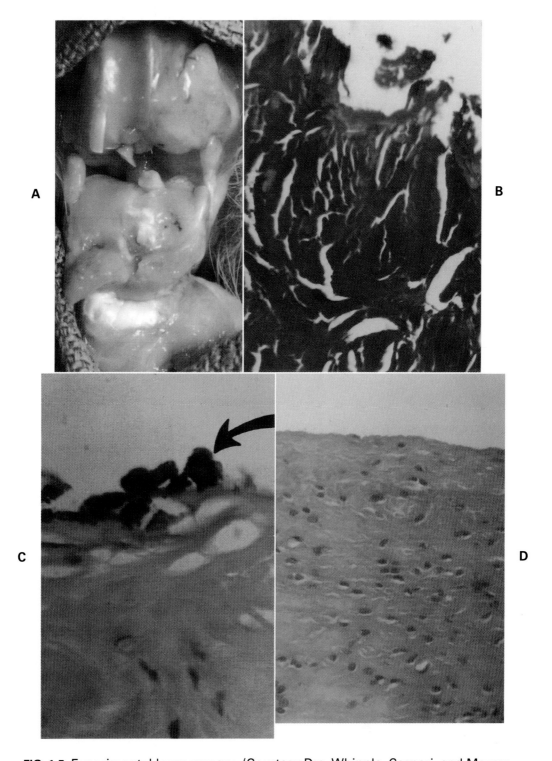

FIG. 1-5. Experimental laser surgery. (Courtesy Drs. Whipple, Caspari, and Meyers, Richmond, Virginia.) **A,** Gross photograph shows char on and adjacent to meniscus. **B,** Photomicrograph of minimal debris immediately postoperative. **C,** High-power photomicrograph of char on surface. **D,** Photomicrograph of healed surface at 6 weeks.

laser aims the invisible CO_2 beam at the meniscus. A foot switch activates the laser shutter. The laser energy strikes precisely at the point indicated by the red dot visualized through the arthroscopic image transmission system. Care is necessary to avoid hitting the articular cartilage on either side; if hit, it would be destroyed. Smoke, water, and carbon, the major by-products of laser surgery, must be washed out intermittently from the joint. The procedure is not performed in as short a time as it would be by conventional means in experienced hands.

As of August 1983, Smith and Nancst had performed at least 75 partial meniscectomies and reported only one complication of septic arthritis. Subcutaneous emphysema developed in 5 patients. A period of 1 to 10 days was necessary for gaseous absorption.

They are careful to point out that an improperly directed laser would also damage articular cartilage. I agree on the importance of this point. Also, second-look arthroscopy showed that carbon debris was present in the synovium longer than 3 months after the procedure.

An arthroscopic laser surgical procedure is cumbersome and more difficult than standard procedures. It takes a longer time to surgically perform and requires more skill, experience, and expensive equipment. Smith and Nancst reported their first cases at the 1983 annual meeting of the North American Arthroscopy Association. They have instituted a moratorium on new cases as of 1984 to accurately follow up their existing cases.

Glick and Kapany reported on the experimental use of the argon laser on laboratory cases at the International Arthroscopy Meeting in Rio de Janiero in August 1981.[20] Basically, they pointed out their early experiences and the difficulties involved.

My opinion concerning high-energy sources in arthroscopic surgery is that their general application is still in the future. The main advantage of electrosurgery would be the use of electrocoagulation for the benefit of hemostasis. The potential for the use of laser exists especially if procedures can be done faster, better, more safely, and less expensively with it. To date this has not been shown to be the case. I believe the existing mechanical instrumentation is adequate, safe, less costly, and more expedient.

DOCUMENTATION

Documentation for the initial arthroscopic procedures was done in the form of a dictated, typewritten operative record. I now use a computer-synthesized system that increases accuracy and decreases work time (see Chapter 5).

Metcalf introduced the concept of routine slide photography. He took 35 mm photographs before and after all arthroscopic cases. With the growth and availability of video, documentation could be done on videotape. Since 1976 it has been my practice to save all videotapes for before and after comparisons. These documents are intended by "second looks" to allow exact comparison of areas previously operated on. Inspection and comparison of videotapes demonstrate the tissue's response to injury and disease as well as to surgical intervention. It also provides an opportunity to review areas that were not previously operated on that may have subsequently developed a lesion.

LEARNING ARTHROSCOPY

Learning arthroscopic surgery is an enormous task for practicing orthopedic surgeons, most of whom were not trained in or even familiarized with endoscopic work during their residency. This has necessitated an abundance of continuing education courses. Originally these courses involved lectures and slides, but they rapidly evolved into elaborate audiovisual productions for television.

Perhaps the most important development for the learning of arthroscopic surgery was Eilert's introduction of a dry knee model for instructional purposes.[16] This model allowed the orthopedic surgeon to practice eye-hand coordination and triangulation before any patient experience. Another quantum leap was made with Sweeney's arthroscopic surgical knee simulator,[49] which provided an opportunity to perform arthroscopic techniques in a fluid medium and learn the disciplines necessary for live surgery, including motorized instrumentation (Fig. 1-6).

McGinty advocated the use of video equipment as a teaching aid in arthroscopic surgery.[36] I agree and advocate television as an integral part of routine arthroscopic surgery. The surgeon is able to teach others as well as himself or herself by reviewing cases on videotape.

Literature

The opportunity for study of arthroscopic surgery has been provided in textbooks,[10,28,29] including those by O'Connor (now continued by Shahriaree)[41,46] Dandy,[13] Watanabe et al.,[50] Hencke,[24] and Glinz.[21] In addition, there has been

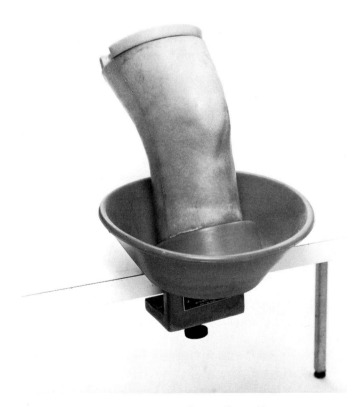

FIG. 1-6. The "Swee-Knee."

gradual acceptance of arthroscopic papers in contemporary literature. The most conservative journals generally limit themselves to anatomical and pathological descriptions or articles that demonstrate the misuse of the technique.[23,33,44] The official publication of the Arthroscopy Association of North America and the International Arthroscopy Association, *Arthroscopy: the Journal of Arthroscopic and Related Surgery,* was published in 1985.

The *Arthroscopic Video Journal,** the first journal committed totally to arthroscopy, was published through the initiative of Dr. David Shneider of East Lansing, Michigan. Uniquely and appropriately enough, this is a videotaped journal. It has gained popularity in the United States not only for the information it contains but also because of the technical quality in the video production. Video is especially well suited for arthroscopic description.

Courses

The American Academy of Orthopaedic Surgeons, under the leadership of Dr. Jack McGinty, has given many courses on arthroscopy and arthroscopic surgery over the years. The North American Arthroscopy Association, the International Arthroscopy Association, and numerous universities, clinics, and individuals have sponsored symposiums on arthroscopic surgery. These meetings have provided these organizations' membership with an introduction to the arthroscopic techniques. Laboratory experiences provide opportunities to test all of the instrumentation. By 1984 popularity and attendance was on the decline for most arthroscopy meetings in the United States, perhaps an indication of the need having been met.

ORGANIZATIONS

The International Arthroscopy Association (IAA) was started in 1973 in Philadelphia under the initiative of Dr. John C. Joyce. Watanabe was the first president, Dr. Robert Jackson the second, Dr. Isao Abe the third, and Dr. John McGinty the most recent. Their biannual meetings are held in conjunction with the Société Internationale de Chirurgie Orthopedique et de Traumatologie (SICOT).

Recently a reorganization of the North American chapter of the IAA, under McGinty's direction, created the Arthroscopy Association of North America (AANA) to serve those with interest in this subspecialty on the North American continent. The American Academy of Orthopaedic Surgeons has also developed an education committee in the area of arthroscopy.

RESEARCH

The opportunity for research by arthroscopic means is enormous. Preservation of the videotapes and microbiopsies of various intraarticular tissues add to our understanding. Second-look arthroscopies, as I did in 15% of my first 200 meniscectomies and 33% of my first 100 abrasion arthroplasties, permit exact comparison of operative and repairative areas. Arthroscopic research can certainly be expanded in the future to give us a better understanding of the various processes, both mechanical and biochemical, that occur not only with age but also with injury and/or disease.

---

*2950 Mt. Hope, Okemos, MI 48864.

"New" arthroscopic procedures are a result of conversion of previous open surgical principles and procedures. My first such experience was with arthroscopic patellar debridement in chondromalacia patella. This was undertaken solely as a pathological model to develop motorized instrumentation for arthroscopic surgery. To my surprise, based on previous open surgical shaving procedures, the patients expressed significant reduction in pain, crepitus, and swelling. Second-look arthroscopic examinations showed fibrous tissue healing of these partial-thickness lesions (see Chapters 8 and 10).

The Magnuson "housecleaning"[35] was modified with the minimally invasive approach of arthroscopy. Bone drilling was replaced by superficial abrasion when surface vascularity was recognized in the arthroscopic environment. The remainder of the debridement procedures, meniscectomy, synovectomy, and osteophyte resection, became more exacting, with preservation of healthy tissue.

The arthroscopically monitored reconstruction of the anterior cruciate ligament with semitendinosis grafting is similar to a Mott procedure[40] (see Chapter 12). The principles of Feagin and Mott to harvest the cruciate ligament and augment with patient's tendinous tissue are followed without the extensive joint capsule disruption of the arthrotomy. Drill hole imbedding is used with metallic staple fixation. The magnification factor enhances the anatomical placement of the graft attachments. X-ray films confirm placement.

Arthroscopic reconstruction for recurrent dislocation of the shoulder is a combination of Bankart's principles[5] and Dutoit and Roux's concept[14] of metallic staple fixation. The time required for the surgical exposure and closure is reduced by an arthroscopic approach.

More recently, the rotator cuff tears and anterior impingement syndromes have been shown to lend themselves to arthroscopic inspection and debridement procedures.

The area of most interest at present is the healing potential of meniscal tissue. Originally meniscal disease was managed by total resection. Partial meniscectomy became popular, especially after arthroscopic techniques were developed. The lesser resection was supported by arthroscopic evidence and clinical patient response. The enhanced respect for meniscal function resulted in preservation and surgical repair. Recognition that a bucket-handle tear reduced, sutured, and healed is truly a free meniscus graft supported the notion of both pedicle and free meniscal grafting procedures.

In June 1984 I performed my first rotational pedicle meniscal graft. I reasoned that a pedicle would preserve the all-important vascularity. Postoperative biopsy confirmed this; however, the vascularity was so abundant the tissue did not resemble avascular fibrocartilage but rather hypervascular fibrosis tissue (see Fig. 8-66).

By accident, my third meniscal pedicle rotation case resulted in severing of the pedicle at the base while it was being positioned. It was sutured as a free pedicle graft. The resultant biopsy showed normal appearing meniscal tissue in the graft. At this point I abandoned vascular pedicle grafting for free grafts.

The first cases were patients with totally absent meniscal tissue, at least in the area of the tibial collateral ligament, and with exposed bone of osteoarthritis on both sides of the compartment. The patients were usually elderly, which seemingly reduced the opportunity for healing. The patient risk was reduced to failure of healing and fragment removal. This occurred once, in my first case, in a patient who fell down on the fifth postoperative day and tore loose the pedicle graft. No other case has been symptomatic for fragment impingement or motion. All second looks to date have shown healing and amalgamation of the graft.

The issue is not whether a free graft will "take," but whether the patient will benefit.

The project will continue with ipsilateral and contralateral homografts. Arnoczky's recent work on dog meniscal allografts suggests this possibility should be considered in humans.

Arthroscopic observations have challenged accepted truths. The most notable is the healing response of joint surfaces. Hyaline cartilage does respond to disease or injury, but there is no evidence that hyaline cartilage will heal or replace itself with like tissue. Partial thickness articular cartilage lesions have been shown to heal with fibrous tissue and subsequent fibrocartilage by second-look photographic documentation and exact correlative site biopsy. Our recent experimental work shows that this response is related to saline's depression of cartilage metabolism and the effects of proteoglycan reduction on blood clot formation (see Chapter 8).

The idea that it is necessary to drill or decorticate to subchondral bone to reach the blood supply has been dispelled by arthroscopic observation (see Chapter 8). The tissue response to deep bone cutting is fibrous in nature. The superficial debridement of abrasion arthroplasty established by arthroscopic techniques shows a fibrous tissue conversion to fibrocartilage by 4 to 6 months. Biopsies show re-establishment of the tidemark at 4 years. No biopsy to date has shown any type II collagen in the cartilaginous repair tissue. It should be noted that Salter's 2 mm drill hole lesions in normal animal articular cartilage subjected to continuous passive motion showed histochemical staining properties suggestive of hyaline cartilage; however, no test was reported concerning critical evidence of type II collagen to establish hyaline cartilage properties. Firbrocartilage has similar histological staining properties, especially when seen in small areas.

Recent experimental work in dogs by Richmond et al. has supported my arthroscopic observation in humans that cartilage cells are produced with intracortical abrasion, but only primitive fibrous tissue results with deeper resections into cancellous bone.[45]

Many inconsistencies and controversies, which were so often "apples and oranges" comparisons of open surgical experiences or animal experiments, are being resolved under the illumination of the arthroscope.

As exciting as recent arthroscopic observations have been, this experience seems to indicate that arthroscopists have barely scratched the surface; there is much more knowledge to be gained.

THE FUTURE

The acceptance and integration of arthroscopy into orthopedics were well underway in 1985. It appears that most orthopedic surgeons desire to perform these procedures, and there are some whose practices are entirely devoted to arthroscopic surgery. Whether arthroscopy will continue to be a discipline within orthopedic surgery or will become a subspecialty is yet to be seen.

I believe that we are moving toward a point at which endoscopic techniques will be a part of every type of orthopedic procedure. Procedures not only in joints but also in other areas will be performed using an endoscope with image transmission or magnification. This will minimize the surgical exposure necessary and maximize the visualization and accurate observation of abnormalities. Subsequently, debridements, resections, and repairs of both synovial joints and intraosseous structures will be enhanced as well.

Meniscal repairs and autografts are already being evaluated. Anterior cruciate ligament substitutions are performed arthroscopically. At present shoulder reconstruction for traumatic dislocation is regularly performed. Rotator cuff disease lends itself to debridement procedures. Cuff repairs are being performed by arthroscopic techniques.

Arthroscopic techniques of debridement and repair will be extended to the hip, ankle, and wrist. Joint fusion will be an arthroscopic routine. Intraosseous debridement of bone cysts and benign tumors will be achieved. Eventually, ablation of malignant tumors by intraosseous endoscopic laser techniques will be attempted. Selective staining of tumor tissue will facilitate exact resection of the full extent of lesions; this is already done in urology.

Some long bone fractures will lend themselves to endoscopic inspection, reduction, and internal fixation. Certain intraarticular fractures are already treated in this manner.[26a]

The future belongs to those who have an intense interest in arthroscopy. New innovations will come along with technical advances and understanding of pathology.

REFERENCES

1. American Academy of Orthopaedic Surgeons Symposium on arthroscopy and arthrography of the knee, St. Louis, 1978, The C.V. Mosby Co.
2. Andrews, J.R., Carson, W.G., Jr., Ortega, K.: Arthroscopy of the shoulder: technique and normal anatomy, Am. J. Sports Med. 12:1, 1984.
3. Arnoczky, S.D., and Warren, R.F.: The microvasculature of the meniscus and its response to injury: an experimental study in the dog, Am. J. Sports Med. 11:131, 1983.
4. Austin, M.: Personal communication, 1979.
5. Bankart, A.S.B.: The pathology and treatment of recurrent dislocation of the shoulder joint, Br. J. Surg. 26:23, 1938.
6. Bircher, E.: Beitrag zur Pathologie und Diagnose der Meniscusverletzungen (Arthroendoskopie), Beitr. Klin. Chir. 127:239, 1922.
7. Burman, M.S.: Arthroscopy on direct visualization of joints, and experimental cadaver study, J. Bone Joint Surg. 13:669, 1931.
8. Burman, M.S., Finkelstein, H., and Mayer, L.: Arthroscopy of the knee joint, J. Bone Joint Surg. 16:255, 1934.
9. Caspari, R.: Personal communication, 1984.
10. Casscells, S.W.: Arthroscopy: Diagnostic and surgical practice, Philadelphia, 1984, Lea & Febiger.
11. Casscells, S.W.: Arthroscopy of the knee joint: a review of 150 cases, J. Bone Joint Surg. 53A:287, 1971.
11a. Clancy, W., and Graf, B.: Arthroscopic meniscal repair, Orthopedics 6:1125, 1983.
12. Clayton, M.: Personal communication, 1979.
13. Dandy, D.J., Arthroscopic surgery of the knee, Edinburgh, 1981, Churchill-Livingstone, 1981.
13a. DeHaven, K.E.: Peripheral meniscus repair as an alternative to meniscectomy, J. Bone Joint Surg. 63B:463, 1981.

14. Dutoit, G.T., and Roux, D.: Recurrent dislocation of shoulder: the Johannesburg stapling operation, J. Bone Joint Surg. **37A**:633, 1955.

15. Eikelaar, H.R.: Arthroscopy of the knee, Groningen, Holland, 1975, Royal United Printers, Hoitsema B.V.

16. Eilert, R.: Laboratory aid in the teaching of arthroscopy. In American Academy of Orthopaedic Surgeons Symposium on arthroscopy and arthrography of the knee, St. Louis, 1978, The C.V. Mosby Co.

17. Ewing, J.W.: Personal communication, 1984.

18. Fox, J.M., et al.: Electrosurgery in orthopaedics. Part 1. Principles, Contemp. Orthop. 8:21, 1984.

19. Fraider, C.T.: Arthroscopic surgery of the knee: history and state of the art, J. Am. Osteopath. Assoc. **80**:817, 1981.

20. Glick, J.M., and Kapany, N.S.: Laser for potential use in arthroscopic surgery, Presented at International Arthroscopic Association meeting, Aug. 29, 1981, Rio de Janiero.

21. Glinz, W., Arthroscopic partial meniscectomy, Helv. Chir. Acta **47**:115, 1980.

22. Gross, R.M., and Fitzgibbons, T.C.: Shoulder arthroscopy: a modified approach, Arthroscopy **3**:156, 1985.

23. Hadied, A.M.: An unusual complication of arthroscopy: a fistula between the knee and the prepatellar bursa, case report, J. Bone Joint Surg., **66A**:624, 1984.

23a. Hamberg, P., Gillquist, J., and Lysholm, J.: Suture of new and old peripheral meniscus tears, J. Bone Joint Surg. **65A**:193, 1983.

24. Hencke, H.R.: Arthroscopy of the knee joint, Berlin, 1980, Springer-Verlag.

24a. Hergenroder, P.: Personal communication, 1985.

24b. Hughston, J.C.: A simple meniscectomy, J. Sports Med. **3**:179, 1975.

25. Jackson, R.W., and Abe, I.: The role of arthroscopy in the management of disorders of the knee: an analysis of 200 consecutive examinations, J. Bone Joint Surg. **54B**:310, 1972.

26. Jackson, R.W., Dandy, D.J.: Arthroscopy of the knee, New York, 1980, Grune & Stratton, Inc.

26a. Jennings, J.E.: Arthroscopic management of tibial plateau fractures, Arthroscopy **1**:160, 1985.

27. Johnson, L.L.: Arthroscopy of the knee using local anesthesia: a review of 400 patients, J. Bone Joint Surg. **58A**:736, 1976.

28. Johnson, L.L.: Comprehensive arthroscopic examination of the knee, St. Louis, 1977, The C.V. Mosby Co.

29. Johnson, L.L., Diagnostic arthroscopy of the knee joint. In Excerpta Medica, New York, 1974, American Elsevier Publishing Co., pp. 131-139.

30. Johnson, L.L.: Diagnostic and surgical arthroscopy, ed. 2, St. Louis, 1981, The C.V. Mosby Co.

31. Johnson, L.L., and Fu, F.: Status of arthroscopic training in orthopedic residency programs, Orthop. Surv. **6**:225, 1983.

32. Joyce, J.J., III, and Jackson, R.W.: History of arthroscopy. In American Academy of Orthopaedic Surgeons Symposium on arthroscopy and arthrography of the knee, St. Louis, 1978, The C.V. Mosby Co.

33. Joyce, M.J., and Mankin, H.J., Caveat Arthroscopos: extraarticular lesions of bone simulating intra-articular pathology of the knee, J. Bone Joint Surg. **65A**:289, 1983.

34. Kreuscher, P.H.: Semilunar cartilage disease: plea for early recognition by means of arthroscope and early treatment of this condition, Illinois Med. J. **47**:290, 1925.

35. Magnuson, P.B., Technic of debridement of the knee joint for arthritis, Surg. Clin. North Am. **26**:249, 1946.

36. McGinty, J.B.: Closed circuit television in arthroscopy, Int. Rev. Rhematd. pp. 45-49, 1976, special edition devoted to arthroscopy.

37. McGinty, J.B., and Freedman, P.A.: Arthroscopy of the knee, Clin. Orthop. **121**:173, 1976.

37a. McGinty, J.B., Geuss, L.F., and Marvin, R.A.: Partial or total meniscectomy, J. Bone Joint Surg. **59A**:763, 1977.

38. McGinty, J.B., and Mapza, R.A.: Evaluation of an outpatient procedure under local anesthesia, J. Bone Joint Surg. **60A**:787, 1978.

39. Metcalf, R.W.: An arthroscopic method for lateral release of the subluxating or dislocating patella, Clin. Orthop. 167, pp. 9-18, July 1982.

40. Mott, W.H.: Semitendinosus anatomic reconstruction for cruciate ligament insufficiency, Clin. Orthop. **172**:9, 1983.
41. O'Connor, R.L.: Arthroscopy, Philadelphia, 1977, J.B. Lippincott Co., 1977.
42. O'Connor, R.L.: Arthroscopy in the diagnosis and treatment of acute ligament injuries of the knee, J. Bone Joint Surg. **56A**:333, 1974.
43. Orbon, R.J., and Poehling, G.G.: Arthroscopic meniscectomy, South Med. J. **74**:1238, 1981.
44. Reagan, B.F., McInery, U.K., Treadwell, B.U., Zarins, B., and Mankin, H.J.: Irrigating solutions for arthroscopy: a metabolic study, **65A**:629, 1983.
45. Richmond, J.C., et al.: A canine model of osteoarthritis with histologic study of repair tissue following abrasion arthroplasty, Presented at the Annual Meeting of the North American Arthroscopy Association, Boston, 1985.
45a. Salter, R.B., et al.: The biological effect of continuous passive motion on healing of full thickness defects in articular cartilage: An experimental investigation in the rabbit, J. Bone Joint Surg. **62A**:1232, 1980.
46. Shahriaree, H.: O'Connor's textbook of arthroscopic surgery, Philadelphia, 1984, J.B. Lippincott Co.
47. Shneider, D.: Personal communication, 1983.
48. Smith, James B.: Personal communication, 1983.
49. Sweeny, H.J.: Teaching arthroscopic surgery at the residency level, Orthop. Clin. North Am. **13**:255, 1982.
50. Watanabe, M., Takeda, S., and Ikeuchi, H.: Atlas of arthroscopy, ed. 3, Berlin, 1979, Springer-Verlag.
51. Whipple, T.L., Caspari, R.B., and Meyers, J.F.: Arthroscopic laser meniscectomy in a gas medium, Arthroscopy **1**:2, 1985.
52. Whipple, T.L., Caspari, R.B., and Meyers, J.F.: Laser energy in arthroscopic meniscectomy, Orthopedics, **6**:1165, 1983.
53. Wiley, A.M., and Older, M.W.: Shoulder arthroscopy investigations with a fibro-optic instrument, Am. J. Sports Med. **8**:31, 1980.
54. Yamamoto, R.: Personal communication, 1979.

CHAPTER 2

Clinical practice of arthroscopic surgery

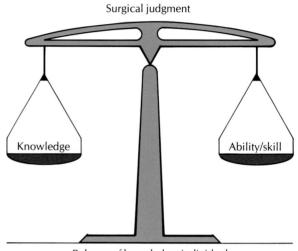

Balance of knowledge, individual ability, and skill

REVIEW OF STATUS IN THE UNITED STATES

Arthroscopy has found its way into most orthopedic surgical care. It is not a stand-alone technical exercise. Arthroscopic surgical techniques must be placed in their proper perspective in orthopedics.

This chapter deals with the history of arthroscopy in the United States and offers a means of properly integrating arthroscopy into the clinical practice of orthopedic surgery.

1978 AAOS questionnaire

In 1978, the American Academy of Orthopaedic Surgeons (AAOS) sent out a questionnaire to its members concerning their educational needs. The results indicated that 50% of the respondents used arthroscopy in their practice, 10% performed arthroscopy using a local anesthetic, and 6% had performed arthroscopy in a joint other than the knee. There were no questions to differentiate between diagnostic and operative arthroscopy, and no correlative demographics performed on the information.

1981 practice review
Material and methods

In 1982, I, Dr. Albert Ferguson, and Dr. Freddie Fu published the results of a survey reflecting the status of arthroscopy in the United States in September of 1981.[26] The data used in the study were derived from anonymous questionnaires mailed to a 10% random sample of orthopedic surgeons. The universe from which the sample was selected consisted of those 11,463 physicians in the American Medical Association (AMA) physician membership file who indicated that their primary speciality was orthopedic surgery and who were office based, hospital based, or involved in medical teaching as defined by the AMA records. A total of 1,148 questionnaires were mailed, of which 9 were undeliverable. A total of 590 completed questionnaires were received for a response of 52%. While there was a substantial variation in the response rate by state, the response rate did not vary significantly by census region. After the responses were edited for any inconsistencies, the data were keypunched and tabulated by a computer using a statistical package for social sciences.

Results

The results showed that 90% of the respondents were members of the American Board of Orthopaedic Surgeons (ABOS). The same percentage were members of the AAOS. Four percent of the respondents were members of the International Arthroscopy Association (IAA), which in 1985 would basically reflect membership of the Arthroscopic Association of North America (AANA).

Of the respondents, 76% said that they performed diagnostic arthroscopy, and 53% stated that they performed operative arthroscopy (see Fig. 1-2 and Table 2-1). At that time the average total case experience for both diagnostic and operative arthroscopy was 176 cases, and the range was between 1 and 2,000 cases. For individuals who did only diagnostic arthroscopy, the average case experience was 76, with a range of 2 to 724. For those who did operative arthroscopy, the average case experience was greater: 227 cases, with a range of 3 to 2,000 procedures.

It was significant that half of the respondents had performed fewer than 100 cases by September 1981, and 12.7 percent had performed more than 300.

There was no statistically significant relationship between the number of years the surgeon had been in practice and the inclusion of either diagnostic or operative arthroscopy in his or her practice. For instance, those who had been in practice between 1 and 5 years accounted for 23% of the total number of arthroscopists, and those in practice longer than 21 years accounted for 18.4%. I would

TABLE 2-1. Professional affiliation related to frequency of arthroscopy practiced

	Diagnostic (%)	Operative (%)
American Board of Orthopaedic Surgeons	76	51
American Academy of Orthopaedic Surgeons	77	52
International Arthroscopy Association	78	54
Doctor of Orthopaedics	76	53

From Johnson, L.L., Ferguson, A.B., Jr., and Fu, F.: Orthop. Surv. **5**:400, 1982, © 1982 The Williams & Wilkins Co., Baltimore.

have thought that the younger people performed more of these procedures.

The study further indicated that the frequency of use of operative arthroscopy varied by region. The Pacific region of the United States had the highest frequency, followed by the Mountain region, the Central South, and finally New England. Conversely, those areas which reported high in diagnostic arthroscopy ranged from east to west, the reverse of the operative experience, not yet embracing surgical techniques.

By September 1981, operative arthroscopy was being performed by 72% of the responding surgeons in the Mountain region, with a lower percentage indicating they did only diagnostic arthroscopy. In the East, about 50% said that they did diagnostic arthroscopy only and were just beginning operative work.

One of the most interesting observations was lack of difference in the frequency of either diagnostic or operative arthroscopy performed when tabulated by professional affiliation (see Table 2-1). For instance, for those affiliated with the American Board of Orthopaedic Surgeons or the AAOS or for doctors of osteopathy, the statistics were all basically the same: approximately 75% performed diagnostic and 52% performed operative arthroscopy only.

It was especially interesting to note that 20% of the responding American membership of the IAA did not perform either diagnostic or operative arthroscopy. It should be noted that there were no membership requirements at the time of its formation beyond interest in arthroscopy, an application, and a $50 membership fee. Restructuring of this organization has occurred with the establishment of the AANA. Membership qualifications now require a documented 25% of practice in arthroscopic surgery.

Extrapolating from the responses regarding the number of cases performed, the national total of diagnostic arthroscopies in the month of September 1981 would have been 87,118. The number of operative arthroscopic procedures performed in that same month would have been 91,130.

The surgeons indicated that their operative time for a diagnostic arthroscopy averaged 29 minutes. For arthroscopic surgery their average operative times were as follows: for plica resection or loose bodies, 40 minutes; for patellar shave, 47 minutes; for meniscectomy, 67 minutes; for chondroplasty, 51 minutes; and for operative arthroscopy of other joints, approximately 50 minutes (Tables 2-2 and 2-3). The operative times were less for respondents who were members of the IAA.

TABLE 2-2. Frequency of diagnostic arthroscopy: average number and operative time of diagnostic arthroscopies performed in September 1981 by all respondents

	Number	Average operative time (minutes)
Knee	8	29
Other joints	2	33
Local anesthesia	7	29
Prior to arthrotomy	5	29

From Johnson, L.L., Ferguson, A.B., Jr., and Fu, F.: Orthop. Surv. **5**:400, 1982, © 1982 The Williams & Wilkins Co.

TABLE 2-3. Frequency of operative arthroscopy: average number and operative time of operative arthroscopies performed in September 1981 by all respondents

	Number	Average operative time (minutes)
Plica	2	40
Loose body	2	40
Patellar shave	3	47
Meniscectomy	5	67
Chondroplasty	2	51
Other joints	1	50
TOTAL	15	

From Johnson, L.L., Ferguson, A.B., Jr., and Fu, F.: Orthop. Surv. **5**:400, 1982, © 1982 The Williams & Wilkins Co.

TABLE 2-4. Correlation between the number of arthroscopy case experiences and the average time to perform diagnostic arthroscopy of the knee

Number of arthroscopy case experiences	Average time for diagnosis of knee (minutes)
1 to 50	33.7
51 to 100	32.4
101 to 150	31.6
151 to 200	27.2
201 to 300	22.5
301 to 400	21.9
401 to 500	17.7
501 to 1000	22.9
1001 to 1500	16.2
Entire population	29.6

From Johnson, L.L., Ferguson, A.B., Jr., and Fu, F.: Orthop. Surv. **5**:400, 1982, © 1982 The Williams & Wilkins Co.

The average number of case experiences necessary to achieve an average diagnostic arthroscopy time of 29 minutes was 200, which actually exceeded the average case experience (Table 2-4). The same number of cases were required to obtain the average operative time for meniscectomy.

The use of television was considered a measure of sophistication of the equipment used for arthroscopic procedures. Of all respondents, 25% used television. Those doing only diagnostic arthroscopy used television 8% of the time, those doing operative arthroscopy 33%, those who had a 300-case experience 44%, and those who had performed more than 1,000 cases used television all of the time.

In 1981, 81% of the respondents believed that the use of diagnostic and operative arthroscopy would increase, 16% thought it would stay the same, and 3% thought it would decrease as a discipline within orthopedic surgery.

TABLE 2-5. Self-assessment of arthroscopic skills: 1981

Diagnostic experience: 473 cases (average)
67% See well, trust what they see
11% Diagnostic experts
90% accuracy (average)
91% competent (average)
Operative experience: 205 cases (average)
26% Able to do any case
Technical success 83% of time
13% of cases aborted

1981 Shneider survey

Data are also available from a questionnaire that was answered in September 1981 by 127 surgeons attending an arthroscopy meeting in Lansing, Michigan hosted by Dr. David Shneider. The surgeons were invited to this meeting on the basis of known or demonstrated interest in arthroscopic surgery and therefore were a select group.

They were asked questions on a variety of topics, including their level of proficiency for both diagnostic and operative arthroscopy (Table 2-5). The 127 responding surgeons had an average case experience of 473 cases as compared to the average of 176 cases reported by me, Ferguson, and Fu. In response to questions about diagnostic arthroscopy, 67% said they could see well and could trust what they saw, and 11% considered themselves to be diagnostic experts. The average competence level was 91%, and the average accuracy rating was 90%.

The same group indicated that they had performed 205 operative arthroscopies, averaging two a day, and procedures averaging 67 minutes per case. Twenty six percent said they could do any operative arthroscopic technique they desired, and self-assessment of results indicated they were technically successful in 83% of their cases. Thirteen percent of their cases were abandoned arthroscopically and required open procedures.

When comparing the previous 1981 study with this select group, it again emphasizes that confidence and expertise increase with more than 200 case experiences. Even the more experienced group abandoned 13% of their 473 cases for open surgical completion.

1982 residency review
Materials and methods

In April 1982, an anonymous questionnaire was mailed to a 25% random sample of orthopedic residents.[27] The sample was selected on March 19, 1982, from an AMA list of residents in orthopedic surgery as maintained by their marketing representative, Marketing Mailing Services, Inc., of Chicago. As of that day there were 2,669 residents in their file.

TABLE 2-6. Classification of those practicing or teaching arthroscopy in residency programs

Specialty	Percentage	Academic rank	Percentage
General orthopedist	74	Senior staff	52
Sports medicine expert	53	Junior staff	52
Arthroscopic surgeon	38	Chairperson	20
		Other	4

From Johnson, L.L., and Fu, F.: Orthop. Surv. **6:**225, 1983. © 1983 The Williams & Wilkins Co., Baltimore.

TABLE 2-7. Residents' rating of teachers' proficiency at arthroscopy (1982)

Rating	Diagnostic (%)	Operative (%)
1 Poor	3	11
2	6	9
3	18 (3.9 mean)	27 (3.4) mean
4	37	30
5 Excellent	36	22

From Johnson, L.L., and Fu, F.: Orthop. Surv. **6:**225, 1983. © 1983 The Williams & Wilkins Co., Baltimore.

We used a technique of nth selection where every fourth resident was selected. This yielded a sample of 667 residents.

A total of 256 questionnaires were returned, and after we discarded those which were unusable or were internally inconsistent, 243, or 36%, of the questionnaires were available for analysis.

All but 12 states were represented in this survey, and we received responses from 134 of the 190 accredited residency programs. After editing, the data were keypunched and tabulated by computer using a statistical package for social sciences.

Results

The results were all from medical doctors. Most responses were from university-based programs (66%), followed by affiliating programs (23%), and free-standing programs (12%) (see Table 2-5). Arthroscopic teaching was universal in free-standing programs. Some university programs did not teach in this area of orthopedics in 1982.

In the typical program, a general orthopedic surgeon or sports medicine specialist most commonly performs or teaches arthroscopic surgical procedures, and the program chairmen are least involved (20%) (Table 2-6). The senior and junior residents were equal in their participation.

The average time for diagnostic arthroscopy was 31 minutes and for operative meniscectomy 66 minutes. Television was used in these residency programs for diagnostic arthroscopy 49% of the time and operative arthroscopy 56% of the time. Arthrograms were regularly performed before arthroscopy in 28% of the reporting programs.

TABLE 2-8. Program year of diagnostic training

Year (postgraduate)	Percentage of programs
1	12
2	54
3	63
4	47
5	25

From Johnson, L.L., and Fu, F.: Orthop. Surv. **6**:225, 1983. © 1983 The Williams & Wilkins Co., Baltimore.

TABLE 2-9. Program year of operative training (1982)

Year (postgraduate)	Percentage of programs
1	7.5
2	34
3	58
4	52
5	30

From Johnson, L.L., and Fu, F.: Orthop. Surv. **6**:225, 1983. © 1983 The Williams & Wilkins Co., Baltimore.

TABLE 2-10. Instructional methods used in diagnostic arthroscopic training (1982)

Method	Percentage of programs
Live surgery participation	94
Live surgery observation	83
Videotape	57
Lecture	42
Knee model	18

From Johnson, L.L., and Fu, F.: Orthop. Surv. **6**:225, 1983. © 1983 The Williams & Wilkins Co., Baltimore.

The residents rated their teachers' proficiency just above average on a scale of 1 to 5, with 5 being excellent (Table 2-7).

Eighty-one percent of the respondents had received training specifically devoted to diagnostic arthroscopy (Table 2-8). Of these, 93% received their training in residency programs and 18% in seminars or continuing education courses; 23% taught themselves.

Most of the residents received their arthroscopic training in the early years of their residency program (Table 2-9). Live surgery participation with observations was the most common method employed in teaching diagnostic arthroscopy. Practice on a knee model or simulator was the least used method (Tables 2-10 and 2-11).

In regard to arthroscopic surgical training, 76% of residents responding to the questionnaire had training specifically devoted to arthroscopic skills. Of these, 93% got their training in residency programs and 18% in seminars or continuing education courses; 23% taught themselves. The method of teaching used was similar to that of teaching diagnostic arthroscopy (see Table 2-11).

TABLE 2-11. Instructional methods used in operative arthroscopic training (1982)

Method	Percentage of programs
Live surgery participation	93
Live surgery observation	85
Videotape	56
Lecture	34
Knee model	16

From Johnson, L.L., and Fu, F.: Orthop. Surv. **6**:225, 1983. © 1983 The Williams & Wilkins Co., Baltimore.

TABLE 2-12. Residents' self-rating of proficiency (1982)

Rating	Diagnostic (%)	Operative (%)
1 Poor	10	40
2	19	28
3	34 (2.9 mean)	26 (1.9 mean)
4	32	6
5 Excellent	4	1

From Johnson, L.L., and Fu, F.: Orthop. Surv. **6**:225, 1983. © 1983 The Williams & Wilkins Co., Baltimore.

The residents were asked to estimate the total number of arthroscopies in which they had participated. Their diagnostic experience averaged 23 cases, with a range of 0 to 300 cases; 6% had done none. The operative arthroscopy participation also ranged from 0 to 300 cases with an average of 23 cases, and in this group, 19% had no operative arthroscopic experience. The residents rated their current proficiency in both diagnostic and operative arthroscopy as just slightly lower than that of their teachers (Tables 2-7 and 2-12). Most of these same resident surgeons anticipated incorporating both diagnostic (96%) and operative (90%) arthroscopy into their future practices.

In the 2 years before the survey, 4% of these residents had personally had an arthrotomy, 6% a diagnostic arthroscopy, and 3% arthroscopic surgery.

Discussion

The results of this survey indicate that orthopedic training programs were just starting to give attention to the discipline of arthroscopy and arthroscopic surgery in March, 1982. The fact that only 20% of program chairmen participated in the arthroscopic training is perhaps an indication of why such training was in its infancy.

The average experience of 23 cases each of diagnostic and surgical arthroscopy, with 19% of respondents having had no arthroscopic experience, indicates that the average resident has very little experience. Yet, they anticipated incorporating arthroscopy—96% for diagnostic and 90% for surgical—into their subsequent practices.

It seems good that 38% reported that their arthroscopic training was done under somebody who specialized in that particular technique. I was also somewhat surprised that the diagnostic and operative experience was learned in the middle part of the residency program rather than in the latter part or, even more ideally, throughout the entire program.

This would seem to indicate a need for continuing education in the area of arthroscopic surgery, especially from the standpoint of developing motor skills. The residents reported that a minimal amount of participation time was received in their programs, and yet so many anticipate including it in their practices. I was especially surprised that the use of a knee model or simulator was the least used method of training. This may be the result either of a lack of knowledge or a lack of appreciation for the value of these simulators.

Video would seem to be underused as a teaching and educational device, both at the time of surgery and for review of case experience. Video was used in just over 56% of the surgical cases.

Arthroscopic surgical training had made a good start in American residency programs as of April 1982. However, these programs were not fully using the training materials, such as arthroscopic knee simulators or video, that were readily available to them in 1982.

It would appear that the future of arthroscopy and arthroscopic surgery in the United States is strong, since 90% of the residents anticipated including that discipline within their practice. This was even higher than the actual percentage of practicing surgeons using arthroscopy at that time.

With all this information in mind, it was our desire to review and update the status of arthroscopy in September, 1983, for comparison.

1983 practice review
Materials and methods

The data used in the 1983 practice review were derived from anonymous questionnaires mailed to a 10% random sample of physicians. The universe from which the sample was selected was physicians in the AMA's physician member file who indicated that their primary specialty was orthopedic surgery and who were office based, hospital based, or involved in medical teaching as defined by the AMA records. Residents and physicians who were retired or otherwise inactive were specifically excluded from the universe. The universe consisted of 11,463 physicians. A total of 1,275 questionnaires were mailed, of which 9 were undeliverable and 3 were returned after the cut-off date. A total of 257 completed questionnaires were received, resulting in a rate response of 20%. While there was substantial variation in the rate response by state, the rate response did not vary significantly by census region.

The responses from the questionnaires returned were first edited for internal consistency. (For example, if a response indicated that the physician did not perform arthroscopy but used a television monitor while performing arthroscopy, the response was viewed as inconsistent and treated as a nonresponse to that particular question.) After editing, the data were keypunched and tabulated by a computer, using a statistical package for social sciences.

Results

Of the respondents, ninety-eight percent indicated that they had performed diagnostic arthroscopy and 75% that they had performed arthroscopic surgery as of September 1983 (Fig. 1-2). The average total case experience was 491 pro-

TABLE 2-13. Practitioners' method of learning: 1983

Method	Percentage
Seminar	39
Observation	34
Self-taught	26
Literature	1

cedures, with a range between 9 and 5,000 cases. For individuals who reported performing only diagnostic arthroscopy, the average case experience was 260, with a range of between 2 and 3,000. For those who did operative arthroscopy, the average case experience was 248, with a range of 1 to 3,000 total experiences.

Of the respondents, 31% had 100 or fewer case experiences, 42% had performed 150 or fewer arthroscopies, 50% had 300 or more cases, and 30% had more than 500 case experiences.

Respondents who were members of an arthroscopy association reported an average of more than 1,000 case experiences, while those who were only members of either the ABOS or the AAOS had just under 300 cases.

When asked which was the best method by which they learned arthroscopic surgery, 39% said by seminar, 34% by observation of another surgeon, 26% self-taught, and 1% by the literature (Table 2-13). This survey showed that American surgeons first performed their diagnostic procedures around 1978, and their operative work started in 1981.

During the month of September 1983, the average operative time was 42 minutes. There was an average of 3 diagnostic procedures performed on joints other than the knee in an average time of 43 minutes, and 14 diagnostic procedures performed using a local anesthesic in an average time of 44 minutes.

The operative profile showed that 78% of the surgeons performed arthroscopic work. The average distribution of cases was 4 plicas, 2 loose body removals, 4 patellar shaves, 13 meniscectomies, 4 chondroplasties, 2 operative procedures in other joints, 3 abrasion arthroplasties, and 2 meniscal repairs.

The average operative times of the respondents were as follows: plica, 44 minutes; loose body removal, 40 minutes; patellar shave, 46 minutes; meniscectomy, 55 minutes; chondroplasty, 61 minutes; abrasion arthroscopy, 59 minutes; and meniscal repair, 70 minutes. The average case experience necessary for a surgeon to achieve the average time for both diagnostic (44 minutes) and operative (55 minutes) arthroscopy was 200 case experiences (Table 2-14). Those with longer than average times had less than 200 case experiences.

Video was used on a regular basis by 80% of the respondents.

In the 4 years previous to the survey (1979 to 1983), 5% of the respondents had had an arthrotomy, 4.8% a diagnostic arthroscopy, and 5.2% an operative arthroscopy.

When asked to anticipate the future of arthroscopic surgery, 76% said that they believed its use would increase, 22% that it would stay the same, and 2% that it would decrease.

The respondents were also provided an opportunity for self-assessment.

TABLE 2-14. Average operative times: 1983

Procedure	Time (minutes)
Plica	44
Loose body	40
Patellar shave	46
Meniscectomy	55
Chondroplasty	61
Abrasion arthroplasty	59
Meniscal repair	70

TABLE 2-15. Summary of growth of arthroscopic surgery

	1978	1981	1983
Diagnostic	50%*	76%	98%
Operative	—	53%	75%
Local anesthesia	10%	—	—
Other joints	6%	5%	26%
Average case experience	—	176	491
Under 100 cases	—	50%	31%
Television	—	25%	80%
Operating times			
Diagnostic	30 minutes	26 minutes	42 minutes
Meniscectomy	—	67 minutes	55 minutes

*The 1978 AAOS survey made no distinction between diagnostic and surgical arthroscopy.

They were asked to judge their present level of expertise, and 11% said they were just getting started, 60% said they were at the intermediate level, and 29% said they were experts.

Of the respondents, 87.6% said they were diagnostically accurate. They described their surgical skill as follows: 8% said they were not yet surgically successful, 67% said they were able to do most cases, and 25% said they were able to do any case.

The future

When the data available from the four surveys are compared, it is clear that the most valid results would be those from the AAOS questionnaire in 1978. The percentage of respondents was high, and the questions were not specifically aimed at arthroscopic surgery but were varied in a general educational format. The 1981 and 1983 surveys were aimed toward arthroscopic surgeons and would probably elicit a response from those interested in this discipline, as compared to a general orthopedist or someone who had no interest in arthroscopy. Therefore if the statistics were used to compare growth between 1978, 1981, and 1983, the rate of growth would probably seem to be greater than it really is because of the special interest of the respondents on the more recent questionnaires (Table 2-15).

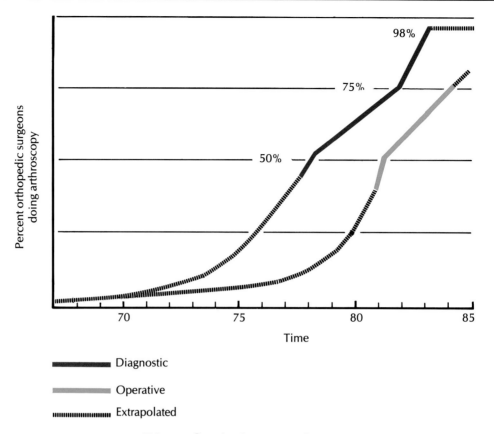

FIG. 2-1. Graph of growth of procedure.

That consideration aside, it certainly would be valid to compare the near-identical questionnaires of 1981 and 1983 to show the relative increase of arthroscopic surgery, if not the raw numbers. The only disappointment in the response to the 1983 survey was that it was lower than that in 1981, and therefore, perhaps does not reflect the same statistical validity.

At any rate, the following observations can be made (Fig. 2-1). Since 1978, when most orthopedic surgeons commenced practicing diagnostic arthroscopy, there has been a rather significant growth in the use of the procedure. By 1983 operative arthroscopy was performed by 78% of respondents. The total case experiences for the average surgeon increased from 176 to 491.

It was interesting to note that the average diagnostic times were not reduced between the reports of 1981 and 1983, even though case experiences increased. The average time for diagnostic arthroscopy in 1981 was 30 minutes, while in 1983 it was 42 minutes. For arthroscopic meniscectomy the average time was reduced below 1 hour.

The most significant change was the increase in the use of television during arthroscopy, from 25% in 1981 to 80% general use by 1983 (see Fig. 2-1).

The respondents to the two surveys felt basically the same concerning the volume of arthroscopic surgery that might be in their practices in the next 5 years, 75% of them believing that it would increase.

The method of learning arthroscopic surgery basically remained the same, with the emphasis on the seminar, observation, and self-taught methods, with fewer than 1% indicating that there was any information in the literature by which to learn arthroscopic surgical principles.

The self-assessment showed that the surgeons were gaining confidence. They considered their overall percentage of diagnostic accuracy to be 87.6%. A minority of surgeons, fewer than one third, consider themselves to be in the expert category. Only 25% believe they have the ability to handle almost any case.

It was interesting to note that the number of case experiences necessary to achieve the average operative time was exactly the same in the 1981 and the 1983 questionnaires, at 200 case experiences.

Orthopedic surgeons can be characterized into two typical groups. First there is the board-certified orthopedic surgeon who performs arthroscopy as a part of his or her general practice and has an overall experience of under 200 cases. Second there is the member of an arthroscopic association who has more than 1,000 case experiences and whose operative times are somewhat shorter than those in the first group.

The 1983 questionnaire indicated that none of the respondents referred even a single case. I would anticipate that the vast majority of practicing orthopedic surgeons are adding and/or planning to add this discipline to their surgical armamentarium without referring cases on a routine basis, thereby adding to their case experience.

CLINICAL EVALUATION
Medical history

The medical history of the candidate for arthroscopy can be obtained in a traditional way by physician inquiry and patient response. I have learned from experience that the use of a patient information questionnaire assists in completeness (see Fig. 5-3). The questionnaire allows the patient to go through a more inclusive medical history in the relaxed atmosphere of the waiting room. It also helps reduce anxiety. It helps prevent the deletion of questions from the surgeon's standpoint and provides a permanent record that is available to the surgeon at the time of the patient interview. The questionnaire should not be a substitute for the physician interview, nor should it interfere with establishment of a physician-patient relationship. In addition, the use of the questionnaire appears to shorten long or rambling stories, maximizing physician-patient interaction time.

The arthroscopic information questionnaire I use was developed over the past several years (see Fig. 5-3). It initially was developed for the knee joint, and recently one was devised for the shoulder. There is space for the physician to emphasize or elaborate on various questions. It can easily be constructed into a narrative through the use of computer synthesis (see Fig. 5-3, C). This allows the information to be stored for future reports or research purposes.

The key points for arthroscopic surgery are the patient's height-weight ratio and the workmen's compensation insurance or third-person liability dimension. The chief complaints are important, as is the duration of the problem. The exact location of the problem and how it manifests itself are also important. The opportunity to see previous x-ray films may reveal comparison changes. A review of any previous arthrograms is also helpful. Knowledge of the results of any previous diagnostic or operative arthroscopy adds to a diagnostic conclusion, as do videotapes of previous arthroscopies. The nature and frequency of any open surgery should be considered as well.

Other medical conditions, medications, or known allergies that might interfere with any recommended therapeutic course should be detailed. The most common medication to interfere with scheduling of surgery is an antihypertension medication with resultant hypokalemia. Even if the patient is taking a potassium supplement, a serum potassium level of 3.5 mEq or above should be established before the risks of anesthesia should be undertaken. This reduces the chance of cardiac arrythmias.

The ultimate medical history questions for a patient are: To what extent is this problem interfering with your life? Are you able to do what you need or desire to do? Will you be able to be gainfully employed or do your work?

The last portion of the patient interview includes the following questions. What have you been told about arthroscopic surgery? What is your understanding of the procedure? What are your expectations concerning the results?

Physical examination

One of the first areas of physical diagnosis to be stressed in a medical student's training is the examination of the heart and lungs. The emphasis is on inspection, palpation, percussion, and auscultation. I like to think of the examination of the knee joint in a similar manner. Of course, the designations are changed somewhat; examination of the knee includes inspection, palpation, manipulation, auscultation, and measurements. I use a computerized form for physical examination (see Fig. 5-4).

Inspection

Inspection of a patient with a knee joint problem includes observation of the patient's entire body during the time of the interview as well as the physical examination (Fig. 2-2).

The patients are observed directly during the examination to observe how they get out of a chair, particularly whether they use their arms or good leg first and at what pace they are able to raise up into the walking position.

Inspection of their gait can show whether they walk with a limp or with their knee straight or bent, or whether they are able to put full weight on their foot. Possible aids to ambulation include a cane, a walker, crutches, or a wheelchair. In evaluating patients' medical histories and/or physical examination reliability, inspection may be made of their hands to determine whether or not they demonstrate wear or callouses consistent with prolonged crutch walking or use of a walker. The bottom of the shoe may be worn when the patient says he has not been walking on it for a long time. The shoe may be wet or dirty if it has been in a weight-bearing position recently. The physician may also check to see that the crutches or cane demonstrate wear to reflect the use of such aids in ambulation.

Perhaps one of the more important observations, especially in medicolegal or workmen's compensation cases, is indirect observation. Those opportunities can be provided when the patient is entering or leaving the room or being transferred to the x-ray department. On some occasions, I have observed patients as they left the office and entered the hallway or parking lot. Unstaged, environ-

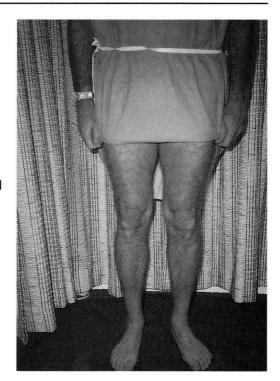

FIG. 2-2. Inspection of patient and joint involved.

mental observations may give important information. The patient's gait pattern and joint protection may not be the same as portrayed under direct observation.

Inspection of the knee includes visualization of the entire extremity, starting with the skin to see if it is of normal consistency, texture, color, and temperature. It should be noted that the skin over the normal knee joint is cooler than either the thigh or the leg on the same or opposite extremity. A knee joint that is as warm as the thigh or leg reflects increased intraarticular vascularity or inflammation.

Documentation of the presence of any skin incisions, whether arthroscopic or open, single or multiple, healed, draining, tender, or swollen is essential. Relative positions can be documented, and conventional incision length can be measured.

Palpation

Palpation of the extremity provides the surgeon with an opportunity to ascertain the areas of tenderness, whether anterior, posterior, medial, lateral along the joint line, or related to one of the bony structures (Fig. 2-3). It is also possible to palpate the areas of either suprapatellar or medical plicae when they exist in normal patients. Areas of tenderness can be palpated along the femoral condyles, or areas of thickened synovium can be identified. Further palpation for tenderness in the area of the calf, quadriceps muscle, pes anserinus bursa, patellar tendon, and peroneal nerve may ascertain whether these structures are contributing to the patient's symptoms. In acute ligamentous injury, the exact site of the lesion is palpable by defect and local tenderness. This is especially so in torn

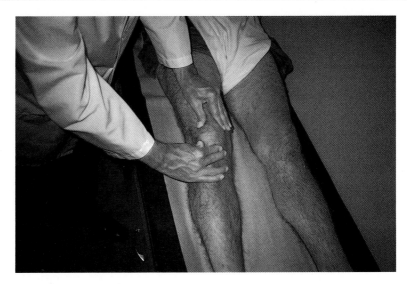

FIG. 2-3. Palpation of knee for tenderness, stability, and smoothness of gliding.

tibial collateral ligament and avulsion of the insertion of the lateral capsular ligament from the tibial condyle.

Palpation for a mass about the knee in the area of the popliteal fossa could be a Baker's cyst, vascular aneurysm, or tumor. Obese patients may have a false positive mass with bulging popliteal fat. Palpation along the area of the peroneal nerve itself could reveal a ganglion of nerve origin or a ganglion cyst of the proximal tibiofibular joint.

Palpation along the joint lines demonstrates thickness or induration as well as inflamed or degenerative meniscus. Cystic structures may be palpated along the meniscal areas.

A common cystic structure posteromedially, not associated with a meniscus, can be that along or adjacent to the semimembranosus tendon or bursa.

Palpation along the pes anserinus can show a bursitis. There can be an area of thickened bursa over the patellar tendon or the prepatellar area.

It should be noted that, in some patients who are very sensitive to their knee problem, it is possible to palpate a rubbing sensation with flexion or extension or with motion of the examiner's fingers over the patella or the tibial tubercle, where there is a normal anatomical bursa. A normal bursa may give a sense of a deep rubbing or vibration.

Examination of the quadriceps, hamstring, calf, and anterior thigh musculature is carried out by palpation for any areas of tenderness, atrophy, or muscular weakness. Palpation of the popliteal pulse at the knee or the dorsalis pedis posterior tibial pulse at the ankle can be evaluated, as well as cutaneous innervation over the knee of the knee joint or lower extremity.

Characteristically, neurological deficit of the skin is related to incisions or interruption of the neurovascular structures of the lower extremity most commonly associated with an open incision. The infrapatellar branch of the saphenous nerve and the main saphenous nerve down the medial aspect of the leg are commonly interrupted.

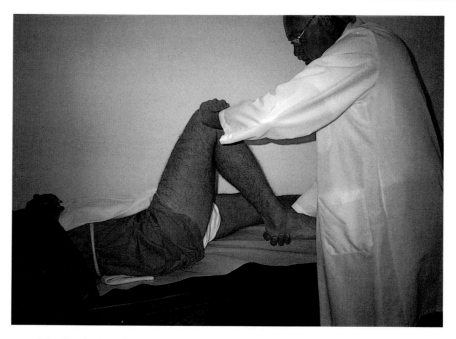

FIG. 2-4. Manipulation for range of motion, stability, and smoothness of gliding.

Manipulation

Manipulation of the extremity affords an opportunity to examine the full range of motion of the knee as well as to palpate the patella in its relative motion (Fig. 2-4). Examination of the patella specifically can show crepitus with flexion-extension or occasional catch. Compression of the patella with flexion-extension will cause the more subtle catches or crepitus to be accentuated. Pain with compression may be of some significance. Pain with distal push, or holding the patella distally and advising the patient to very gently contract their quadraceps against a fixed, distally pushed patella may elicit patellofemoral problems. A plica syndrome may produce the same signs.

Manipulation of the patella, such as a lateral push, may cause the patient to grimace. Subluxable or dislocatable patella should be correlated with the patient's expression and confirmed with reproduction of the actual symptoms. The quadriceps mechanism is more relaxed and the patella more movable when the patient is in a prone position.

A McMurray test along with auscultation should be performed (Fig. 2-5). An Apley test with compression will show subtle lesions. It is a painful test for patients with major alterations of knee function.

Routinely, the Lachman test; pivot shift test; and anteromedial, neutral, and lateral Slocum tests are performed on ligamentous and capsular structures.[18,48,49,55] Other tests to perform on suspicion of a specific lesion are outlined in the physical examination form (see Fig. 5-4).

Evaluation of the tibial collateral ligament is more isolated with 15 to 30 degrees of flexion. This differentiates between the posterior capsule and posterior cruciate ligament integrity. The latter is tested with valgus force in extension. When only the tibial collateral ligament is torn, the extension test is stable.

Direct lateral examination in extension and slight flexion is carried out. Palpation identifies the fibular collateral ligament with the knee in the figure-4 position.

Posterior instability is evaluated in the posteromedial, neutral posterior, and posterolateral planes with a position of passive rotation established before posterior displacement.

The manipulative drawer sign test of the posterior cruciate ligament might be interpreted as anterior cruciate ligament insufficiency. When the tibia is sitting posterior to the femur, the anterior drawer test moves the tibia from a posterior to a neutral position. Looking at the lateral aspect of the femur, with the tibia on the femur with the knee at 90 degrees, can reveal the initial posterior site of the tibia and reduce this examination error (see Fig. 12-79).

When the tibia sits posterior on the femur in extension because of posterolateral ligamentous insufficiency, a valgus force and flexion produces a "pivot shift." The tibia moves from posterior to anterior to reduced position with flexion. This is the reverse or posterior pivot shift. The anterior pivot shift has the tibia in an anteriorly subluxed position with valgus, and the tibia moves from anterior to a reduced position with flexion.

Auscultation

Auscultation can greatly enhance a physical examination of the knee. By auscultating during manipulation of the knee, the surgeon can differentiate various abnormalities within the knee joint (see Fig. 2-4).

The combination of manipulation and auscultation helps to locate areas of lesion. For instance, straight flexion and extension moves both the patellofemoral surfaces and the femoral tibial compartment surfaces. The combination of listening and feeling correlates sound with vibration to locate the site of the lesion.

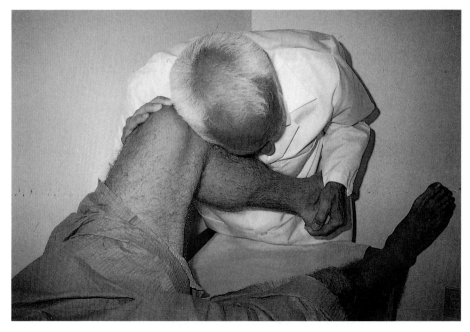

FIG. 2-5. McMurray test with auscultation

To further differentiate the location, the knee is taken into 90 degrees of flexion. No extension-flexion motion is used. The tibia is rotated back and forth internally and externally. Both listening and feeling isolate perception to intercondylar spaces. The patellofemoral joint is not involved.

Correlation of sounds and vibrations isolates the source of a problem to one or both compartments.

It is possible, especially in young people with hypermobile knees, to differentiate by auscultation the hypermobile meniscus from the typical meniscal tear or degenerative articular surfaces.

Gradishar's work has shown some differentiations between various pathological conditions by high technology and audiology (Fig. 2-6).

Measurements

Various measurements are important in preoperative evaluations and certainly in measuring the progress or deterioration of a patient's condition following

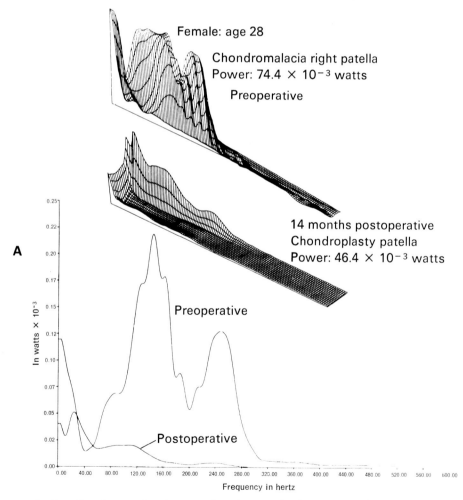

FIG. 2-6. A, Gradisar's results 1 year after intraarticular shave of patella show before and after computerized reduction and noise spectrum of crepitus.

Continued.

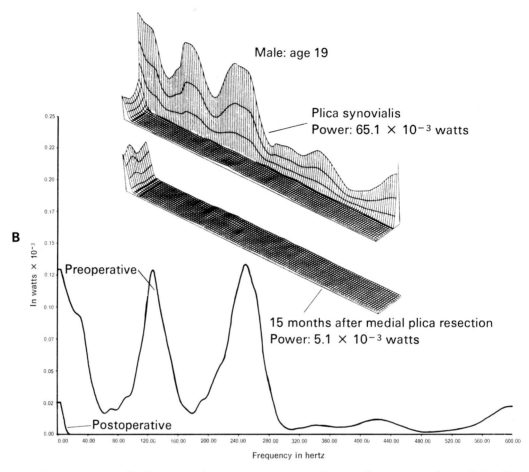

Male: age 19

Plica synovialis
Power: 65.1 × 10^{-3} watts

15 months after medial plica resection
Power: 5.1 × 10^{-3} watts

B

Preoperative

Postoperative

In watts × 10^{-3}

Frequency in hertz

FIG. 2-6, cont'd. B, Preoperative and postoperative audiographs of medial plica resection. (Courtesy Dr. Ivan A. Gradisar.)

conservative and/or operative intervention. The routine measurements include varus-valgus alignment angle. The Q angle is measured with the fulcrum of the goniometer over the patella. Lines are drawn from the anterior superior iliac spine to the tibial tubercle (Fig. 2-7, *A*).

Only recently have I started to make actual measurements of displacement, anterior or posterior, with a knee laxity tester. Originally, Daniels came out with his KT-1000. More recently, a knee ligament tester designed by W. Dilworth Cannon has been marketed by Stryker[7,8] (Fig. 2-7, *E*). It is less expensive and secures the leg for 30- and 90-degree measurements. There still are some inconsistencies by patient and examiner, but these are minimized with experience.

It should be mentioned that although these devices do give a measurement, it is related to the ability of the surgeon to reproduce the measurement in his or her own hands. I have noticed that familiarity with the instrument is important. The patient's level of cooperation results in considerable variables. With experience, comparisons are possible between preoperative and postoperative evaluations for any progression or benefit from surgery.

Range of motion can be measured next with flexion and extension. My estimates with or without a goniometer are inconsistent (Fig. 2-7, *C*). It should also

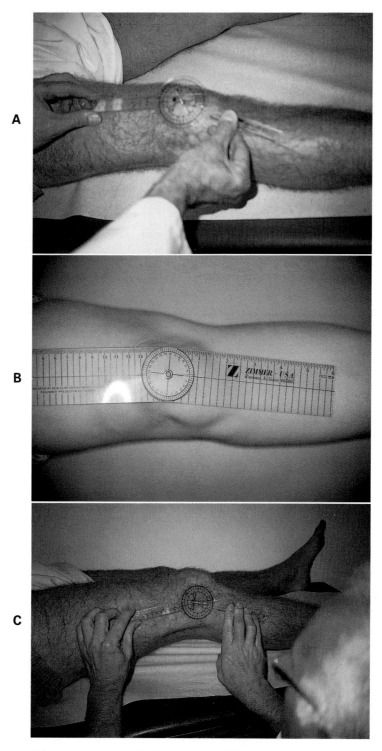

FIG. 2-7. Measurements. **A,** Q angle. **B,** Alignment. **C,** Range of motion.
Continued.

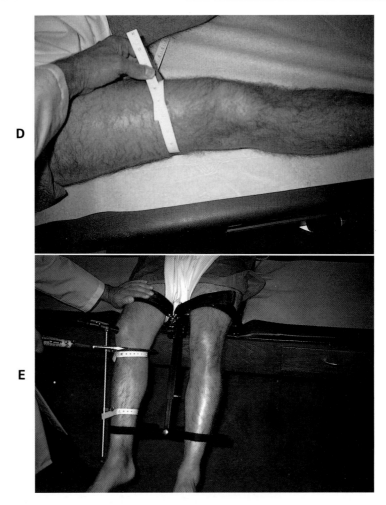

FIG. 2-7, cont'd. D, Circumference. **E,** Knee ligament tester.

be mentioned that getting accurate measurements can be a problem, even when a goniometer is used, and especially in obese patients. An attempt at measurement certainly offers a higher opportunity of accuracy than no measurement at all.

Circumferential measurements of the thigh and calf can be carried out and one side compared to the other (Fig. 2-7, *D*). Although these are a routine, they are not of great significance in an obese or edematous extremity. They only document extremity size, not specifically the musculature. The muscle bulk and power are tested separately.

At this time, the surgeon should evaluate for any pitting edema in the extremity, especially in the elderly person with degenerative arthritis. This may be a tip-off to hypertension and cardiac, renal, or liver failure, and may indicate a medical work-up for hypokalemia. In cases of thrombophlebitis, one leg may be larger than the other.

Evaluations of muscle strength can be done. The usual standard polio measurements can be instituted.

The neurovascular status is observed and recorded. Evaluation of whether amputation exists on one side or another would be a rare circumstance.

The patient's cooperation should be recorded as "good," "failed to relax," or "failed to cooperate."

Other considerations in the physical examination would involve the opposite knee or extremity and the patient's ability, if he is anticipating surgery or some rehabilitation period, to protect the injured knee by use of the good knee. In addition, upper extremity strength must be evaluated as to whether it is sufficient to allow the use of crutches, a cane, or a walker.

Does the patient have neurological disease or lack of balance? Is their strength adequate to allow ambulation with crutches, a cane, or a walker? Is the heart and lung capacity sufficient for either the ambulation or rehabilitative process that may be necessary following surgery?

These factors certainly have to be considered to allow adequate rehabilitation.

The physical examination of the knee lends itself well to computerized synthesis of data (see Fig. 5-4). The forms allow for completeness of the medical record and also simplify the narrative reproduction of this information without dictation or typing. Its accuracy is enhanced by the fact that it is done right at the time of the examination; a completed physical examination sheet with its computer-synthesized printout is immediately available.

X-ray evaluation
Standard x-ray films

The routine x-ray examinations of the knee should include a supine and standing anteroposterior view to compare loss of joint space, alignment, or mechanical shift problems with weight bearing and gravity loading (Fig. 2-8). Rosenberg has recently emphasized the importance of the standing anteroposterior x-ray film in 45 degrees of flexion (Fig. 2-9). He points out that if the loss of articular surface is posterior on the tibia (which is common) then the x-ray film with the knee straight does not demonstrate the critical area of loss. A false negative interpretation may result from a single-angle anteroposterior x-ray film.

A notch view in slight flexion plus a standard lateral view should also be performed.

The patellar position in the lateral view can be taken at 30 degrees of flexion to evaluate patella alta by the Insall-Salvati Method (Fig. 2-10).

Comparison lateral x-ray films of both knees in maximal extension with active quadriceps contraction have been proposed by Norman et al.[41] to accurately assess patella alta (Fig. 2-11).

The axial view of the patella is taken with both knees at 45 degrees of flexion after the method of Merchant[9] (Fig. 2-12). Rarely are 20-, 30-, 60-, or 90-degree films necessary, because the 45-degree view correlates best with actual dynamics as shown by arthroscopy (see Chapter 10). Multiple positions often result in confusion or poor technique on the part of technicians.

A patellar tangential view with flexion and weight bearing may be helpful in diagnosing the subtle patellar malposition problem.

I encourage especially the standing anteroposterior and Merchant patellar x-ray views. My case review experience shows that neither view has been taken

Text continued on p. 49.

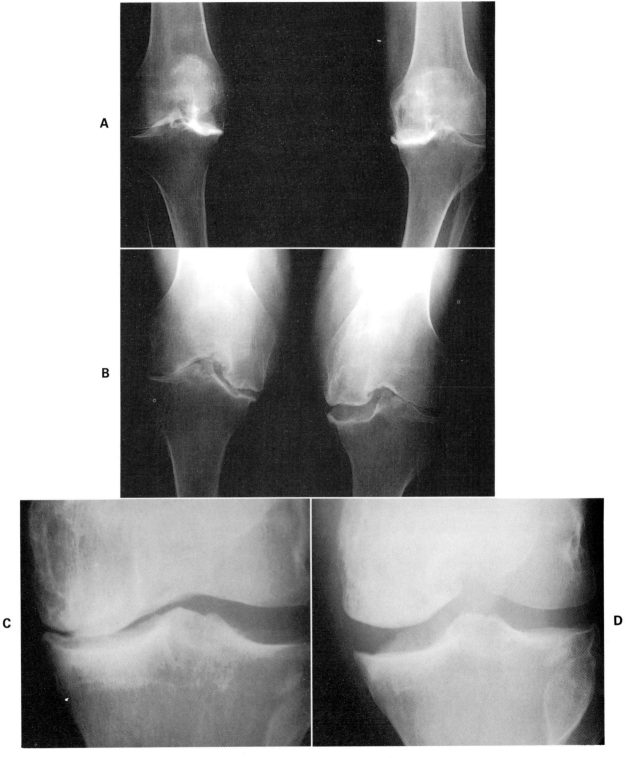

FIG. 2-8. Comparison supine and standing films are important to demonstrate joint space. **A,** Standing anteroposterior film with both knees in extension. **B,** Supine x-ray film shows wider joint space. **C,** Close-up standing film. **D,** Supine film of patient in **C** shows false negative widened joint space.

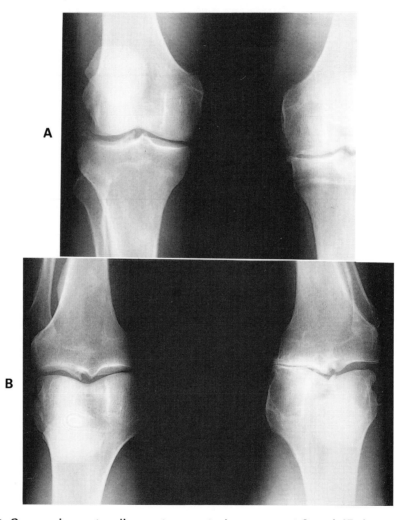

FIG. 2-9. Comparison standing anteroposterior x-rays at 0 and 45 degrees of flexion. **A,** 0 degrees. **B,** 45 degrees. Notice similar joint space in flexion. *Continued.*

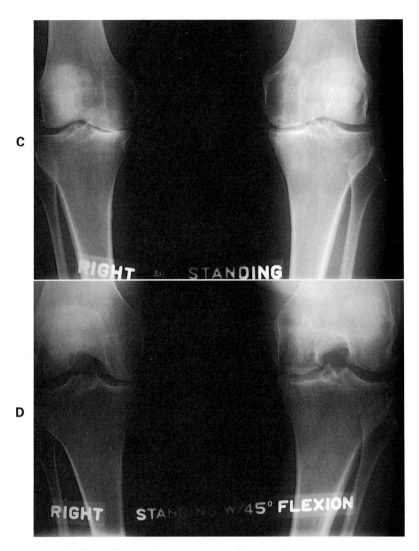

FIG. 2-9, cont'd. **C,** Standing anteroposterior film at 0 degrees shows narrow right medial joint space. **D,** Same knee at 45 degrees shows wider joint space. (Contrast with **A** and **B**).

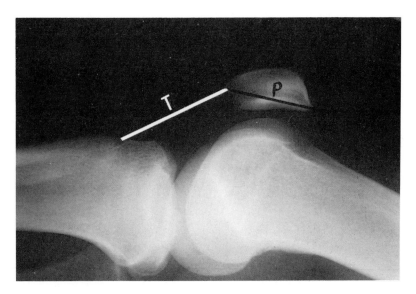

FIG. 2-10. Insall-Salvati method of assessing patella alta.

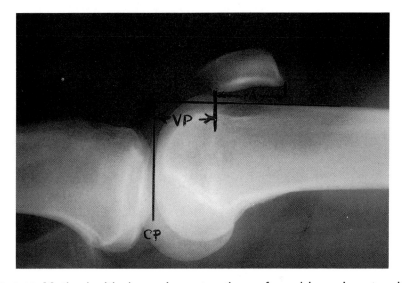

FIG. 2-11. Method with dynamic contractions of quadriceps in extension.

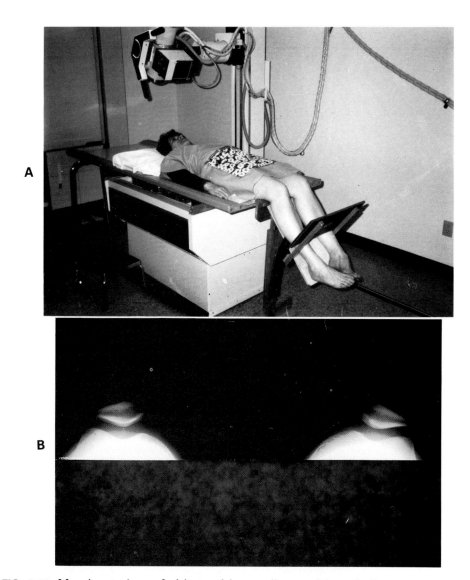

FIG. 2-12. Merchant view of side-to-side patellar position. **A,** Proper patient position with both knees flexed 45 degrees, tube angled 30 degrees, 48 inches proximal to knees. **B,** Normal Merchant views of both knees.

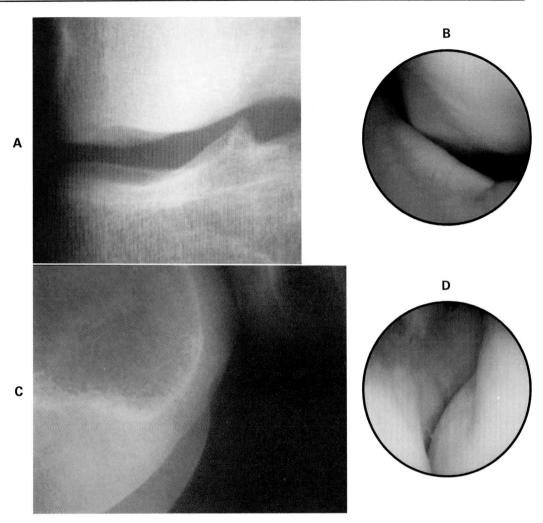

FIG. 2-13. Variations in x-ray films. **A,** Normal depression of lateral femoral condyle seen in anteroposterior view. **B,** Arthroscopic view of atraumatic depression of lateral femoral condyle. **C,** Lateral x-ray view of femoral depression. **D,** Arthroscopic view of same patient.

in most cases (95%), even when the knee has been previously evaluated or operated on. The taking of these views should be a standard practice.

The evaluations of the knee can be done very rapidly with a checklist x-ray evaluation form (see Fig. 5-5). Any special x-ray films taken, such as arthrograms, tomograms, or bone scans can be included on the form and become part of the computer-synthesized medical record, easily retrievable for any patient. This form will allow for comparison studies.

Variations in plain films

Variations in plain x-ray films must be recognized and combined with arthroscopic observations to properly diagnose and treat patients. A lateral femoral condylar depression is a normal arthroscopic finding (Fig. 2-13). In some pa-

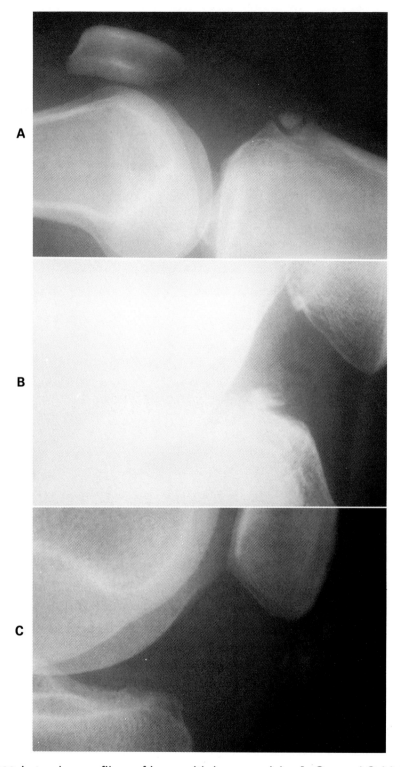

FIG. 2-14. Lateral x-ray films of knee with bony ossicle. **A,** Osgood-Schlatter's disease, old. **B,** Extrasynovial loose body in fat pad. **C,** Patella tendon calcification.

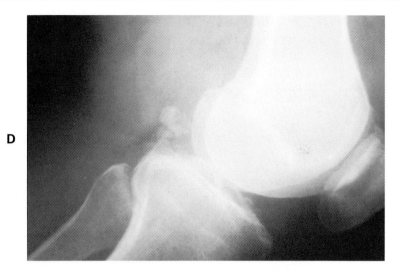

FIG. 2-14, cont'd. D, Intraarticular posterior loose body.

tients, the condition is so prominent that it is obvious on x-ray film and produces symptoms of catching and popping on lateral joint line. It is atraumatic. No treatment has been instituted. Symptoms may persist without progression or destruction.

Juxtaarticular radiopaque ossicles and calcifications must be evaluated for pathological significance (Fig. 2-14). If there is a loose body, it may be located inside or outside of the joint. Repeat x-ray films may reveal change of loose body position, confirming intraarticular mobility.

Other ossicles may represent avulsion of ligament or tendinous insertion. (Fig. 2-15)

Stress x-ray films can identify joint laxity and differentiate ligament tear from epiphyseal injury (Fig. 2-16).

Specific x-ray evaluations for joints other than the knee can be found in the chapters on those joints.

Special tests

Arthrography. Arthrography has been of considerable benefit in advancing the art of diagnosis of joint diseases. At present, I limit the use of arthrography in my practice to unusual problem cases about the knee joint, such as a mass adjacent to the joint with the possibility of communication with the joint. A Baker's cyst or a popliteal fossa tumor may require arthrography for differentiation. In some cases, juxtaarticular masses and cysts of menisci and/or of the proximal tibiofibular joint can be evaluated by this means.

Arthrography is used in suspected meniscus tears to determine location of tear and suitability for repair (Fig. 2-17, *A*). This meniscus evaluation affects indication for arthroscopy in acute hemarthrosis with clinical evidence of an "isolated" tear of the anterior cruciate ligament or a tear of the tibial collateral ligament (Fig. 2-18).

In the shoulder, arthrography is used to determine the existence of a rotator cuff tear; however, small tears may seal over. Acute tears may be filled with blood

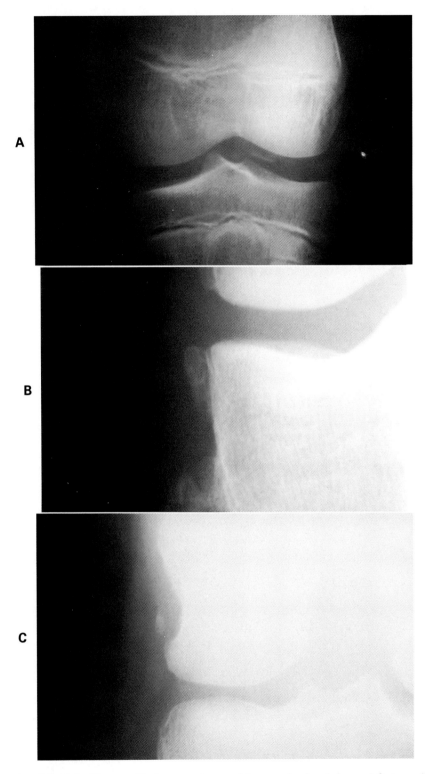

FIG. 2-15. AP plain films with loose piece of bone. **A,** Avulsion of femoral attachment of ACL. **B,** Avulsion of insertion of lateral capsular ligament. **C,** Avulsion of popliteus tendon insertion on femur.

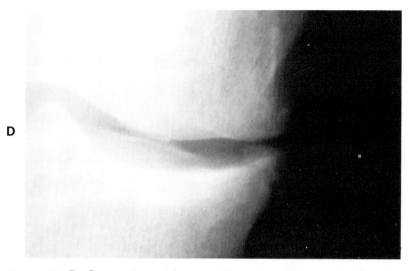

FIG. 2-15, cont'd. D, Sequestrated bone adjacent to TCL caused by degenerative fracture of tibia.

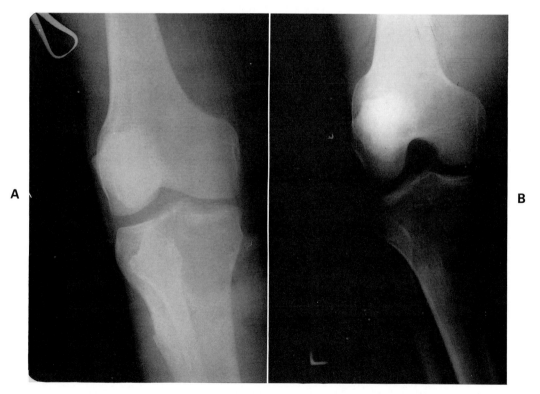

FIG. 2-16. Stress films. **A,** Resting AP film taken in OR. **B,** Application of varus force shows opening of lateral joint line.

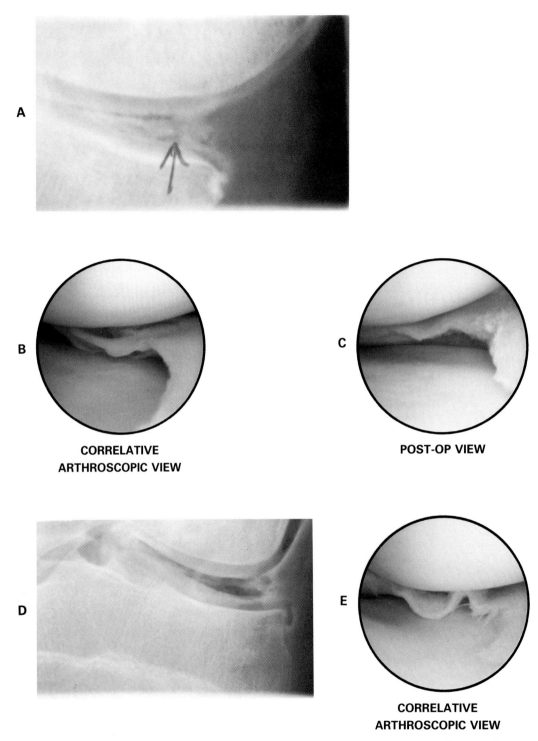

FIG. 2-17. Arthrography in meniscal tears. **A,** Arthrogram of torn medial meniscus. **B,** Arthroscopic view. **C,** After arthroscopic resection. **D,** Arthrogram of complex tear. **E,** Arthroscopic view of complex tear.

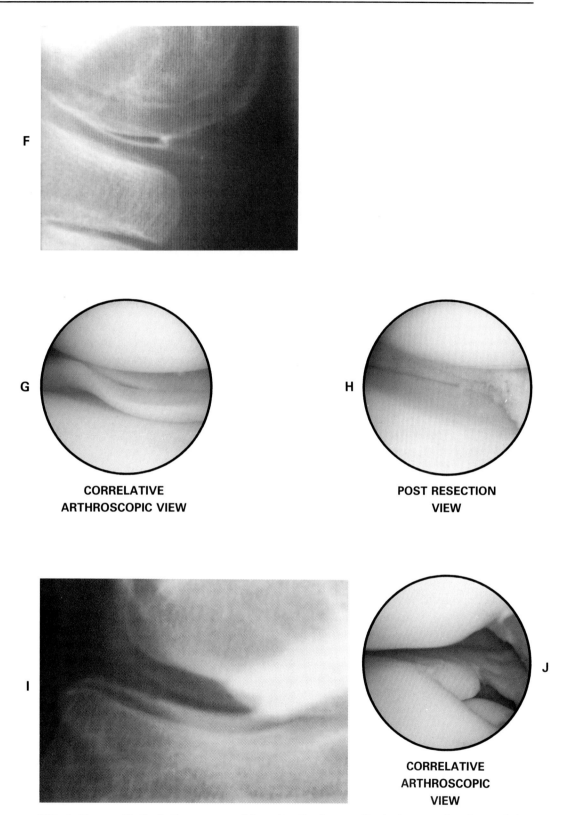

FIG. 2-17, cont'd. F, Arthrogram of longitudinal tear. **G,** Arthroscopic view of the tear in **E. H,** Arthroscopic view after resection. **I,** Arthrogram of diskoid meniscus. **J,** Arthroscopic view of patient in **I.**

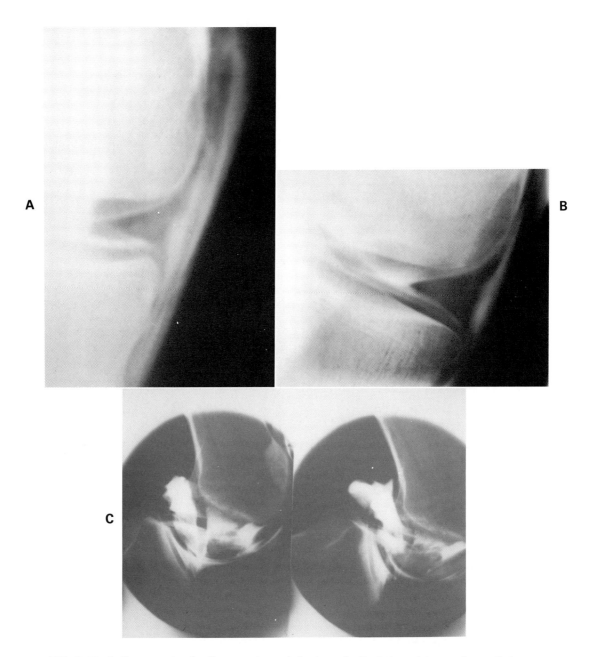

FIG. 2-18. Arthrography in ligamentous injuries. **A,** Peripheral tear of medial meniscus adjacent to TCL. **B,** TCL tear with medial extravasation of dye. **C,** ACL tear. Nomal left, torn right. (Courtesy Drs. F. Deltour and C. Miremad, Paris.)

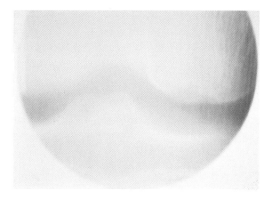

FIG. 2-19. Tomogram shows osteochondritic lesion in medial femoral condyle without sequestration.

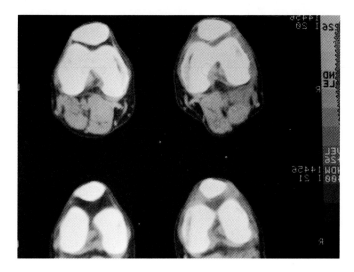

FIG. 2-20. Computed tomography of patellofemoral joint.

or fibrous exudate. Chronic tears with synovial coverings give false negative results.

In any event, the best arthrographic examination does not compare to the direct visualization possible by arthroscopic means. In addition, arthroscopy provides an opportunity for simultaneous diagnosis and operative correction.

Tomography. Tomography can be helpful in cases of bony lesions. It is most helpful in determining separation in osteochondritis dissecans (Fig. 2-19).

Computed tomography. Computed tomography has been used to evaluate the patellofemoral articulation (Fig. 2-20). It is, however, an expensive and elaborate means, considering that problems in this area can be assessed clinically by plain x-ray film and arthroscopic inspection. Computed tomography is rarely used in the knee except in unusual lesions about the joint, such as complex fractures of the articular surface and/or tumors.

Bone imaging by radionuclides. Technetium-99m polyphosphate bone scans are used in problem cases. In patients with knee joint complaints but no positive physical findings, operative intervention might be indicated if there is a positive scan (Fig. 2-21). The bone scan may localize the lesion in cases of postsurgical problem knees (Fig. 2-22). If the bone scan is normal in a patient who has physical complaints but a normal physical examination, it is highly unlikely that there is any intraarticular abnormality in my experience.

It is possible for a bone scan to be normal in a case of chronic subluxation of the patella if it is in its quiescent stage. The diagnosis would show up clinically and/or by x-ray examination.

FIG. 2-21. Bone imaging by radionuclides

A Normal knees with open epiphyseal plates show increased uptake.
B Plain film showing disuse osteoporosis.
C Bone scan shows increase uptake at joint on focal lesion of previous infection of medial diaphysis.
D X-ray film showing osteochondritis dissecans.
E Bone scan showing osteochondritis dissecans

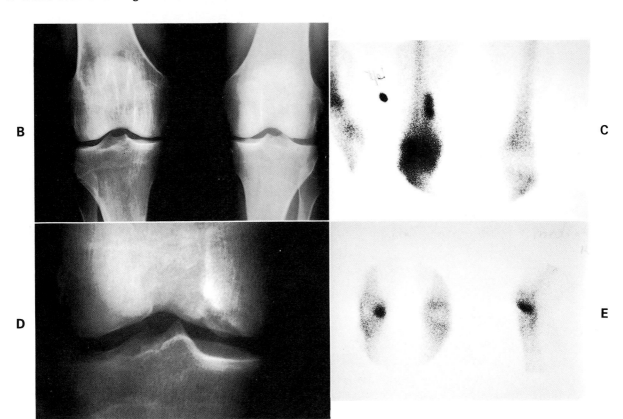

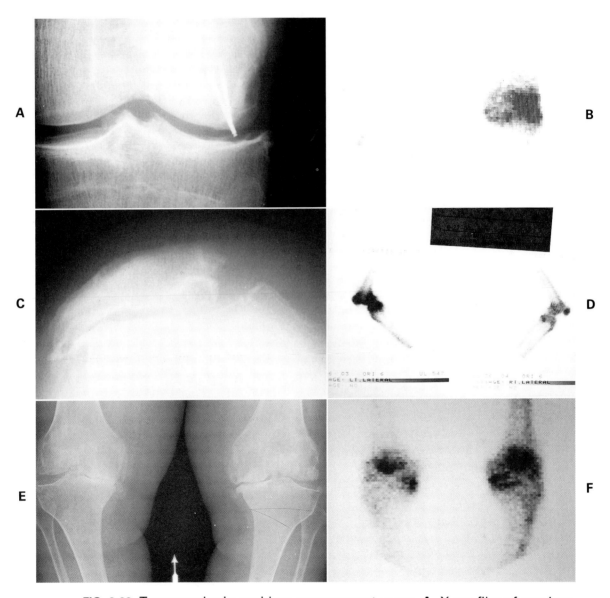

FIG. 2-22. Tomography in problem management cases. **A,** X-ray film of previous open reduction of osteochondral fracture. **B,** Bone scan of same patient shows both femoral and tibial involvement (see Fig. 9-22). **C,** X-ray film of degenerative patellofemoral joint. **D,** Lateral bone scan (left) shows increased uptake by patella and joint compared to right side. **E,** X-ray film of patient with degenerative arthritis. **F,** Bone scan shows increased uptake in medial compartment and patella on both sides. Osteotomy could be considered.

Continued.

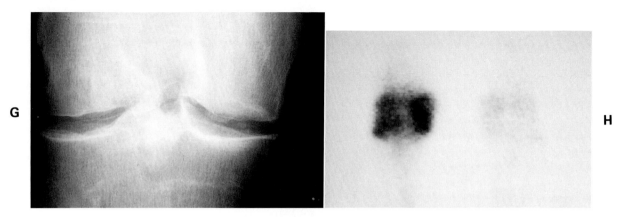

Fig. 2-22, cont'd. G, X-ray film of osteoarthritic knee. **H,** Bone scan of knee in **G** shows diffuse uptake. Osteotomy is ruled out.

A normal knee joint usually shows symmetrical activity in both knees on bone scan. If anteroposterior and lateral scans have been done in both knees, a total body scan is usually not done, unless there is some other indication. If total body scan is taken, one should know that there is some increase in uptake in the dominant hand and shoulder. This should be noted, especially when comparing one shoulder to the other shoulder. The uptake is also increased by epiphysis. The uptake by bony masses increases in proportion to the size of the mass. For instance, the medial femoral condyle is larger than the lateral, so it generally will have a greater uptake than the lateral femoral condyle.

Soft tissue uptake increases where there are areas of synovitis or infections, or even where there have been previous injection sites in or about a joint. There is evidence that postoperative abdominal scars can increase uptake of this particular radionuclide. The test is basically related to the blood flow in or about tissues, including the knee.

The usual dose of nuclide is 15 to 20 mCi and the scintigraphy is performed 2½ hours after the IV injection. The technique involves computerized manipulation of data to show both minimal and maximal densities (Fig. 2-23). The time necessary for this test is sometimes inconvenient for the patient.

Thomas et al.[54] reported the use of radionuclide in evaluating osteoarthritis of the knee before possible tibial osteotomy. He noted that radionuclide joint imaging correlated more closely with the actual pathological findings than other x-ray modalities. On direct inspection, he found intensive uptake to be related to both the extent and severity of the actual pathological abnormality. Further, he found that the results of valgus-producing high tibial osteotomy were better if the lateral compartment was negative on bone scan (see Fig. 2-22, *E* and *F*). If there was an increased uptake in the lateral tibial compartment, then the patient was probably a poor candidate for high tibial osteotomy (see Fig. 2-22, *G* and *H*). This finding is of value in planning combined procedures with arthroscopy.

My own observations with bone scans in degenerative arthritis indicate that what Thomas reports is true: there is a direct relationship between the uptake of the radionuclide and the extent and severity of the lesion. Radionuclide uptake

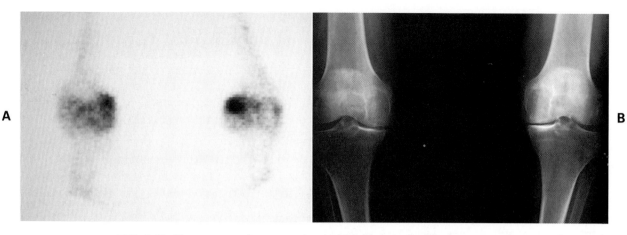

FIG. 2-23. Bone scan shows various densities to facilitate comparison and magnitude of uptake. **A,** Anteroposterior bone scan of both knees shows bilateral medial compartment uptake. **B,** Anteroposterior standing x-ray film of same patient shows mild varus and joint space still open.

of great intensity related to the articular surfaces indicates exposed sclerotic bone with increased vascularity at the surface. The patient would probably be a candidate for abrasion arthroplasty, osteotomy, or even total knee replacement in severe cases.

I also use the bone scan with patients who have had previous multiple surgical procedures to delineate the problem area. A bone scan may reveal involvement of previously operated sites and/or involvement of a previously unoperated site in patients who have had open or arthroscopic surgery in one or more compartments of the joint (see Fig. 2-6, *A* and *B*). A site may be involved that would have been unsuspected clinically or by plain x-ray film. Special attention could be given to palpation of the articular surfaces in areas of increased uptake.

The presence of bone reaction is a prognostic indicator that is of value in certain cases. The disease may have progressed to such an extent that the prognosis is poor. These patients should know that their joints and the tissues adjacent to their joints are responding to an extent beyond that seen on the surface. An operation on the joint surfaces alone would not deal with the basic underlying pathology in these cases.

Repeat annual bone scans may be used to follow the progression or recession of the arthritic processes.

Cahill and Berg have shown the value of the bone scan in conservative management of osteochondritis dissecans in the knee.[2]

Laboratory tests

On hospital admission, the patient should have routine multiphasic laboratory tests, including complete blood count and urinalysis. Some specific tests are of importance to surgeons caring for patients who have joint diseases. Although these tests are not absolutely diagnostic, they are helpful. In diagnosing and profiling the patient with synovitis, I measure the sedimentation rate, perform the latex agglutination test, do the lupus erythematosus prep three times, and do the antinuclear antibody test. However, if all these tests are normal, it does not rule out rheumatological or collagen problems. They establish a baseline by which to profile patient progress or measure the therapeutic benefits of a treatment program.

Surprisingly enough, the most common and necessary laboratory test is the serum potassium level. This is because many patients are hypertensive in the United States. The standard of practice in the United States is not to give any potassium supplement to patients receiving antihypertensive medications. Serum potassium levels are not regularly monitored. For any patient taking hypertensive medication, I do not schedule surgery until the serum potassium level has been established at 3.5 mEq or above. After this level has been achieved, the patient can safely be scheduled for anesthetic administration.

Joint fluid analysis can be helpful, including a cell count, differential, and mucin test. The most common laboratory test on synovial fluid is a culture, including aerobic and anaerobic tests. This is usually best done at the hospital or an immediately adjacent laboratory. Performing this test in conjunction with the laboratory technician permits immediate placement in the culture tubes, which is especially important for the anaerobic culture. A culture and sensitivity report is obtained. When infection is suspected, a gram stain on a smear of centifuged joint fluid can be helpful. A test that is of diagnostic importance but infrequently done is inspection for intercellular crystalline material, indicating gout or pseudogout. As with many other joint conditions, the diagnosis of gout or pseudogout ends up being made more often by medical history, physical examination, and x-ray films.

Psychological tests

The Minnesota Multiphasic Personality Inventory (MMPI) is a valuable test for gaining some objectivity by third-party interview and examination (Fig. 2-24). Performing this test can give the orthopedic surgeon some input that he or she would not otherwise have. In general, I reserve the MMPI for patients who have had multiple surgeries or those who have, in my opinion, some type of personality disorder. It does not matter whether they have intraarticular disease; a significant aberration in their emotional dimension will affect the overall success of any treatment, including arthroscopy.

Gaining acceptance of this test may encounter resistance. In the interview I explain to the patient that the emotions do affect the body. I never deny that the patient has pain. Pain is subjective and not otherwise measurable. I usually illustrate this to patients by asking if they are aware of peptic ulcers, which are actual pathological conditions that can bleed, obstruct, and perforate. I ask them if they know that stress can cause an ulcer, a physical abnormality. This type of discussion seems to enlighten some patients concerning their own joint problem.

I explain to these patients that, although it is just my opinion, I feel that their psychological state is a significant enough issue that it ought to be addressed. I suggest that a third-party interview and MMPI can help establish this.

I do not try to either confront or bludgeon the patient with this information. I represent it as a matter of data collection and patient profiling, just like that we would get by x-ray or laboratory evaluation.

I do not electively accept third-party liability or workmen's compensation

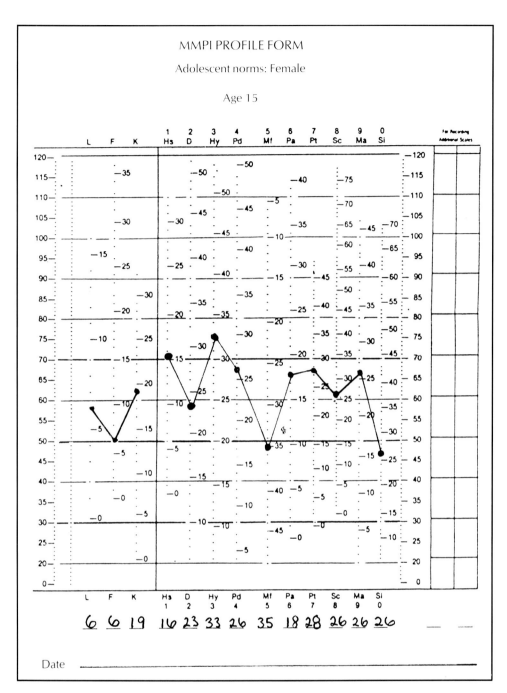

FIG. 2-24. The most common scale for adolescent knee pain patients who lack evidence of organic pathology is shown here. This is technically called a 3-1 profile. This means there is a moderate elevation in hysteria and to a lesser degree an elevation in hypochondriasis. Depression is not evident and this profile is rightly termed the "conversion V" profile. These pattern of scores suggest complaints of pain and preoccupation with somatic symptoms as an unconscious strategy to cope with emotional conflict. Conflicts in the adolescent knee pain patient are often in the form of control over solicitous parents. (See Lachar, D.: The MMPI: clinical assessment and automated interpretation, Detroit, 1971, Western Psychological Services, Lafayette Clinic; and Marks, P.A., and Seeman W.: The actuarial use of the MMPI with adolescents and adults, Baltimore, 1974, Williams & Wilkins.) (Courtesy John Jerome, Ph. D.)

patients in my practice, except by referral from a physician. If one chose to treat these patients, the MMPI would be of benefit, at least from the physician's standpoint, to know what type of emotional character one was treating. MMPI profiling may offer a better opportunity for success in this type of patient.

Surprisingly, some patients do not want to be well, in spite of the fact that they have come to see a physician. Complex secondary gain factors are involved in these cases. I approach this potential problem by direct inquiry.

Often I ask patients if they would have a desire to be successful if we made the right diagnosis and did the correct operation. If they answer yes, I confirm that this is also my desire. If they answer no, I say "good-bye."

Patient expectations

Expectations need to be discussed with the patient. Most patients who come for arthroscopic surgery are interested in how it will allow them to be more effective or efficient in sports. They frequently have lost all perspective on the other dimensions in their lives. Many patients, even some who undergo technically successful arthroscopic surgery and rehabilitation, will require activity modification. They must be informed of the consequences of their injury or disease and the possible extent of benefit from surgery.

The patient must weigh the consequences of hospitalization, immobilization, recovery time, crutches, time off work, and return to sports. These considerations are as important as effects of diseases process. The patient will need answers to many questions. Will reoperations be necessary? What about future open surgery? Should open surgery be performed now? If not, when?

The one-treatment-cures-all approach, although desired by both the patient and the physician, can rarely occur. Patients with a joint condition should understand they have entered into a lifelong management problem. Some conditions are simpler than others; for example, a loose body from a small osteochondritic lesion is of less future consequence than a large lesion, a dislocated patella, or degenerative arthritis. Taking out the loose body is balanced against its underlying cause. The patient with a torn tibial collateral ligament has a better prognosis and shorter rehabilitation than the patient with a torn anterior cruciate ligament.

The patient education or informed consent assist the patient in the decision-making process.

PATIENT MANAGEMENT
Pathological clinical impression

I believe the patient treats himself with the help of the physician. The late Dr. John Dorsey, professor of psychiatry at Wayne State College of Medicine, introduced me to this concept. My subsequent years of practice have convinced me of the validity of the statement. Any physician who disagrees should think back on his or her recent patient experience.

The course of events in patient management is not as simple as rendering a specific diagnosis with a specific cure; I wish it were. Much of what follows in this section may seem obvious. My own practice observations and those of other surgeons demand inclusion of a section on patient management in a text on the practice of arthroscopic surgery. A number of my colleagues have asked that this information, previously delivered in lectures, be printed.

Events of recent years are even more convincing, especially the increasing consumer knowledge of and participation in medicine, supported by information in the media. Many patients even research the literature, and some have brought lists of references to my office on controversial subjects. Some patients desire a dialogue on unresolved medical issues.

Answering patients' questions—including their families', neighbors', and associates' questions—often takes longer than the anticipated surgery. I try to provide enough information and time for the patient to decide what course of treatment he wishes. Some patients require more time than office hours provide. I suggest decisions be deferred until after the visit and after family conferences. I encourage patients to obtain other medical opinions. I provide any and all information I have gathered. *In the final analysis, the physician informs the patient, who makes most therapeutic decisions.*

Following the customary medical history, physical examination, x-ray review, and laboratory tests, the physician has a clinical impression of the patient's problem. An exact pathological diagnosis would be confirmed only by time, disease progression, direct inspection, or confirmation at surgery. Histological or even chemical analysis may be necessary.

Many other factors affect the anticipated treatment. Of what significance is the problem to the patient, his family, and associates? The physician could not possibly learn of all these factors. Many questions are left unanswered or problems denied by patients. The physician must gather as much information as possible. The presentation of clinical impression must be understandable. Patients must comprehend their problem well enough to make a decision concerning *their condition* and the treatment alternatives. Except in life-threatening conditions, the prerogative should rest solely with the patient and his family or associates. This is a way of addressing the legal issue of informed consent.

Patient management is a judgment call. A patient's personality, character, employment, and recreational desires affect any treatment recommendation. The longer recovery period of one treatment method over another may have economic impact in terms of work loss.

The surgeon's personality, as matched or mismatched to the patient and his family or associates, affects the physician-patient relationship. The surgeon's skill and confidence in arthroscopy affects what procedures might be recommended.

In spite of these types of considerations, some determination and/or action is desirable. The surgeon and patient should recognize that the physician is rendering a medical opinion based on his or her training and experience. Neither party should be insecure with this situation, and it could not be otherwise. The surgeon's responsibility is to be honest in appraisal and deliberate in exercising judgment. The patient's welfare is of paramount importance.

A benefit to the patient and his family or associates should be objective. The benefit may be advice, treatment, or referral. It may be arrived at by medical means, physical therapy, or activity modification. Surgery may also render a benefit. Reasons must be formulated for treatment recommendation, and I call these reasons surgical indications.

Indications for arthroscopy
General indications

The indications for *diagnostic* arthroscopy are as follows:
1. A diagnosis has not been made by other more simple, less expensive, noninvasive, or safer means.
2. Information will be obtained that could benefit the patient or affect treatment.
3. A complete diagnostic arthroscopy is to precede anticipated surgical intervention.

The indications for *operative* arthroscopy are as follows:
1. A disease condition or process exists that is treatable by arthroscopic or combined techniques with possible patient benefit.
2. There is reasonable medical certainty that the surgeon is able to perform the necessary surgery arthroscopically.

Contraindications

General contraindications for arthroscopy are as follows:
1. No meaningful information or patient benefit can be expected.
2. The patient is uncooperative, especially under local anesthesia, but also concerning preoperative and postoperative instructions.
3. The surgeon is unable to perform the procedure.

Absolute contraindications for arthroscopy are as follows:
1. No indications are present.
2. Surgical ability or proper equipment is absent.

Relative contraindications to arthroscopy include the following:
1. The joint space is occupied by fibrous or bony growth.
2. There are general medical or anesthetic contraindications.
3. There is infection in skin or subcutaneous areas in an otherwise uninfected knee.
4. There is active (acute) thrombophlebitis.
5. There is wide capsular disruption demonstrated by physical examination of joint or recognized extravasation of fluid at the time of arthroscopy.
6. The joint is normal, unless all parties agree to arthroscopy for medicolegal or psychological treatment purposes.

Judgment calls

Beyond lists of indications and contraindications, surgical judgment is necessary in individual cases and conditions.[25] This is particularly true in some cases of hemarthrosis, chronic conditions, infections, and ankylosis. If a treatable diagnosis is suspected, then same-day or prompt arthroscopic examination is valid.

Hemarthrosis. It has been stated that hemarthrosis is a contradication to arthroscopy because of lack of visualization and low yield of meaningful or treatable diagnosis. Neither reason is valid.

This controversy dates back to early 1970s, but techniques of simple joint lavage and vacuuming changed that teaching. Some physicians still say that many knees with hemarthrosis get better without these procedures. Others suggest that ligament injuries require no early surgery, including torn anterior cru-

---

```
Differential diagnosis in hemarthrosis
• Torn anterior cruciate ligament
• Torn meniscus
• Dislocated patella
• Torn tibial collateral ligament
• Articular injury
• Contusion
```

FIG. 2-25. Differential diagnosis of hemarthrosis.

ciate ligament, even when combined with torn tibial collateral ligament.

If there is no evidence of gross capsular disruption to prevent joint distention or cleansing or to permit excessive fluid extravasation, then hemarthrosis itself is not a contraindication.

The patient with an acute hemarthrosis has a torn anterior cruciate or tibial collateral ligament, a torn meniscus, dislocated patella, articular bony disruption, and/or contusion of synovium.[7,42] Only contusion does not require surgical inspection (Fig. 2-25).

The differential diagnosis of hemarthrosis includes the following (see Fig. 2-25):

1. Torn anterior cruciate ligament
2. Torn meniscus
3. Dislocated patella
4. Torn tibial collateral ligament
5. Intraarticular fracture or avulsion
6. Contusion

Contusion can usually be diagnosed by history and physical examination. Simple aspiration would confirm hemarthrosis and provide comfort by decompressing the swollen joint. The other diagnoses listed are probably treatable with arthroscopic or combined methods.

Arthroscopy provides a means of rendering a judgment as to pathologic lesion, prospective treatment, and prognosis. At least, the patient management is outlined or instituted based on accurate information. For instance, a fracture or osteochondral fracture may be repaired with reduction and internal fixation. This otherwise undiagnosed lesion would prolong recovery or adversely affect the outcome.

If the meniscus is torn or displaced, removal or repair is indicated. Removal allows for restoration of normal joint motion. If repair is possible, repair and immobilization decrease the chance of complete disruption or articular injury.

Dislocated patella often produces loose bodies of cartilage, often nonradiolucent or undetected. An arthroscopic repair will not lengthen the recovery time of the existing injury. Reduction of repeat injury and restoration of normal patellofemoral mechanics is possible. The benefit reduces subsequent morbidity and recurrence.

Tibial collateral ligament tear with hemarthrosis suggests greater magnitude of disruption or even other intraarticular lesions. A tear with no effusion but positive abduction stress test suggests anterior cruciate ligament tear. Small tibial collateral ligament disruptions that are palpable or demonstrable on testing are amenable to transcutaneous arthroscopically monitored suture repair.

This leaves only the question of repair of acute tears of the anterior cruciate ligament. First, the examination of the patient who is under anesthesia may show capsular instability which requires open surgery. Next, the extent of all accompanying damage may be assessed. The amenability of the anterior cruciate ligament to repair can be determined. Removal of joint-blocking ligament fragments has been suggested. I do not do this anymore; I prefer to save all anterior cruciate ligament tissue. Presently, either primary repair or harvest with augmentation reconstruction is performed (see Chapter 12).

Chronic conditions. The diagnosis is usually established clinically in patients with chronic conditions. Still there may be a benefit of intermediate surgical care before "definitive" open surgery. Arthroscopy can determine the extent of chronic conditions. Lavage and debridement procedures improve the degenerative joint environment (see Chapters 8 and 9) and benefit the patient. Staging of more formal procedures is advised.

Infections. Certainly an uninfected joint should not be arthroscoped if adjacent skin, bursae, or subcutaneous tissues are infected. I defer operative arthroscopy on referral cases until previous arthroscopic puncture wounds are healed (approximately 10 days). There should be no scabs.

Joint infection is not a contraindication. In fact arthroscopic diagnosis with culture, lavage, and debridement synovectomy is beneficial.

Ankylosis. A bony, fused joint would be impossible to enter with the arthroscope, but if any space exists arthroscopic adhesiolysis may be a treatment choice. Ankylosis increases the difficulty of arthroscopy, but these techniques can be useful in adhesion resection and quadriceps mechanism release, often accompanied by gentle manipulation and followed by postoperative continuous passive motion and physical therapy.

Physician education

Some have suggested that no fee should be submitted if arthroscopy is being performed for the educational benefit of the surgeon. The inference is that the procedure would be beneficial solely to the beginning arthroscopist and not the patient. I take exception to that concept. Every operative procedure should be educational to the surgeon. In fact that is why our profession is called the "practice of medicine." No surgeon would testify that practicing the profession of medicine did not enhance his or her knowledge. Review of videotapes, done soon after the surgical procedure, is an excellent means of self-assessment and study.

Physician selection

Physicians erroneously believe that the selection process begins with them, during the patient interview and examination. In fact, the patient has first selected the the physician, based on his knowledge of the physician's reputation.

Factors such as proximity to home or relatives, expense, HMO contracts, insurance, and even personality also affect the selection.

Specifically, patients who are aware of alternative treatments will select a surgeon who performs procedures arthroscopically. The reconstructive surgeon who does not fully use arthroscopic techniques will be sought out by patients who, for whatever reason, desire open procedures.

The physician must keep in mind that he or she was first selected by the patient. Only afterward does the physician become involved in selection of the patient. This important factor is often not realized.

Patient selection

After the physician has formulated a clinical impression in the quest for a pathological diagnosis and while reviewing the indication for treatment, the physician must figuratively step aside and consider the matter of patient selection. Patient selection is the final and highest plane in surgical judgment.

Patient selection plays a major role in the success of the treatment and the patient benefits to be derived. In the patient interview, contact, and examination, the surgeon should establish rapport and gain the confidence of the patient. This is achieved by sufficient interaction with the patient. Sitting down and writing notes during the patient interview helps both parties in this new relationship. Involvement in the patient's problem to the extent of understanding how it is affecting his life will direct subsequent judgment.

The surgeon should also be aware of how he or she feels about a given patient's problem and of how the patient is reacting to the physician-patient relationship. Is the patient reacting favorably toward the physician, the office environment, the practice, and the physician's demeanor and appearance? All these things are quite an added responsibility for the physician. He or she tries to meet the needs of many different people within limited time, including interruptions for different types of emergencies. With all these different demands on the surgeon, he or she must arrive at a conclusion concerning the patient's diagnosis. If it is not possible to proceed on the basis of history, physical examination, and x-ray findings, the surgeon has to proceed with necessary adjunct tests such as laboratory studies, bone scan, and MMPI. Enough data must be collected to arrive at a conclusion and disposition, a diagnosis, and a recommended treatment.

After the surgeon has arrived at a conclusion, he or she has to synthesize all of this information and decide whether it is possible to make a therapeutic recommendation. It is important for the patient not only to know the physician's impression but how it was arrived at. The spectrum of the patient's alternatives ranges from doing nothing to doing something. If the patient plans to do something, there may be some course of medication, physical therapy, rehabilitation, or bracing to follow. There may be a place for diagnostic arthroscopy, operative arthroscopy, and/or conventional surgery, and there is also the question of the best timing.

After the patient is fully informed concerning diagnosis, alternatives, and expectations for both immediate and long-term results, it is possible to consider engaging in a contractual agreement concerning the treatment. The surgeon must also consent.

There is one criterion that I have found to encompass all the other criteria of whether I should continue as the treating physician: *will I enjoy my office hours after I have carried out the course of treatment with this patient?* If the answer is no, there is no reason to consider entering into any form of treatment with the patient. If the answer is yes, I can treat without reservation.

This question is actually asking numerous questions. Do I get along with the patient and vice versa? Can I meet the patient's expectations? Have I made the correct diagnosis? Can I satisfactorily perform technically the necessary diagnostic and operative work indicated? Am I able to manage any complications that might be anticipated with my surgical recommendation? Am I willing to see the patient through the rehabilitation process to a conclusion that meets our expectations?

Sometimes the overall picture (as it were, the forest) can be lost (for the trees). The issue of enjoying my office hours can truly assist in patient selection. As a bonus, my office hours are more pleasant.

This also leads to the possibility of not wanting to accept a patient for treatment for reasons related to interpersonal relations, diagnosis, or anticipated treatment. I believe that it is legitimate to explain to patients that it is your belief that you would not be able to meet their expectations. Suggesting that they seek another opinion is legitimate. You may wish to elaborate, or you may not. Just stating "for personal reasons" is enough and avoids unpleasant discussion. Explain that both the physician and the patient have a choice in these matters. Even if you showed desire to treat, the patients would also be free to go somewhere else. Either way, physicians do not take this option often enough. It is important both medically and legally to make these decisions ahead of time if you perceive that there may be any potential problems either with you or with the patient. The patient can very well go on to success with some other physician and some other environment.

The fact that you tell patients that you are unable to meet their expectations or that the surgery could in no way do what they are expecting it to might give them a better sense of reality and prepare them to meet another surgeon. The patient's expectations are better in line, and the results will be more satisfactory for both you and the patient.

HOSPITAL CREDENTIALS

In most states a physician licensed to practice medicine may perform or render medical care in any area encompassed by his profession. In the case of a medical doctor or doctor of osteopathy in the State of Michigan, he or she would be able when licensed, to practice any surgical or medical discipline, be it open heart surgery, neurosurgery, or arthroscopic surgery. As a practical matter, of course, this does not occur. Physicians usually function within the realm of their training or experience and are designated as specialists on that basis. Further, they may be certified by the AMA or the American Osteopathic Association board within any given specialty and present themselves to a community and/or hospital with those credentials for the purpose of practicing within the area of their medical or surgical expertise.

Hospitals in the past have routinely requested physicians to fill out a questionnaire indicating procedures they desire to perform. After a peer review by medical doctors and/or administrators, privileges are granted.

Furthermore, in large part, what the physician asks to do is conditioned by his or her special interest and/or experience. In common practice many orthopedic surgeons design their practices into subspecialty areas at the exclusion of others, although most orthopedic surgeons still consider themselves general orthopedists. In addition, there are still-developing subspecialties within orthopedic surgery. Societies and journals are now dedicated to the hip, the shoulder and elbow, scoliosis, the hand, and even arthroscopic surgery.

With the advent of arthroscopic surgery, a discipline that is performed in an environment completely different from other orthopedic surgical procedures, there is concern over what criteria should be used to grant hospital privileges in the area of diagnostic and operative arthroscopy.

The Arthroscopy Association of North America has established guidelines for the practice of arthroscopy (see p. 72).

The orthopedic department of Ingham Medical Center in Lansing, Michigan, under the chairmanship of Dr. James G. Bullock, established a subcommittee to study this issue. The subcommittee presented to orthopedic surgeons practicing at the hospital the following criteria for privileges or credentials to perform arthroscopy at the Ingham Medical Center. These criteria were approved by the orthopedic department, the medical executive board, the hospital administration, and the board of trustees. These criteria are outlined in the box on pp. 73-74.

These criteria are logical and provide a sequence for demonstrating knowledge and experience as well as acquaintance with equipment. These skills must be demonstrated to the satisfaction of the observers or subcommittee.

Certain numbers of case experiences were established as reasonable. They are below the average case experience for an orthopedic surgeon in the United States. We felt these were minimal standards for granting privileges.

There was a transition period of credentialing in the area of arthroscopic surgery to recognize the difficulty of procedures progressing from levels 1 to 4. Level 4 includes virtually all of the more complicated cases.

This concept was well received by hospital administration and the medical executive committee. However, it was not universally well accepted by practicing orthopedic surgeons at Ingham. First, as might be expected, they wanted to have a grandfather clause that included everybody; this idea was rejected. However, compliance by the subcommittee members was instituted. The arthroscopic credentialing subcommittee consisted of two experienced and one relatively inexperienced arthroscopist.

After acceptance of these credentials by the executive committee and the hospital board of trustees, 3 months were allowed for the physicians to comply.

As may have been expected, two members of the subcommittee complied the week before the deadline. Two more weeks were given for all other staff members to comply.

One surgeon asked for diagnostic arthroscopic credentials only. He does not participate or intend to become involved in arthroscopic surgery. Five members complied with the requirements. Level 4 surgical arthroscopic privileges without reservation were granted to four surgeons. One surgeon was given privileges with reservation, providing for upgrading of motorized and surgical instrumentation as a result of observation of his videotapes. It was determined that the equipment he used did not reflect the current state of the art.

SUGGESTED GUIDELINES FOR THE
PRACTICE OF ARTHROSCOPY

This statement was prepared by the Committee on Ethics and Standards of the Arthroscopy Association of North America.

Privileges

The decision to grant and renew privileges in arthroscopy is typically made by individual hospitals with input from medical staff committees and appropriate department chairpersons in accordance with individual hospital and medical staff bylaws, rules, and regulations. It is desirable to include in the decision-making process individuals who have a working knowledge of arthroscopy as well as board certification or its equivalent in orthopaedic surgery.

Training

Adequate training for the practice of arthroscopy may be evidenced by regular attendance at arthroscopic educational courses and/or successful completion of a fellowship training program in arthroscopy and/or experience with skilled arthroscopists. Experience in any or all of the above should be documented and skills may be demonstrated by observed performance, patient records, and peer review.

Practice

The arthroscopist should:
1. Perform an adequate history and physical examination as well as laboratory workup of the patient or determine that these have already been performed.
2. Explain the procedure to the patient, including its benefits, possible risks, and complications.
3. Exercise due consideration in selecting the correct arthroscopic procedure for a particular condition.
4. Prepare a report of the procedure that includes the operation itself and the findings.

Continuing education

The arthroscopist should maintain a high level of expertise in arthroscopy. In order to remain informed the arthroscopist may update his or her knowledge and skill by regular attendance at postgraduate arthroscopic meetings, collaboration with arthroscopists, and continual review of current arthroscopy literature. The arthroscopist should obtain necessary training before undertaking a new procedure.

Performance review

The performance of the arthroscopist should be reviewed regularly. The numbers of procedures, indications, results, and complications should be made available to appropriate medical staff members of individual hospitals which are charged with granting, reviewing, and renewing clinical privileges.

From The Committee on Ethics and Standards of the Arthroscopy Association of North America: Arthroscopy 1(3):A-14, 1985.

CREDENTIALS FOR ARTHROSCOPY, INGHAM MEDICAL CENTER, LANSING, MICHIGAN

Diagnostic arthroscopy

I. Medical doctor or osteopathic physician: preferably with training in joint surgery.

II. Demonstrated knowledge of joint disease and arthroscopic techniques in the following categories:
   A. Literature (reference list)
      1. Textbooks
      2. Periodicals
   B. Course attendance with reports
   C. Experience
      1. Observation
      2. Preceptors confirmed with letter
      3. Residency supported with letters
      4. Fellowship supported with letters
   D. Equipment
      1. Demonstrated knowledge of personal and hospital equipment
   E. Skills
      1. Demonstration on arthroscopic simulator of basic technical skills of insertion and manipulation including triangulation and probing of major structures.

After satisfactory completion of above criteria, the surgeon may schedule a case with observation by a credentialed arthroscopist or committee member.

After 10 cases with satisfaction of the observer, operative notes and operative times are to be submitted to the subcommittee. The subcommittee makes recommendations to the Chief of Orthopedics. He, in turn, writes a letter of approval. Copies are sent to the operating room supervisor and administration.

Surgical arthroscopy

I. Surgeon satisfactorily met criteria for diagnostic arthroscopy, having performed no fewer than fifty (50) cases. This may be waived if the surgeon has previous experience, i.e., fellowship, practice, etc.

II. Satisfactory review of diagnostic work including a review of unedited videotape documenting comprehensive diagnostic examination, multiple portals, if necessary, plus triangulation and successful probing of all structures.

III. Demonstrated
   A. Surgical course attendance
   B. Observation
      Preceptor-resident experience
      Fellowship
   C. Familiarity with personal and hospital arthroscopic instrumentation necessary for comprehensive arthroscopic surgery, including television

Continued.

Surgical arthroscopy—cont'd

    D. Demonstrated competence with all instruments (hand and motorized) on arthroscopic surgical simulator.

       1. Perform bucket-handle tear resection

       2. Perform posterior complex tear resection

       3. Perform synovectomy on plant or vegetable material

       4. Perform chondroplasty on condyles.

When the above criteria are met, the applicant has approval for scheduling cases. Operative cases to include, with candidate responsible for:

    1. Compulsary video documentation—unedited

    2. Both hand and motorized instrumentation at disposal in working condition

    3. Experienced observer for a minimum of six (6) cases for each level, but unsupervised privileges for level 1 or 2 may be granted by recommendation of the Credentialing Committee transmitted by letter to the applicant with a copy to the department chairman, operating room supervisor, and hospital administration.

The level of approval is granted by the Department Chief after documentation by monitors and videotape. Approval for subsequent levels should require satisfactory accomplishments of previous levels of cases documented by operative notes.

Annual certification by hospital Credentialing Committee upon recommendation of Orthopedic Department Chief includes review of number of cases, technical levels, and videotape observation.

    Level 1 approval

       Loose body

       Plica

       Patellar shaving

    Level 2 approval

       Lateral release

       Bucket-handle and flap

       Simple meniscus

    Level 3 approval

       Combination of above

       Complex meniscus tears

       Chondroplasty

    Level 4 approval

       Abrasion arthroplasty

       Synovectomy

       Patellar realignments

       Ligament repair

       Meniscus repair

       Other joint surgery

          Shoulder reconstruction

The other five orthopedic surgeons who practice at the hospital did not apply for privileges in arthroscopic surgery. They choose to perform their procedures at another community hospital that has not established criteria for diagnostic or operative arthroscopy.

One new physician joined the staff during the period in which the credentials were established. He had been given full privileges in orthopedic surgery through the normal monitoring procedure based on his training and experience. He complied with both the letter and the spirit of the law in the area of diagnostic and operative arthroscopy and was granted privileges within 8 months. He received considerable assistance in fulfilling the criteria from the remainder of the active credentialed orthopedic surgeons in the medical center.

One member of the subcommittee fulfilled only a portion of his credentials and chose not to complete his credentialing. He performs arthroscopic procedures at his primary hospital, which is not the Ingham Medical Center.

In my opinion the credentials established at Ingham Medical Center were reasonable. The requirements are easily fulfilled by those who have the necessary arthroscopic experience and ability. We undertook credentialing as something of an adventure. It was successful at Ingham. This program could serve as a model for centers that face the same challenges in their communities.

LEARNING ARTHROSCOPIC SURGERY
Philosophy

Future orthopedists will be adequately trained to perform arthroscopy during their residencies or fellowships, but most practicing orthopedists receive this training in postresidency continuing education programs. To avoid the common frustrations and pitfalls of considering inclusion of arthroscopic surgery in your practice, I recommend the following approach. First you must have the desire to perform arthroscopic surgery. Second, to avoid frustration, you must make an honest appraisal of your own technical abilities. Last but not least you must be able to create an environment at your institution that will allow successfully implementation of learning and maximization of your technical skills.

Expectations

The experience and training of the surgeon is of first and foremost importance. Open joint surgery can be the basis of anatomical and pathological knowledge necessary to begin arthroscopic procedures. The arthroscope has allowed access to areas of the living synovial joint not before seen by open methods and has increased appreciation of anatomical relationships not before recognized. Arthroscopic technique should enhance or build on the experience of any orthopedic surgeon who cares for patients with synovial joint problems.

The surgeon, no matter what or how vast his or her experience in open surgery, will require specialized knowledge and training in arthroscopy. A gradual, staged experience is necessary for successful progression in technique.

I recommend a logical progression of training. Prepare yourself with the appropriate experience and abilities to undertake surgery on any patient. You must possess the level of surgical know-how and ability that you anticipate the patient's condition will require.

The old adage of allowing oneself a choice—"Be humble going in, or humbled coming out"—is especially true in arthroscopic surgery.

You have certain expectations of your own abilities. There tends to be a lot of discouragement while learning arthroscopic surgery, especially for a surgeon who has performed well in general orthopedics for many years. Even those who have specialized in knee joint surgery find themselves frustrated by the inability to see, expose, and resect or repair areas, whereas they could have performed these tasks much more quickly by opening the joint.

I recommend that you only expect as much of yourself as is realistic. Arthroscopic surgery is a new discipline, and you can anticipate that time and experience will be required to develop the skills. Those willing to put in the necessary energy will be well satisfied and rewarded. Those who try to perform arthroscopic procedures beyond their surgical experience will experience frustration and discouragement.

I-beams for success

The I-beams for success demonstrate the progression of experience necessary to learn arthroscopy (Fig. 2-26). The I-beams are in a logical progression based on existing knowledge.

Like any building, the foundation must be on firm footings (knowledge). The ability of the building to stand is based on the superstructure, which I call the I-beams. Each I-beam is a word starting with the letter *I*. The absence of any I-beam results in collapse.

Integrity of the surgeon's character includes honesty and consistency. Attention to operative indications, willingness to demonstrate surgical cases on a television monitor, and reasonable operating times make up this I-beam.

Interest must be high. Arthroscopic techniques are too difficult to master with a casual interest. This I-beam is made up of desire for knowledge and evaluation of case experiences.

Intensity may in itself require discipline and control. It is not possible to be successful with a casual pass at these techniques. This I-beam is made up of quiet patience and persistence.

Intimacy is necessary in the educational experience. As important as reading and viewing education tapes might be, hands-on experience is paramount. Personal visits, one-on-one observation, and questioning solidify this I-beam. Attention moves from the television screen to how the teacher's hands and body move. By another name, this is attention to detail.

The horizontal connecting rods or floors of the I-beams building for success are composed of the logical progression of educational experience.

Courses, reading, and laboratory work

When you are considering whether to include arthroscopic surgery in your practice, I recommend exploring the field by attending a course, reading some papers, talking with others, watching an expert, or studying a textbook. Success in arthroscopic surgery is accomplished by a serious intent, rather than by dabbling for a time. Many survey courses are available almost every month in the United States. These courses allow you to get an overview of what is going on in the field of arthroscopic surgery. If you are determined after that review to move

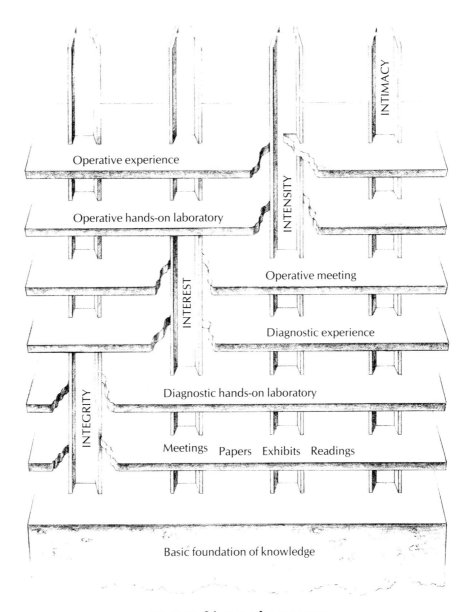

FIG. 2-26. I-beams for success.

ahead, then you must attend a course that includes a laboratory experience of at least 8 hours. In my opinion, a laboratory experience of 1½ hours divided between two or three different attendees in a room with 50 other surgeons is not the optimal atmosphere to gain the intimacy necessary for success in this endeavor.

The ideal laboratory course includes individual instruction. It should start with the absolute basics of the arthroscope: instrumentation and assemblage. The knowledge and use of the arthroscope is most important. The arthroscope will be your eyes for the operation. Your exposure is based primarily on the ability to construct a clear, bright image with the arthroscope.

You should be provided with not only a working knowledge and understanding of the instrumentation but also a hands-on experience with each individual device.

Use one system—perfect it

As in so many other disciplines, it is advantageous to get off on the right foot and follow a given system in arthroscopy. Generally mixing and matching of approaches to arthroscopic surgery leads more to confusion than success. That is one reason I have written about a single method in this textbook and not a compilation of a variety of methodologies. In the early planning stages of arthroscopic surgery, it is important to follow a given school of thought. Once you reach a point of success, you may either continue with that method or design one of your own.

You should read Chapter 6, Techniques, before attempting the following exercises.

Arthroscopic surgical simulator

An arthroscopic knee simulator is essential to learning arthroscopic surgery. The first dry knee model was developed by Robert Eilert.[11] The first wet knee practice device was developed by Howard Sweeney.[53] He used a plastic pitcher with dampered portals. Various vegetables provided the material for resection. Subsequently, under Sweeney's direction, the Arthroscopic Surgical Simulator was developed for more sophisticated surgical work, including meniscectomy and abrasion arthroplasty (see Fig. 1-6).

This particular model has the advantage of allowing the observer to not only work arthroscopically in a place that cannot be seen but also to look over the top of the model to obtain a perspective that could be obtained in no other way (Fig. 2-27). Obviously, this luxury is not possible during live surgery. Simulators are available commercially from several sources for home study.[17,47]

Conception

Conception necessitates transforming the two-dimensional image of the arthroscope or video into a three-dimensional image. This step in conception is assisted by motion of the arthroscope to yield positional sensation and comparative size relationships. Appreciation of the three dimensions is facilitated by entry of a second instrument for probing and triangulation. The palpation, visualization, and the known size of the probing instrument add further to the artistic conception. An appreciation of the anatomy or pathological composition results.

Composition

In arthroscopy the surgeon must mentally compose a picture of the joint. You will quickly learn that visualization is not automatic after the arthroscope is placed. The resultant inside image is a product of many factors (i.e., joint distention, illumination, arthroscopic manipulation, reflective surfaces, and contour of the joint).

Information is obtained technically but conceived in the surgeon's mind.

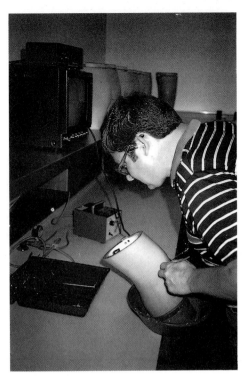

FIG. 2-27. Looking over top of simulator for perspective.

Not all areas can be seen at once, and the composite picture of the joint is constructed from various portals and pictures.

Each and every arthroscopic picture requires conception of maneuvers that will yield a composition from excellent surgical exposure.

The manipulated end (eyepiece) of the arthroscope is outside the joint. Within the joint, the visual end (objective) is out of direct sight or feel. An outside move to the right makes the inside picture go left. If the scope is moved up, the resultant image goes downward. Penetration increases magnification; retraction gives a larger overview. A rotational motion with the standard 30-degree inclined view causes the image to move toward the inclination with a positional distortion of 30 degrees from the axial alignment of the scope.

You must automatically conceive a mixture of these maneuvers to produce successful composition. Practice will replace the step-by-step thought process with smooth, orchestrated motion.

Conception and composition are necessary to arthroscopic success. These skills develop with time and meaningful experience. The following exercises are designed to develop expertise in conception and composition.

Exercises for the arthroscopic surgical simulator

For a better understanding of spacial relationships, it is helpful to look into the top of the canister to visualize the contents (see Fig. 2-27), and study the actual sizes, shapes and relationships. Adding fluid to the system via suprapatellar cannula route is a matter of student discretion during exercises.

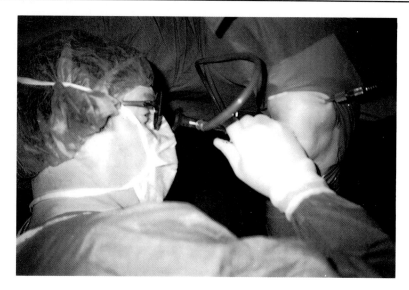

FIG. 2-28. Direct viewing with arthroscope.

DIRECT SCOPE VIEWING

EXERCISE 1: Place the arthroscopic cannula and obturator in the anterolateral inferior portal. (This is a right knee.) A trial insertion with a No. 18 spinal needle may be of assistance.

After the cannula enters the joint, remove the obturator and place the arthroscope.

Direct viewing through the arthroscope aids in positional and tactile sense (Fig. 2-28).

Observe all the structures systematically from medial to lateral.

SCOPE MANIPULATION

EXERCISE 2: Draw a crooked line within the simulator with a pencil, for instance, on the tibial plateau (Fig. 2-29). The line should be curved or squiggly. Identify one end by the arthroscope.

Follow the line first at a distance then up close. When going along its course, make necessary scope manipulations to follow the irregular line across the plateau. Do this slowly, then retrace the course with retraction of the scope. Perform this exercise both right- and left-handed. Also perform it with the left eye and then the right eye at the scope.

Perform the exercise with your best hand and then your best eye. Then follow the line with your nondominant hand and eye, until you can perform it in every possible combination.

Following a squiggly line necessitates scope rotation and angulation with pistoning. All factors involved in conception are necessary to obtain a picture in your mind. If you cannot conceive it, you cannot make a composition.

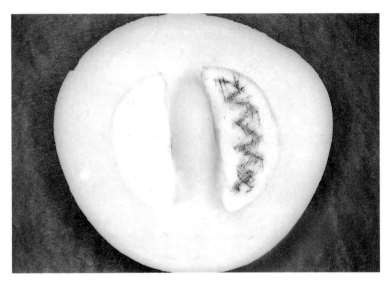

FIG. 2-29. Crooked line drawn on tibial plateau.

SIZE AND SHAPE PERCEPTION

EXERCISE 3: Evaluation of size is an important factor in arthroscopic surgery. Have another person drop unknown objects of various sizes and shapes into the simulator.

Look for these objects arthroscopically. Draw them on a piece of paper, and then remove them from the simulator and compare the pieces to your drawings.

Continue this exercise until you learn to perceive the various sizes and shapes with the arthroscope alone. The techniques of pistoning in and out and comparing adjacent objects within the knee or simulator are important in size determination.

PLACEMENT AND REPLACEMENT

EXERCISE 4: The arthroscope provides a view of the medial compartment from anteriolateral portal. Introduce a No. 18 spinal needle via an anteromedial portal. Identify the needle with the arthroscope. If it is not seen, replace or redirect the needle. Remove the needle and reposition it, up, down, or side-to-side until you have achieved a proper placement site. This will determine the proper cannula and instrumentation entry site to gain access to all areas of the medial compartment.

TRIANGULATION

EXERCISE 5: After introduction, manipulate the needle so as to touch each anatomical structure of the medial compartment.

If you cannot locate the needle, look at the instruments on the outside and triangulate or aim them at each other. Touch them together with palpation. Move the needle down into view (Fig. 2-30). As a last resort you may look over the top of the simulator.

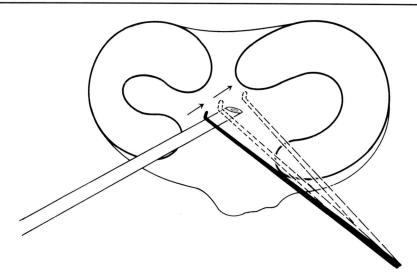

FIG. 2-30. Drawing of touching and moving so ends meet.

BIMANUAL MANIPULATION

EXERCISE 6:   The arthroscope is positioned to view the medial compartment, and the needle is held out of view. Move the needle in front of the arthroscope.

Place the needle tip up close to and in front of the scope. Then, leave the needle stationary in the medial compartment. Remove and reinsert the arthroscope to find the needle. Move the arthroscope up close to the needle tip.

ORCHESTRATION

EXERCISE 7:   As in music, the instruments must be moved or played together in a coordinated and meaningful fashion according to a plan. Improvisation should be reserved for musicians.

Place the scope in the joint and visualize the medial compartment. Insert the needle at the optimal site for the medial compartment and bring it into view of the arthroscope.

Bring the end of the needle into view at the posterior horn of the meniscus. Move the tip of the needle along the inner edge of the meniscus and follow with the arthroscope, thus orchestrating the two instruments. Repeat until action is smooth.

CANNULA PLACEMENT

EXERCISE 8:   After you have determined the proper placement site with the No. 18 spinal needle, remove the needle and incise the rubber skin at the same site.

Remembering the placement and angulation of the needle, place a cannula and obturator in the same plane. The tip of the cannula-obturator will come into view of the arthroscope.

PROBING

EXERCISE 9:   Holding the cannula, remove the obturator and place a probe through the cannula and into view of the arthroscope that is focusing on the end of the cannula. Leaving the probe in place, remove the cannula and place it on table. This avoids unnecessary leakage during triangulation.

EXERCISE 10:   Repeat Exercises 1 to 9 using the probe.

EXERCISE 11:   Reverse the entry sites of the arthroscope and the probe. Repeat Exercises 1 to 9. This necessitates use of both hands for manipulation.

EXERCISE 12:   Repeat exercises 1 to 9 on the lateral compartment.

Triangulation requires conceptualization of sizes, shapes, and lengths of instrumentation. Also, you must appreciate the positions or planes in space, especially if you are looking at a video monitor and away from your hands.

Palpation. After the concept of triangulation is mastered, emphasis may be given to palpation. The probe manipulation of the various structures increases the appreciation of size, shape, and consistency. The probe may be used for manipulation of objects and elevation or depression of various parts. The meniscus may be elevated and the scope passed under for a better view.

Attention should be given to the different manipulative and proprioceptive information gained by touching with the tip and then the knuckle of the probe.

OPTIMAL POSITION FOR ARTHROSCOPIC VISUALIZATION

EXERCISE 13:   By trial and error, find the "optimal" position for the posterior horn medial meniscus. Then find the optimal position for the anterior horn, the lateral meniscus, and the anterior cruciate area.

The optimal position is one which gives the largest actual field of view possible of a structure without compromising illumination. Although arthroscopic motions are necessary, most surgical manipulation should be performed with the arthroscope held at a distance from the object to be viewed. Maximal illumination of the largest field of view possible, is essential for surgical instrumentation. To achieve this, preliminary manipulation of the scope to an optimal position is necessary.

ROLE OF ILLUMINATION IN COMPOSITION

EXERCISE 14:   Place the arthroscope into the joint and identify a structure within the joint, such as a tear of the meniscus, a foreign body, or a probe.

Retract the arthroscope back for an overview of the entire compartment. At that time, gradually dim the illumination to see the effect of the lack of light in a major compartment. Then brighten and visualize that compartment. Notice the effect of light on clarity.

With the light dimmed, move the arthroscope up close to the femoral condyle. Note that the femoral condyle can be seen with the dim light. Holding that position, slowly increase the brightness of the light so that you have a "whiteout," showing no structure.

Gradually dim the light so that you are again able to see the condylar details.

Move the arthroscope back for an overview with a dim light. Penetrate the scope all the way down to the posterior aspect, up to the meniscus, and notice that the closeness of the arthroscope to an object will compensate for the lack of brightness.

SPATIAL RELATIONSHIPS

EXERCISE 15: Look through the arthroscope directly and without looking at the outside of the knee joint or the instrument tray. Pick up a No. 18 spinal needle and place the needle within the joint.

Remove the needle, insert a cannula then a probe, and then set the cannula back on the table, leaving the probe in the knee. This exercise expands appreciation of the surrounding environment and the necessary ability to find and work with instrumentation without having to interrupt visualization.

VARIOUS PORTALS

Normal operative arthroscopy requires access to posterior and superior portals for both visualization and instrumentation.

The superior (medial or lateral) portal above the patellar area is entered with relative ease because of the large space. Still, a preliminary trial with a No. 18 spinal needle will identify the best position. This is the site of the inflow cannula for "wet knee" experience.

EXERCISE 16: Enter the posteromedial portal by palpation and then insert a No. 18 spinal needle to an area posterior to the condyle, superior to the meniscus, and anterior to the posterior wall of the joint (medial head of gastrocnemius). Place a cannula at the site after needle determination.

Identify posterolateral portal in a similar way.

Cannulas with obturators will now be in all portals. Visualize each with the arthroscope from the anterolateral portal.

CHANGING PORTALS

EXERCISE 17: Change portals by leaving the cannulas in place, removing the scope or obturators, and then placing metallic rods (switching sticks) in each cannula. Remove the cannulas. You can now interchange cannulas of various diameters and lengths without losing position and without the trouble of repeat puncture.

Place a cannula of the appropriate size for the arthroscope or instrument over the switching stick. Remove the rod. Place the arthroscope or instrument in the joint. Repeat this for the various portals.

MIRROR IMAGE MANIPULATION

EXERCISE 18: With the arthroscope inserted from anterolateral, enter the posteromedial compartment via the intercondylar notch. View the transcutaneous cannula entering from posteromedial. Place a probe in the posteromedial compartment.

Viewing from one side, touch various spots from the other side, recognizing coordination of the motions that are seen when operating directly toward the arthroscope.

Interchange the scope and probe with the switching sticks and repeat. Repeat for posterolateral and superior compartments as well.

TELEVISION

The exercises up to this point are all performed with direct viewing to increase the intimacy, palpation, and position sense. To skip this step is a mistake.

Television is an integral part of arthroscopic surgery. Direct viewing through the scope gives a clearer optical image, but the loss of optimal body position and the loss of freedom of both hands for instrumentation outweigh any advantage gained by putting the eye to the scope.

Knowledge of television's role in arthroscopy and comfort with its operation are essential for successful progression to more complex operative arthroscopy. Discipline yourself to the use of video.

EXERCISE 19:   Attach the television camera and repeat Exercises 1 to 18. Start with the basic scope motions, noting the interaction of the scope with the television camera attachment, especially with rotation. A hand-held chip camera will require two hands to rotate the scope in the camera mount. Always keep the image horizontal on the monitor.

Notice the image is not as clear or bright as with direct viewing. You can readily accommodate to the image to gain body position and comfort.

TEAM PRACTICE

During instrumentation and especially portal interchange an assistant is necessary for best execution. At this stage, the operating room team can profit from performing the exercises. In fact, the model can be set up in the operating room after hours for an entire environment and instrumentation check.

Play with the various video camera and monitor dials and connections to enhance complete familiarity. This is important, because the camera will be your eyes.

Finally, complete all the variables of composition with the video camera.

FINAL ORCHESTRATION

After individual training with each instrument or technique, it is time for combining the skills and procedures in a coordinated fashion: orchestration.

EXERCISE 20:   Start by placing the arthroscope in the lateral portal and viewing the medial compartment. Commence with positioning and add angulation.

Bring in the probe and follow it up close to the posterior horn of the meniscus. Dim the light if it is too bright. Elevate the meniscus and pass the scope underneath. Rotate the scope to look down in the sulcus behind the tibial plateau.

Retract the arthroscope. Brighten the light. Rotate the scope to the right, following the inner edge of meniscus as you retract the probe along the inner meniscus to the anterior horn. To continue to see both meniscus and probe at the anterior horn, both scope angulation and retraction will have to come into play.

Why are all these exercises necessary for surgeons? We call our profession the practice of medicine and surgery, so let's practice. Also, arthroscopic surgery demands a different skill than open surgery, even a different discipline of manner and execution of surgical principles.

I have often said, not so much in jest, that when professional golfers finish a competitive round, they practice golf, and when doctors finish their day, they practice golf. Arthroscopic techniques will develop faster and more surely if you repeat your case or cases of the day on a simulator while the experience is still fresh in your mind.

The so-called tricks of arthroscopy are really fundamentals. No trick will convert error to success when basic surgical techniques and principles have been violated. The foregoing exercises are the basics of which even the most complicated arthroscopic surgical procedure is composed.

Surgical manipulations. Following is a series of surgical manipulations in order of difficulty, starting with the simpler manipulations. The femur is placed in the top of the simulator. The top encloses the cannister, which reduces space in the simulated joint and eliminates looking over the top.

LOOSE BODY RETRIEVAL

Have another person place a loose body in the simulator. Place the arthroscope in the routine portal. Identify and remove the object with forceps via an established portal.

Place the object in each compartment and use all portals and a variety of approaches for removal.

METALLIC FRAGMENT

Because intraoperative instrument breakage can occur, this exercise should be performed to increase your preparedness for such an event.

Ask your partner to place a metallic fragment in the simulator. Place a scope in the joint and identify the fragment. Place a cannula down to the fragment and remove the obturator.

Using the Golden Retriever magnetic attraction attachment and manipulation of the cannula, remove the fragment. Do not remove the fragment through tissue; always move the fragment inside the cannula and remove it with the cannula.

ADVANCED OPERATIVE EXERCISES

Create a series of meniscal lesions within the simulator. (You may wish to have another person create the lesions as unknowns.)

A logical progression would be meniscal flap tears through bucket-handle tears, complex posterior horn tears, and double bucket-handle tears.

Debridement procedures on the condyles may include use of abrasion instrumentation.

Finally, devise and perform repair procedures of the meniscus and anterior or posterior cruciate ligaments.

A combination of these conditions may be created, lengthening the operative time to increase endurance.

Human material

Beyond artificial simulators, the use of fresh cadavers is satisfactory when available. Embalmed cadaver material is not suitable; it is not supple and tends to absorb saline into adjacent tissue. I did my original operative work on surgical amputation specimens. After the necessary pathological studies, knee specimens were stored in deep freeze. This allowed the freedom to choose an optimal time to practice surgical procedure at my office laboratory (in the basement). The laboratory experience included all the equipment and simulated the operating room. The operating room staff was also included in this training.

If at all possible, I highly recommend this exercise before live surgical practice. Nothing can simulate a human knee exactly in space, size, configuration, and color.

Personal visits

If the opportunity presents itself, it is beneficial to observe another surgeon performing the procedure within one's own hospital environment. If that is not possible and the surgeon is establishing arthroscopic surgery at the institution, a visit should be made to a surgeon who regularly practices arthroscopy. This will not only allow a chance to observe the techniques but also to see an arthroscopic environment.

If you did not have an opportunity for hands-on experience during a residency program or as a fellow, then an opportunity to participate in surgery might be provided by a colleague.

Personal experience

Live case experience should be preceded by as much preparation as possible. Eventually, the opportunity to schedule your first diagnostic case will arrive. Years ago most surgeons did diagnostic arthroscopy and performed the necessary operations by open methods. The consumer demand for and wide acceptance of arthroscopic surgery now restrict this option. The reasonable options are to have associates of adequate skill and experience complete the anticipated work by arthroscopic means or to perform diagnostic arthroscopy and then refer the patient. The first case experience should be carefully selected. The patient should understand your skill level and what to expect. From a diagnostic standpoint, it should be an operation that is within the realm of your current ability.

Many arthroscopists had the benefit of performing thousands of diagnostic arthroscopies before the development of operative arthroscopy. Now the basic arthroscopic techniques should be performed in the laboratory. They can give you the conception and the composition necessary to performing a successful diagnostic case. Operative experience should also be initiated in the laboratory.

Self-study (video and charts)

Video recording is important because it provides an opportunity for review. I recommend that the surgeon who is really serious about arthroscopy review his or her cases, preferably on the same day they were performed. If possible the entire surgical team should review the case(s). The opportunity to study not only your own technical ability but also your own results certainly exists in arthroscopy as in no other area of orthopedic surgery. Television documentation of your cases and teaching tapes should be studied. The occassional opportunity for a second look into the knee of a patient who has had previous surgery provides a comparison study of the areas of resection of menisci and/or other debridements. Further, studying your case experiences will assist you in your development as an arthroscopic surgeon. The results of surgery will affect future diagnostic and operative judgments.

Progression of skills

Arthroscopic surgery demands that the orthopedic surgeon give increased consideration to technical skill level. The restricted parameters of arthroscopic surgery dictate smaller, more delicate instruments. Also, the surgical exposure is limited.

Viewing through an arthroscope or viewing a projected video image gives a two-dimensional perspective. It is up to you to add the third dimensional perspective in your mind. Palpation and/or other manipulative skills must be learned to perceive the actual shapes and sizes of various tissues. Also, the interpretation of variations from normal in this new medium can only be learned with time and experience.

The basic technical principles of asepsis, hemostasis, and gentleness are important, as in open procedures. The medium of expression has changed; it is like switching art media from charcoal drawing to sculpture. Time is necessary to be successful, as in open surgery. You must be patient and diligent.

A level of diagnostic confidence is achieved when you can be assured that a negative diagnostic examination will be confirmed by subsequent patient recovery.

It is presumed that you have prepared yourself intellectually and technically for operative arthroscopy. The organization requires thorough knowledge of all the instruments and of television in your surgical environment. You will usually be responsible for training, or at least preparing, the surgical team for his or her method.

You should have backups of equipment and possibly surgical experience in the form of an available surgical colleague.

Surgical skills will develop gradually for everyone involved. Growth in arthroscopy can be likened to compound interest. The accumulation of principal is slow at first. With passage of time, however, the principal grows rapidly (Fig. 2-31).

Simple operative procedures

An appropriate patient for your first operative/diagnostic case is one who has a degenerative flap tear or symptomatic moderate degeneration. A bucket-handle tear, although relatively easy to handle by open methods, is not always easy arthroscopically. The fragment is within the notch and accompanied by synovitis. Frequently there are secondary tears in the posterior horn that may be difficult to expose or resect.

Other simple arthroscopic procedures include removal of loose bodies and

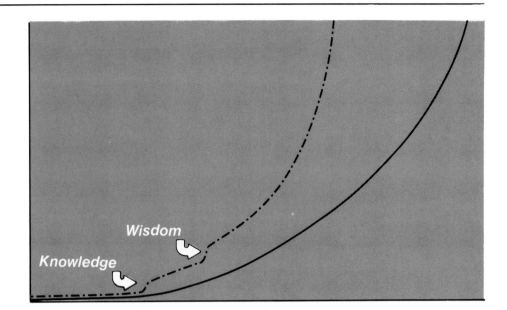

FIG. 2-31. Learning curve in arthroscopy is likened to growth of principal at 6% compound interest. Knowledge and wisdom add to principal growth.

sectioning of a plica. Arthroscopic lateral release alone is simple but rarely sufficient to correct patellar malalignment (see Chapter 10).

Make a progression to procedures involving the menisci as well as chondroplastic debridements of degenerative compartments. More complicated procedures would involve abrasion arthroplasty, meniscal repair, cruciate ligament reconstruction, and arthroscopy of other joints.

Growing in operative skills

At present arthroscopic procedures are performed by most orthopedic surgeons, but there is a dilution factor reducing any individual surgeon's experience. After you have had some operative experience, I recommend repeating every procedure on a simulator. Although you may have perfected the removal of a bucket-handle tear, a patellar shave, or some other procedure, the more complicated procedures and technical know-how will not be in your armamentarium. Also, after you have gained a certain amount of experience, you will have a better appreciation of factors affecting improvements. Return to the seminar or personal observation of others. To gain experience you might plan to operate together with an associate.

In addition, if you anticipate a certain case you can use an arthroscopic surgical simulator to run through that case beforehand with your own instrumentation. The operating room, on a Saturday when it is not in use, is a good place to check the operative instrumentation and facilities as well as your own skills.

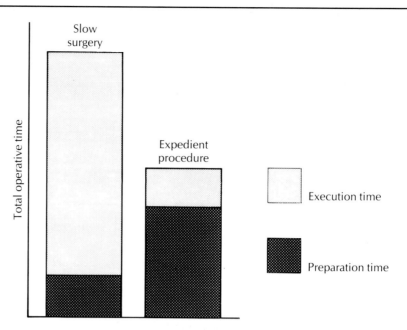

FIG. 2-32. Relationship of operative time to organization and planning.

Operative time is a product of intraoperative organization and planning followed by actual execution, that is, cutting or repairing. Preliminary organization of the environment, instruments, and staff beneficially affect the operative time.

The environment must be suitable for arthroscopic procedures (see Chapter 3). It will require continual attention and upgrading.

You should train and encourage the staff. Do not expect them to be more of anything than you are. If you are enthusiastic they will become that way sooner or later. The same rule applies for interest, patience, and satisfaction. Negative attitudes, all too easily, are also adopted.

The staff must be participants in the procedures, including observation of television. The instrumentation must be sharp, clean, and operational, including cutting instruments and video systems. You must be prepared intellectually. You must have eye-hand coordination techniques mastered and have a ready knowledge of anatomy and pathology. You must also understand the mode of operation of the instrumentation.

Not devoting time to organization and planning makes for a slow surgical procedure; the time is consumed in the execution phase. If more time is used for organization and planning phases, the operation can be performed with dispatch. The total operative time is also reduced (Fig. 2-32).

After gradually increasing your case experience, you will note a logical progression of ability and knowledge in arthroscopic surgery (see Fig. 2-31). If you continue to be successful, your intensity and interest will branch out into reviewing your cases, into research, and into a desire to exchange information with other practitioners.

Organization and planning chart. You can study and review your own practice of arthroscopic surgery using an arthroscopic organization and planning

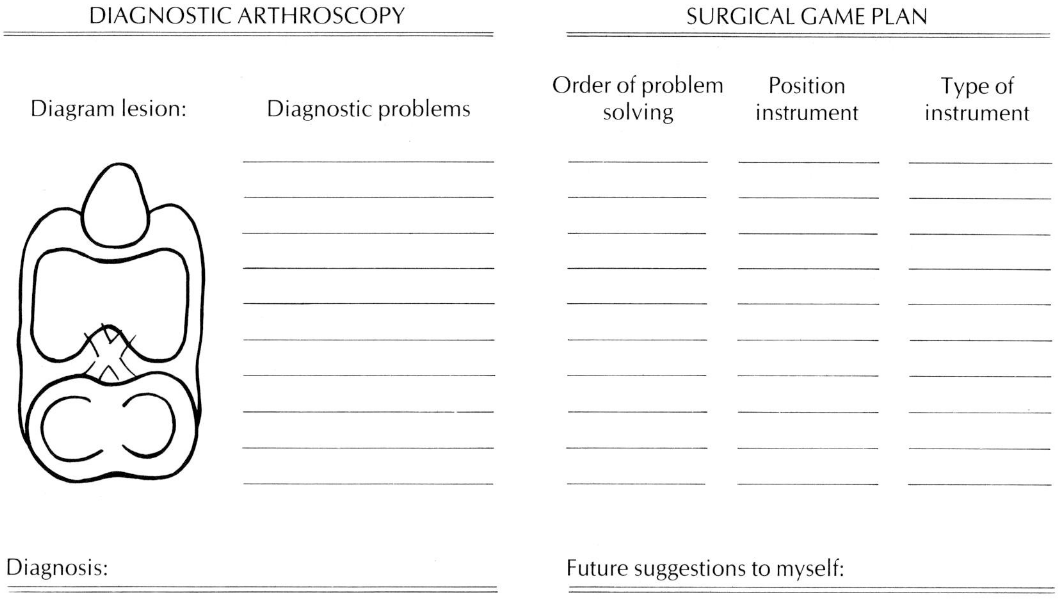

DIAGNOSTIC ARTHROSCOPY   SURGICAL GAME PLAN

Diagram lesion:	Diagnostic problems	Order of problem solving	Position instrument	Type of instrument

Diagnosis: Future suggestions to myself:

FIG. 2-33. Arthroscopic organization and planning chart.

chart (Fig. 2-33). This particular chart can be used to state the diagnosis, diagram the lesion, state the diagnostic problems, and draw up a surgical "game plan": the order of your problem solving, your positioning of instruments, your reasoning for this response, and the type of instrument. Extra space is provided for notations and suggestions for future operations.

How *not* to be successful technically

Dr. Howard J. Sweeney has listed 16 rules for a talk he calls "How to be Unsuccessful in Arthroscopic Surgery."[52]

1. Set up the operating room differently each time.
2. Use new nurses each case.
3. Use only local anesthesia.
4. Never use a leg holder.
5. Ignore standards of sterile technique.
6. Use inflow (always inadequate) on scope.
7. Limit system to gravity suction.
8. Use small diameter or straight viewing scopes.
9. Use inadequate light.
10. Use dull cutting instruments.
11. Obtain poor exposure.
12. Do not have an operative plan.
13. Be unfamiliar with equipment.
14. Fail to take courses.
15. Assume an arrogant "I know it all" attitude.
16. Fail to develop motor skills.

This entire text is devoted to the opposite outcome. In short, more than lip service must be paid to organization and planning before the procedure.

MECHANICS OF SURGICAL SCHEDULING

It is important to schedule your first case at a time near the end of the day. This precludes limitations either by office hours or another operative procedure, and you will not be holding up the rest of the operating room activities. As you begin to schedule cases, it is good to group them together at an appropriate time in your schedule that will allow relaxed time constraints, considering all parties involved.

The orthopedist should schedule arthroscopic cases in groups. Initially arthroscopic cases will take longer than anticipated. If the cases are scheduled as a group in the afternoon, the beginning arthroscopist will cause the least disruption of other surgeon's operative schedules. Another advantage of grouping arthroscopic cases is that it allows a block of time to focus on arthroscopic techniques uninterrupted by open surgery. This helps both staff and surgeon.

The beginning surgeon should avoid interspersing arthroscopic cases with other appointments or office hours because of the inability to predict operative time initially. This also provides the necessary relaxed environment for arthroscopic surgical success.

Similar recommendations should be incorporated for the hospital or clinic surgical suite. A room should be dedicated for arthroscopic surgery, and certain days or times should be reserved for these procedures. This provides for proper environmental set-up and surgical assistants' assignments. The designated time will expand with demand. Grouping of arthroscopic cases will facilitate scheduling of room use, the physician's time, and staff assignments.

Inpatient-outpatient status

Most arthroscopic surgical patients maintain an outpatient or same-day surgical status.[44] Preoperative crutch training by physical therapists can usually be accomplished on the day of surgery.

Hospital admission is reserved for patients with medical conditions best managed in that environment. This may be for cardiopulmonary problems, debilitating diseases such as advanced rheumatoid arthritis, or advanced age necessitating extensive preoperative instructions in ambulation and/or occupational therapy concerning home care. In some cases unusual insurance contracts require hospitalization for reimbursement.

The possibility of postoperative hospitalization always exists. The rare anesthetic or surgical complication might be an indication for hospitalization. Postoperative admission is usually a result of the magnitude of the surgery and resultant pain or special postoperative care, intensive physical therapy, uncontrolled pain, or vomiting. Often, a great distance to travel home is the reason the patient stays for local observation for possible complications.

Use of continuous passive motion has resulted in hospitalization for patients undergoing combined debridement procedures and osteotomy. Patients having procedures for anklyosis have the same postoperative requirements.

ARTHROSCOPY IN CHILDREN

Conditions in children that necessitate arthroscopic techniques are not as common as in adults.[10,38,39,51,59] Participation in competitive sports during pre-

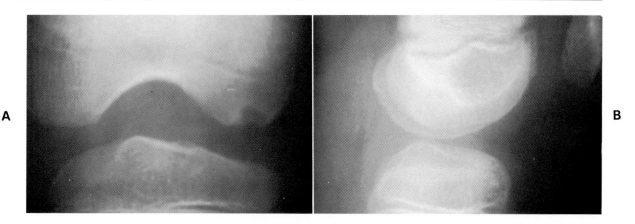

FIG. 2-34. Epiphyseal articular growth defects. Not to be confused with osteochondritis dissecans. The lesion is posterior on condyle. **A,** AP x-ray film. **B,** Lateral x-ray film.

adolescence has increased, causing adult problems in children. The value of arthroscopy in children should not be overlooked.

Congenital abnormalities are uncommon causes of intraarticular problems. My youngest arthroscopic patient (18 months) had hemangioma of the knee. Diskoid meniscus often produces symptoms in children. I have seen one case of congenital band in a shoulder joint that caused locking in abducted position.

Congenital dislocation of the hip could be an area of investigation, but I have no experience. Dr. David Shneider investigated arthroscopy in Legg-Perthes disease of the hip but abandoned these procedures because the information gained added nothing to management of the condition.

The traumatic injuries of children usually involve a penetrating foreign body. I have seen glass, wood, and metal needles or nails within the knee joint.

Torn menisci or ligaments are unusual before adolescence. Intraarticular fractures may be managed by arthroscopy. Patellar dislocation with patella alta and hyperelastic diathesis may be another indication for arthroscopic surgery.

Osteochondritis dissecans of the knee and elbow may occur in preadolescence. Arthroscopy provides an opportunity for repair and preservation of tissue. Osteochondritis should not be confused with epiphyseal articular growth defects (Fig. 2-34). These are more posterior on the femoral condyle, and the lesion fills in without treatment. Serial x-ray films confirm the diagnosis. The synovial conditions of rheumatoid arthritis and hemophilia are suitable for arthroscopic treatment. An occasional synovial biopsy may help in diagnostic problems.

ANESTHESIA
Choice of anesthesia

The type of anesthetic used for arthroscopic procedures is determined by the patient's joint problem, medical condition, and personal preference.[24,36,46,57] The choice is conditioned by the surgeon's ability and the anesthesiologist's judgment. Even the existing environmental conditions at the host health facility may affect the choice, based primarily on familiarity of the team and equipment available, especially as they affect operative time.

Originally most of my arthroscopic procedures were performed with the patient under local anesthesia. In 1972 arthroscopic surgical techniques were not developed beyond basket forcep resection of meniscal tissue, and most of the instrumentation pictured in this textbook had not been conceived. The state of the art was clinical diagnosis sufficient for an exploratory arthrotomy.

Local anesthesia for arthroscopic diagnosis provided an alternative. It was used to confirm a clinical impression and direct the anticipated surgical approach. I performed thousands of such cases, usually for another orthopedist who would subsequently perform the necessary open surgery. I functioned somewhat like a consulting radiologist would, only not with arthrography but diagnostic arthroscopy.

In recent years as arthroscopic surgery has developed, pure diagnostic arthroscopy has become less common. If there is an intraarticular problem, the diagnostic and operative procedures are combined using one anesthetic. The techniques and instrumentation are such that the operative times are under 90 minutes (safe tourniquet times), and the morbidity is little more than in diagnostic arthroscopy.

Because the diagnostic and operative procedures are combined, general anesthesia is often selected. This provides comfort during the somewhat longer procedure, allows use of the tourniquet and extremity-securing device, and aids in relaxation for joint manipulation to provide adequate exposure.

Local anesthesia is used in selected patients for diagnostic arthroscopy, especially for a second look for investigational purposes related to status of tissue repair or progression of disease process. Local anesthesia is used in some problem cases, patients with previous failed surgery, pain syndromes, medicolegal evaluations, or plica syndromes. When the arthroscopy is performed with skin and capsular infiltration, without intraarticular instillation, it is possible to palpate sensitive intraarticular structures. Careful correlation is possible by means of direct patient inquiry concerning the exact areas of discomfort or disease.

I have performed operative procedures of patellar debridement, loose body removal, meniscectomy, lateral release, and even abrasion arthroplasty on patients under local anesthesia. This was done at the patient's or consulting physician's recommendation.

As a routine, I use general anesthesia because the complexity of the operation cannot always be accurately determined preoperatively. There then are no anesthetic, time, or magnitude limitations to the accuracy of diagnosis or thoroughness of the operative arthroscopy.

Local anesthesia

Because there are still indications for local anesthesia, I will review the factors involved in the technique.

Success factors

Several factors facilitate arthroscopy with the patient under local anesthesia.[30] First and foremost is the confidence and ability of the surgeon to portray a calm attitude while technically performing the procedure gently but with dispatch. The patient's comfort is facilitated by his perception of the surgeon's ability, often learned from another patient's experience with the local anesthetic technique.

Once informed of anesthetic alternatives, the patient may choose the local anesthetic, but should not be persuaded.

The surgeon's explanation of the procedure should be reinforced by a written information sheet (see Fig. 2-39). At first reading this may produce anxiety, but at the time of the procedure apprehension is reduced considerably, as the patient is pleased to find the procedure is performed as outlined.

The circulating nurse can comfort, reassure, and even distract the patient during the procedure. The circulating nurse should appraise the surgeon of the patient's comfort and sometimes encourages the surgeon to finish; this usually gains the patient's agreement.

Initially I administered a narcotic or sedative intramuscularly or intravenously. Often the patient became drowsy and frequently nauseated, even with vomiting. The patient's stay in the hospital was often prolonged. Also, premedicated patients were requested not to operate a motor vehicle on the day of surgery. This required that another person accompany the patient home. Therefore I abandoned the premedication and have rarely found it necessary.

Technique

An operating room environment is recommended. This can be in a general hospital, outpatient surgical center, or clinic, but it must provide necessary equipment for patient safety.

The skin prep with antiseptic solution and sterile surgical draping is no different than for open surgery. The anesthetic administration must be adequate at the anticipated puncture sites, and sufficient time must be provided to achieve anesthesia before the incision is made for the arthroscope.

Local anesthetic agents

My local anesthetic agent of choice has been 1% plain lidocaine (Xylocaine). I do not combine it with epinephrine (Adrenalin), because the hemostatic effect is minimal and a tourniquet is used. Epinephrine does potentiate the duration of anesthetic effect.

I have used 0.25% bupivacaine (Marcaine) for lateral release. I inject along the fascia to be incised. I do not use it intraarticularly or intramuscularly because of deleterious effects.

Nole et al. have reported inhibition of glycosaminoglycans synthesis within articular cartilage caused by the saline vehicle, not the reagent, bupivacaine.[40] They point out there is a dose-related effect, so a 0.25% solution is my choice. The preservative methylparaben potentiates ill effects so solutions without it, such as those for epidural anesthesia, are preferred. Bupivacaine is damaging to muscle and has serious central nervous and cardiac complications if administered intravenously. Obviously, bupivacaine should be used judiciously.

Lidocaine, 1% plain, is injected at the anticipated portal of entry (Fig. 2-35, A). Blockage of the infrapatellar branch of the saphenous nerve has reduced patient apprehension with decreased propioception over the anterior skin surfaces (Fig. 2-35, B).

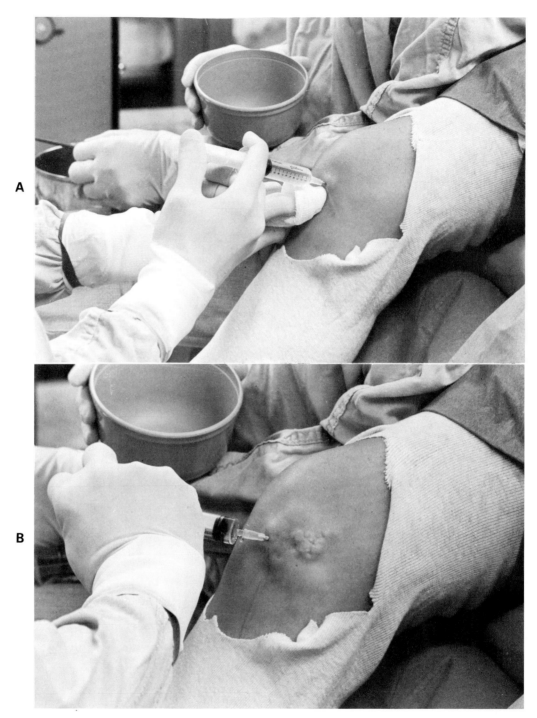

FIG. 2-35. Local infiltrative 1% plain lidocaine. **A,** Plain lidocaine, 1%, is placed within knee along course of anticipated penetration of joint. Surgeon places index finger against patellar tendon and onto tibial plateau to palpate for entry one fingerbreadth above tibial plateau and approximately one-half fingerbreadth medial to inner border of patellar tendon. In some overweight patients, position may be considerably more lateral because knee tends to rotate externally. **B,** Infrapatellar branch of saphenous nerve is blocked by local infiltration in three to four directions medially from the initial puncture. This decreases proprioception during manipulation of knee and therefore reduces apprehension.

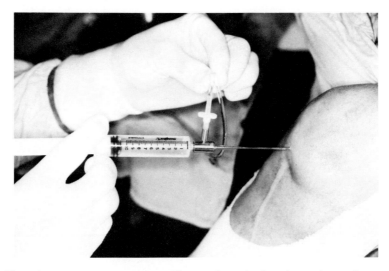

FIG. 2-36. If patient expresses some discomfort during insertion of scope, rather than withdraw cannula and reinsert needle, it is possible to pinch off K-52 catheter and infiltrate 1% plain lidocaine directly through cannula to tip exact site where patient is having discomfort.

Normally 10 to 12 ml of 1% lidocaine are used per puncture. Occasionally more is added in a sensitive patient or a prolonged procedure.

No intraarticular anesthetic has been necessary with the small diameter arthroscopes. When a scope of 5 mm cannula sheath is used, the intraarticular anesthetic will reduce the sensation of the larger instrument in the joint.

After the physician-patient relationship is established, the procedure must be performed with dispatch; it should not exceed 15 minutes for multiple puncture diagnostic arthroscopy. If it will take longer I advise a general anesthetic. In some cases a stand-by anesthesiologist may assist if time and comfort requirements are not met.

It is essential that the patient not be in pain or be apprehensive. A dialogue between the patient and surgeon or circulating nurse can monitor and prevent this. If there is any possibility of discomfort, the patient should be warned. If the cannula or trocar is in place when the discomfort occurs, remove the trocar, bend the K-52 catheter at the entry site, and place lidocaine through the cannula to that exact area (Fig. 2-36). This delivers the anesthetic directly to the area of discomfort and works better than withdrawing the cannula or trying to pass a needle adjacent to the cannula to achieve anesthesia in the area.

Patient monitoring

The arthroscopist can anticipate any sudden moves by the patient by being sensitive to his reactions. During the procedure with local anesthesia, the arthroscopist can monitor the patient's discomfort or anxiety by observing his breathing or deep sighing. The anxious patient will tighten his Achilles tendon. This can be monitored easily by the surgeon by placing a hand on the patient's ankle (Fig. 2-37). It should be noted that when the patient is under local anesthesia and there is pain in the quadriceps muscle the capsular tissues will be compressed,

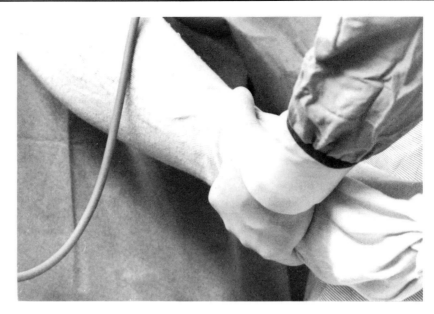

FIG. 2-37. With free hand, arthroscopist can hold patient's ankle and monitor tightening of Achilles tendon. Any tightening of knee or apprehension of patient is quickly discerned through Achilles tendon tenseness, allowing arthroscopist to be sensitive to patient's comfort under local anesthesia. In addition, with internal and external rotation, flexion and extension abduction and adduction, arthroscopist can compose clear-cut endoscopic picture.

making it difficult to puncture the fascia let alone obtain joint distention or manipulate the arthroscope.

In certain cases it is possible to determine the patient's relative pain threshold at the time of arthroscopy. If a patient complains of severe pain when the skin is touched, even with a finger or the tip of a needle, his pain threshold can be perceived as being different from that of another patient who does not complain with a similar maneuver.

It is possible to palpate internal structures to check for sensitivity or insensitivity in the course of the arthroscopic examination. This palpation can be done by anesthetic needle placement. Intraarticular nonanesthetized areas may be probed.

The small-diameter scopes leave minimal scars of scope entry (Fig. 2-38).

POSTOPERATIVE PATIENT MANAGEMENT FORMS

As for preoperative patients, it is important to write instructions for postoperative patients. (Fig. 2-39). The excitement of surgery combined with the anesthetic frequently leads to misunderstandings with instructions and even amnesia. I have developed postoperative instruction forms. Other forms are illustrated after specific operative procedures in this textbook. The forms are similar in content but each has a different message and color for the specific procedure. Space is provided for additional or specific handwritten instructions. Instruction in cast care is added when appropriate (Fig. 2-39, C).

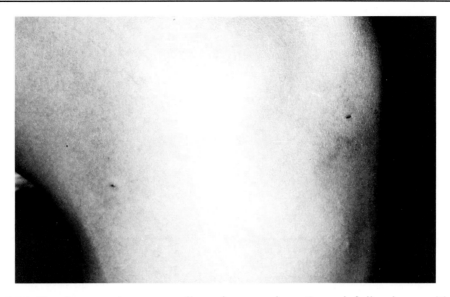

FIG. 2-38. Needlescope leaves small marks, seen here 1 week following multiple-puncture technique arthroscopy. Punctures are so small that no suture is required, and adhesive bandage is all that is indicated after second day. Surgery can be performed any day after arthroscopy without risk of infection.

Most important to me is color coding of instruction forms for each procedure. Since arthroscopic incisions give no clue to the procedure, color coding provides a means of identifying a given patient's operation in the absence of a medical record. This is most valuable when responding to calls at home or other places away from the office medical record. The patient will usually remember the color of the instruction sheet even if it was lost. This method has allowed me to provide intelligent medical advice for individual patients even without recalling their specific surgical procedure.

Most patients appreciate the written reminder of the various events of the postoperative course. Anticipating an event makes its occurrence less threatening and directs the patient to reasons for concern while removing the frightening unknowns. A few patients still call and ask questions to which the answers are Already printed in the instructions.

CONVALESCENCE

Convalescence (from the Latin convalescere: to become strong) is defined as, "the stage of recovery following an attack of disease, a surgical operation, or an injury." The concept of convalescence has been ignored by an impatient society, but still is necessary. The period of convalescence provides the opportunity for rest, comfort, renewed confidence, and, most important, tissue healing.

To ignore this stage of recovery results in reaggravation of the injury or poor surgical result. If the rehabilitation exercise program is initiated too soon, areas of incomplete tissue healing may be damaged.

On the other hand, prolonged convalescence could result in failure to mobilize a joint or return to previous function status. Convalescence must be properly reintroduced to postoperative management. *Text continued on p. 105.*

ARTHROSCOPIC SURGERY INFORMATION

Arthroscopic surgery has become a standard method for diagnosing and treating many joint problems. The word "arthro" means joint. "Scopic" means to look into. In practice, the procedure is performed in an operating room under anesthesia and sterile techniques. The joint is distended with saline (salt water) via a small tube to facilitate visualization. A second puncture wound is utilized for the arthroscope (small telescope) which is attached via an elaborate lens system to a television camera. The interior of the joint is projected upon a video monitor to facilitate the technical maneuvers necessary with miniature cutting instruments. The three of four puncture wounds replace the conventional open incision.

Just as miniaturization has come into electronics, i.e., small calculators, radios, and TVs, the same is so in surgery. In fact, it comprises a subspecialty known as microsurgery.

Continually developing technology has extended arthroscopic procedures beyond the knee to other joints as well, including shoulder, elbow, wrist, hip, and ankle.

Unfortunately, not every condition is amenable to arthroscopic surgery. A review of medical records, preoperative evaluation, and examination will determine the suitability for each patient. The magnitude of surgery possible in the joint includes diagnostic arthroscopy, simple cartilage removal, major surface cleaning in arthritis, kneecap realignment procedures, plus some acute ligament or dislocation repairs. Ligamentous reconstruction, including grafting, is now possible in certain circumstances.

The advantages of this method include the opportunity for exacting diagnosis plus an operative procedure of less morbidity (less patient discomfort). In addition, the miniature punctures are cosmetically more acceptable than conventional incisions.

The convalescence will vary with the magnitude of the disease rather than the surgical procedure itself. The healing process inside the joint is not necessarily accelerated with these techniques.

It is possible, in some cases, to predict the postoperative course. Crutches will be necessary in lower extremity surgery from a few days (simple cartilage removal) to 8 weeks in the most severe arthritic patient, or even casting with major ligamentous repairs. A sling may be required for shoulder, elbow, or wrist surgery yet with the hand free for use.

Most procedures are performed on an out-patient basis or "same day" surgery. In case of certain existing medical conditions, type of insurance, out of town patients, or personal preference, hospitalization may be elected. Occasionally, events surrounding the surgery, anesthesia, or postoperative conditions may necessitate admission for someone anticipating "same day" surgery.

A

FIG. 2-39. Patient information forms. **A,** Preoperative information.

Our medical facility, Ingham Medical Center, has a surgical suite and staff dedicated to the specialty of arthroscopic surgery, the first such facility within a general hospital. The Medical Center also offers a full complement of medical specialists for consultation plus the customary diagnostic and treatment facilities of a general hospital (see enclosed map).

Lansing Anesthesiologists, P.C., includes all types of anesthesia in their practice; local regional blocks, spinal, and general anesthesia. Your anesthetic will be designed for your needs, your medical condition, and the requirements of the surgery. Their practice experience ranges for outpatient anesthesia to the more difficult open heart procedures at Ingham Medical Center. In short, they are very well qualified. They will see you before your surgery and postoperatively if you are hospitalized. Their offices are adjacent to Ingham Medical Center, 405 West Greenlawn, Lansing, Michigan. (517) 482-2118.

The objective of surgery is to accurately diagnose your problem at the onset, properly treat your condition, and appropriately advise you of your anticipated recovery and future functions that could benefit or adversely affect your condition. In short, every effort will be made to obtain the best, long-lasting result for everyday life.

With any surgery or penetration of the body, even in drawing a sample of blood from the arm, there is some discomfort. It is no different with arthroscopic surgery. In spite of the discomfort you may experience, you may be assured that it is less than by open surgery. Every reasonable attempt will be made to perform the surgery arthroscopically, but when indicated, open surgery by conventional methods may be performed.

Your cooperation will facilitate your care. A careful reading of all materials presented, plus completing the questionnaire material, assists us in evaluating your problem and answering your questions.

Enclosed are directions to the Ingham Medical Center and general instructions concerning your preparation. Please hold on to this and other information for future reference.

MEDICAL RECORD: A dictated medical record is filed at Ingham Medical Center and our office. A copy will be forwarded routinely to the referring doctor when identified or to your own home on request.

Thank you,

Lanny L. Johnson, M.D.

Continued.

POSTOPERATIVE PATIENT INFORMATION
DIAGNOSTIC ARTHROSCOPY

After a thorough arthroscopic inspection, the diagnosis was
_____.
No surgical procedure was performed in the absence of identifiable reason. It did not seem you would benefit from surgery at
this time.

A silent video recording was made of arthroscopic findings.
As previously indicated, a copy (½-inch) can be produced at your
request (charge $50.00). Please indicate so in writing, identify-
ing video format (VHS, Beta I, II) and include payment of $50 to
cover labor and materials.

DRESSING: A soft dressing covers your knee. This compression
dressing should be comfortable and absorb any leakage of fluid
and/or blood. Although the dressing may become moist or blood
stained, this is not usually a cause for alarm. We have not experienced any hemorrhage or excessive bleeding in our patients.

The dressing may be removed safely at any time. Routinely,
the dressing is removed the day after surgery, and the appropriate number of Band-Aids are applied. The Band-Aids may be used
over the next several days.

PAIN: On discharge you should secure a prescription for pain
medication. Usually this will be an analgesic with codeine.
Please inform us of any known drug allergy. Codeine may produce
nausea and/or a fine skin rash. In that case, the medication
should be discontinued and our office contacted for an alternate medication. The application of an ice pack to the knee
will decrease swelling and discomfort in the first 48 hours.

WOUNDS: The small points of entry may be sore and develop bruising over the next several days. This bruising will eventually
disappear and does not require any special care.

BATHING: The sensation of "splashing" of fluid in the joint is
not a cause for concern. It represents residual fluids from
surgery and they will absorb. It will be safe to shower 48 hours
following surgery. Bathing or soaking should be delayed for several days. Cleansing of the skin adjacent to the small wounds
with soap and water may be performed with the first dressing
change.

ACTIVITY: You may walk on the leg with or without crutches as a
matter of comfort. Muscle tightening exercises will "milk"
swelling out of the extremity and assist recovery. Bending of
the knee should commence at once.

Swimming and recreational bicycling may be possible after
1 week. Expect 3 to 6 weeks to return to more vigorous sports.

RE-EXAMINATION: You should contact our office (or the referring
physician's office for out-of-town patients) for evaluation and
consultation in 10 days to 2 weeks.

B

FIG. 2-39, cont'd. Patient information forms. **B,** Postdiagnostic arthroscopy.

PRECAUTIONS: Early postoperative problems could be manifested by unusual pain, unrelieved by prescriptions, temperature elevation (101 degrees or above), or progressive swelling or bleeding. These are uncommon, but if presented you should seek consultation at our office, your own physician, or even an emergency room in some instances. Our telephone: (517) 351-7450.

MEDICAL RECORD: A dictated medical record is filed at Ingham Medical Center and our office. A copy will be forwarded routinely to the referring doctor when identified, or to your own home on request.

OFFICE APPOINTMENT: Call now for an appointment in 2 to 3 weeks.

Thank you,

Lanny L. Johnson, M.D.

NOTE: Although this is a postoperative form, it is specific for your condition unless otherwise noted in writing.

Continued.

C

CAST CARE

Cast immobilization was necessary to protect the repair performed during your surgery. This cast may require some attention on your part.

The cast takes up to 72 hours to dry and should be protected from damage.

You should not remove or loosen the cast without medical attention or approval.

While in the cast, frequent wiggling of toes or ankle (if free) stimulate circulation, and the muscle contraction reduces potential swelling. Elevation of the cast on pillows at or above the level of your heart assists with fluid movement out of the extremity.

The following instructions are basic rules for casts that should be followed:

1. DO NOT physically abuse your cast. If cracks or breaks occur, contact your physician.

2. DO NOT decorate your cast with enamel, shellac, or oil base paints because they seal the cast and prevent air exchange.

3. DO NOT get your cast wet.

4. If your cast feels uncomfortable, or if the padding is not right, contact our office or your own physician for instructions. DO NOT try to rearrange it yourself.

5. Itching is a common occurrence with casts. If this occurs, try scratching it with air! Use a cool blow dryer. You may find that scratching another part of your body may help to relieve the itch. DO NOT stick anything into the cast to scratch.

6. Keep extremity elevated at all times except for walking.

7. Notify our office (517) 351-7450 or your physician if you have:

    a. Severe pain that is prolonged and unrelieved by prescribed pain medication.

    b. Toes or fingers which are cold, swollen, bluish in color, difficult to move, numb, tingling, or in pain.

    c. Local pain or burning under the cast. This may indicate a pressure area underneath the cast where a sore may be developing.

    d. Unusual or foul odors, other than body odor, from the cast. This may indicate an infection underneath.

If you have a problem, and are unable to reach me or your family physician, go to any emergency room for evaluation.

Thank you.

Lanny L. Johnson, M.D.

FIG. 2-39, cont'd. Patient information forms. **C,** Cast care.

SUCCESSFUL REHABILITATION

Dorland's Illustrated Medical Dictionary defines rehabilitation as, "the restoration of normal form and function after injury or illness," or "the restoration of an ill or injured patient to self-sufficiency or to gainful employment at his highest attainable skill in the shortest possible time."

Successful rehabilitation depends on the realization that maximal functional potential is in the patient's best interest. It is a process that centers around patient education and is never concluded (Fig. 2-40, *A*). It is highly individualized for each patient.

With arthroscopy the small puncture wounds minimize surgical morbidity. The customary set-back of open surgery is avoided and rehabilitation is minimized. Many patients require crutches or a sling for a few days but return to activity before experiencing loss of motion or muscular atrophy.

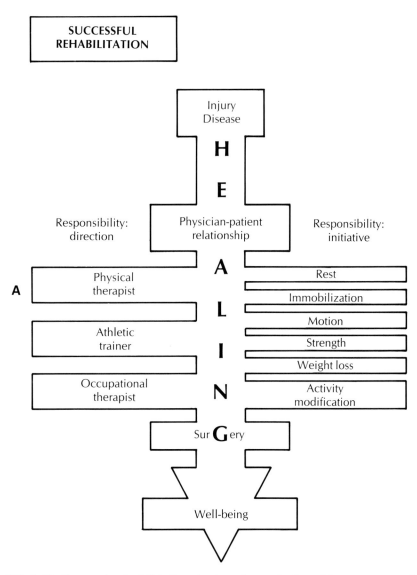

FIG. 2-40. General rehabilitation instructions. **A,** Graphic representation.

Continued.

CONVALESCENCE THEN REHABILITATION

Convalescence is a period of rest and recovery for the surgical area as well as for the total patient. There is time under pain medication, and perhaps immobilization of the injured or surgically treated extremity. The patient may be in bed, have restricted activities, use crutches or an arm sling. Convalescence cannot be eliminated or substituted for by rehabilitation. Rehabilitation follows convalescence.

Let's understand rehabilitation. A dictionary definition: "the restoration of an ill or injured patient to self sufficiency or to gainful employment at their highest attainable skill in the shortest possible time." A second definition, "restoration of normal form and function after injury or illness," is not possible in the strictest sense. Once there has been a joint injury or disease, restoration to normalcy is not achievable. The process is one of repair, not restoration, of diseased or injured tissues to normal. The healed tissue usually does not have the same strength or resiliency as normal. This is usually reflected in some loss of full motion, strength, or stability.

What then can you expect from treatment? First, every consideration will be made concerning nonoperative measures, i.e., rest, medication, bracing, activity modification, and/or physical therapy. Rehabilitation does not mean you have to have surgery or just a process that follows surgery.

In some cases, the surgery may be deferred until a certain level of power or motion is achieved by physical therapy.

Rehabilitation starts before your surgical procedure scheduling. It begins with your understanding of your condition, anticipated surgery; and expectations for postoperative conditioning and activities.

The single most important event in rehabilitation is HEALING of the tissues. Generally, the skin appears healed in 7 to 10 days. It is longer before the complete maturation of the tissues on the inside. Therefore, the skin healing is not the critical measure of the actual healing of areas operated on. Studies have shown that even the simplest surgical procedure requires 3 months for early tissue maturation. The more extensive arthritis and ligamentous procedure requires 6 to 12 months for strong mature tissue to develop.

Only mature healed cells can tolerate normal activities let alone weight lifting and vigorous activities. The signals of an aggra-

FIG. 2-40, cont'd. General rehabilitation instructions. **B** Patient information form.

vated joint that has not yet healed are heat, swelling, and pain. Let's avoid these and stage activities in your best interests, maximizing HEALING.

While healing is occurring, it is safe and important to initiate range of motion of your joint with regular daily activity.

Walking and swimming are advised in the early phase. Bicycling may follow, but hold off on stationary bikes with resistance.

Avoid undue sudden pressure, loads, and range of motion, even sudden hard auto braking in early phases.

Rehabilitation is not limited to weight lifting. Weight lifting programs vary with each individual, their own joint problem, and their physical activity goals. We will advise each patient individually. In general it is better to do less rather than more until healing is complete. The indiscriminate loading of healing joints to gain muscle power may even be detrimental. Rehabilitation is best done by the physician s instruction and patient's initiative. In some cases physical therapy may be prescribed.

Briefly, the rehabilitative process for joints starts with gaining range of motion, then muscle power. After MOTION and MUSCLE, then MOBILIZATION can start. The last M is MOTIVATION, which must be applied throughout the rehabilitation.

Return to activities will be gradual, depending on the severity of your problem. Unfortunately, most patients requiring surgery (abnormal knee) cannot technically be returned to normal (see above definition). Most, however, may become active again, whether employment or recreation is the object.

Some few patients will require a temporary or even permanent modification of activity. Their conditions, even with successful surgery, will not permit aggressive sports activity again, obviously in the patients' interest. Those with arthritic problems will have to modify running, handball, racketball, and tennis. Still others with ligamentous instability will probably never have the pre-injury level of speed, acceleration, deceleration, or jumping ability.

Please save this information for future reference.

Thank you,

Lanny L. Johnson, M.D.

However, with the expansion of arthroscopic techniques to include degenerative conditions or ligamentous injuries, rehabilitative processes must be addressed.

The rehabilitation process is affected by the patient's condition and the healing process. In general the injury or repair must be protected from adverse conditions that would impede healing. For example, a ligamentous repair may be initially casted and/or restricted in range of motion by bracing. Protection of the repair with gradual motion, except for extremes of flexion and extension, may be used.

The articular surface condition affects the rehabilitative process. If there is no articular cartilage injury or disease, early weight bearing is possible. When a partial-thickness loss of articular cartilage exists over a significant area of weight-bearing surface, up to 1 month of non-weight-bearing crutch protection will reduce the chance of postoperative effusion and discomfort. Loading of the joint with weights and motion should be delayed several months. A full-thickness area of sclerotic bone debrided (abrasion arthroplasty) requires 2 months of strict non-weight bearing to provide the proper environment for conversion of blood clot to avascular spindle cell. Partial weight bearing thereafter facilitates the transition to a fibrocartilage cell by 4 to 6 months.

Arthroscopic meniscectomy requires no immobilization and minimal joint protection. Crutches may be used for a few days for comfort.

Meniscal repair, whether arthroscopic or open, requires 4 to 6 weeks of cast immobilization with crutches. Temporary stiffness and muscle atrophy occur. Athletes who undergo meniscal repair are withheld from sports for 6 months for tissue maturation. This illustrates that a similar condition, in this case torn meniscus, treated differently, can have different postoperative rehabilitation requirements.

A compromised neurovascular status of the extremity reduces the stress that should be applied during the rehabilitative process. When the neurovascular condition reduces the functional capacity of a limb, then a slower rehabilitation process is chosen.

Proper rehabilitation is an integral part of surgical success. Rehabilitation should be based on the physician's instruction and the patient's initiative (Fig. 2-40, B). If either is lacking supervised physical therapy may be indicated. Most patients are rehabilitated successfully without machines and modalities. Often the so-called intensive physical therapy regimen only gives the patient something to do while healing is being realized, hopefully without jeopardizing the surgical repair.

The most frequent benefit of formal physical therapy is in previously injured, previously operated on, or debilitated patients. Maximizing muscle power and motion is important before another surgical setback. Proper rehabilitation may also salvage an otherwise failed surgery, avoiding a subsequent operation.

Strength is not everything

Strength is only one dimension of well-being. Well-being includes comfort, motion, mobility, and confidence. Patients often inquire, "Will my knee be just as strong after surgery?" I believe they are asking, "Will my knee be well after surgery?" Most patients equate strength with well-being; that is why they inquire so often about lifting weights. Dispelling this notion requires physician instruction and patient education.

With understanding, the surgeon must fully explain these considerations in the restoration of "strength" for the patient. Thinking only of strength is analogous to considering only the gasoline octane rating and engine horsepower in evaluating an automobile. In the absence of tie-rods (ligaments), tires and shock absorbers (articular surfaces), steering mechanisms (range of motion), or the electrical (neurovascular) system, the octane rating and engine horsepower are of little value.

Serious recreational or competitive athletes derive the most benefit from intensive physical therapy and its sophisticated machines and modalities. Such treatment should be directed and monitored by the physician. Care should be taken to avoid any activities that would be contraindicated by the specific patient's condition.

The ideal environment for rehabilitation is in the same location as the physician and with the treating therapists responsible to the surgical staff. This results in clear communication, a cooperative effort, and mutual respect and satisfaction. The patient's geographical mobility, parental and coaching pressures and influences, and therapist initiatives often prevent this. Too often rehabilitation is reduced to more repetitions or more weight, with little regard for the specific needs of the patient, his diagnosis, or surgical correction. "The more, the better" does not apply here anymore than "If one pill is good, two would be better" does with drug therapy.

Patient education is continuous and repetitious. Patients usually do not hear or want to hear the consequences of their condition or treatment; no one does. Therefore continued reminders of nature of injury or condition, factors and time necessary for healing, and probable results are necessary. Written instructions serve as a reminder.

Patients must therefore understand the nature of their condition and its consequences. Still, there is the insistent emphasis on equating weight-lifting with rehabilitation. I shift this emphasis to healing, range of motion, and maximization of strength without jeopardizing repair.

Most patients require weight loss and activity modification to achieve their rehabilitation potential. For other patients rehabilitation may mean occupational retraining.

Sometimes successful rehabilitation requires rest, not activity. Tissue healing is accompanied by decreased signs of inflammation and improved voluntary motion. Second-look arthroscopic studies have clearly illustrated that internal joint healing lags behind the outwardly observed signs.

The physician's instructions concerning the nature of the disease or injury, its natural history, surgical treatment, and consequences in terms of life-style, educate patients so that they may take the proper initiative in treating and rehabilitating themselves.

Patient responsibility

It is important that patients recognize the responsibility for their own well-being rests not with any agency or person but with themselves. At that point they can move away from the dependency of injury or illness to the freedom and independence that accompany well-being.

Patients should be the most interested person in their problem. The physician's role can only be that of advisor, helper, and comforter. If the advice or help is rejected or refused, the responsibility remains with the patient.

During the rehabilitative process, the surgeon may find that the patient did nothing or too much. The surgeon must adapt the same attitude as a cardiologist would if the patient took none or double the prescription of digitalis. The consequences of the patient's initiative must be reiterated. These matters demonstrate the continuing balance between the physician's instructions and the patient's initiative.

Rehabilitation processes are highly individualized, not just by conditions, but by patient age, personality type, and activity goals. This is the art of medicine. For one patient you might outline too much to do, realizing that if he does anything it will be good; for another patient you might give instructions to do absolutely nothing, realizing that she will try every machine in the gym.

One last point: the patient is always tempted to test what the doctor says could not or should not be done. Many times a patient hopes to prove the physician wrong and returns with problems. Avoid telling such a patient, "I told you so." Instead, start over.

Specific modalities

If I was quick to recognize the value of arthroscopy, I have been equally slow to recognize the value of various machines and modalities in rehabilitation.

The ability to measure and assign values to specific muscles, motions, or combined activities has the most value. The measured monitoring of deficits and progress is of benefit in the problem case and the high-performance athlete. If it is not happening already, evaluation measurement will be the next area of rapid growth in orthopedics.

The intense interest in physical fitness along with the international incentive to greater athletic performance has changed the emphasis from simple weight lifting to the concept of strength training in all sports. This concept emphasizes individual muscles and gives attention to the fast and slow responses of muscle fibers by histochemical analysis.

Machines now measure muscular strength and endurance at both fixed and variable speeds. Exercises are also available at fixed and variable resistances.

A few definitions can help clarify the complexity of strength-training modalities available. I am not qualified to evaluate the benefits of the various systems available but rather I rely on others' opinions and research.

Muscular strength:	The contractile force created by a muscle group in one brief, maximal effort.
Muscular endurance:	The ability of a muscle to perform at a submaximal level to fatigue or hold a maximal contraction.
Isometric contraction:	A muscular contraction with no accompanying movement of limbs or torso in which constant length or position is maintained. Recommended are six repetitions of 6

seconds each. Maximal contraction at different joint angles is the customary routine.

Isotonic contraction: A contraction to move a constant load. This is best done
at submaximal load. Two or three sets of 6 to 12 repeti-
tions each is a recommended routine.

Isokinetic contraction: A contraction in which the limbs move at a constant ve-
locity. The shortening speed of the contracting muscle is
not constant. Isokinetic devices frequently alter the resistance they offer in proportion to the changing output of
muscles. They include Cybex and are popular for knee extension-flexion.

Concentric contraction: Any contraction in which the muscle shortens while creating movement.

Eccentric contraction: Any contraction in which the muscle length increases despite efforts of the contractile proteins to shorten.

Variable resistance: Changes in the effective force placed on a muscle. It may
happen randomly by effects of gravity and movement of
limbs through space, as in free weight-lifting. It may be
applied through electronically or mechanically driven machines.

Principles of various modalities

Most strength training devices work on the principle of concentric contraction followed by eccentric contraction of the antagonist group or muscle. These
include Nautilus, CAM II, Total Gym, and free weights. Some machines hold
speed of movement constant and effectively accommodate changing muscular
output (Hydrafitness).

Most machines offer variable resistance through cam or mechanical link-
ages. Free weights do not offer a constant load, because position in space with
motion of body part and resultant load on a given muscle change with this activity.

I present this review as much for myself as the reader. Many kinds of devices require our inspection. They are described in language not common to our
discipline, but they require our input concerning their use in patient management.

Specific rehabilitation measures are outlined by condition and treatment in
each specific chapter. I follow this outline.

Physician instruction
Patient initiative and responsibilities
Conservative measures
    Preoperative program
    Postoperative program
        Rest and immobilization
        Restoration of motion
        Restoration of healing
        Restoration of strength
        Restoration to activity
Activity modification

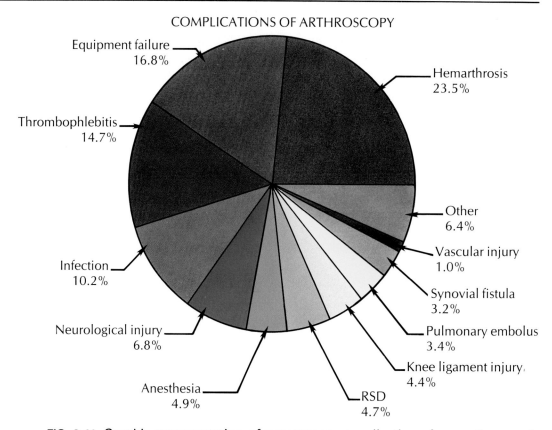

COMPLICATIONS OF ARTHROSCOPY

Equipment failure
16.8%

Hemarthrosis
23.5%

Thrombophlebitis
14.7%

Other
6.4%

Vascular injury
1.0%

Infection
10.2%

Synovial fistula
3.2%

Neurological injury
6.8%

Pulmonary embolus
3.4%

Knee ligament injury
4.4%

Anesthesia
4.9%

RSD
4.7%

FIG. 2-41. Graphic representation of percentage complications from arthroscopic surgery. (Courtesy Arthroscopy Association of North America and Committee Chairman Dr. Jesse DeLee.)

COMPLICATIONS

The potential complications of arthroscopic surgery are those common to any surgery. They include anesthetic problems, technical problems, postoperative infection, and thromboembolic phenomena (Fig. 2-41).

Complications related to arthroscopic surgery are minimal because of the small incision, continuous irrigation diluting and cleansing the wound, and the potentially short operative time. This low morbidity often makes hospitalization unnecessary and promotes early ambulation.*

Still it would be unrealistic to think a zero complication rate could be realized. Anesthetic risks are inherent to any operation. Although the infection rate is low with arthroscopic procedures, infections do occur. Host resistance is a factor. Any break in the skin, in or out of the operating room, has a potential for infection.

The incidence of thromboembolic phenomena is low because of decreased anesthesia time, minimal tissue disruption, and early ambulation after arthroscopic procedures.

Intraoperative instrument breakdown or breakage is the most common com-

*References 4, 9, 16, 18, 21, 23, 29, 33, 43, 45, 56, and 58.

plication. Instrument failure resulting in disruption of a procedure is avoided by having back-ups of all types. The small, delicate instruments used in arthroscopic surgery by their very nature have the potential for intraoperative breakage. A free portion loose in the joint is a possibility.

I liken the surgical procedure to the sport of golf. A complication, like the hazard of a sand trap, is a factor that results in a problem, no matter what the intent or skill of the golfer (or surgeon). Virtually all surgeons will experience a complication unless they stop practicing. The issues become recognition of the potential hazards, their avoidance, and recovery measures necessary to deal with them.

These problems may be grouped by their time of occurrence or recognition, either operative or postoperative.

Operative complications

The intraoperative complications involve anatomical structural or tissue injury or problems with instrumentation.

The skin and subcutaneous tissues are rarely the object of a problem. Occasionally a cutaneous nerve or vessel may be lacerated. In spite of efforts to avoid the subcutaneous neurovascular structures by transillumination, small vessels or nerves may be transected. If bleeding is active, suture ligation is necessary. A lacerated cutaneous (infrapatellar or saphenous) nerve may result in a small residual area of anesthesia. I have not found repair necessary, because patients usually adapt with crossover of dermal innervation. I have seen no postoperative neuroma or need for neurectomy following arthroscopic procedures.

Scuffing, gouges, and lacerations

The most common surgical injury to tissue is "scuffing" of the articular cartilage. A scuff is a permanent injury with loss of articular hyaline cartilage (see Fig. 6-23). Small areas of articular surface may be elevated even by smooth-surfaced instruments. Scuffing is more prone to occur in compartments with edematous articular cartilage. The injured surface becomes smooth with fibrous tissue repair or matrix flow. Still, technical means should be employed to minimize or avoid these injuries.

Obtaining adequate exposure with distention, mechanically securing the body part, and taking care in handling instrumentation should avoid these problems. If the articular cartilage is gouged or elevated, the elevated or loose fragments should be debrided.

An articular cartilage laceration should not be altered. Further shaping or debridement causes further tissue loss. Animal studies show minimal or no reactivity or degeneration up to 1 year following laceration.

Ligament injury

Lacerations of the tibial collateral and posterior or anterior cruciate ligaments are uncommon. Avoiding these injuries is a matter of gentle, adequate exposure and control of the cutting instruments.

The tibial collateral ligament is most vulnerable during meniscectomy. It may be torn with valgus stress on the knee. A small tear need not be treated or immobilized. A larger laceration may be amenable to transcutaneous suturing.

Immobilization may be considered but is not imperative with good repair in an otherwise stable joint.

Anterior or posterior cruciate ligament laceration represents a more difficult problem. A highly individualized judgment call will determine amenability to and advisability of primary repair, even with augmentation. Reconstruction may be deferred for evaluation of subsequent knee function.

The lateral collateral ligament is not vulnerable to stress tear or laceration. If this occurred surgical repair would be indicated.

Vessel injury

The potential for genicular artery and/or vein injury exists with transcutaneous approaches, but I have not seen any acute bleeding or false aneurysm from these vessels from routine arthroscopic approaches. The use of limited skin incisions and cannula approaches may minimize this complication.

Arthroscopic lateral release has the potential for significant bleeding from the superolateral geniculate artery. The chance of a bleeding problem is minimized if the retinacular incision courses are near the patella and across the tendinous portion of the vastus lateralis insertion. Posterior incisions, especially those releasing the muscle from the lateral intermuscular septum, will cut the vessels where their diameter is greater and thus result in more bleeding. This is not recommended. Routine lateral release bleeding is managed by compression dressing.

Hemarthrosis may be aspirated after arthroscopy, although much of the swelling may be tissue extravasation or clot, especially after lateral release. Continued bleeding should be managed by reoperation and ligation or electrocoagulation of the vessel. Fox and his associates have used electrical cutting and coagulation methods to reduce routine bleeding in lateral release. I believe the techniques described in this textbook makes electrosurgical methods unnecessary.

The superolateral genicular artery may be partially lacerated, and this can result in a false aneurysm. It is recognized not so much by bleeding but by the onset of severe pain unexplained by other causes and localized to the anatomical site. The typical case develops several days after surgery. False aneurysm is managed by surgical exposure, often open, with resection and ligation. The pain relief is dramatic (Fig. 2-42).

Injury to the popliteal vessels or nerves results from passage of cutting instruments into the popliteal fossa. Anatomical cross-section (see Fig. 7-11, *A*) shows these structures almost an inch from the joint cavity at the joint line. The loss of cutting instruments from the field of view is the most common cause. Major vessel laceration has accompanied lateral meniscal repair when the needle was passed from same compartment as tear and too posterior. Surgical approaches to the posterior compartments, even to the Baker's cyst, require special care in both entry and surgical manipulation to avoid this complication. Although vessel laceration occurs intraoperatively, routine use of the tourniquet during arthroscopic procedures may delay its recognition until the postoperative phase.

Recognition of major vessel injury requires prompt action and even vascular surgical consultation. Surgical exploration and repair or grafting may be necessary. Exposure of the adjacent nerves allows inspection and repair as indicated.

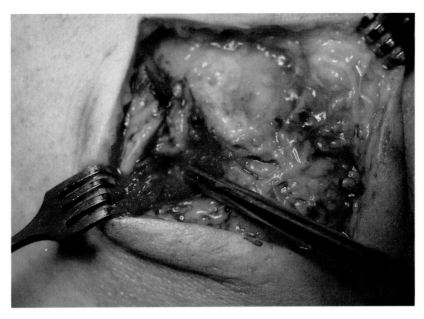

FIG. 2-42. False aneurysm.

Vascular injury from compression of the pneumatic tourniquet of the Surgical Assistant mechanical device is unknown to me. I had a patient with arteriosclerosis in whom the pneumatic tourniquet would not compress the pipelike vessel and the distal tourniquet effect could not be obtained. I have had no cases of intravascular plaque dislodgement.

Manipulation problems

I have had experience with two cases of partial tibial collateral ligament disruption during valgus stress application with the thigh secured mechanically. Both patients were over 70 years of age. Both occurred in 1978, when I first used the Surgical Assistant. Both were partial lesions and healed without treatment. No episode has occurred since.

I am aware of operative manipulative tears of the tibial collateral ligament that occurred without using a mechanical securing device. Two surgeons assisting one another, pulling in opposite directions, had this experience. The technique of the surgeon controlling the joint opening should avoid this complication. It is more difficult for two people to coordinate the effort than for the individual surgeon using a mechanical device.

Traction

Andrews et al. reported upper extremity neuropraxia while using static traction for shoulder arthroscopy.[1] The upper extremity was tied to the operating table after passing over a pulley system. The problems resolved spontaneously. A pulley suspension system with balanced traction avoids this potential complication.

One patient of mine had transient tenderness of the radial nerve at the wrist caused by compression of elastic wrap used to secure traction.

Tourniquet effects

I am not acquainted with tourniquet paralysis related solely to the Surgical Assistant mechanical clamping device.

Tourniquet paralysis may occur with tourniquet time that exceed 2 hours. This is avoidable. Some surgeons avoid use of the tourniquet to have longer operative times. As experience is gained, procedures should not last 2 hours.[31,32] The tourniquet control minimizes bleeding, facilitates clarity of view, and eliminates the necessity of altering surgical techniques to accommodate small bleeding areas. The tourniquet may be released at the end of the procedure to inspect synovium or control hemostasis, but this is not done routinely.

An idiosyncratic type of tourniquet paralysis has been reported in the literature that is unrelated to tourniquet time. I have had one case. It was a 25-minute open operation, and the symptoms resolved completely in 6 months.

Nerve paralysis occurs in 1 out of 8,000 cases with use of pneumatic tourniquet.[31] The cause is high cuff pressure rather than duration, unless over 3 hours.

The lesion is a localized nerve conduction block produced by direct mechanical deformation of nerve fibers. It affects the large myelinated nerves and displaces the Ranvier's nodes. This explains the relative sparing of sensation. It takes 500 to 1,000 mm Hg to produce tourniquet paralysis in baboons.

Recommendations for tourniquet use include regular calibration of the system, use of a pneumatic cuff, and short operative time. The tourniquet pressure should be two to three times the systolic pressure. Extremity compression with Esmarch elastic wrap should be used except in tumors or swollen extremities. Do not use bilateral tourniquets if the patient has poor cardiac reserve.

There is no benefit to releasing and reinflating the tourniquet if operative time is under 2 hours. With longer tourniquet times there is postischemic edema. In some cases tourniquet release before vessel ligature or cast application may be indicated.

Instrumentation problems

The greatest potential for intraoperative problems is related to instrumentation. Initially arthroscopic instruments were borrowed from other endoscopic disciplines. The surgical technique was new to surgeons, and the operative tools and spaces were small.

Instrumentation that takes the arthroscopist and the joint environment into consideration has now been developed. Still, problems may occur (Fig. 2-43). I have experienced fracture of disposable knife blades (the early models), basket forceps, and cutting tips of motorized instruments. To date, all these have been retrieved at the same surgery by arthroscopic means.

Fractured instrumentation may be lodged outside the joint cavity. I was referred a patient who had a basket forceps tip within the popliteus tendon (Fig. 2-44). This required open surgery to identify and remove the tip. I know of two cases of lateral release with knife blade breakage that left a fragment in the tissue.

I have consulted on a case with portions of the arthroscope remaining in the joint after breakage. It was discovered 1 year later, when postoperative effusion would not subside. This probably resulted from assembly without the cannula

A   B

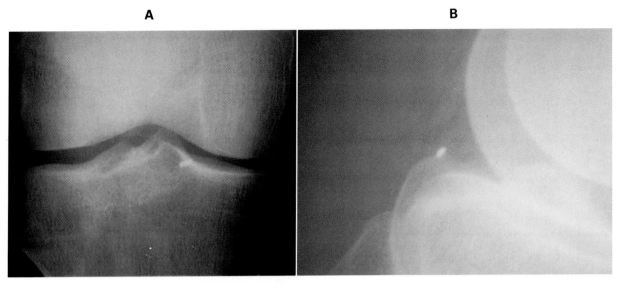

FIG. 2-43. Instrument breakage. **A** AP x-ray film of tip of basket forceps resting in posterior cruciate sheath. **B** Lateral x-ray film of same patient.

A 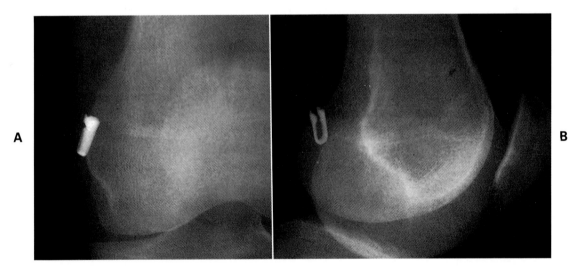 B

FIG. 2-44. Instrument breakage within popliteus tendon tissue. **A,** AP x-ray film. **B,** Lateral x-ray film.

bridge, with the short cannula acting as a lever when forcefully manipulated. I presume arthroscopic visualization was lost during the end of the procedure.

The "ounce of prevention" is to use instrumentation that is small and resistant to breakage. The metallic material should be magnetic to facilitate removal. A magnetic-suction device should be available for immediate identification and insertion. Surgical technique should include keeping instrumentation in view at all times, being continually conscious of gentle manipulations, and obtaining adequate exposure.

At the moment of the instrument breakage, *freeze!* Do not move, and keep the fragment in view. Check the inflow so that the bags do not empty, causing joint collapse and obscuring vision. Call for a Golden Retriever or similar instrument. Keeping the fragment in view, *think!* Formulate a plan. Usually your first attempt will be your best. If you use a method of inflow on the arthroscope, turn it off; it will move the piece out of sight. Establish another inflow portal.

Tell your team what your plans are and allow them time to give opinions and help. Often the event has taxed your emotions. There may be periarticular edema or no clear location of the fragment. Obtain an x-ray film of the joint. If the piece is seen, you can try to identify and remove it. Most pieces can be removed by a magnetic section device via a cannula. Some fragments may lend themselves to forceps removal.

Open surgery will be beneficial only if the piece has been located. An open surgical exploration to "parts unknown" in a postarthroscopic edematous knee may just end in frustration.

If the piece is not identifiable and tourniquet operative time is expiring, I recommend completion of the intended surgery and deferral of fragment retrieval.

In my opinion, the major issue is exercising reasonable and good judgment, and that may mean leaving the fragment. Repeat the surgery on another day, preferably 7 to 10 days later. If the fragment is shown to be extraarticular by arthrogram, it can be followed by clinical evaluations and x-ray films to confirm its innocuous position.

Instrument breakage is a potential complication, unavoidable even by industrial quality control or surgical technique. The issue is the safe and judicious management of the problem. That may mean removal, immediately or later, or clinical observation.

Postoperative complications
Bleeding

Bleeding accompanies every incision, even the small punctures of arthroscopic procedures (Fig. 2-45). These wounds normally seal over in a matter of hours. Little bleeding occurs from the lacerations after the first day. Most is controlled by pressure or collects on the surgical dressing.

Bleeding to a greater extent in either time or volume suggests an open vascular source. Inspection of the wound may show a small skin vessel or a vessel in the subcutaneous area. Most are controlled by pressure. The small "pumper" may be controlled by transcutaneous needle suture ligation.

On two occasions, ligation of the saphenous vein was necessary when it was lacerated during a posteromedial approach to the knee.

In shoulder arthroscopy I have experienced one intraoperative cephalic vein laceration. Another manifested itself 1 day postoperatively. Both were managed by suture ligation, which is routine with open surgical approaches. No sequelae have occurred.

Technically speaking, hemarthrosis follows every surgery. Intraarticular sources of bleeding may result in postoperative hemarthrosis. The problem cases cause painful distention. However, problem hemarthrosis is not common, even

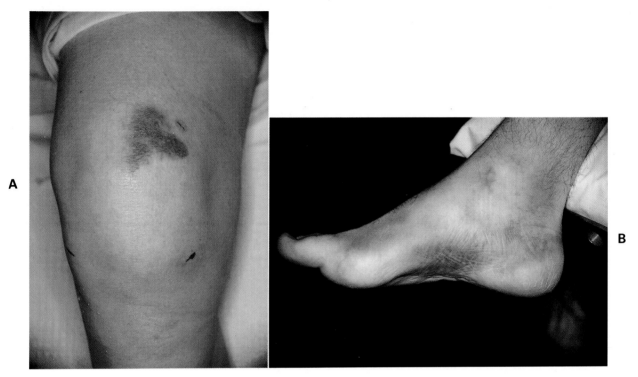

FIG. 2-45. Postoperative bleeding. **A,** Adjacent to arthroscopic portal. **B,** Dependent drainage to foot and ankle.

with abrasion arthroplasty and osteophyte resection, because of the clotting mechanisms and compression dressing.

I rarely use sutures to close the operative sites. This permits normal drainage for 2 days. I have seen no need for routine drains of any type.

In a rare case the patient may flex the knee, even up to the seventh day postoperatively, and experience a sudden gush of blood. Aside from the inconvenience, there has been no other problem.

Recognition of the hemarthrosis and early aspiration result in resolution. Multiple aspirations are rarely needed. Aspirations at later dates will yield little fluid because of intraarticular clotting or capsular extravasation rather than intraarticular blood.

A hemarthrosis associated with active vascular bleeding after lateral release may require open clot evacuation and vascular ligation. The same would be so with a false aneurysm.

Patients with a bleeding diathesis must have supportive medical care to reduce the chance of bleeding.

The use of epinephrine (Adrenalin) solutions has been a benefit in controlling intraoperative bleeding during shoulder and hip arthroscopy, because bleeding from these joints cannot be controlled with a tourniquet. A solution of 1 mg epinephrine to 1,000 ml of fluid is used judiciously and intermittently. It is used during the initial diagnostic phase for distention and cleansing. Subsequent use is only with anesthesiological approval. Under no circumstances should a continuous epinephrine drip be used, because the amount cannot be monitored and delayed absorption phenomena may result from extravasated fluid. I do not use epinephrine in the knee, because tourniquet control is routine.

I believe it should not be used in the elbow, wrist or beyond in the upper extremities because of possible adverse peripheral vascular constriction. I do not use it in the ankle for the same reason. The ankle and foot tissues are slow to recover circulation, even with distention of extravasated normal saline.

Noninfectous effusion

Postoperative effusion is common. It resolves within a few days and is serosanguineous in nature. Any effusion persisting over 3 weeks in a properly protected joint is reason for review of the patient's diagnosis, operation, and postoperative activity level. Synovial diseases, especially rhuematoid arthritis and hemophilia, cause prolonged postoperative effusions. Some reactive degenerative knees will do the same.

Operative procedures that include extensive synovectomy or bony debridement are prone to longer resolution time. Failure to adequately remove loose particles, for example, in basket forceps meniscectomy, or inadequate lavage during or on completion of the case will cause synovitis and effusion.[28,35]

The most common cause of postoperative effusion is resumption of patient activity before intraarticular healing has occurred. The patient starts "trying out" the joint too soon or takes initiative in physical therapy. The patient who undergoes joint surface debridement must protect the joint with non-weight bearing. As a rule, it is required for 4 weeks for partial-thickness surgery and 8 weeks for full-thickness abrasion arthroplasty (see Chapter 9). Failure to comply results in effusion and even undesirable vascular hypermic fibrous repair. Repeat surgery may be required for repair, debridement, and lavage followed by mandatory joint protection.

Most effusions will resolve with rest or non-weight bearing. If rest is successful, it establishes the cause as overactivity. A persistent (6 weeks) effusion may be aspirated, but if rest is instituted this is rarely necessary. Cortisone injection would be the final nonoperative modality to try, but not in the absence of the patient's willingness to protect and rest the joint. Antiinflammatory medicines have not been of any more dramatic help for postoperative effusion than rest. Salicylates may be used for pain.

If the effusion persists for more than 3 months, there is probably articular debris in the joint. This is most common following arthroscopic debridement of a degenerative compartment with a complex posterior horn meniscal tear in an active middle-aged man. Another typical case for persistent effusion is the overweight patient with a valgus deformity and degenerative meniscal and compartment disease.

Persistent effusion calls for aspiration cell block. A pathological study will prove the intraarticular debris. If aspiration fails, repeat arthroscopy through lavage, rest, and medical treatment (antiinflammatory) is indicated.

The most difficult to manage of all cases in this category is the degenerative arthritic knee with an inflammatory component. This should be recognized at arthroscopy because of its poor prognostic implication. These patients are usually too young for total knee replacement, and they may have had multiple arthroscopies. In my experience, they are no better following open synovectomy. Rheumatological consultation and treatment has not reversed any disease course in my experience. After a year or so, the patient goes on about activities as tolerated. A few patients have spontaneously improved after a few years. No evidence of rheumatoid arthritis was determined by either laboratory test or clinical course. Fortunately, these cases are rare.

An effusion that develops some months after surgery without new injury probably is caused by progression of degenerative changes, especially related to failure to modify activity in accordance with postoperative instructions. An overlooked or underresected meniscus may be the cause. Patients with cruciate instability may develop subsequent effusion. The postoperative development of transarticular adhesions may produce late effusion, especially following lateral release or anterior cruciate ligament repairs.

Conservative measures are reinstituted, but a prolonged unsuccessful course should be avoided. Repeat arthroscopy and appropriate treatment should be performed.

Persistent effusion should not be accepted. However, the patient should know that this is a signal of joint problems and subsequent irreversible changes.

Synovial fistula

Leakage from arthroscopic puncture sites is common for a few days. I have had one case continue for a week before spontaneous closure. I have not seen a persistent synovial fistula.

My puncture wounds are small. Multiple approaches through the same or adjacent incisions are minimized. Arthroscopic portals should be preselected by needle placement. Cannula systems are used whenever possible to minimize tissue trauma. The incision size is smaller than the cannula system (4 to 6 mm outside diameter).

Suture closure is not routine. Only a large incision should be sutured, such as with a large loose body removal. The rationale for abandoning suture closure is that it is unnecessary. Suturing prevents natural joint drainage in immediate postoperative days and may cause subcutaneous infection.

Infection

Infection is a known complication of any surgery, although it is infrequent following arthroscopic procedures. This complication occurs despite precautions. Contributing factors to infection are penetration of the skin, operative instrumentation, postincisional bleeding, and presence of normal skin or pharyngeal bacterial flora. Minimal incisional trauma and coupious lavage routine, causing dilution of any organisms, are the main factors in the low infection rate in arthroscopic surgery.

We reviewed 12,000 arthroscopic cases from our institution up to 1981. The overall infection rate was .04%. The infections that did occur were related to direct viewing arthroscopy followed by open surgery without repeat skin preparation and sterile draping. This technique is no longer practiced.

It was only recently that I have again experienced any infections. There were three cases within 1 year. There were one *Streptococcus* and two *Staphylococcus aureus* gram positive infections. After the third case, the common denominator was obvious; all the patients had a meniscal repair with transcutaneous sutures tied outside or over the skin. All were treated by prompt arthroscopic lavage and synovectomy plus antibiotics and continuous passive motion. All recovered without permanent sequalae or joint damage. I abandoned transcutaneous suturing and now tie the sutures beneath the skin. There have been no subsequent infections.

One patient developed an infection following arthroscopic quadricepsplasty. The operation involved medial and lateral retinacular releases and resection of scar tissue between quadriceps tendon to the femur. Although monitored arthroscopically, the incision sites were close to 1 inch in length to facilitate the large resection. Subcutaneous suture closure was used on these "arthrotomies." A postoperative infection developed with massive hematoma and wound separation. Arthroscopic debridement, antibiotic treatment, and continuous passive motion resulted in prompt resolution and maintenance of the original surgical benefit. The quadricepsplasty procedure should be considered a combined operation rather than a routine arthroscopic case because of its magnitude. I have performed similar procedures without infection. I believe the large amount of cutting and resultant hemarthrosis in a quadricepsplasty merit prophylactic antibiotic therapy.

The minimization of infection rests with sterile technique, gentle surgical manipulation, and hemostasis or its management.

I do not routinely use prophylactic antibiotics. Prophylactic antibiotics are used in debilitated, diabetic, and infection-prone patients. Those with a known procedural potential for hemarthrosis, implant surgery following recent arthroscopy (10 days), and history of furunculosis may also require antibiotic prophylaxis.

Fibrous adhesions

Injury and/or surgery initiates a fibrous tissue repair (see Fig. 13-6). Intracapsular and intraarticular fibrous adhesions are commonly seen at second-look arthroscopy. They are surprisingly common after even simple arthroscopic meniscectomy. Procedures such as lateral release and anterior cruciate ligament repair frequently cause adhesions that span the intraarticular space. Adhesions are rarely symptomatic. Clinically symptomatic fibrous bands may follow wide resections of medial plicae. They are also seen in lateral release and cruciate ligament repairs. The symptoms may be swelling, pain, popping, or even a loose body shown by a palpable mass.

On one occasion, I identified a painful adhesion inside and adjacent to an arthroscopic portal. I have seen one case of painful meniscotibial adhesion following arthroscopic meniscectomy and abrasion of an adjacent sclerotic lesion. Local anesthesia helped confirm the exact area of symptoms in both patients. Simple resection to the joint wall relieves the symptoms.

Ankylosis

Ankylosis following arthroscopic procedures is uncommon. I have seen two cases that followed a lateral release procedure performed with sterile water medium for electrosurgery. Both patients experienced severe postoperative pain in the quadriceps area and were slow to regain motion. They both required repeat surgery with adhesiolysis and manipulation.

I have experienced three cases of ankylosis following arthroscopic repair of acute tear of anterior cruciate ligaments. The repair was held with a metallic staple, and the knee was casted at a 45-degree angle for 6 weeks. All three patients were women between 18 and 22 years of age. All are active in recreational sports. There were no infections.

Second-look arthroscopy was necessary. The fibrous tissue was abundant to and through the notch from the entire anterior chamber. Adhesiolysis with staple removal, including release of the superior notch attachments of the repair, was successful in all patients.

Except for the fact that all of these cases were women, there was no common denominator or reason for these patients to have the same conditions and operations. A shorter period of immobilization (3 to 4 weeks) should be considered in young women having this surgery.

Thromboembolic phenomenon

Thromboembolic phenomenon is a rare problem following arthroscopic surgery, with an incidence of perhaps 0.1% in my practice.[9] The three cases I knew of previously occurred in men. Two patients had torn menisci with degenerative joint disease, and the third case followed a lateral release procedure. I recently experienced a fourth case in an elderly woman after joint debridement.

The first two were treated in their home city with medication without sequelae. The lateral release patient developed pulmonary embolism, necessitating a vena cava plication. A satisfactory result was achieved. The woman responded to anticoagulant therapy.

Although many of the predisposing factors exist for thromboembolic phenomenon (extremity surgery, immobilization, obesity, varicose veins) the incidence in arthroscopic surgery is low. This may be related to the minimization of incisions, relatively short operative times (under 1 hour), and immediate ambulation.

I use prophylactic anticoagulation when the medical history indicates a previous problem.[19] Complicated cases may require medical consultation. The existence of varicose veins or previous vein stripping surgeries requires prophylaxis only if there is a previous thromboembolic episode.

This complication is unfortunately unpredictable in otherwise healthy patients.[23] Routine postoperative instructions contain information that the onset of pain, swelling, fever, and chest pain or the coughing of blood, merit medical attention. (See Fig. 2-39, *B*)

Neurological complications

I have not had experience with traction neuropraxia or tourniquet paralysis. Aside from cutaneous nerve contusion or interruption, I have had no other problems of this type.

Sudeck's atrophy

I had one patient who developed Sudeck's atrophy in both lower extremities from the knee down, although an arthroscopic procedure was performed on only one knee (a minimal articular debridement). The patient was treated with diazepam (Valium), moderate activity, and gradual return to recreation. The event could not have been related to the magnitude or length of the procedure; 1 year was necessary for a return to normal.

Probably more important than the postoperative incidence of Sudeck's atrophy is its preoperative recognition. The condition may be localized to the knee joint or even the patella.[14] Surgical intervention in the presence of Sudeck's atrophy may exacerbate the condition and even result in ankylosis.[6]

Physician hazards

Possible damage to the surgeon's eye by visible light has been discussed[13,22]. Data indicate that visual radiation can cause injury to the photoreceptors in the macula. This is probably not a thermal effect, but visual radiation may accelerate inherent retinal degeneration. These photochemical changes are most severe in the center of the retina and can affect visual accuracy.

Some studies indicate that the ultraviolet ray is a risk in an increased incidence of cataracts, especially the senile type. However, there is not accompanying senile macular degeneration.

The possibility of existing light sources causing retinal injury has been reported by Drs. Thomas Rosenberg and J. Whitaker Ewing. It has been reported to me by industrial engineers that such injury would not be possible when using the normal halogen light source. The possibility of retinal damage could exist as a result of irradiation over prolonged exposure times. Absolute documentation of retinal injury related to direct viewing is lacking.

At present, the chance of injury is low, because most surgeons use video for their visualization.

JOINTS OTHER THAN THE KNEE: SHOULDER

The shoulder joint has been an area of considerable interest over the years to orthopedic surgeons, based on patient's complaints of the pathological abnormalities that develop in and around that joint. Previous investigations included physical examinations, x-ray films, and open surgical explorations. The opportunity to visualize arthroscopically the glenohumeral joint, the subacromial bursa, and the acromioclavicular joint not only allows a better understanding of the anatomy and pathology of the shoulder joint but also opens a completely new avenue for exploration of new surgical procedures.

In Chapter 15, a discussion of the debridement of condylar surfaces and synovectomy by arthroscopy is included, as well as the repair of glenohumeral ligaments in acute and chronic recurrent dislocation, the ability to carry out acromioplasty endoscopically, and the potential to resect well-defined meniscal lesions with synovitis and degenerative change inside the acromioclavicular joint.

The future certainly holds the opportunity for repair of rotator cuff injuries when necessary.

MEDICAL MARKET CHANGES AND ARTHROSCOPY

Arthroscopic surgical procedures are here to stay and are growing steadily.

Arthroscopy has an enormous impact on the practice of orthopedic surgery, especially in the area of medical economics. A discipline started in the 1960s, when it was considered a curiosity with perhaps some diagnostic possibilities, arthroscopy rapidly became a service with consumer demand fueled by the media by the 1970s. In the early 1980s, it is becoming the standard of practice both diagnostically and therapeutically in the United States. Surgeons with arthroscopic skills enjoy an increased demand for their services.

Arthroscopic techniques developed in the private practice sector of the orthopedic community. Most of the advocates were private practitioners with clinical appointments in various medical schools. Even by 1982 only 20% of orthopedic department chairmen were involved in arthroscopic teaching. The only orthopedic programs not teaching arthroscopy in 1982 were university programs (see Table 2-5). This development was in contrast to the history of joint replacement surgery, which required a greater academic support team to accomplish.

The first organizational meetings for arthroscopy attracted so little interest that many joined out of curiosity, never having performed the procedure. Results of a survey taken in 1981 showed that 20% of IAA members did not perform arthroscopy.

As stated earlier in this chapter, one half of AAOS members said they used arthroscopy in their practice in 1978. By 1981 the percentage grew to 75% and to over 90% by 1983. Operative work was performed by 75% of respondents as of that date. Most surgeons in resident training plan to incorporate arthroscopic surgery in their practices.

At present there are at least 600 orthopedists with 25% or more of their practice designated for arthroscopic surgery (present membership number and basic criteria for AANA). Many have practices limited to arthroscopic disciplines. Most orthopedists have incorporated basic diagnostic and operative methods into their practices.

Between 1974, the date of the first arthroscopic organization meeting, and 1986 arthroscopic surgery has grown from a procedure of dubious value to an integral part of most orthopedic surgeons' practices.

Consumer demand

The individual orthopedist has been significantly affected by arthroscopy. Those who had early arthroscopic experience watched their practices grow because of consumer demand and media coverage. This is not to mention the now-established lower morbidity, more accurate diagnosis, and increased success of treatment.

The nonarthroscopist often clashed ideologically with the arthroscopic surgeon. Early arthroscopists were criticized for performing unnecessary surgery, taking too long, holding up surgery schedules, damaging joints, doing incomplete jobs, and adding unnecessary risks during the learning process. The nonarthroscopist contended that he or she could make a more accurate diagnosis clinically and see better in the joint, perform operations faster, and do a more thorough job with arthrotomy.

This controversy has waned with time and exposure to the procedure. I often wonder what the discussion would have been like if arthroscopic techniques been easily mastered by every orthopedic surgeon.

The consumer demand and news media exposure created a shift in patient populations away from the nonarthroscopist, whatever the merits of the procedure. As a result many surgeons were motivated to perform arthroscopic surgery by economic necessity. This movement was supported by growing clinical evidence of the benefits of arthroscopic surgery.

Professional response and effects

The increased use of arthroscopic surgery by the orthopedic surgeons in the United States from 1979 to 1986 presents its own unique problems. There was a great increase in course attendance, equipment purchase, and clinical practice. Arthroscopes were scarce in 1981. The medical industry responded; at first there were a few small companies, but now most every major orthopedic supplier offers its version of what was seen at the last exhibition.

Television became as common in the arthroscopic surgical suite as in the home. The use of video for arthroscopic procedures grew from 25% in 1981 to 80% in 1983. Orthopedists rapidly moved from direct viewing to video surgery.

Questions of hospital credentials for arthroscopic practice were now challenged. The question was, what constitutes privileges to perform this new procedure?

The early arthroscopists had the luxury of a slow, step-by-step progression from direct view diagnostic arthroscopy to simple operative resection. The uses of video were introduced slowly and developed along with the arthroscopic instrumentation. The 50% of orthopedic surgeons who began arthroscopy after 1978 were faced with learning basic skills amid a multitude of sophisticated equipment. For some reason it was thought that arthroscopy was not so important for diagnostic purposes but that its surgical possibilities validated the procedure. Many surgeons tried to bypass basic principles and launched their arthroscopic surgical careers, but not without difficulty and frustration.

A second major impact on practice profiles occurred with the dilution of available surgical cases. When virtually all orthopedists became arthroscopists, the patient population was spread over more physicians. Hence fewer surgical experiences were available for the large number of orthopedists who sought to develop their skills. Arthroscopy requires a constant flow of technical experience to maintain skills, let alone advance them. The opportunity probably will not exist again to gain the number of case experiences enjoyed by the pioneers of arthroscopy. The reduction in case experiences will continue to present a problem as the number of orthopedic surgeons in the United States grows. As a result I expect a shift of practice profiles. Diagnostic and simple operative procedures will be a part of most practices. There will also be arthroscopic surgical centers where the more complex or previously complicated cases will be managed.

The original arthroscopist purchased equipment at great expense: $40,000 in the late 1970s. This was the result of intense interest, often accompanied by colleagues' opposite opinions. By 1981 most purchases of equipment were made by hospitals or group practices. Institutional interest was prompted by concern over loss of market share to those institutions at which the procedure was performed. The summation of these events was probably that learning surgeons worked with suboptimal instrumentation, teaching staff as they performed new procedures.

The personality of the surgeon was severely tested by having to learn this new technique while continuing a practice; the time away from practice to learn the surgical techniques of the new medium led to many demands on the surgeon's patience and precision. A surgeon who was successful in open surgery may become frustrated to encounter difficulty in learning the arthroscopic technique.

The pluses for many orthopedists include the excitement of a rapidly developing discipline within their own specialty and the meeting of new challenges. A sense of satisfaction is derived from being a part of a discipline that is growing so rapidly. And there are other benefits: reduced hospital rounds, fewer suture removals, and fewer multiple office visits. There are also patient benefits: less discomfort, less time off work, quicker recovery and little or no interruption in personal plans.

Government and insurance industry effects

The development of arthroscopy coincided with the overhaul of the national medical-economic picture.[12,20,50] Insurance company directives toward outpatient surgery only serve to promote arthroscopic procedures. With recent medical reimbursement programs, it may not be economical for the physician or institution to render treatment in any other way than arthroscopically, when applicable.

It appears that arthroscopy has benefited by two economic incentives. First, consumer demand has effected physicians' willingness to provide the service; and second, the changes in governmental reimbursement and insurance procedural changes have promoted it.

Insurance

If George Orwell had written a chapter on orthopedic surgery in his book *1984* he would have recognized every person's right to an annual arthroscopic procedure at society's expense. The insurance companies were not prepared for the onset, extent of use, or growth of this discipline.

The insurance companies struggled with the increased use of arthroscopy but rapidly recognized the cost benefits of same-day surgery, minimal morbidity, and resultant rapid return to work.

In 1973 Michigan Blue Shield responded with a code and fee for diagnostic arthroscopy based on reimbursement for other endoscopic procedures, that is, gastroscopy and bronchoscopy. After 2½ years of petitioning, Michigan Blue Shield responded with limited operative arthroscopy codes in 1978. Other states followed suit.

Michigan Blue Shield agreed to pay the full fee for diagnostic arthroscopy and the operative procedure as if they had been performed by open means. Their previous practice was to pay one-half of the lesser fee and the full amount on the larger fee. The summation of the two full fees recognized the difficulty and value of the arthroscopic methods.

Recently Michigan Blue Shield was presented with a more comprehensive provider service profile and a relative value scale (Table 2-16). The purpose was to identify more specifically the service and appropriate reimbursement. As arthroscopic procedures are perfected, the entire spectrum of diagnostic complexity, time, technical difficulty, postoperative management, and potential complications needs to be addressed.

No price values are given here; the letter designation indicates my opinion

TABLE 2-16. Arthroscopic surgical relative value scale

Procedure	Relative value
Diagnostic arthroscopy	
Single procedure	F
Multiple compartment	E
Operative arthroscopy (multicompartmental and diagnostic procedures and therapeutic lavage)	D
Biopsy	D
Loose body	
Single	C
Multiple complex	B
Meniscectomy	
Simple	C
Complex medial or lateral	B
Both	B
Degenerative arthritis (multicompartmental)	B
Cruciate instability	A
Meniscal repair (closed or open)	B
Chondroplasty	
Single surface (patella or condyle)	C
Multiple surfaces	B
Abrasion	A
Synovectomy	
Simple—plica	D
Multiple compartments	B
Alignment procedure	
Lateral release	C
With medial imbrication	B
Ligament repair (arthroscopically monitored)	
Tibial collateral	C
Medial patellar retinacular	C
Anterior cruciate (delayed primary)	B
Reconstruction with graft	A
Combined with open surgery	Arthroscopic fee plus 50% of conventional fee
Other joints	
Diagnostic	D
Shoulder	
Glenohumeral joint	
Loose body	C
Multiple	B
Chondroplasty	B
Synovectomy	B
Reconstruction	A
Subchondral bursa	
Synovectomy	B
Acromioplasty	A
Acromioclavicular joint	
Meniscectomy	B
Chondroplasty	B

TABLE 2-16. Arthroscopic surgical relative value scale—cont'd

Procedure	Relative value
Elbow	
Lavage (loose bodies)	D
Loose body removal (motorized forceps)	C
Multiple	B
Chondroplasty	B
Synovectomy	B
Hip	
Lavage	D
Loose body removal	C
Multiple	B
Chondroplasty	B
Abrasion arthroplasty	A
Synovectomy	B
Ankle	
Lavage	D
Loose body removal	C
Multiple	B
Chondroplasty	B
Abrasion arthroplasty	A
Synovectomy	B
Fingers, toes, etc.	
Diagnostic	C
Any operative	B

of relative value. *A* has the highest value, *B* is next lower, and *C*, *D*, *E*, and *F* follow. Payment would be based on the highest single service rendered. Multiple payments for single joint procedures would be eliminated. Bilateral cases would pay full on the first extremity and one half on the second, as with open surgery.

An attempt was made to grade the procedures by disease category and technical difficulty. No accounting was made for patient or insurance carrier benefits.

This relative value scale does not favor arthroscopic methods. The same fee is paid for meniscectomy or meniscal repair, whether open or conventional. This removes any possible financial incentive that could interfere with the treatment options of any given patient.

MEDICAL ECONOMICS
Supply and demand

When I was in training in the early 1960s the emphasis was on *a*bility, *a*vailability, and *a*ppearance. In addition to the "triple *A*s," some added affability. In those days the demand for orthopedic services far outweighed the supply of orthopedic surgeons. The resolution of the "doctor shortage" also applied to orthopedic surgery. Now orthopedic surgeons are practicing in virtually every rural community. The supply side was compensated for by the expansion of orthopedics into total joint replacement, electrostimulation, and chymopapain treatment for disk problems.

Arthroscopy also provides a new service and creates new demands. Expansion of the technique beyond meniscectomy to repair, treatment of the arthritis, and to synovial joints other than the knee further increased the demand side. However, with ever-increasing numbers of orthopedists offering the service of arthroscopy, the demand was met.

The new ball game

The cost of health care is a matter of public concern.[12,20,50] The development of sophisticated treatment modalities, public demand for these services, and industry and/or government's past willingness to meet these spiraling costs had to be re-evaluated. The system provided the patient with "best is none too good" service at no or little out-of-pocket cost. The cost was "hidden" in the costs of services or taxes, into which society (the patient) paid. Health care was just his fringe benefit. Physicians enjoyed virtually unlimited hospital or personal budgets for the latest in technology to treat patients. They were well compensated financially. The insurance companies could just increase the premiums to employers and the government increase the taxes.

Now the rules have changed. Hospitals and physicians have less input; the company paying the bill has more. The automobile industry estimates that $600 of the cost of an automobile goes for medical care benefits. Some say employee medical care costs more than the steel to build the car, since many parts of modern cars are plastic.

I have addressed this topic because if one is going to be an arthroscopic surgeon, it will result as much from his or her response to this new system as it will from knowledge and ability in arthroscopic surgery. Also, I believe arthroscopic techniques are especially well positioned to render better health care at a cost savings.

Administrative setbacks

In October, 1983, Michigan Blue Shield discontinued reimbursement on all arthroscopic procedures except those on the knee joint. It would fully reimburse any open procedure on other joints. It had paid for the arthroscopic procedures for 8 years under individual consideration codes. At this same time, 26% of American orthopedists were performing arthroscopies on joints other than the knee joint. Arthroscopic shoulder reconstructive surgery was 1 year old at the time. No rationale was offered, and no change in policy was rendered for 2 years.

I mention this to illustrate the impact of medical economic decisions on medical care and advancement of technology.

Michigan Blue Shield will pay for open shoulder reconstruction, with its increased hospital and facilities cost, but not outpatient arthroscopic techniques. Furthermore, the failure to reimburse carries with it the implication of unacceptable or experimental procedure. The expertise and technological advances of the medical profession are now challenged by society's inability or unwillingness to afford them.

The new direction

Originally surgeons established fees based on the patient's ability to pay. Some patients paid, some did not, and others were unable. The third-party payment system introduced the concept of reasonable, usual, and prevailing fee schedules. "Usual" means the fee the individual physician charged. "Prevailing" applied to what was customary in his or her area. "Reasonable" was determined by the insurance company. The insurance company then paid what was then called "relative value;" it was the lowest of the three other categories.

The second dimension of the physician–insurance company relationship was designation as "participant" or "nonparticipant" in the insurance company plan. Originally this could even be designated upon an individual case basis, and subsequently on an annual basis. To participate meant the physician accepted what the insurance company's fee as payment in full. Nonparticipation indicated the money was sent to the patient, and the patient was responsible for paying the physician's designated fee. This often required additional outlay for the patient and collection problems for the physician.

The term *relative value* is a misnomer. There was no discrimination of payment based on experience, ability, or results or value to patient, carrier, or society.

Within the past few years, the terms health maintenance organization (HMO), preferred provider (PPO, PPP), and diagnosis related group (DRG) have become common. To adjust to the changing medical economic environment, I offer the following definitions.

Carrier: Insurance company, governmental agency or insured company.
Consumer: Patient
Provider: Physician/hospital or HMO

Health maintenance organizations

An HMO is an organization established either by a hospital, clinic, group of physicians, or even an insurance company. The most familiar ones are the Kaiser-Permente organizations on the west coast, which have existed for years. This concept is growing in popularity, because the member pays a single fee and is guaranteed any and all medical care. The fee is established after evaluating potential costs. The incentive for the organization is to maintain the client's health in such a state that he has a higher level of well-being and a reduction of disease. These groups hope for a profit. The physician's incentive is to reduce the medical costs to his or her patients through good treatment and reduction of costs for excessive tests and/or treatment modalities without compromising good care. This would result in physician bonuses based on the overall financial performance of the organization. At the time of this writing, the community with the largest percentage of people participating in HMOs is Minneapolis, with approximately 25% of the population participating in this method of health care.

Preferred providers

To reduce its Medicare, Medicaid, or CalMed costs, the state of California introduced the concept of preferred provider. This allowed designation of the physicians and hospitals that will provide the treatments for the state patients. This was done on a competitive basis to receive the best possible medical care at the lowest price. The desire was to have a resultant premium savings of between 10% and 20%. The effects of that arrangement are certainly under evaluation. The concept has been widely accepted and is either under study or being instituted in most states at the present time.

Preferred provider organizations

A PPO consists of one or more providers (physicians and/or hospitals) that take the initiative to contract on a low-cost basis with an employer or insurer. In return the employer or insurer uses benefit program incentives to channel employees to the preferred providers. This is currently the most common type of preferred provider arrangement. These PPOs are usually established by physicians practicing in a large multispecialty group or at a given hospital.

Preferred provider products

A PPP is a case of the carrier offering and administering a product that integrates benefit incentives and selective provider contracting. The carrier identifies and secures a preferred panel of providers (physicians).

There are three basic models for PPPs:
1. Open Choice. This model covers the services of all qualified providers and also carries explicit incentives, such as higher benefits, for subscribers who use any preferred provider.
2. Designated Choice. This model also covers the services of all qualified providers but carries explicit incentives for subscribers whose care is performed or ordered by a single preferred provider, designated by the subscriber in advance. This model begins to capitalize on patient case management concepts.
3. Limited Choice. This model gives subscribers the option to enroll in a program that only covers services performed or ordered by a designated provider.

Diagnostic related groups

In October, 1983, the federal government began a prospective system of reimbursement for hospitals caring for Medicare patients based on diagnostic related groups (DRGs). This is similar to the system pioneered in New Jersey to improve management for hospital administrators. All possible admitting diagnoses are divided into 468 different categories based on the anatomical system, the age of the patient, and the degree of complication or other morbidity involved.

Under the DRG system hospitals are reimbursed by a fixed, predictable amount for each DRG, regardless of the funds expended to provide care for the Medicare recipient. Theoretically hospitals that were more efficient could "win" by being reimbursed for more than their costs; less efficient hospitals would "lose" by being reimbursed less than their actual costs. There is a single code for arthroscopy.

At present physician fees are not currently covered by this program.

Near-future practices

In my opinion the concepts of preferred provider and DRG will be commonplace in medical practice. It behooves the surgeon to clearly understand, anticipate, and respond to these changes in a positive way. There is nothing practition-

TABLE 2-17. Benefits of true preferred provider

	Economic benefit	Good result	Good relation	Benefit
Consumer (patient)	X	X	X	Result
Carrier (insurance company)	X	X	X	Expense
Provider (physician or hospital)	X	X	X	Professional

ers can do to prevent the full implementation of this system of contract medicine. Therefore the response has to be understanding of and positive about the new medical economic environment. This means taking initiative.

Physicians must also be in a position to provide a full, timely, and accurate diagnosis for the medical record. This diagnosis must be accurate and also be what is known as a resource-intensive diagnosis. That means that it must accurately portray the extent of the diagnosis and any complicating medical factors. The physician undoubtedly will be responsible for establishing the diagnosis, and will probably have to do so before any reimbursement is initiated either at the hospital or by the physician. This means more paperwork.

To understate the severity of a diagnosis could result in a financial loss to either hospital or physician. To overstate it would probably mean a subsequent necessary reimbursement and the mandatory audits that will be part of this program.

Physicians' input should come in the area of clearer identification of the training and experience necessary to render certain medical treatments as well as the extent of the complexity of the various diagnoses to clearly delineate and establish relative value of the services rendered.

We must be very patient, especially with the hospital administration, in working out problems with third-party payment by insurance or government agencies.

If you like your hospital and its administration, join with them in offering services.

Last, we have to be alert to our own possible wasteful practices and those of our colleagues. We should set a standard not only for them but for the hospital and society by our increasing high level of practice. I believe that the arthroscopic surgeon is in a favorable position because of his or her ability to render a service with minimal hospitalization, expense, and morbidity to a patient and subsequent rapid return to work.

New definition of preferred provider

I submit the following definition of a preferred provider of medical care (Table 2-17). The provider (physician or hospital) would render such care that there would be an economic benefit for the consumer (patient) and carrier (insurance company) as well as the physician.

New system and arthroscopic procedures

Medical advances in orthopedics provided arthroscopic techniques before but just in time for the new system of decreased hospitalization policies (prior authorization) and reimbursement based on DRGs. The surgeon with arthroscopic surgical skills is well positioned to participate in the "new ball game."

The treatment result is good for all parties. The patient will be treated with minimal discomfort and without complications or repeat operations. The good result translates to minimal costs to the insurance carrier. The treating physician gains professional satisfaction from the good result.

Advantages of arthroscopic surgery

As the arthroscopic surgeon gains time and experience, it is becoming increasingly evident that arthroscopic surgery reduces the hospital stay, usually to the same day. The reduced morbidity translates into decreased time off work, and arthroscopy produces a result equal to if not better than conventional methods. From the standpoint of the insurer or underwriter, either the insurance company or employer, this translates into reduced initial costs for the medical care.

The issue of a good result is based on an accurate diagnosis, the physician's judgment, and successful rehabilitation. These factors should lead to good results and decreased future costs. For instance, the case of patient with a severely degenerative arthritic knee who otherwise would be a candidate for high tibial osteotomy and/or total knee abrasion arthroplasty could be considered. Both procedures are conventional and carry a greater risk than arthroscopic surgery for complication and even major reoperation.

When arthroscopic abrasion arthroplasty was performed in 100 patients, 3 total knee operations and 3 high tibial osteotomies were necessary within the first 3 year minimal follow-up. Arthroscopic surgery at least deferred the major conventional reconstructive surgery in 94% of that patient population. There was a minimum of complications and reoperations, including arthroscopic procedures.

I believe that industry, government, consumer, and providers ultimately will participate in more clearly identifying what is a "good dollar value" in medical care. The technique of arthroscopic surgery and those who perform it are well positioned to offer the optimal result with a maximal economic benefit to both carriers and consumers in this new ball game.

REFERENCES

1. Andrews, J.R., Carson, W.G., and Ortega, K.: Arthroscopy of the shoulder: technique and normal anatomy, Am. J. Sports Med. **12**:1, 1984.
2. Cahill, B.R., and Berg, B.C.: 99m-Technetium phosphate compound joint scintigraphy in the management of juvenile osteochondritis dissecans of the femoral condyles, Am. J. Sports Med. **11**:329, 1983.
3. Cannon, H.D.: Personal communication, 1984.
4. Christopher, G.W., et al.: Meningococcal arthritis, bacteremia, and osteomyelitis following arthroscopy (report of a case), Clin. Orthop. **171**:127, 1982.
5. Daniels, D.: Personal communication, 1983.
6. DeHaven, K.E.: Personal communication, 1984.
7. DeHaven, K.E.: Diagnosis of acute knee injuries with hemarthrosis, Am. J. Sports Med. **8**:9, 1980.
8. Delgado, M.H.: A study of the position of the patella using computerized tomography, J. Bone Joint Surg. **61B**:443, 1979.
9. Dunn, P.M., Post, R.H., and Jones, S.R.: Thromboembolic complications of knee arthroscopy (letter) West. J. Med. **140**:291, 1984.
10. Eilert, R.E.: Arthroscopy and arthrography in children and adolescents; arthroscopy. In

American Academy of Orthopaedic Surgeons Symposium on arthroscopy and arthrography of the knee, St. Louis, 1978, The C.V. Mosby Co.

11. Eilert, R.E.: Laboratory aids in the teaching of arthroscopy. In American Academy of Orthopaedic Surgeons Symposium on arthroscopy and arthrography of the knee, St. Louis, 1978, The C.V. Mosby Co.

12. Council on Long Range Planning and Development: The environment of medicine, 1984.

13. Ewing, J.W.: Personal communication, 1983.

14. Ficat, R.P., and Hungerford, D.S.: Disorders of the patello-femoral joint, Baltimore, 1977, The Williams & Wilkins Co.

15. Galway, H.R., and MacIntosh, D.L.: The lateral pivot shift: a symptom and sign of anterior cruciate ligament, Clin. Orthop. **147**:45, 1980.

16. Gambardella, R.A., and Tibone, J.E.: Knife blade in the knee joint: a complication of arthroscopic surgery. A case report, Am. J. Sports Med. **11**:267, 1983.

17. Goldberg, D.: No-knee learning process for arthroscopic instrumentation, Ortho. Rev. **1**:121, 1982.

18. Hadied, A.M.: An unusual complication of arthroscopy: a fistula between the knee and the prepatellar bursa. Case report, J. Bone Joint Surg. **66A**:624, 1984.

19. Harris, W.H., et al.: Comparison of warfarin, low molecular weight dextran, aspirin, subcutaneous heparin in prevention of venous thromboembolism following total hip replacement, J. Bone Joint Surg. **56A**:1552, 1974.

20. Hejna, W.F.: Saving shacks and building empires, Orthopedics **8**:348, 1985.

21. Henderson, C.E., and Hopson, C.N.: Pneumoscrotum as a complication of arthroscopy (a case report) J. Bone Joint Surg. **64A**:1232, 1982.

22. Hochheimer, et al.: Invest. Ophthal. Vis. Sci. **19**:1009, 1980.

23. Hotmann, A.A., and Wyatt, W.B.: Fatal pulmonary embolism following tourniquet inflation, J. Bone Joint Surg. **67A**:633, 1985.

23a. Jacob, R.P.: Observations on rotary instability of the lateral compartment. Acta Orthop. Scand. **52**, suppl. 191, 1981.

24. Johnson, L.L.: Arthroscopy of the knee using local anesthesia: a review of 400 patients, J. Bone Joint Surg. **58A**:736, 1976.

25. Johnson, L.L.: Impact of diagnostic arthroscopy on the clinical judgement of an experienced arthroscopist, Clin. Orthop. **167**:75, 1982.

26. Johnson, L.L., Ferguson, A.B., Jr., and Fu, F.: Present status of arthroscopy in the United States: September, 1981, Orthop. Surv. **5**:400, 1982.

27. Johnson, L.L., and Fu, F.: States of arthroscopic training in orthopaedic residency programs: September, 1982, Orthop. Surv. **6**:225, 1983.

28. Joyce, J.J. III, and Farqhver, H.: Arthroscopy: the previously operated knee, American Academy of Orthopaedic Surgeons Symposium on arthroscopy and arthrography of the knee, St. Louis, 1978, The C.V. Mosby Co.

29. Joyce, M.J., and Mankin, H.J.: Caveat arthroscopos: extra-articular lesions of bone simulating extra-articular pathology of the knee, J. Bone Joint Surg. **65A**:289, 1983.

30. Klein, W., and Schulitz, K.P.: Outpatient arthroscopy under local anesthesia, Arch. Orthop. Trauma Surg. **96**:131, 1980.

31. Klenerman, L.: The tourniquet in orthopedic surgery. In Harris, H.: Postgraduate textbook of clinical orthopedics, Bristol, England, John Wright & Sons, Ltd., 1983.

32. Klenerman, L.: The tourniquet in surgery, J. Bone Joint Surg. **44B**:937, 1962.

33. Lindenbaum, B.L.: Complications of knee joint arthroscopy, Clin. Orthop. **160**:158, 1981.

34. Marymont, J.V., Lynch, M.A., and Henning, C.E.: Evaluation of meniscus tears of the knee by radio nuclide imaging, Am. J. Sports Med. **11**:432, 1983.

35. Matsui, N., Moriya, H., and Kitahara, H.: The use of arthroscopy for follow-up in the knee joint surgery, Orthop. Clin. North Am. **10**:697, 1979.

36. McGinty, J.B., and Mapza, R.A.: Evaluation of an out-patient procedure under local anesthesia, J. Bone Joint Surg. **60**:787, 1978.

37. Merchant, A.C., et al.: Roentgenographic analysis of patellofemoral congruence, J. Bone Joint Surg. **56A**:1391, 1974.

38. Mital, M.A., and Hayden, J., Pain in the knee in children: the medial plica shelf syndrome, Orthop. Clin. North Am. **10**:713, 1979.

39. Morrissey, R.T., et al.: Arthroscopy of the knee in children, Clin. Orthop. **162**:103, 1982.
40. Nole, R., Munson, M.L., and Fulkerson, J.P. Bupi-vacaine and saline effects on articular cartilage, Arthroscopy, **1**:123, 1985.
41. Norman, O., et al.: The vertical position of the patella, Acta Orthop. Scand. **54**:908, 1983.
42. Noyes, F.R., et al.: Arthroscopy in acute hemarthrosis of the knee, J. Bone Joint Surg. **62A**:687, 1980.
43. Noyes, F.R., and Spievack, E.S.: Extraarticular fluid dissection in tissues during arthroscopy: a report of clinical cases and a study of intraarticular and thigh pressures in cadavers, Am. J. Sports Med. **10**:346, 1982.
44. Older, J., and Cardoso, T.: First year's experience of day-case arthroscopy in diagnosis and management of disorders of the knee joint, Lancet **2**:264, 1983.
45. Peek, R.D., and Haynes, D.W.: Compartment syndrome as a complication of arthroscopy: a case report and a study of intersitial pressures, Am. J. Sports Med. **12**:464, 1984.
46. Pevey, J.K.: Outpatient arthroscopy of the knee under local anesthesia, Am. J. Sports Med. **6**:122, 1978.
47. Poehling, G.G.: Arthroscopic teaching technique, South. Med. J. **71**:1067, 1978.
48. Slocum, D.B., et al.: Clinical test for anterolateral rotary instability of the knee, Clin. Orthop. **118**:63, 1976.
49. Slocum, D.B., and Larson, R.L.: Rotatory instability of the knee, J. Bone Joint Surg. **50A**:211, 1968.
50. Starr, P.: The social transformation of American medicine, New York, 1983, Basic Books.
51. Suman, R.K., Stother, K.G., and Illingworth, G.: Diagnostic arthroscopy of the knee in children, J. Bone Joint Surg. **66B**:535, 1984.
52. Sweeny, H.J.: Personal communication, 1983.
53. Sweeney, H.J.: Teaching arthroscopic surgery at the residency level. Orthop. Clin. North Am. **13**:255, 1982.
54. Thomas, R.H., et al.: Compartmental evaluation of osteoarthritis of the knee: a comparative study of available diagnostic modalities, Radiology **116**:585, 1975.
55. Torq, J.S., Conrad, A.B., and Kalen, A.B.: Clinical diagnosis of anterior cruciate ligament instability in the athlete, Am. J. Sports Med. **7**:34, 1979.
56. Walker, R.H., and Dillingham, M.: Thrombophlebitis following arthroscopic surgery, Contemp. Orthop. **6**:29, 1983.
57. Wred, M.T., and Lundh, R.: Arthroscopy under local anaesthesia using controlled pressure-irrigation with prilocaine, J. Bone Joint Surg. **64B**:583, 1982.
58. Young, R.W.: A theory of central retinal disease. In Sears, M.L., ed.: New direction of ophthalmic research, New Haven, Conn., 1981, Yale University Press, pp. 237-270.
59. Ziv, I., and Carroll, N.C.: The role of arthroscopy in children, J. Pediatr. Orthop. **2**:243, 1982.

Environment

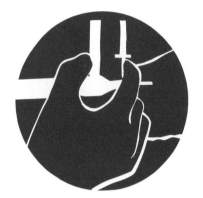

CREATING THE ENVIRONMENT

The environment in which the arthroscopic surgical procedures are performed always surprises our visitors at Ingham Medical Center, Lansing, Michigan. The arthroscopic suite is a separate surgical unit within a general hospital setting (Fig. 3-1). We presently have two operating rooms, a recovery room, and all the ancillary support systems in one location dedicated to arthroscopic surgery. The operating room personnel have primary responsibility in arthroscopic surgery.

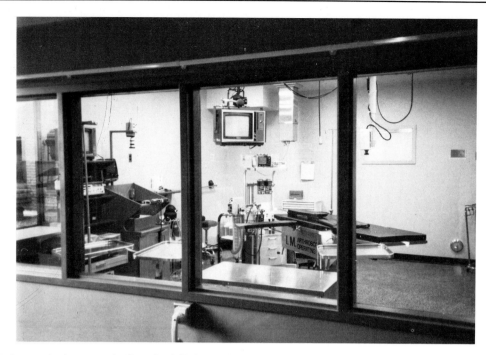

FIG. 3-1. Arthroscopic Surgical Suite at Ingham Medical Center, Lansing, Michigan, as seen from viewing room.

Our visitors immediately reflect on their own situation, which they describe as less than ideal. I remind them that we used to work in similar circumstances and faced all the same problems that they are presently facing. I also tell them that the ideal operating room environment is only created by the persistence of the surgeon or orthopedic staff. This is not a one-time task but a continuous effort that takes place in many different areas. Attention to the proper environment continues throughout the surgeon's practice lifetime.

Of course arthroscopic surgery is a new discipline within orthopedic surgery, and those who perform this surgery must give attention to the details of the obvious, the not-so-obvious, and the invisible factors. Doing so maximizes success while exercising the most delicate, even frustrating arthroscopic techniques (see the box on p. 139).

As with other endeavors, time and energy must be given to organization and planning to be successful. There must be a willingness to invest money, because beginning in arthroscopy is expensive.

In the past an orthopedic surgeon was expected to perform surgical procedures in whatever operating room might be available at whatever time it was available. In addition, it was customary to work with a different untrained assistant for every surgical procedure. Subspecialization now is common in orthopedic surgery, as well as arthroscopy. The surgical environment is no less important for the orthopedic surgeon than it is for the cardiac surgeon or organ transplant team.

Getting started

The orthopedist who uses arthroscopic surgical techniques must organize, plan, and insist on the proper environment to maximize his or her skills in the care of the patient. As previously discussed, some orthopedic surgeon–arthroscop-

---

FACTORS IMPORTANT TO THE SURGICAL ENVIRONMENT

Obvious	Not so obvious	Unseen
Patient	OR furniture	Administration
Evaluation	OR table	Hospital policy
Preparation	Other tables	Insurance
Comfort	Cast cart	Hospital
Confidence	Stool	Physician
Surgeon	Power sources	Central supply
Knowledge	Tourniquet	Outpatient service
Comfort	Suction	Physical therapy
Confidence	Collection bottles	Therapists
Leadership	Tobacco bag	X-ray
Attitude	Anesthesiologist	Laboratory
Technical skills	Staff surgeons	Electrical
Image transmission	Orthopedic	Microwave
Scope	Others	Radiowave
Video	OR team approach	Bovie
Instruments	Instrument care	Electrocautery
Lighting	Surgical	Air conditioning
Room dimmer	Television	
Scope	Suction	
Draping	Floor	

ists' requests for a proper environment have been met with a lack of understanding from administrators, some bewilderment on the part of the operating room personnel, and, all too often, hostility from staff orthopedists who have no interest in arthroscopic surgery. This is changing gradually.

Success in arthroscopic surgery requires that the surgeon have complete freedom within a proper environment. The surgeon must concentrate intensely over the period necessary to resect pathological intraarticular structures through miniature incisions in restricted joint spaces. To accomplish this, the surgeon must embark on both an educational and essentially promotional effort on behalf of himself or herself and arthroscopic surgery within the institution.

Hospital personnel

The major sales job has to be done with the personnel within the hospital. This starts with other orthopedic surgeons. If they have the same interest, a coalition may be formed. Only in recent years have there been enough orthopedic surgeons with an interest in arthroscopic surgery to make this possible. A coalition has both its benefits and its disadvantages. One of the benefits is the safety found in numbers. A disadvantage is that it may be difficult to get agreement by all the surgeons concerning how something ought to be done, what ought to be purchased, and especially what their "perceived needs" are.

The concept of "perceived needs" means that the uninitiated, inexperienced

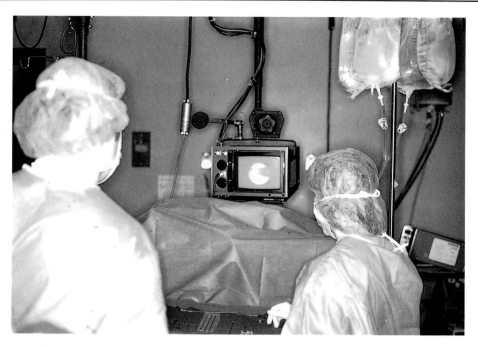

FIG. 3-2. Surgeon and surgical team observe live television monitoring of surgical procedure.

arthroscopist will project his or her needs based on a previous experience or concept. Having had no actual arthroscopic experience, these surgeons can only "perceive" their needs. Consultation with experienced arthroscopists can reshape perceived needs before actual purchases are made.

There may be some resistance from the operating room supervisor and personnel; they may not like change. All too often the first arthroscopic procedures done at an institution consume more time than those done by previous methods. Coworkers must be educated to the ultimate patient benefits provided by arthroscopic methods.

Another way to encourage the operating room personnel is to communicate the idea of the adventure and excitement of these techniques. A tangible way to encourage this sense is with the use of intraoperative television viewing. Video allows each person to experience what is going on arthroscopically and in that way allows them to participate (Fig. 3-2).

The best way to select people for the arthroscopic surgical team is on a volunteer basis. Several factors come into play. Interest in the new procedure is essential. The personality of both the potential team members and the surgeons must be compatible. If arthroscopic surgery is being introduced at a hospital, I suggest that borrowing instructional videotapes from the American Academy of Orthopaedic Surgeons or the *Arthroscopic Video Journal*. These programs show the surgical techniques in action. These materials will both encourage and educate the staff. A number of individuals may participate in the early arthroscopic cases. After group exposure the arthroscopic surgical team may be selected.

Unfortunately, operating room personnel and specifically supervisors traditionally want every individual in the operating room to know every possible procedure and discipline. Their reasoning, of course, is to provide ample coverage for all procedures in case of an off-hours emergency.

In practice, emergencies remain emergencies and require finding keys and equipment and preparing the room. There is therefore no actual benefit to this preparation; 99% of emergency procedures are performed under less than optimal conditions.

I recommend just the opposite approach, having people with similar interests working in teams in general surgery, urology, ENT, and so on, with limited overlap where it is practical. The hospital does not think twice about having an organ transplant team or a cardiac surgical team. There could just as easily be teams established for arthroscopic surgery.

An orthopedist requests this not because of a personality quirk or an ego trip but because arthroscopic surgery is a procedure as demanding as any performed in the hospital. A successful arthroscopic service demands a proper environment with interested, actively participating, knowledgeable personnel. Patient benefit must be the primary motivating factor.

Arthroscopic surgery is not a simple technique to learn, and as a result the initial cases will consume more time than procedures performed conventionally. Arthroscopic procedures will be performed more rapidly as time goes by.

Because other surgeons on the staff, orthopedists or otherwise, wish to avoid delays within operating room schedules, arthroscopic cases should be scheduled at the end of a single day. This is a courtesy to other members of the staff and a means of avoiding conflicts or resistance to arthroscopic surgery within the institution.

The physician-patient relationship

The surgeon has to be especially sensitive in "reading" the patient. Is the patient comfortable with the diagnosis, the anticipated treatment and outcome, and the explanations? If the surgeon does not perceive this comfort, he or she should make every effort to provide it; otherwise the patient must be advised to get a second opinion or to defer surgery until confident. The patient should be prepared for the possibility of an open procedure.

The surgeon

The surgeon is as much a part of the environment as the patient, the operating room personnel, or the equipment. Ideally the surgeon should be comfortable with the diagnosis, the patient, and the anticipated postoperative care. The surgeon should have confidence that he or she can execute the procedure by wise application of knowledge.

The surgeon must assume a position of leadership and responsibility. If the surgeon does not like a part of the operating room environment, be it personnel, hospital, or equipment, then it is that surgeon's responsibility, not someone else's, to make changes.

The care of the patient is directly related to the leadership role that the surgeon takes in creating the ideal environment. If the surgeon is lax in personal discipline, the other people in the operating room will be the same. If the surgeon is disciplined, careful, and attentive and works with dispatch, this will be reflected in the environment.

Arthroscopic surgery, more so than any other orthopedic discipline, requires a great deal of patience. One cannot force one's way through it. I have often said, "If things are not going fast enough for you arthroscopically. then slow down." In some situations it is a good idea to stop altogether, even for 5 minutes by the clock. If the surgeon has been operating under frustrating circumstances, time out allows him or her to regroup, reconsider a surgical approach, plan the conclusion, or even abort the procedure.

Last, but certainly not least important, the surgeon must be confident that his or her technical skills are equal to the anticipated level of surgery. Nothing is more discouraging to the surgeon, alarming to the personnel, and potentially injurious to the patient than an operation on a condition or in an area that is beyond the surgeon's training or experience. I liken this to skiing out of control; it is risky. I believe that every surgeon should operate at a level that is below his or her ability, so that if any unforeseen problem occurs there is an extra capacity to meet the challenge. Like skiing under control, it can be enjoyable and safe!

Hospital administration

The hospital administration should be apprised of the arthroscopic surgeon's needs, both financially and for personnel. Administrators usually come to a greater understanding when the surgeon talks in terms of patient volume and cash flow. If the necessary capital expenditures are not made and arthroscopic surgery is not performed at the facility, administrators can be well advised that those cases will be performed elsewhere.

They should know that the arthroscopic surgical procedure will be, if it is not already, the most common procedure within orthopedics. If orthopedics is a major specialty within a hospital, arthroscopy and its combined procedures will be the most common operative procedures performed within the operating room suite.[3,4] Administrators rapidly calculate this in terms of cash flow, especially when they understand that arthroscopy brings a large outpatient volume, with its potential cost effectiveness. This is especially convincing with today's medical-economic reimbursement policies.

Recent legislative and administrative actions by group health carriers have accelerated the use of outpatient surgery. Arthroscopy is now the most common procedure for knee joint problems. There is a financial motive for both the surgeon and the hospital to deliver outpatient surgical health care in the knee and even the shoulder joint.

PATIENT CONSIDERATIONS AND RELATIONSHIPS

The most important focus is the care, comfort, and treatment of the patient. This can be facilitated in several ways. First the patient should be given directions and a map of the hospital. The entrance to the hospital and the designated parking areas should be marked. The hospital corridors should either be outlined or well marked for the patient's travel through the maze of the hospital. This may seem silly or simple, but it is not to the patient.

Preoperative and postoperative instructions are important. Patients' friends and relatives generally do not remember what they have been told before or after surgery. Often they will call back and ask the same questions; therefore written instructions are an absolute necessity. Patient instruction sheets should be different colors, one for each type of surgery. The instructions should explain what the patient can anticipate. I have separate instruction sheets for postoperative care, physical therapy, and return visits. These instructions include specifics about dressings and postoperative medications.

The environment of the patients' waiting area should be pleasant and comfortable. Noise is probably the most aggravating problem in the hospital. Hospital personnel and equipment are responsible for much of the noise. They should be reminded that laughter and loud talking can be somewhat disturbing to a patient who is contemplating surgery. I recently had a patient express great concern over the hammering and pounding he heard while in the waiting room. He was relieved to be told that it came from a nearby construction area and not the operating room.

Hospital personnel should be discouraged from handling equipment casually. Laughter in an operating room or casual attitudes of the part of personnel can create apprehension and discomfort. Recent studies show that the anesthetized patient remembers communications that take place during surgery.

Whether in the office, clinic, or hospital, the attitude of the receptionist is of great importance. The first impression that a patient receives can affect his confidence in the surgeon.

Laboratory personnel can greatly affect the patient's stay in the hospital. Comfort, privacy, and attention to detail are important to the patient's well-being.

Nurses probably affect the way the patient feels more than the surgeon does, because nurses have more personal contact in the presurgical holding area and recovery room. Their demeanor and attitude tremendously affect the patient's comfort and confidence during these times.

The orderly, although frequently thought to be "low on the totem pole," is the person responsible for the important job of moving the patient on the cart or litter. The manner in which the move is made affects the patient's comfort and feelings of apprehension. Therefore the orderly's demeanor and conversation should be well disciplined and within the limitations of his or her knowledge of the procedure.

Finally, there is the unbelievable billing maze: insurance and hospital forms. It takes a highly educated person to handle the complex procedures. Every effort should be made to assist the patient in his handling of financial matters.

So often with higher technology comes greater opportunity to lose track of one's objectives. With all the many facets of arthroscopic surgery, surgeons sometimes forget that they are treating people. In a busy practice, it is easy to think in terms of operations, office hours, and paperwork. Therefore I believe it is important for everyone to recognize that the focus of the treatment is one individual, the patient, and every possible effort should be made to make each procedure the most important one performed.

A good indication of how good a job the surgeon has done is gained through feedback from the patient. The surgeon should inquire about any difficulties the patient encountered in or out of the hospital. Were there any unpleasant confrontations along the way? Once their surgery is behind them, some patients may be critical and consider it a bad experience. Occasional monitoring of patient experiences can catch any trouble spots in personnel or procedures.

THE OPERATING ROOM
Operating room construction

Every construction decision should allow for ease of future modification to accommodate the many changes that occur in arthroscopic surgery. Ideally a room should be dedicated to arthroscopic and associated procedures. The specific requirements of arthroscopic surgical techniques justify a designated specialized space.

Space, viewing, and ceiling mounts

An arthroscopic surgical suite was established at Ingham Medical Center in 1981. It includes two operating rooms, one with an observation/viewing room (see Fig. 3-1). A recovery room, nurses' station, nurses' offices, instrumentation and sterilization rooms, and storage and locker facilities are adjacent to the suite. In this institution an existing obstetrics/gynecology suite was remodeled. An outpatient holding area and waiting room were placed next to the suite to facilitate patient transportation.

The deficiencies of the suite at Ingham Medical Center are lack of storage area and small room size. These problems were created by the proliferation of arthroscopic equipment and the performance of various combined procedures.

I would suggest a room measuring 24 × 24 feet as the minimum size for an arthroscopic surgical suite. The ceiling should be 15 to 16 feet high to accommodate a drop ceiling. This allows for electrical and television cables as well as suspension systems. If the space above the drop ceiling is limited, any repairs or revisions will be difficult to perform.

The ceiling serves as a mount for various suspension systems (Fig. 3-3). The television monitor and camera are commonly suspended, thus eliminating cables on the floor. Suspended systems facilitate personnel and patient movement within the room as well as cleaning. Permanent installation avoids the wear and tear of electronic equipment caused by handling. The camera or monitor can be easily moved, elevated, or rotated without having to lift it each time.

At one time, we installed multiple pullies in the ceiling for shoulder and elbow work. However, we now use the suspension system attached to the table (see Fig. 3-18).

The observation/viewing room was built in response to the daily continuing education programs for in-service and visiting physicians, nurses, and administrators (see Fig. 3-1). It also has been used by the hospital in public relations and promotional activities to provide a rather innocuous view of "high-tech" surgery for those involved in hospital development programs (i.e., fund raising).

Electrical system

Ideally the electrical system of an arthroscopic room or suite should be isolated from all other systems. This is because microwave, electrocautery, or x-ray equipment running adjacent to or on the same circuits as the equipment in the suite will cause considerable interference with the video picture. Loss of visualization can stop an operation. The room should be lead-lined or be set off by distance and thick cement walls.

Radio wave frequencies (RF) can also affect the operating room video picture. Sources of radio waves are the emergency room's radio dispatch system and

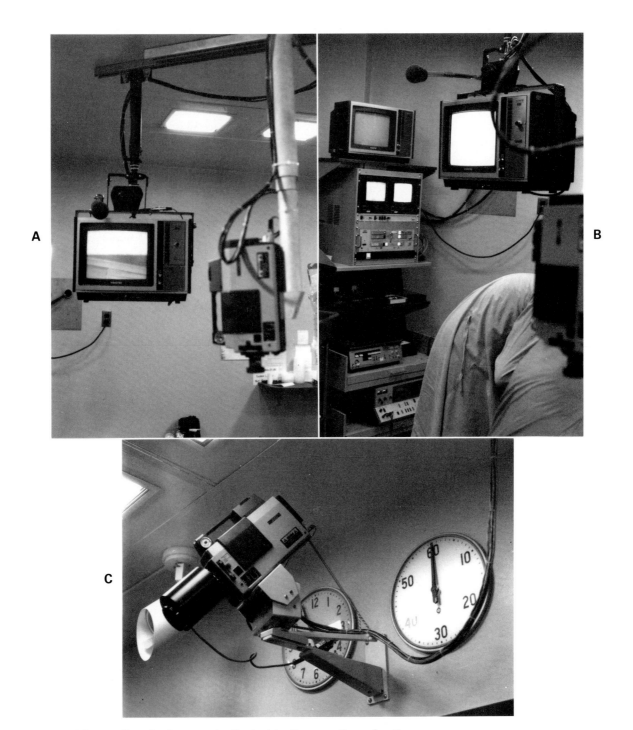

FIG. 3-3. Surgical room dedicated to the practice of arthroscopy.

A Ceiling-mounted television camera and monitor on balanced pistoning support system.
B Suspended monitor and simultaneous editing system.
C Wall-mounted outside camera for construction of teaching tapes.

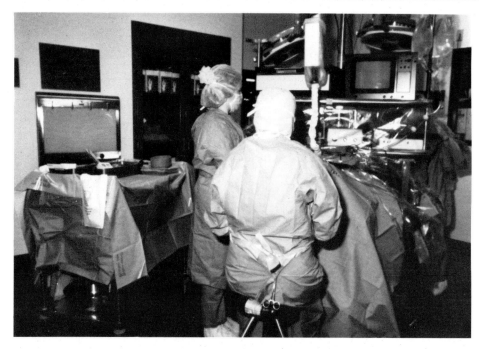

FIG. 3-4. Surgeon sitting comfortably with over-the-top table holding power source. Sterile plastic drape permits viewing of instruments (Courtesy Dr. Howard Sweeney, Evanston Hospital Arthroscopic Surgical Center)

the arthroscopic lights. The electrical light sources should be shielded from RF waves. Some video cameras are shielded from radio wave interference (see Fig. 5-19).

Electrical cords should drop from the ceiling for a single connection to the power source at the table. This is preferable to cords running from side to side across the floor.

The power sources should be conveniently placed in front of the surgeon (Fig. 3-4). They should also be of such design and style that they will offer easy recharging overnight or over the weekend.

Lighting

The operating room lights should be on a rheostat dimmer so that a spectrum of illumination is possible. It is important that the lighting system for arthroscopic procedures does not allow bright lights to reflect on the video monitor, which makes visualization more difficult. If there is a designated arthroscopic room, there should be spotlights available for the combined surgical cases. If an operating room is equipped only for arthroscopic procedures, the light cable detached from the arthroscope can be used as a light source during an open procedure. It will be adequate for most surgeries.

Air conditioning

The matter of supplying hot or cool air is taken for granted by architects and engineers. However, this does not constitute air conditioning. Calculations must also be made for the heat of people, lights, and power sources. A consider-

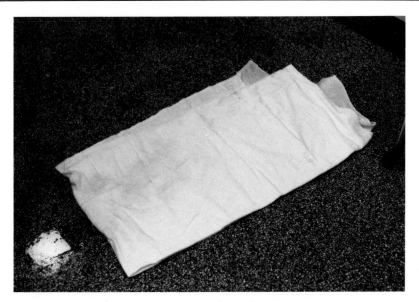

FIG. 3-5. Bath blankets used to absorb abundant spillage of water on floor.

ation must be made for gown-covered personnel and the patient covered with surgical drapes.

The matter of hot or cool air supply is not as critical as the circulation or exchange of air, which is usually neglected. It is the most critical factor for a pleasant, comfortable environment. Humidity control is especially challenging in an arthroscopic suite because of the "water, water, everywhere" syndrome experienced during this type of surgical procedure (see Fig. 3-7). A separate air circulation system allows for better control of these factors.

Floor

The floor should be a terrazzo surface. The direction of drainage should be away from or toward the end of the operating room table. Drains are not permitted by law in some states. It would be ideal to have the drain directly under the operating room table so that all the water flowed to an area where no one was walking or standing.

The use of bath blankets is most effective to handle extra water on the floor, because they are quite absorbent and bigger than towels (Fig. 3-5). Other methods are not usually acceptable within standard operating room protocol.

Room arrangement

The furniture arrangement for routine knee joint arthroscopy is shown in Fig. 3-6. Arrangements for combined procedures and joints other than the knee are discussed in specific chapters of this text.

Each assistant is located in the same position every time, with positions reversed for the opposite knee. Assistants perform the same designated tasks in each case, without overlap, to avoid confusion in assignments.

The surgeon stands and/or sits at the end of the table, controlling the patient's leg and foot (see Fig. 3-4). Some surgeons have an assistant perform this task, but this increases the need for communication and complicates coordina-

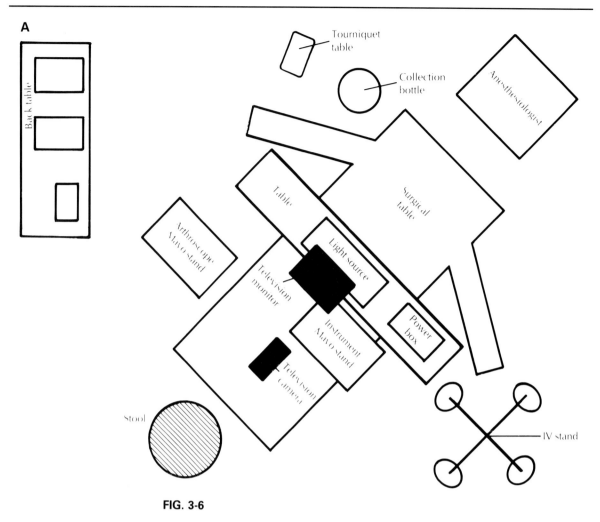

FIG. 3-6

A Diagram of room arrangement for knee joint arthroscopy.

tion, especially of the fine-tuning of motions needed for tight knees or complicated exposures.

Ideally the television monitor is suspended and movable, including side-to-side, up-and-down, and rotating movements. The need for additional monitors for simultaneous editing, viewing by the anesthesiologist, or teaching purposes may be determined on an individual basis (see Fig. 5-18).

The operating room patient table need not be elaborate; kidney rests, side tilting, and motorization are not necessary (Fig. 3-7, *A*). The table should have the capacity to be lowered more than the normal tables (27 inches from the floor). Work in the lateral compartment often requires varus, hyperextension, or figure-4 flexion positions. This results in rotation of the thigh, which necessitates pushing toward the ceiling on the leg. If the table is not low enough, pushing up on the leg is either awkward or tiring or both. Exposure is not gained or maintained. The ideal arthroscopic table lowers to 22 inches from the floor to accommodate this and other manipulations.

In the absence of such a table, reverse Trendelenburg's position may be

B

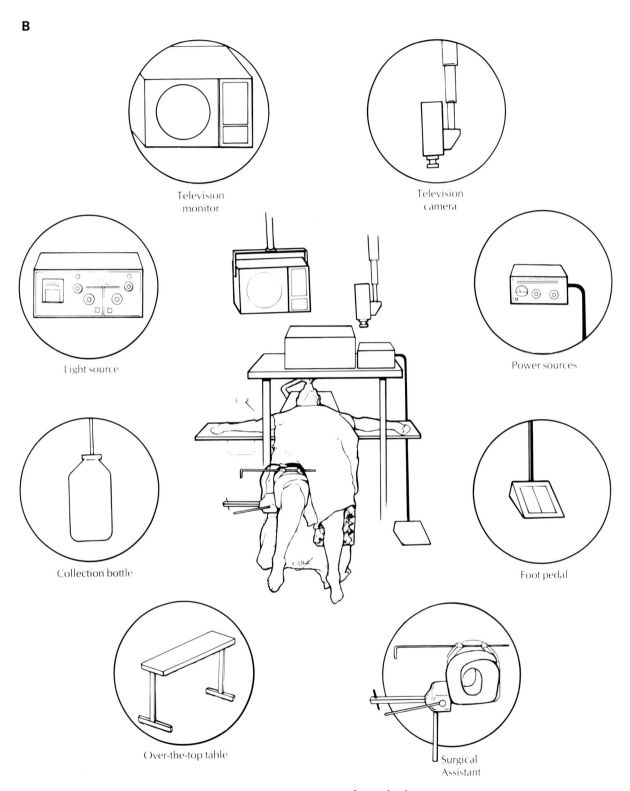

Television
monitor

Television
camera

Light source

Power sources

Collection bottle

Foot pedal

Over-the-top table

Surgical
Assistant

FIG. 3-6, cont'd. B, Diagram of surgical set-up.

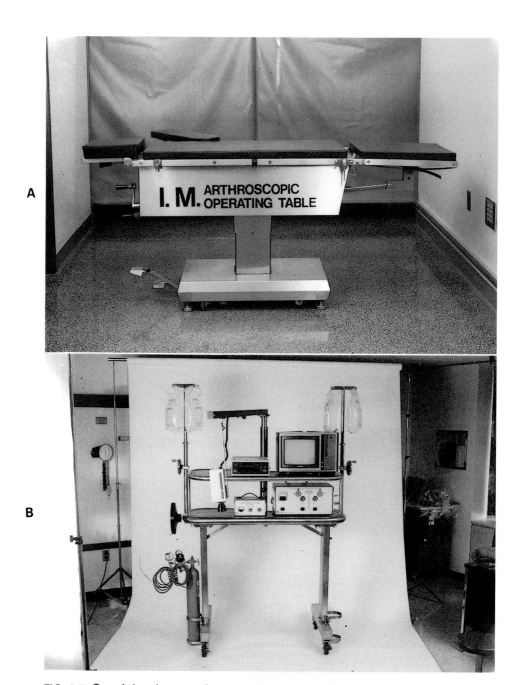

FIG. 3-7. Special arthroscopic operating room tables.

A Patient table lowers to 22 inches above floor.
B Surgicenter holds all equipment plus boom for television camera.

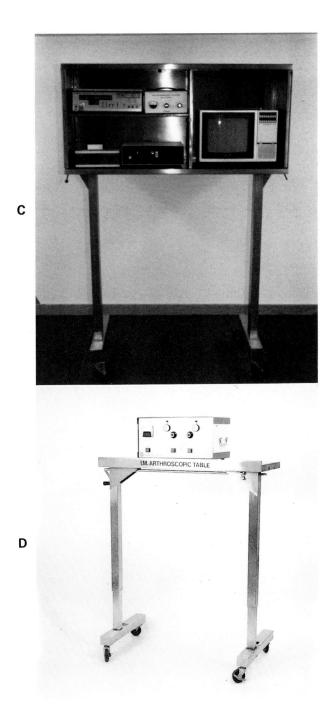

FIG. 3-7, cont'd

C Treasure Chest holds and stores all arthroscopic equipment.

D Simple over-the-top table is cantilevered over patient to hold power sources and clear room for staff at operative site.

used with the anesthesiologist's approval. Otherwise the surgeon will be straining for balance on his or her toes or lacking exposure.

The surgeon's stool should sit securely on the floor. If it has rollers, a simple locking mechanism should be included. The seat should be firm. The stool should be secure, because it often serves as the platform against which the surgeon pushes to manipulate the extremity or arthroscope. The wetness of the floor increases the necessity for security. The stool should occupy little space and be easily movable with the surgeon's foot. The sitting position is used for the suprapatellar and posterior approaches.

The over-the-top table is a modified neurosurgical table (see Fig. 3-7, *D*). It has been narrowed and cantilevered to allow the anesthesiologist as well as the surgical assistants access to patient's head and chest. It holds the light source and power supply for motorized instruments. In some cases, in the absence of a suspended system, a small television monitor is placed on the light source (see Fig. 3-4, *B*).

There are two other, more elaborate types of over-the-top tables, which were designed for the undesignated operating room without ceiling mounting. The first is an enlarged version of the original over-the-top table. It also has locking doors for secure off-hours storage (see Fig. 3-7, *C*). The table holds all power sources. It is especially adapted to hand-held camera use and facilitates room-to-room changes.

The second, known as a Surgicenter, incorporates all of the necessary spaces and structures for a stand-alone system (see Fig. 3-7, *B*). It is constructed of stainless steel for operating room standards. There is shelf space for all power sources. A suspension bar is cantilevered for television camera suspension. Mechanically operated poles are included for saline bag suspension. There is a place for both tourniquet and thigh holder storage. This table converts any room into an arthroscopic surgical center. Mounted on wheels, it can be moved from room to room or from storage without the need for carrying each piece of heavy equipment.

The back table is any customary stainless steel operating room table with wheels. It serves for initial instrument gathering. It holds the less frequently used instruments and various trays and containers (Fig. 3-8, *A*).

Two Mayo stands are routinely used. One holds the arthroscopic equipment, the television, the drapes, and the large forceps. It remains to side of operative field (Figs. 3-8, *B*, and 3-9, *A*). It is under the control of the first assistant.

The second Mayo stand holds the operative instrumentation. In knee arthroscopies, it is located over the top of the patient's knee or to the side in arthroscopy of other joints. It is under control of the second assistant. The power cables and light guides come under it to the operative field (see Figs. 3-8, *C*, and 3-9, *B*).

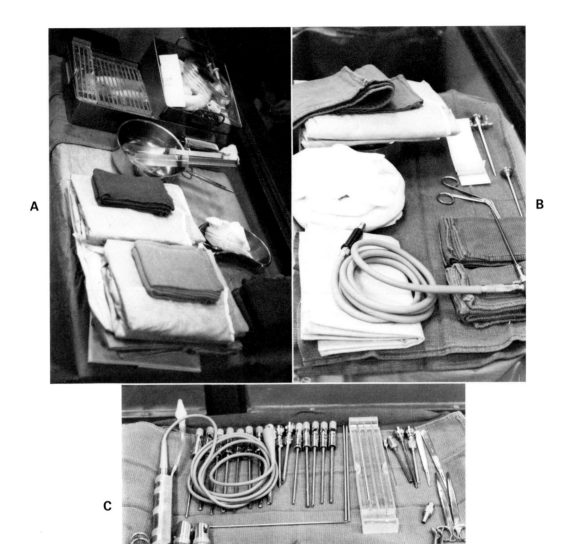

FIG. 3-8. Various tables with specific instruments

A Back table with drapings, dressings, syringes, accessory instruments.
B First Mayo stand has arthroscope, forceps, basin, and television drapes.
C Instrument Mayo stand has orderly arrangement of equipment.

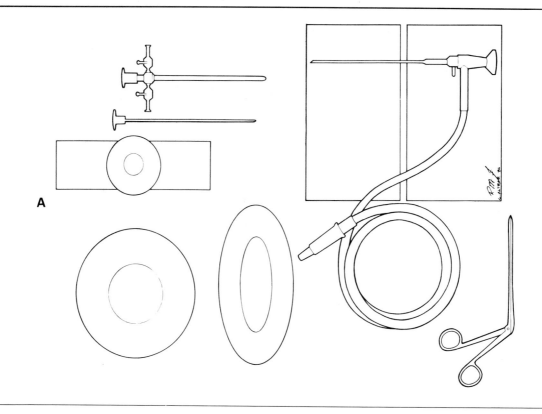

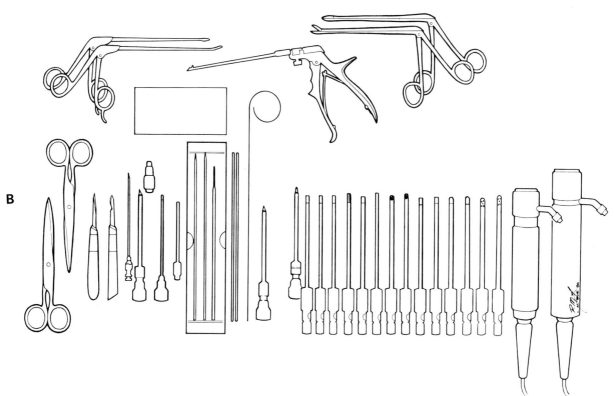

FIG. 3-9. Diagrams of instrument placement used in OR for set-up.

A Arthroscopic Mayo stand.
B Instrument stand.

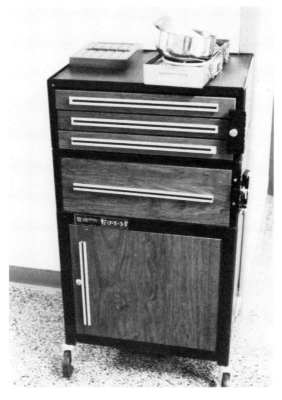

FIG. 3-10. Storage case for instruments.

Storage and warehousing

A separate lockable storage case on wheels facilitates availability and security of expensive instruments (Fig. 3-10) and keeps instruments in one place. The less frequently used or back-up instruments are kept in storage, sterile-wrapped and ready on request. This system eliminates searching from cupboard to cupboard or room to room at a crucial time during the arthroscopic procedure. The case also serves as a storage area at the end of the day.

Any space that is not filled means an instrument is missing. A list of contents may be placed inside each drawer or door as a reminder.

In addition to the areas of table and case storage, it is important to consider a tertiary area in which to store certain instruments. From time to time, manufacturers' supplies or loaner services cannot meet the needs of our center. Therefore we purchase extra arthroscopes, cables, and knife blades that experience has shown may not be available on request. This method eliminates any disruption in the surgical schedule.

Instrumentation

Image transmission

A good, clear image is a necessity for arthroscopic surgery. The factors that are involved in a good picture are not limited to the arthroscope. In other sections I have discussed the distention, the security of the thigh, and the amount of light on the object and returning back through the arthroscope. Even with all of these technical factors taken care of, a poor image can still result unless the surgeon is able to make arthroscopic composition (see Chapters 2 and 6).

The maintenance of a clear, bright image requires constant checks on the many potential problem areas. There must be a powerful light source with a new bulb. The light cable must be of adequate size (5 mm in diameter and 6 feet long) and be without breaks and free from corrosion or debris at both ends. The arthroscope's fiberglass conduit should be uninterrupted and clean at both ends. The objective should be polished without scratches or fracture. There should be no disruption of the lens system alignment or seals. The ocular should be inspected for dirt, dust, or water droplets, especially before it is coupled with an articulated viewing device or camera. The coupling to the articulated viewing device or camera should be properly focused. The result should be an optimal size of apparent image (focal length) on the television screen. The television monitor should be in proper functioning order and image balance. Every interface must be clean, including the monitor screen.

Potential sources of diminished light are as follows:
1. Light source
   a. Bulb
2. Cable
   a. Each end
   b. Fibers
3. Arthroscope
   a. Fibers
   b. Objective lens
   c. Glass lens system
   d. Ocular
4. Articulated viewing device
   a. C-mount adaptor
5. Television monitor

Organization of instruments

A list of the instruments used should be compiled. Instruments should be organized into groups according to their end-of-the-day storage or means of sterilization. For example, the arthroscope and cannulas are put together for ethylene oxide gas sterilization. The hand and motorized instruments are in containers for steam autoclaving. The television camera and power sources are both secured in another area. The less used equipment is in a movable storage cupboard. The instrument list should include the exact place of storage.

A map of the operating room with the specific placement of instruments on Mayo stands should be mounted within the operating room for reference as the surgical team mobilizes the equipment for the surgical procedure.

The final step in the organization process separates the instruments based on their frequency of use. The most-used instruments are kept closer to the operative field.

The instruments are also grouped by type. The arthroscope, cables, cannula, and so on are placed on one Mayo stand. The hand and motorized instruments are placed on a Mayo stand located over the patient, above and adjacent to the knee.

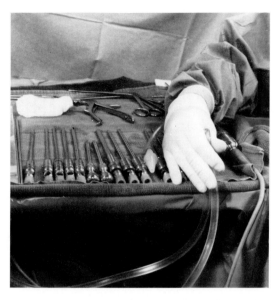

FIG. 3-11. Second assistant controls outflow suction with variable pinching of tubing.

Finally, the individual responsibilities of the team members must be considered. The first assistant controls the arthroscope; his or her table is adjacent to this position (Fig. 3-9, *B*). The second assistant controls the passing of instruments and the outflow suction (Fig. 3-11).

The following lists reflect the organization of instruments and are invaluable for training purposes and with substitute assistants.

INSTRUMENTS FOR OPERATIVE FIELD (BY TABLE)
1. Scissors (two)
2. No. 11 knife blade on No. 3 knife handle
3. No. 15 knife blade on No. 3 knife handle
4. No. 18 spinal needle
5. Intra-articular Shaver (IAS) cannula, with holes, on sharp trocar
6. Blunt IAS trocar
7. IAS cannula
8. Probe
9. IM 761 knife blade
10. No. 64 Beaver blade on Beaver handle
11. IM knife holder
12. Switching sticks (two)
13. IAS stylet
14. Arthroplasty cannula on sharp trocar
15. Arthroplasty cannula on blunt trocar

Motorized instruments
1. Surgical electric motor
2. Drain cases
   a. IAS
   b. Arthroplasty
   c. Small joint

IAS heads
1. 3.5 mm meniscal cutter
2. 4.5 mm meniscal cutter
3. 5.5 mm meniscal cutter
4. 3.5 mm trimmer
5. 4.5 mm trimmer
6. 5.5 mm trimmer

Arthroplasty heads
7. Medium burr
8. Large burr
9. 4.5 mm regular synovial resector
10. 5.5 mm regular synovial resector
11. 3.5 mm full-radius synovial resector
12. 4.5 mm full-radius synovial resector
13. 5.5 mm full-radius synovial resector
14. Johnson & Johnson adhesive strip
15. Single inflow adaptor
16. Meniscus graspers (small and large)
17. Basket forcep, 2.7 mm angled
18. Variable-axis scissors/basket forceps
19. Basket forcep 3.5 mm straight
20. 3- × 4-inch gauze (under towel)
21. Basin
22. 6-inch stockinette
23. Dyonics light cord attached to scope
24. Large-jawed forcep
25. Adhesive strip for articulated arm
26. Storz cannula with modified sharp trocar
27. Storz scope with bridge
28. Sharp Storz trocar
29. 2-inch stockinette (for articulated viewing device)

Instrument care

The care of instruments is a behind-the-scenes activity that is not so well appreciated until the surgeon is handed a dull instrument, the television camera or monitor does not work, or the suction does not function because the tubes are clogged with debris.

Instrument care should be the responsibility of a single person, preferably an employee of the owner of the instrumentation. Every individual on the arthroscopic team must be educated as to the importance of maintenance (Fig. 3-12). The kind of care required for arthroscopic surgical instruments, television equipment, suction and flow, equipment, and so on, cannot be handled adequately by a variety of people on a rotational basis or by someone who is not involved in arthroscopic surgery.

Problems will occur if no one at the hospital is specifically assigned to care for arthroscopic instrumentation. The cost of repair and replacement of surgical instrumentation will be exceedingly high, and this is unnecessary; dollar savings

A

B

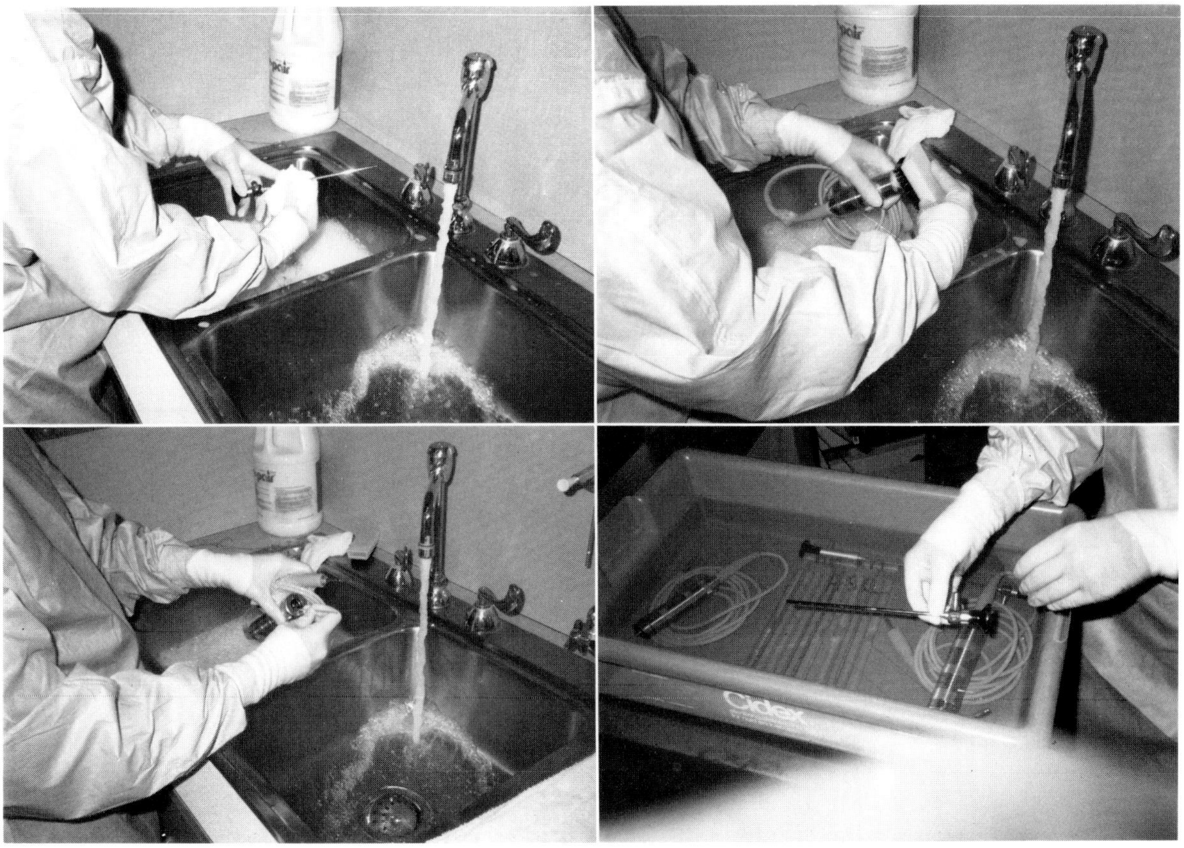

C

D

FIG. 3-12. Care of instruments. **A,** Careful cleansing of arthroscope in soap and water. **B,** Brush scrubbing of hand and motorized instruments. **C,** Careful cleaning of recesses in instruments with cotton swabs. **D,** Cold-soak disinfectant for motors, knife blades, and arthroscopes.

will result from having a team or even one person to care for the instrumentation.

The arthroscope, motors and knife blades are placed in Cidex solution between surgical cases (see Fig. 3-12). This decreases the handling of blades and lessens contact with other metal instruments, which dulls edges. Autoclaving itself does not dull edges.

Electric motors are autoclavable but hold heat, which requires cooling and delays of the start of the next case. Motors are too hot to hold when they are first taken out of the autoclave.

Arthroscopes are soaked between cases and subjected to gas sterilization at the end of each day. Steam autoclaving will injure the cement that holds the lens system.

Sterilization and disinfection of instruments is detailed in Chapter 4.

I own my instruments. Only one person cares for them interoperatively and stores them between surgical days.

Central supply

The instrumentation is most vulnerable in the hospital's central supply. The central supply area is usually situated away from the operating suite, yet the activities that take place there have great bearing on surgical activities. A visit to this facility by the surgeon is well advised. The work at central supply is accomplished by assembly line techniques, with the focus on the total project rather than individual care of instruments.

Education of the central supply staff will help prevent the mishandling of equipment. A videotape of arthroscopic procedures or the opportunity to observe live surgery reinforces the importance of their job.

A system to avoid losing or misplacing instruments is well advised. Having a list and maintaining the same storage assignments every day are helpful.

Draping

Arthroscopic draping must accomodate liquid leakage and spillage. The Surgikos Division of Johnson & Johnson has developed disposable draping packages for the knee and other joints. These packages were developed in conjunction with my nurse, Mrs. Ruth Becker.

The knee package provides a plastic underdrape and a wide, absorbent coverall. Adhesive or rubberized elastic seals provide a tight seal around the thigh. The leg is covered with a plastic stockinette, which is sealed with plastic strips at the knee to prevent collection of fluid inside the drapes that cover the foot. Paper loops on the system hold power supply cords and light cables, as well as inflow/outflow tubing (Fig. 3-13).

The shoulder drape is similar in concept except it provides a wider surgical exposure about the shoulder to facilitate entry to the superior supraspinatus portal (see Fig. 15-30). A sterile plastic drape covers the suspended upper extremity. Various holes hold instrumentation cords and suction tubes.

The shoulder drape is adaptable to elbow and ankle arthroscopy.

Suction system

Suction principles are important to arthroscopic motorized instrumentation. Suction is also used during diagnostic arthroscopy. Most modern operating rooms feature permanently installed suction systems. A measurement of the suction in the operating room pressures must be taken. The Dyonics motorized system is calibrated for 14 to 16 inches of mercury, which is the suction found at Ingham Medical Center. The efficiency of the motorized system depends on adequate suction.

Whether a permanent or temporary suction system is used, the pressure should be known and regulated for arthroscopic work.

The measurement is taken not end-on but with an in-line gauge (Fig. 3-14). This should be inserted in the system just outside the operative field for the best pressure measurement.

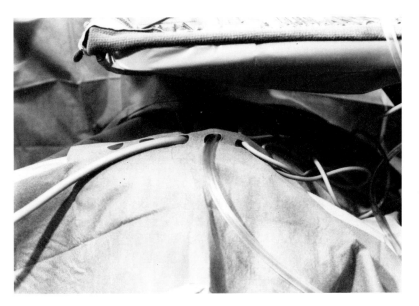

FIG. 3-13. Cords coming under Mayo stand to operative field

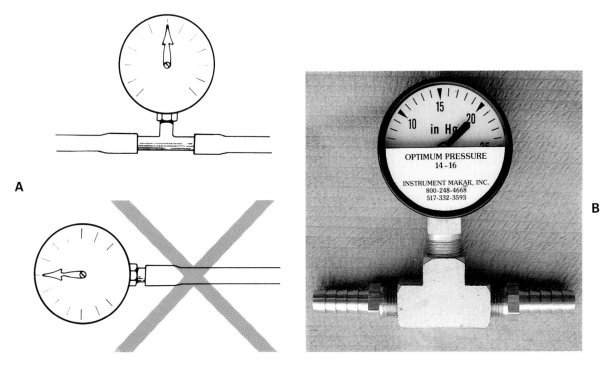

A

B

FIG. 3-14

A Diagram of in-line and end-on suction measurements.
B Instrument.

Collection bottles

A large collection system reduces the necessity for frequent emptying of bottles (Fig. 3-15). A small collection bag, or tobacco bag, can catch the specimen for pathological analysis. This avoids the need to strain large volumes of saline.

Tourniquet

The tourniquet is an environmental instrument that goes unnoticed except when it fails, resulting in bleeding that obscures the surgical view (Fig. 3-16).

We regularly calibrate the tourniquet to verify that the tanks are full and the gauge is working (Fig. 3-16).

The Surgical Assistant

The Surgical Assistant is a metallic mechanical device that secures the patient's thigh, arm, or leg to the operating table. It got its name because it performs a task that was previously performed by a person. It has a closed-cell foam insert to protect soft tissue and is secured by advancing a lever arm by cam action before locking in place. It is attached by a standard Clark clamp to the operating room table.

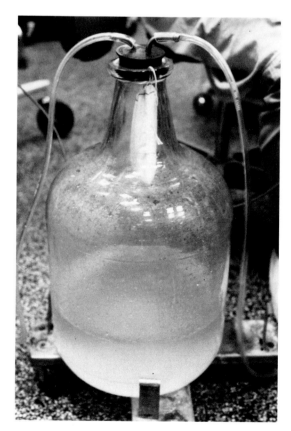

FIG. 3-15. Suction bottle.

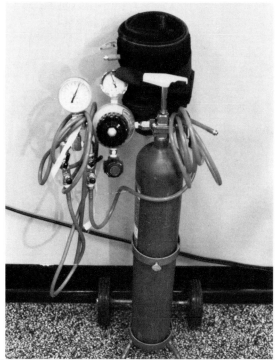

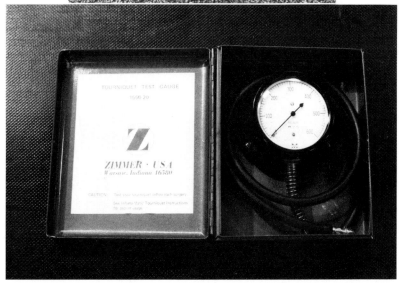

FIG. 3-16. Tourniquet and tourniquet calibration unit.

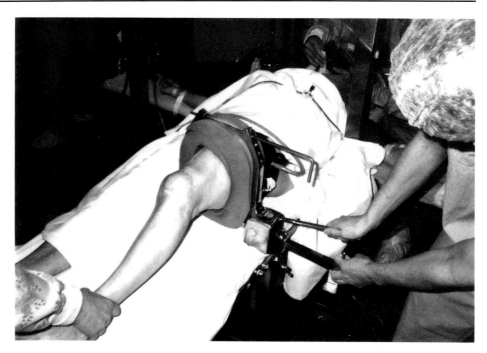

FIG. 3-17. Surgical Assistant being secured by nurse.

It is used in knee, elbow, and ankle arthroscopy (Fig. 3-17) and is described in detail in Chapter 4.

Shoulder Suspension System

A means of securing the upper extremity for shoulder arthroscopy is the Shoulder Suspension System (Fig. 3-18, *A*). It is also used in open rotator cuff repairs. It attaches to the operating table by a Clark clamp (Fig. 3-18, *B*). The desired shoulder abduction is achieved by placement of an upright proximally or distally at the foot of the table. Flexion or extension is achieved by rotating the upright, thereby moving the crossbar in an arc over the patient. Fine-tuning can be achieved by dropping or elevating the foot of the operating room table by increments with controls at the head of the table. The double pulley system provides safe, balanced suspension rather than traction. (See Chapter 15 for further details.)

Plaster cart

Most plaster carts are too high for cast application to the foot or leg when the extremity is in the dependent position. I modified a standard cart with a hole in the top that puts the bucket at the elbow level. This facilitates the mechanics of cast application (Fig. 3-19).

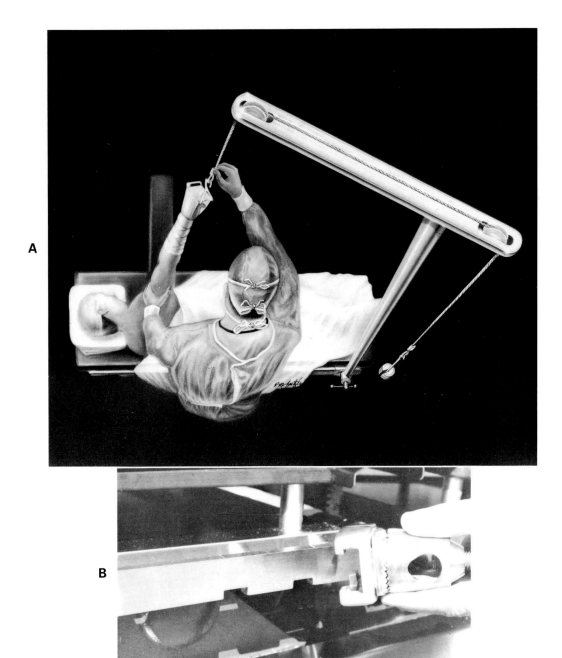

FIG. 3-18. Shoulder Suspension System.

A Drawing of system (Courtesy Instrument Makar).
B Clark attachment is generally used for stirrups suspension but also to accommodate Surgical Assistant and shoulder suspension.

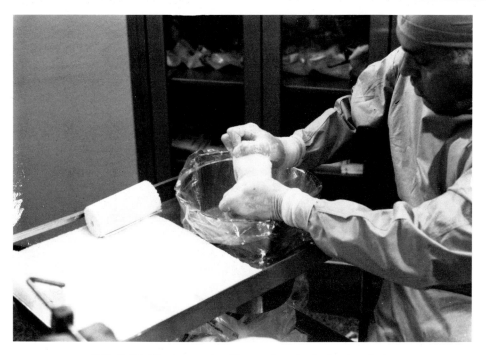

FIG. 3-19. Plaster cart with sunken hole for bucket.

Operating room personnel
The team approach

To be truly successful in arthroscopic surgery, the team approach is a must. It is not a one-person show. Enough cannot be said for the team contribution to the success of arthroscopic surgery. Recent surveys have shown that most arthroscopists have a different untrained assistant for every case. Every effort should be made, either personally or through the hospital administration, to secure well-trained assistants for arthroscopic surgery.

The team should function in a coordinated and cooperative manner. Emphasis is on their primary responsibilities, and overlap of assignments is minimized.

The surgeon directs this orchestra and expects its members to be in tune and on cue; otherwise there is discord. Many simultaneous activities require the attention of each team member, and many details attract the attention of the surgeon. The staff anticipation and participation is a pleasure to be a part of or to observe. These patterns of responsibility, as outlined and carefully observed, result in extreme efficiency.

My team's organization is illustrated in Fig. 3-6, *A*. All personnel, especially the surgeon, must be familiar with each piece of equipment. In all procedures, the instruments, the power sources, the tables, and the people should be in the same position. That way when some measure becomes necessary during surgery, nothing has to be hunted for. Each instrument should be in the same location and on the same table for every case. If each procedure is carried out in a similar manner, the results will be far more satisfying and success will be predictable.

The following sections describe the individual responsibilities. These activities are blended into a coordinated flow.

Anesthesiologist

The anesthesiologist is an integral part of the arthroscopic procedures. In our facility the anesthesiologist participates not only in the preoperative medical evaluation of the patient but also in the postoperative visit. The anesthesiologist's role is particularly important in the control of discomfort following surgery, especially in reconstructive or combined surgical procedures.

The anesthesiologist maximizes the arthroscopic environment with his or her ability to manage same-day surgical cases. Proper skills reduce postoperative recovery time or nausea and vomiting. Regional anesthesia is used on patients with certain medical conditions. Often a stand-by anesthetic is requested for maximization of local anesthesia. General anesthesia is given only if it becomes necessary as the procedure commences.

Circulating nurse

The foremost responsibility of the circulating nurse is the patient's welfare. The circulating nurse answers preoperative questions, identifies the extremity to be operated on, and assists the anesthesiologist.

The circulating nurse converses with the patient who is under local anesthesia. This contributes to the patient's assurance and relaxation by allaying any anxiety or fears. This person's responsibilities are outlined more specifically as follows.

DUTIES OF CIRCULATING NURSE

1. Open sterile supplies and dispense to sterile field
2. Tie scrub nurse's gown
3. Dispense Betadine solution for skin preparation
4. Dispense saline to rinse Cidex from instruments
5. Check patient, bring patient into OR, position on OR table
6. After patient is under anesthesia, assist with the following duties:
   a. Elevate affected leg
   b. Apply tourniquet cuff and connect tubing for pressure
   c. Wrap leg with Esmarch; activate tourniquet, which has been set at 450 mm Hg
7. Bring arthroscopic table over foot of bed to height of arm boards
8. Elevate leg to apply Surgical Assistant
9. Place pad beneath opposite knee
10. While surgeon and assistant are doing hand scrub, do the following:
    a. Plug in light source
    b. Place power box foot pedal on floor near affected knee
    c. Position television over light source
    d. Drop foot of OR table
    e. Make suction tubing available to arthroscopic table
    f. Bring up saline bags to arthroscopic table
11. Tie gowns of surgeon and first assistant

12. Hold extremity for surgeon to do skin prep
13. Hook up suction handed off by scrub nurse
14. Assist in connecting light source; turn on power and light
15. Plug in shaver and arthroscopy cords to power source and turn on
16. Plug sterile Y-tubing to saline bags; unclamp
17. Give articulating viewing device to first assistant (assist with hand-held camera draping)
18. Wait to receive contaminated scissors from surgeon

Surgical assistants

Ideally the assistants are specialists in arthroscopy.[1] In my situation the first assistant has been my employee for the past 18 years.

The responsibilities of the first assistant during set-up are to bring equipment to the back table, assure that all instruments are available in the operating room suite (both sterile and sterilely wrapped in the cupboards), and assist in preparing and draping the patient. During arthroscopy the assistant must control the arthroscope to assist with the inflow and outflow systems, and oversee the second assistant and surgeon. During the take-down, the assistant participates in taking down the instruments. The delicate arthroscopes should be carefully placed in trays for cleansing and sterilization.

The second assistant is responsible for setting up the back table, the Mayo stand, and the skin preparation materials as well as assisting in preparation of the patient, positioning of the Mayo stand, and attachment of the suction tubing and motorized instrument cables. At the end of the procedure the second assistant places the arthroscope and the knife blade in Cidex solution, readies the steam autoclaving tray, and assists in removing and stripping the operating room of laundry and waste to prepare for the next patient. At the end of the day the second assistant cleans, dries, and places other instruments in a secured compartment and prepares the appropriate materials for gas and/or steam autoclaving. At the end of each week the second assistant prepares the arthroscope for gas sterilization.

After each arthroscopic examination, the second assistant carefully cleans the arthroscope with saline solution and then alcohol and places it in activated dyaldehyde solution of Cidex. The interior of the cannula is cleaned by forcing saline through it with the K-52 catheter.

Proper care of endoscopic equipment increases its longevity. With careful handling instrumentation can last more than 3 years.

DUTIES OF FIRST ASSISTANT

Preparation
1. Responsible for bringing all instruments
   a. To back table
   b. Sterile-wrapped in cupboard
2. Assist in set-up of tables
3. Assist in application of tourniquet and Surgical Assistant
4. Organize and position arthroscopic Mayo stand
5. Set up articulated viewing device or hand-held camera

During arthroscopy
1. Control arthroscope and attachment
2. Oversee in coordination with second assistant
3. Assist the surgeon

Take-down care
1. Care for arthroscope and cutting instruments
2. Clean instruments
3. Place appropriate instruments in Cidex solution
4. Prepare metallic instruments for autoclave

Second assistant and circulating nurse

The duties of the second assistant and circulating nurse are listed here.

DUTIES OF SECOND ASSISTANT
1. Scrub
2. Gown and glove
3. Organize back table
4. Prepare prep table
5. Drape Mayo stand
6. Arrange instruments on left Mayo stand with pedestal on left side and arthroscope on right Mayo stand with pedestal on right side
7. Cut sterile drape to wrap around leg and scope and cut rubber end off Y-tubing; cut pieces of suction tubing to attach to drain cases
8. After 10 minutes soaking time, rinse Cidex from instruments
9. Gown and glove surgeon
10. Assist in draping patient by placing sterile stockinette on foot and hold foot during draping
11. Draw instrument Mayo stand to left side and run cords through holes in drape (First assistant brings arthroscope Mayo stand to patient's right side and plugs into light source. Suction tubing goes in the third hole in drape and arthroplasty and shaver motors in first and second holes.)
12. Pass instruments to surgeon during procedures (Also regulating suction to maintain proper distention)
13. Break down draping and assist surgeon with dressing
14. Gather instruments for first assistant to wash
15. Follow usual procedure for turning room over for next case

DUTIES OF CIRCULATING NURSE
1. Circulating nurse opens room; scrub nurse scrubs; surgeon's nurse gets instruments in autoclave and in Cidex (instruments to be soaked: shaver and arthroplasty motors, arthroscope, knives, and holder)
2. Maintain the saline level by adding new saline bags when necessary
3. Apply pressure to saline bags when requested
4. Fill out OR records
5. Control fluid on floor

At end of procedure
1. Replace power source pedal to top of arthroscopic table

2. Unplug shaver and abrasion cords and turn off power box
3. Disconnect suction and place specimen bag into specimen container
4. Disconnect light source
5. Move suspended television off to the side
6. Move saline IV pole off to the side
7. After dressings are applied:
   a. Release tourniquet and disconnect tubing from cuff
   b. Hold leg while surgeon removes leg holder and foam insert
   c. Remove tourniquet cuff
   d. Remove arthroscopic table off to the side
   e. Elevate foot of OR bed
8. Move patient to recovery room cart
9. Transport patient to recovery room
10. Complete OR records
11. Log in specimen and add formalin

RELATED HOSPITAL SERVICES

Outpatient services

A particularly important area in the hospital is outpatient services. It should allow the patient to avoid the ordinary hospital maze of admission and discharge. If arthroscopic surgery is being developed on an outpatient basis at an institution, then attention should be given to and some preferential treatment provided for the patient coming for surgery.

Physical therapy

Physical therapists and the physical therapy department can be a great asset in comforting and instructing the patient.

Strict attention and in-service training are necessary for the physical therapist so that all patients are not treated in exactly the same way. For instance, a patient in a cast would have a different type of activity than a patient who was not. Also, the individual who has had cruciate ligament or patellar realignment procedures will mobilize his knee at a different and slower rate than a person who has had a simple meniscectomy.

A patient who has had abrasion arthroplasty requires active motion and non-weight-bearing crutches, as compared to a patient who has had a patellar-shaved debridement or meniscectomy without articular cartilage changes. Therefore the physical therapist needs to be cognizant of these procedures and their anticipated postoperative courses.

Ideally the physical therapist should have an opportunity to instruct the patient before the surgical procedure. This should be based on the anticipated postoperative course.

Finally, it should be remembered that physical therapy is not a substitute for the physician's instructions and the patient's initiative.

X-ray department

The x-ray department has to cooperate greatly in cases of outpatient surgery. Many patients may arrive at the hospital or center without having had appropriate x-ray films, especially if they have been referred by another physician. Some preference should be given to outpatient surgical patients to facilitate the surgical schedule.

Intraoperative x-ray films may be necessary to confirm internal fixation or to help locate broken metal instruments.

Laboratory

The time spent in the laboratory and the comfort and attention given to the patient there only facilitate his hospital stay. Any delays or anxieties produced in the laboratory can delay the surgery and prolong the patient's anxiety.

REFERENCES

1. Becker, R.L., and Johnson, L.L.: Role of the assistant in arthroscopy. In American Academy of Orthopaedic Surgeons Symposium on arthroscopy and arthrography of the knee, St. Louis, 1978, The C.V. Mosby Co.
2. Johnson, L.L.: Creating the proper environment for arthroscopic surgery, Orthop. Clin. North Am. **13**:283, 1982.
3. Miller, L.B.: Orthopaedic patients in an ambulatory surgery facility. Nurs. Clin. North Am. **16**:749, 1981.
4. Rosenberg, T.D., and Wong, H.C.: Arthroscopic knee surgery in a free-standing outpatient surgery center. Orthop. Clin. North Am. **13**:277, 1982.

CHAPTER 4

Instruments

CHARACTERISTICS OF ARTHROSCOPIC INSTRUMENTATION

The unique environment of arthroscopic surgery places special demands on instruments. Arthroscopy differs from open surgery; operating in a confined space via a two-dimensional projection of the space on a television monitor is a challenge. The instruments must be small and have a shape that conforms to the joint. The edges must be smooth to avoid joint surface injury. Metallic instruments should have magnetic properties to facilitate their removal in case of breakage.

The viewing devices should provide a bright, sharp image with accurate color and no distortion. The light sources should provide a daylight spectrum (5,000° K) of illumination.

The instrumentation for resection and repair must be sharp yet smooth. The working end, whether used for cutting or grasping, should be limited in size and length to maintain its visualization with the arthroscope. The limited fields of view of an arthroscope do not permit viewing of both sides of a wide instrument or the entire length of a long one.

Although miniaturization is important, strength cannot be totally compromised in design or manufacturing. Arthroscopic instruments are weaker than larger, conventional equipment. The surgeon must be aware of this and handle the instruments with respect.

Whenever possible, the instruments should be designed for cannula entry to minimize trauma and to maintain accurate placement during interchange.

The original arthroscopic instruments were adapted from equipment used in other endoscopic disciplines. The original arthroscope, the Watanabe No. 21, permitted visualization of the anterior knee joint chambers only. Miniaturization and the development of fiberoptics resulted in the present high-resolution arthroscopes.

The first operative tools, basket forceps and operating arthroscopes, were adapted from gynecological laparoscopy. At that time arthroscopy was laborious and limited to lavage, loose body removal, and resection of simple meniscal tears.

In 1975 I collaborated with the Dyonics Corporation in the development of an instrument that was probably the first motorized instrument specifically designed for arthroscopic surgery. The Intra-articular Shaver (1976) and the later Arthroplasty System (1980) provided a motorized arthroscopic surgical system.

Since then the need for instrumentation designed for arthroscopy has been met with the introduction of the extremity-holding device, arthroscopic knife blades, arthroscopically deliverable staples, and instruments for transcutaneous suturing. Variations in configurations of basket forceps, with up to 90-degree cutting angles and curved shafts that conform to the joint, adapt to the arthroscopic environment.

PURCHASING EQUIPMENT

The range of instruments available to arthroscopic surgeons is truly amazing. Manufacturers have responded to the increased interest in arthroscopy. There has been a gradual improvement in the instruments and image transmission devices available to the arthroscopic surgeon.

The physician entering the marketplace for arthroscopic instrumentation has to heed the old adage, "Let the buyer beware." Taking advice from other surgeons can be misleading. The physician's relationship with the manufacturer ranges from satisfied purchaser to consultant or ownership. Virtually no instrument or treatment idea develops without the input of an investigative surgeon. The surgeon may be the inventor or consultant, may serve on an advisory board, or may even hold stock in the parent company.

I would advise the surgeon who is considering the purchase of these instruments to evaluate as carefully as possible through his or her own observations. One should talk with as many different people as possible; there is safety in having many counselors. The salesperson should be allowed to detail the equipment carefully, and the surgeon should shop the marketplace for quality and price. When asking the advice of other physicians, the potential buyer should recognize that the most valid opinion would come from a satisfied purchaser.

In 1984 the American Academy of Orthopaedic Surgeons recognized these possibilities and instituted a voluntary commercial interest identification system at its meetings. The audience can be made aware of any possible commercial interest by a designation in the program. Surgeons making presentations were asked to indicate if the subject matter they were presenting was in any way related to a commercial interest. If the presenter agreed to it, an asterisk was placed by his or her name in the program.

I support and cooperate with this method of open communication concerning these matters. Look for the asterisks(*).

Investments

I am often asked, "What is the minimum amount of equipment with which a person can perform arthroscopic surgery?" Arthroscopy can be performed with direct viewing using an arthroscope, a light cable, and a light source. For surgery, one would also need a probe and basket forceps for meniscal work and a knife or scissors for cutting.

Performance of arthroscopic surgery in the absence of any motorized instrumentation severely compromises even the simplest of procedures. Motorized instrumentation, even if it is used for nothing more than vacuuming the joint or debriding synovium for exposure, is very important.

However, one should not enter arthroscopic surgery with a limited perspective. If an expert requires a variety of the best and most sophisticated equipment to maximize technique in patient care, how can a surgeon with less experience and technical skill perform arthroscopy in a lesser environment or without a comprehensive set of instruments?

The beginning arthroscopist has to recognize that there will be a high cost in time, energy, and money. If the surgeon is prepared to expend energy and time learning arthroscopy, it is appropriate to have the best of tools. The adage that a mechanic cannot be better than his tools is never more true than in arthroscopic surgery.

Of course, the investment dollars should be wisely spent. The initial purchase is the most difficult because of lack of knowledge and experience. The first purchase should be deferred until after a fact-finding mission.

The surgical uses of the instrumentation can be learned at arthroscopy courses. The types of equipment purchased should fit some known surgical system approach observed while visiting an established arthroscopic surgeon or learned reading the literature.

Attention should be given to the durability of any instrument. This must be balanced by the inevitable need for quality service for equipment. The availability of loaner equipment or replacements must also be considered. These benefits are weighed against price.

Should purchases be delayed for more advanced models? No! Although we all hope for a perfect machine or tool, waiting for a better one delays learning with the present instrument if the existing one has merit. The benefit of the instrument is also lost. Some purchase mistakes may be made because of antiquation, but they are not made in the learning.

Do most surgical groups buy too many instruments? Yes. Owning every conceivable instrument and variation thereof does not assure success. The surgeon must first recognize that instruments do not perform surgery any more than golf clubs play golf. Having a single, specific instrument for every conceivable surgical maneuver is unnecessary. The integration of instruments to fit a surgical system approach avoids unnecessary purchases.

Who should purchase the instrumentation? I think an individual who plans to be a serious arthroscopic surgeon should consider personal purchase. Many physicians balk at this, because the cost can be over $40,000. The arthroscopic surgeon should look at the investment in arthroscopic instrumentation as an investment in himself or herself. In this area, he or she has the most knowledge and will receive the most satisfaction. The surgeon is the "Chairman of the Board" and will receive the tax benefits of depreciation. No other type of investment can benefit the surgeon to the same extent—most surgeons are well acquainted with investments of lesser benefit.

There are also surgical reasons for the individual surgeon to invest in instruments:

1. The consistent, clear, bright, image on the television is monitored by the owner/surgeon. An overused light source and a dirty, broken, or scratched light guide, let alone a broken arthroscope, are factors eliminated by care and control of one's own image transmission system.
2. Sharp, clean cuts by carefully handled cutting instruments can only be assured by individual attention.
3. Optimal operation of motorized instrumentation depends on careful monitoring of function with care and replacement.

In 1972, within a group practice, I purchased two arthroscopes. Four other partners purchased one arthroscope. "Nobody" broke that one four times in the first month. After that month, each of my partners purchased his own arthroscope and subsequently a second. The incidence of breakage was reduced.

At present, with my practice limited to arthroscopic surgery, I have also purchased a back-up set of instruments. This avoids delays with shipping or stock shortages. I also store as many as four arthroscopes at my office. This way if there is any problem with one arthroscope I do not have any "down time"; I do not have to cancel any surgeries, and there are no patient, surgical, or hospital inconveniences. This clearly demonstrates that it becomes more important to have the equipment readily available as the surgeon becomes more involved. This includes back-ups, not only for daily work but in case of delayed delivery dates.

By having personal instrumentation, the surgeon can be assured that it is always in the highest level of service. With many users of various instruments, optimal condition is not possible. Some surgeons are rougher on equipment than others, usually without recognizing that they are. In addition, these surgeons are likely to be the ones who believe that somebody else caused the problem. Remember our group's experience: "nobody" broke the arthroscope four times!

When it comes to cutting instrumentation, the surgeon may consider the following example. If you come in on Monday and use a motorized cutter, knife blade, or basket forceps, and your next case is on Friday, five other people may have used the same instrumentation by your next surgery. This includes 10 other nurses, 15 shakes during washing, and countless bounces in the instrument pan. When you return for your Friday case, you can expect dull instruments. Owning your own equipment allows you to monitor its sharpness. You control replacement and repair of the instruments. This way you ensure clean, sharp, exacting, and precise resecting tools.

If an institution or group opts for a common instrumentation pool, I make the following recommendations. Each surgeon should be assigned his or her own arthroscope, knives, basket forceps, and motorized instrument cutting heads. In this way each surgeon will be responsible for the care of the critical viewing and cutting portions of the system. The surgeon can monitor any deficiency and make replacement or repair requests. The instrumentation less subject to wear and tear—television, light cables, instrumentation motors, and thigh holders—may be used by all participants.

This system has two major advantages. It eliminates discussion of "who done it" or "who broke the whatever." It also provides a system for monitoring each surgeon's use or abuse of instrumentation for cost-accounting and eventually cost-saving purposes.

There are several major categories of surgical instrumentation. Instruments involved in image transmission include the arthroscope, the light source, and the video system. There are also devices involved in sterility and draping. Devices exist for arthroscopic exposure, palpation, grasping, retrieval, and cutting. Motorized instruments are used for resection and removal via suction. More recently instruments have been introduced for repair and reconstruction, including suture systems and implantation systems.

Individual instruments should be categorized by type and function. This organization avoids unnecessary duplication. Money is better spent for back-up instruments of the same type. As with any mechanical device or technical feat, the opportunity for mechanical or technical failure exists. The patient's surgical care cannot be compromised. I hope that the use of inadequate instrumentation will not be rationalized as means of saving money. The cost to the patient may be too great to support this philosophy.

The following description of instrumentation is in no way exhaustive. It merely reflects the instrumentation that I have played a part in developing or that of which I am a satisfied purchaser. Comparable instruments are sold by many manufacturers.

IMAGE TRANSMISSION

Arthroscopy is really photography, and the film is the surgeon's retina. The camera is the scope or television. The object photographed is within the joint. Simplistic as this sounds, the analogy will aid in problem solving when the surgeon tries to improve the clarity and brightness of the arthroscopic picture.

ARTHROSCOPES
Types

Elliptical thin-lens system

In the classic glass lens system, the lenses are thin in comparison with their diameter[10] (Fig. 4-1, *A*). Air spaces separate the lenses. The objective lens transmits the light from the image, through the relay lens system, to the ocular. This is the original endoscope design.

Rod-lens system

The rod-lens system was designed by Professor H.H. Hopkins of Reading, England. The convex lenses are thick compared with their diameter (see Fig. 4-15). The air spaces between the lenses are relatively small. This system reproduces the concept of the conventional lens, but the air space has the reverse shape of that in the conventional lens. The cylindrical space is glass, rather than air as in the thin-lens relay system.

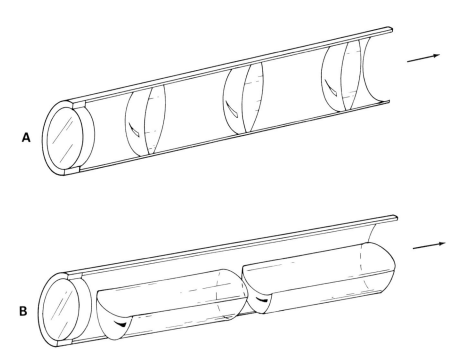

FIG. 4-1. Arthroscope.

A Conventional lens system. Classic thin-lens system is series of small lenses divided by cylinders of air. Image comes through objective lens from left and is transmitted by relay lens system to ocular lens. Light is transmitted in direction of arrow to arthroscopist's eye. The relay lens system varies in different types of endoscopes.

B Rod-lens system is series of glass cylinders separated by small areas of air, the reverse of thin-lens system.

Continued.

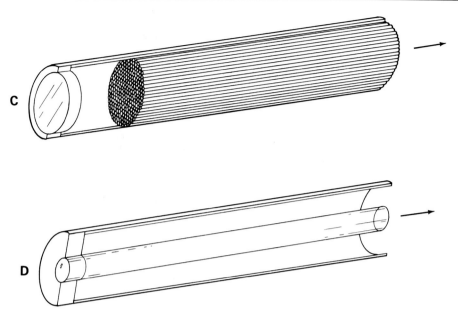

FIG. 4-1, cont'd. Arthroscope.

C Fused coherent bundle system transmits light by individual fibers. Composition consists of many fine dots, each transmitting an element of image.

D Needlescope system consists of two graded refractory index (GRIN) lenses and an ocular lens. Objective lens, about 3 mm in length and 1 mm in diameter, gives a wide field of view. Relay lens, about 134 mm in length and 1 mm in diameter, transfers image from objective lens back to ocular lens, which magnifies it for viewing.

This design was originally manufactured by the Karl Storz Company of West Germany (Fig. 4-2) and is called the Storz Hopkins Rod-Lens System. Subsequently, the design has been used by Thackery in England. The Hopkins patent expired in 1984, so other manufacturers now offer a version of the design.

Coherent bundle system

The coherent bundle system was used in the late 1960s and early 1970s. It had an objective lens to relay the light through a bundle of coherent light fibers

FIG. 4-2. Standard arthroscopes.

A Storz arthroscope, 4 mm, and cannula system.

B Storz rod-lens arthroscope is available in two sizes, with 2.7 or 4 mm telescope. Both provide excellent optical clarity.

C Storz 70-degree inclined view rod-lens telescope is 4 mm in diameter. Its separate cannula is shorter than standard to accommodate greater optical angle and not cover view with metallic sheath. It is used in posterior compartment via Gillquist method.

D *Left to right,* 4 mm diameter Dyonics rod-lens endoscope; 2.2 mm Needlescope seen in end view; 1.7 mm Needlescope; No. 18 needle, shown for relative size comparison.

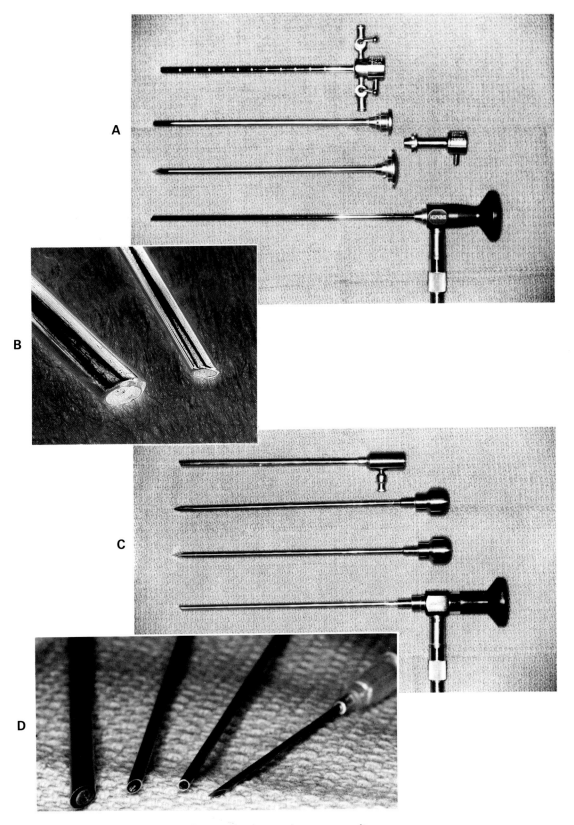

FIG. 4-2. For legend see opposite page.

(see Fig. 4-1, C). The image is transmitted through the ocular lens to the observer's eye. With this system the viewer sees an image that is composed of many fine dots. Each dot transmits an element of the image that is being viewed.

This system was marketed as a No. 24-type arthroscope, but it is no longer available in North America. The advantage of this type of arthroscope was that it relayed a very bright image, even at low light levels. The disadvantage was that it was too fragile for manipulation in arthroscopy.

Graded refractory index (GRIN) system

In the GRIN system, light is transmitted through a slender rod of glass. The refractory index decreases from the center to the periphery according to a specific mathematical relationship[2,6,7] (see Fig. 4-1, D). The lens is processed by an ion-exchange system using cesium. This endoscope is self-focusing and hence its trade name, Selfoc. Rays of light enter the objective lens from a particular point in space, follow helical patterns, and come into focus periodically along the rod. The No. 24 Watanabe arthroscope (1.7 mm diameter) was the precursor of the Dyonics Needlescope, which was made in both 1.7 and 2.7 mm diameters. It was produced in various lengths between 100 and 200 mm. It had an inclined view of 15 degrees in saline.

The Dyonics Needlescope was popular for diagnostic arthroscopy of the knee joint using a local anesthetic (Fig. 4-3). Its use declined with the advent of operative arthroscopy. The necessity for image transmission via television favored the larger arthroscopes with a brighter image. The Needlescope is now limited to use in small joints.

Selection of an arthroscope

There are many factors to take into consideration when selecting an arthroscope. The personality, vision, eye-hand coordination, and technical ability of the arthroscopist, as well as his or her desire to use image transmission systems including video, are important considerations. The various technical aspects of the arthroscope are also very important. These can include brilliance, optical clarity, absence of distortion, field of view, and apparent and inclined view.

No endoscope is ideal for every arthroscopist in every situation. The single and initial purchase is usually difficult, because all arthroscopes and optical systems have limitations that may not be anticipated. Often a second arthroscope will offer advantages that the first purchase lacked.

It is possible in selected patients to carry out a complete arthroscopy of the knee with virtually any endoscope except perhaps the Watanabe No. 21. It is large in diameter, because an eccentrically placed tungsten lightbulb doubles the size.

Originally I preferred the 1.7 mm Dyonics Needlescope which, when housed in a cannula, had an outside diameter (OD) of 2 mm. This allowed easy access to the joint. It was especially well suited for local anesthesia and posterior compartment approaches by transcutaneous puncture. These advantages were not easily achieved with the larger arthroscope. If multiple punctures were made with the larger endoscope, the joint tended to leak and/or deflate through the various entry sites. Distention was then lost without continuous inflow, and dif-

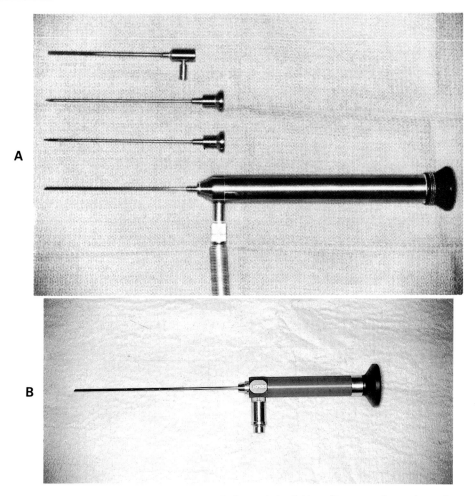

FIG. 4-3. A Dyonics Needlescope. Third model of Needlescope is a closed system with a viewing angle of approximately 70 degrees in saline. Endoscope shown here is 2.2 mm OD. Cannula, which is superior, has sheath of 2.6 mm OD. Sharp and blunt trocars accompany system. **B** Storz small arthroscope.

ficulty in either complete visualization or even manipulation followed. In some patients I used a 2.2 mm Needlescope, with a 2.7 mm OD cannula, and even that size limited visualization into the posterior compartments, especially under or above the menisci.

The desire to obtain good body position and to keep both hands free necessitated attachment of the arthroscope to a video system. However, light is lost in video image transmission, so the imagery is not as clear as with direct viewing. The smaller arthroscope was therefore not applicable to arthroscopic surgery. It is now used for direct visualization of small joints. It should be noted, though, that the 2.2 mm Needlescope can be attached directly to the video system if illumination is adequate or enhanced by a halo light (Fig 4-4). There is still a narrow actual field of view.

Larger arthroscopes are preferred for surgical procedures. A 4 mm scope

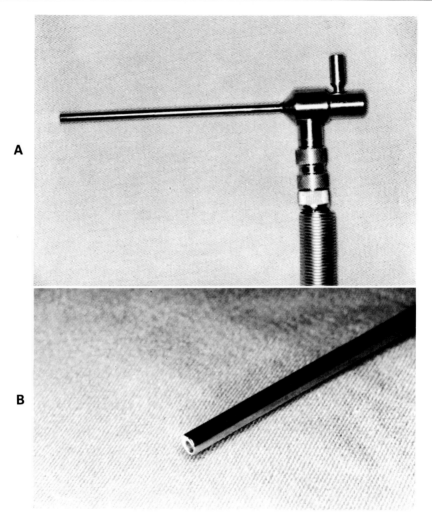

FIG. 4-4. Halo light.

A Halo light is advantageous for photographic work and for protection of small-diameter endoscope when used for training purposes.

B Endo of halo light. Notice central opening that will house 1.7 mm Needlescope. Illumination is up to sixteen times that of endoscope.

with a 30-degree inclined view is standard. The size is compensated for with continuous inflow distention and use of the Surgical Assistant to secure the thigh for manipulation.

Field of view

There are two dimensions to the field of view: the apparent (perceived) field of view and the actual (angle) field of view (Fig. 4-5).

The apparent or perceived field of view is the diameter of the circular image seen at the ocular end of the endoscope. The actual field of view is the measured angle of view the arthroscope visualizes. The apparent field of view is affected by the lens that couples the arthroscope to the television monitor. The placement and size of this lens may create a greater or smaller image. Using television as a

Apparent field of view

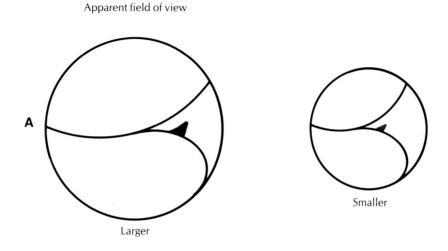

Actual field of view

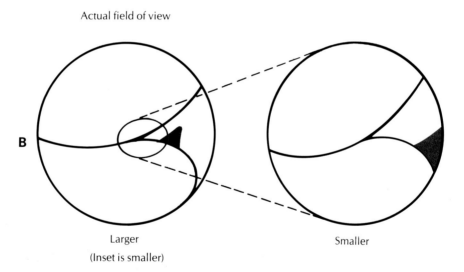

FIG. 4-5. Comparison: field of view.

A Apparent field of view. Circles are different sizes, yet actual image is same. Larger circle gives impression of wider view, hence the designation "apparent" field of view. Actual field of view is same, but apparent view (size of circle) differs.

B Circles are same size, yet image in left circle is far greater than that taken from inset. Apparent fields of view are same, but actual fields of view differ.

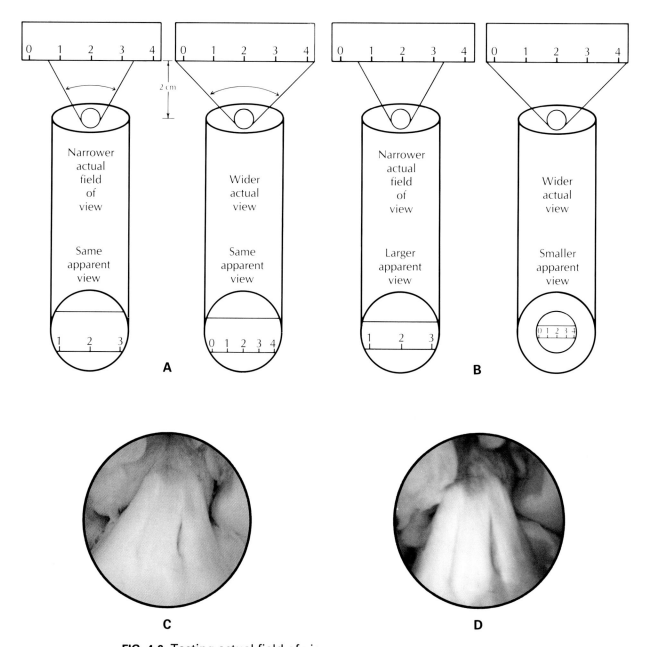

FIG. 4-6. Testing actual field of view.

A Diagram on left shows narrower actual field but equal apparent field of view. Illustration on right shows wider actual field of view, but same apparent field of view.

B Diagram on left shows narrower actual but larger apparent field of view. Diagram on right shows larger actual but smaller apparent field of view.

C Same apparent view as **D**. Larger actual view.

D Same apparent view (circle size) as **C**. Smaller actual view (close-up of **C**).

measuring device is valid only with the same video and C-mount, not from system to system.

A simple means for measuring apparent and actual field of view is accomplished by attaching the arthroscope to the television camera (Fig. 4-6) and following these steps. Lay the scope on a table. Focus on a ruler at distance of 1 to 2 cm. Measure the width of the circle on the monitor (apparent field of view), and record the length of ruler that appears. Draw lines on paper from the center of the end of the arthroscope to the end points seen on the ruler. Measure the angle (actual) field of view. The angle (actual) field of view is the angle of view that the lens design creates. The new Storz arthroscope encompasses an actual field of view of approximately 120 degrees in air.

Various scopes can be compared. It would be possible to produce an arthroscope that had a very large apparent field of view (the large circle seen on the television) and a field of view of 35 degrees. The inspecting surgeon might be impressed with the large apparent field of view. On the other hand, there could be an arthroscope with a small apparent field of view (a small circle on the television), but an actual field of view of about 75 degrees, exceeding the actual field of view of the scope in the first example. The surgeon perceives the smaller circle as the smaller field of view; hence the designation apparent field of view.

The ideal circumstance is the largest apparent view possible without image irregularities at the periphery and a maximal actual (angle width) field of view that is evenly illuminated. Orthopedic surgeons who are learning to become arthroscopists usually are not aware of this distinction.

Inclination of view

The inclination of view is the angle of projection at the objective end of the arthroscope (Fig. 4-7). It is calculated by drawing a line along the axis of the arthroscope that intersects the line drawn from the center of the arthroscopic image to the objective end of the scope.

The incline can be straight or angled (see Fig. 4-7). The 0-degree inclined, or straight-viewing, arthroscope is simple for orientation but not practical for operative arthroscopy. Of the inclined views, the most common are 30, 70, 90, and 120 degrees. The angle permits visualization around corners. The most practical for arthroscopy is the 30-degree inclined view. Most objects seen arthroscopically are either to the side, above, or below. When rotated, the 30-degree inclined view scope provides the best arthroscopic surgical approach. During surgery, it allows eccentric placement of the endoscope away from the instrumentation. Mental adaption to the 30-degree inclined view is accomplished with some practice. Adaption to greater inclined views is more difficult, especially with scope movement. Disorientation may occur. Scopes with a wide inclined view (70, 90, and 120 degrees) are best used for single-placement, stationary viewing.

In some cases a 70-degree inclined view is used for posterior viewing via the transcondylar approach. Orientation is very difficult with a 120-degree scope. There is a place for stationary 70- or 90-degree viewing, especially in work on the patella. Views from the suprapatellar pouch facilitate patellar position tracking, monitoring, and repositioning for a single view. This is more difficult with a 30-degree inclined field of view, especially if there is a thigh holder occupying space.

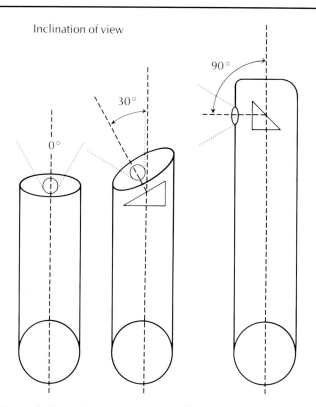

Inclination of view

FIG. 4-7. Inclination of view. The 0-degree inclination views straight ahead. A 30-degree incline views on an angle deviated from axis of arthroscope. A 90-degree scope views at right angle to axis of arthroscope.

If there is no thigh holder, visualization is possible with a 30-degree inclined view. A 90-degree inclined view gives a squared orientation for suprapatellar views of patellar surgery.

Delivery of light

Several factors affect the delivery of light and the subsequent visualization of the image. Two important factors are the amount of light on the object and the quality of the lens system transmitting light back to the ocular.

A large endoscope has a greater capacity to hold glass fibers for carrying light to the object, resulting in a brighter image. A smaller endoscope has less space for fibers; therefore less light is delivered to the image because the light of origin is less. It does not matter how good the lens system is if the amount of light on the object is compromised.

The second factor in delivery of light is the quality of the lens system returning light from the object to the eye. The rod lens system is the highest-quality design for bringing light back to the eye.

Brightness is affected by the number of lenses in the endoscope. The greater number of lenses, the more refraction there is to light transmission. An increased number of lenses decreases the clarity of the image.

The higher the quality of glass, the higher the quality of the image. Although two endoscopes may have the same rod lens optical design, the design of

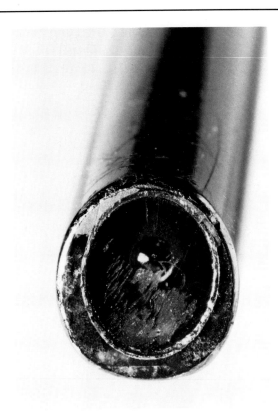

FIG. 4-8. Mechanically injured end of arthroscope may be salvaged by polishing or refurbishing.

the objective lens greatly affects the resultant imagery. Storz's objective lenses have a technological advantage for inclined view arthroscopes (see Fig. 4-2, *A*).

The arthroscope is affected by the technique or the workmanship during assembly. Mechanical security of the lenses and freedom from microscopic particles, accomplished in so-called clean rooms, may be necessary to achieve perfect imagery. A speck of dirt occupies a large part of the surface area of a 1 to 2 mm lens. Any smudge or dirt in the system is magnified many times and interferes with the imagery. Quality control is perfected over years of manufacturer experience.

The most common cause of damage to the endoscope is injury to the ocular surface during arthroscopic surgery or instrumentation, by either banging, cutting, or scratching the end of the arthroscope (Fig. 4-8). Many companies offer polishing services, which are less expensive than so-called exchange programs. An exchange program is one in which the new arthroscope is returned to the company, which sends an exchange arthroscope that has been refurbished. If the continuity of the transmission lens system is intact the ocular can be replaced at a minimum cost to the company, which is in part passed on to the purchaser with an exchange program. In this way it is not necessary to purchase a new arthroscope.

Another issue is how the lenses are cemented in place. To date there is not a perfectly heat-resistant cement. Manufacturers offer arthroscopes that are au-

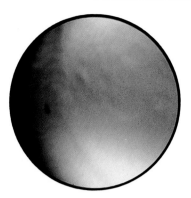

FIG. 4-9. Arthroscopic photograph showing characteristic ellipse of image that occurs with bending of arthroscope.

toclavable, but deterioration occurs in the image transmission capacity when they are subjected to high heat. In fact, the lens systems within the telescope can loosen, resulting in need for repair. Damage is possible by use, by autoclaving, or, of course, by dropping.

As an arthroscope ages there is a yellow coloring to the image. The shelf life should exceed 2 years without alterations in glass or cement.

Mechanical stability

An arthroscope has to be considered from the standpoint of mechanical stability. The larger-diameter arthroscope could be more serviceable than an arthroscope of a smaller diameter. A surgeon with good technique and experience should not break an arthroscope during a procedure. The surgeon should recognize that an elliptical deformation of the image indicates that the arthroscope is bending (Fig. 4-9). At that point, the surgeon should remove pressure on the arthroscope. An arthroscope is a fine surgical instrument and should not be used as a crowbar.

LIGHT SOURCES

Arthroscopy, like photography, depends on light. Many varieties of light sources are available in North America. Most hospitals have several types purchased for other endoscopic procedures, and most light sources produce light of adequate intensity for direct-view arthroscopy. The 150-watt bulbs produce a yellow hue. More powerful light sources have a 300- or 350-watt tungsten bulb, or metallic halogen or xenon arc as a source (Fig. 4-10). The higher-intensity lights are necessary for proper illumination during arthroscopic surgery.

In one environment, the scope is attached directly to the television camera. The direct television attachment conserves light (see Fig. 5-15).

The use of an articulated viewing device (AVD) in the suspended system requires more light because of the many lenses of the AVD (see Fig. 4-14). The three-segment device is preferred over the five-segment device for that reason. A suspended system necessitates no restrictions in camera size. Light loss in the AVD is compensated for by the capacity of the camera to pick up low light levels. There is also the advantage of three tubes for optical resolution.

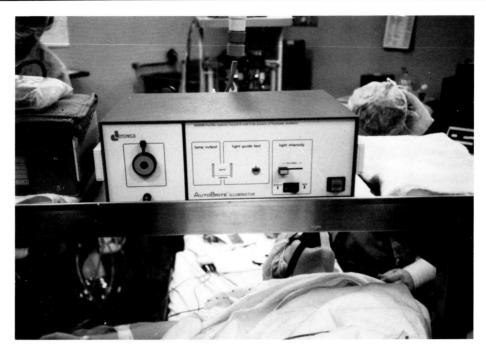

FIG. 4-10. Dyonics Autobrite light source.

Recent light source models have built-in automatic gain controls coordinated with the television system.

In the original Dyonics Model 500 light source and the upgraded Model 510, the Sylvania 300-16 light bulb was favored over the General Electric 300-watt bulb. Recent manufacturer changes have made only the General Electric bulb available. The Model 510 can also use a 350-watt bulb but not without causing increased cable heat, which shortens cable life. The use of this bulb is not recommended.

Other light sources use halogen metallic arc systems to generate effective light levels. Comparison testing in arthroscopic environments shows little perceptible difference on the video screen in any of the aforementioned systems. Manufacturers' reports of actual illumination may indicate increased output when measured on an optical bench. The xenon source produces greater intensity of light but is not necessary for present-day television cameras. It is the most expensive light source.

It should be recognized that a light bulb does not last indefinitely. Its intensity may start to decline even after 6 hours, when light is still coming from the source. The effective light is virtually dissipated after 24 hours in the case of the Dyonics Model 510. The light bulb lasts much longer in the Storz or Dyonics metallic ion arc generator. The loss of level may not be recognized under direct viewing but certainly would result in poor photographic documents. This often surprises the arthroscopist, who sees a good image by eye and then later sees a very dull videotape, movie, or photograph. One must remember that the eye is very forgiving and a better photographic instrument than any man-made arthroscope or television or any other type of camera. Light intensity is most easily appreciated when recording and viewing on television.

The high-intensity light sources are too bright for comfortable, and perhaps safe, direct viewing (see Chapter 2, under Physician Complications). A shading device or rheostat should be used for direct viewing. A less powerful light source within the same unit facilitates direct viewing.

LIGHT GUIDES (CABLES)

A variety of light guides or light cables is available. All manufacturers make adaptors for their competitors' arthroscopes or light sources.

There are two basic types of light guides. The first type is a bundle of fiber-glass encased in a tube. The other is what is known as a liquid light guide.

Bundle light cables

I prefer the bundle cable to the liquid light guide, even though the latter transmits more light. The liquid guides, even in the 3 mm size, which is some-what more flexible than the 5 mm size, do not offer the suppleness of the bundle light guide.

When considering cables it is important to look at the thermal resistance of the plastic covering. My experience indicates that the Dyonics light guides have a long potential lifetime. There has been no deterioration with the outside cover-ing during autoclaving.

Care of the cable is important. Day-to-day handling affects the life of a light cable, as with so many other instruments. Light cables should not be kinked or twisted, although it is technically possible to do so. It results in the breakage of small fibers. As with any other technical equipment, the performance of the light cable should be checked periodically so that gradual deterioration does not com-promise the arthroscopic examination. The passage of light or use over many months does not wear out the cables. However, over time either mechanical breakage or corrosion over the ends of the cables decreases their effectiveness. Finally, with very high-intensity light sources such as a 350-watt bulb or even the Storz xenon arc, the heat generated can deteriorate or injure the end of the cable, diminishing the effective light. Thus the high-intensity light may actually be counterproductive after the cable has been used for some time.

It is important to check for cleanness or injury at each end of the cable. Each end must have a clean, polished surface.

It is also necessary to check for breaks in the conduit. This is accomplished by holding one end of the light cable to a bright light and looking at the other end. If darkened or black areas are seen, this shows that that particular fiber has been broken somewhere along its course. Also, the disrupted fiber can be seen to transmit light at the point of the break along the cable. Repeated checks and replacements are necessary to ensure optimal transmission of light. The Dyonics cable can last for as many as 300 steam autoclavings or surgical cases.

Another factor that affects light transmission is the relative length of the guide. Approximately 8% of light is lost for each foot of cable; therefore 48% of light is lost in the standard 6-foot guide.

Each junction or interface is a source of light loss. The optimal arthroscope is one in which the cable is actually attached to the arthroscope and the light is transmitted without interruption from the light source to the objective lens. How-

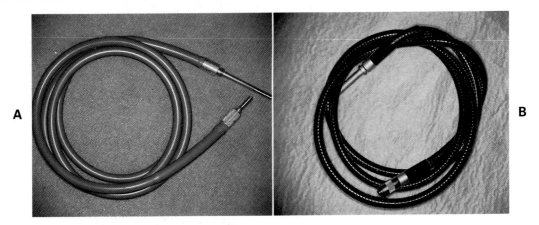

FIG. 4-11. Light guides.

A Fiberglass light cable.
B Liquid light guide.

ever, the life of an arthroscope is longer than that of a light guide, and an integrated system, although it would enhance illumination, would be costly. The breakdown of the light guide would prematurely render the arthroscope useless. Separate systems are most practical. It is important to have a powerful light source to overcome the factors that can decrease the transmission of light.

Liquid light guide

The liquid light guide has been introduced over the last few years. It comes in 3 mm and 5 mm sizes (Fig. 4-11). It transmits considerably more light than the other light cables and appears to have a longer use life. Its major disadvantage is the inflexibility of the guide, which can slow the procedure or limit access. Kinking or rotational limitation can also occur in the guide. Where maximal transmission of light is needed a liquid-type guide should be considered. It is more expensive than conventional cable.

Halo light

Light is diminished when a small-diameter Needlescope is used, so photography is difficult. Fragility is another problem. The halo light compensates for these problems (see Fig. 4-4). This 3.5 mm OD cannula provides 16 times the illumination of the small-diameter scope. A better image is possible for documentation on video or slides. It is not practical for use in arthroscopic surgery. An arthroscope of a larger diameter offers more optical clarity and brightness. However, the halo light allows arthroscopists to become more proficient with a small-diameter scope and yet have the safety, protection, and photographic capacity of a larger-diameter arthroscope.

Light wand

A light wand is used for transillumination in photography (Fig. 4-12). It is placed parallel to the view or may transilluminate tissue from behind, above, or

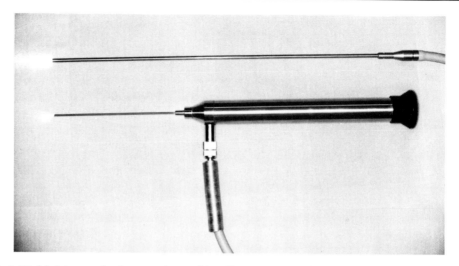

FIG. 4-12. Light wand, shown above Needlescope, can be useful for photographic purposes, especially transillumination. It is brought into knee through separate puncture wound. Photographs are taken through small-diameter endoscope with camera attached to ocular lens.

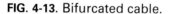

FIG. 4-13. Bifurcated cable.

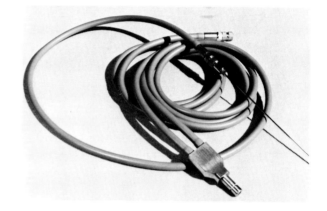

below. Transillumination first showed the engulfing of saline in synovium. Observation of the vascular pattern and morphological characteristics of synovium can be enhanced by transillumination for photographic purposes.

A light cable with a 2 to 3 mm diameter light wand attached may be useful in arthroscopic surgery. The main cable is attached to the viewing arthroscope. The second portion of the cable, with its attached light wand, can be placed in the posterior compartment via a second puncture. This provides backlighting to improve visualization and depth of field.

Bifurcated cable

The bifurcated cable permits one attachment to the endoscope and a second to a separate light source for photographic illumination, improving depth of field and conceptualization during small-scope arthroscopy (Fig. 4-13).

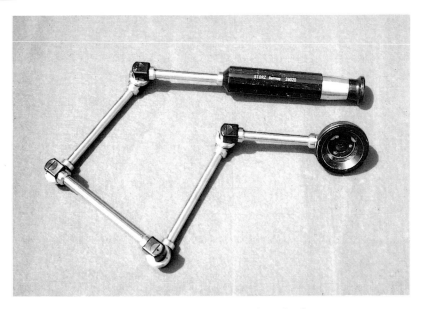

FIG. 4-14. Articulated viewing device.

ARTICULATED VIEWING DEVICE (AVD)

The AVD is a linkage of arthroscopic lenses by glass prisms (Fig. 4-14). It provides angulation and rotation by the mechanical connections. It connects the ocular of the arthroscope to the suspended television camera. It has been used for direct viewing as a teaching device.

In 1976 we attached the video camera (Hitachi 9016, which then weighed about 4½ pounds) directly to the arthroscope. The size and weight of the camera were impractical. Therefore the camera was suspended from the operating room light bracket and connected via an AVD (see Fig. 4-14). It rotated and folded on itself to provide flexibility, not only in knee surgery but also in surgery of the shoulder and especially the elbow with posterior approaches.

My initial experience was with the five-segment device. The AVD was shortened to a three-lens system when a pistoning ceiling mount system was installed, because it gave more light.

I still favor the AVD because of its mobility, relative weightlessness, the small attachment to the arthroscope. (It occupies less space than even the smallest chip camera.) The surgeon is free to remove the hand from the scope without losing position or having the unit fall to the floor.

The major advantage of the AVD is the single hand control for rotation of the arthroscope to create composition. A direct attachment of the television to the scope requires two hands for rotation: one hand for the camera and another to stabilize the camera orientation (Fig. 4-15, *A*). With the AVD the rotation or derotation is controlled by the first assistant (Fig. 4-15, *B*).

The suspended system allows a video camera of any size. The larger three-tube cameras have minimal service problems; I have had no service problems in 8 years.

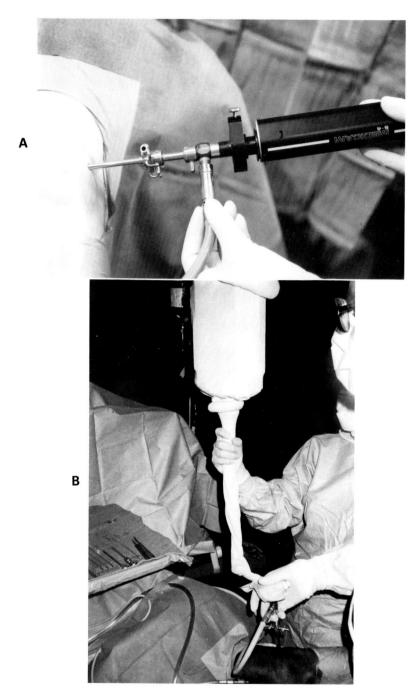

FIG. 4-15. Control of image rotation.

A Hand-held camera requires two hands.
B Articulating viewing device is corrected by first assistant derotating device at suspended camera attachment.

SURGICAL ASSISTANT

The first leg holder was made out of pipes with an Olympic Vacpac insert and secured with a thumbscrew (Fig. 4-16). The second leg holder, or its prototype, was an expensive instrument, costing almost three times the retail price of the most expensive manufactured leg holder (Fig. 4-16, *C*). This prototype required a number of cuts through stainless steel to create the shapes. Today's Surgical Assistant is a 16-pound metallic frame with a closed-cell foam insert. It is secured to the operating table by a Clark clamp (Fig. 4-17, *A*).

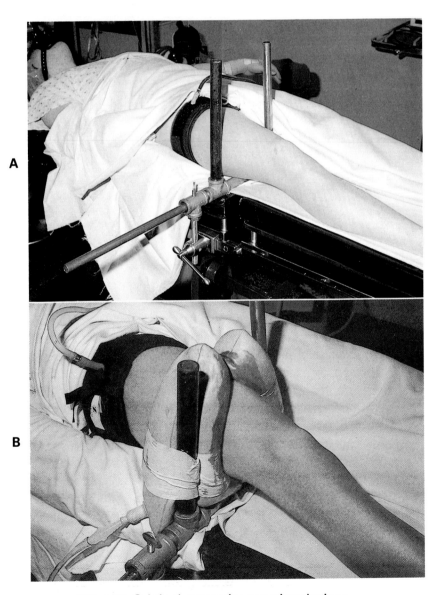

FIG. 4-16. Original extremity-securing devices.

A First model was constructed of pipes.
B Vacuum bag was used to pad and secure thigh.

Continued.

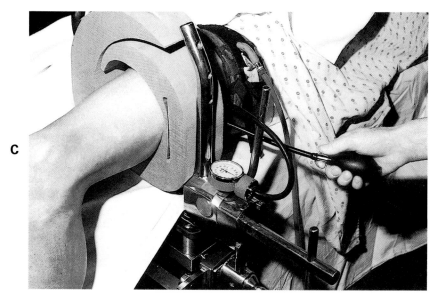

FIG. 4-16, cont'd. Original extremity-securing devices.

C Pressure gauge was used on prototypes to secure maximum pressure at safe 360 mm Hg.

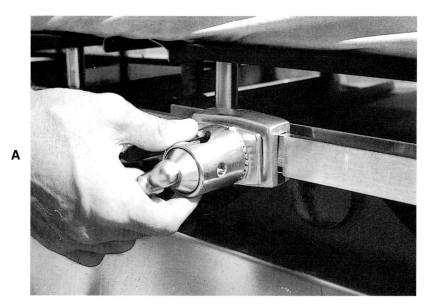

FIG. 4-17. Surgical Assistant extremity-securing device

A Secured to OR table via Clark attachment borrowed from obstetrics/gynecology.

B Closed-cell foam insert protects soft tissues.

C Cam action applied by lever creates quadrilateral shape to thigh.

D Surgical Assistant secures and suspends knee for circumferential approaches when foot of table is lowered. (Courtesy Johnson & Johnson Company.)

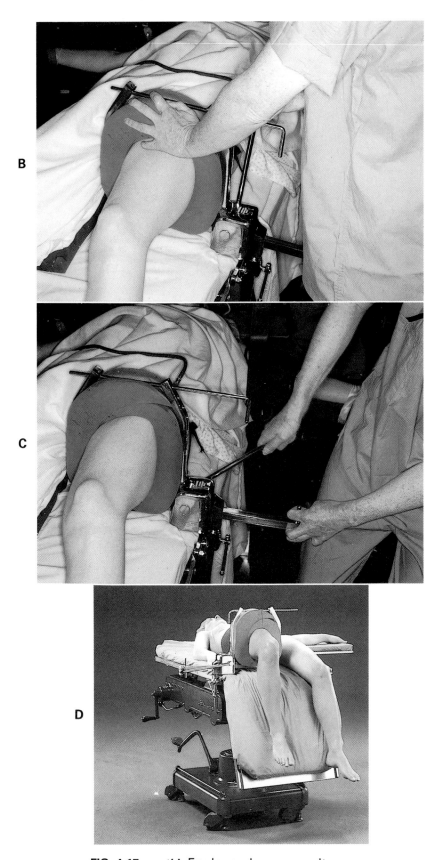

FIG. 4-17, cont'd. For legend see opposite page.

The Surgical Assistant is a valuable instrument. Next to the arthroscope it is most important in my arthroscopic surgical system. A patented locking mechanism on the Surgical Assistant provides safe, secure fixation. Screw mechanisms and ratchet mechanisms were tried before cam action and were considered potentially unsafe; there was no way to calibrate the pressure applied to the thigh. The Surgical Assistant with matching insert will not exceed 350 mm Hg of pressure (Fig. 4-17, B).

The Surgical Assistant is usually applied 6 inches above the superior aspect of the patella with the leg in extension. In some patients the thigh is too short to make that possible, and in some it is longer than necessary. A higher application results in rotation and compromises fixation.

Properly applied, the Surgical Assistant should give a quadrilateral shape to the thigh musculature (Fig. 4-17, C). This is accomplished by placing the transverse bar in the most superior slot. Traction is applied to the T-bar. The cam-action advancement mechanism assists the compression by pumping the lever. After a satisfactory compression, the quadrilateral shape is achieved. Depressing the bar secures the position (Fig. 4-17, D).

It is possible to view patellar tracking from the superomedial portal with the Surgical Assistant in place. This sometimes necessitates pushing the transverse bar to the lateral side to accommodate the arthroscope or AVD. The Surgical Assistant may limit direct viewing or with viewing direct television camera attachment. The surgeon's head may be blocked during direct viewing or the size of attached cameras limited by the thigh holder.

In an alternative application the Surgical Assistant is placed high on the thigh with the tourniquet distal. This removes the Surgical Assistant from the patellar area. In another method the tourniquet is applied in its normal position and the Surgical Assistant applied over the tourniquet. Neither of these methods has been reported to cause any neurovascular complications, but I have not found it necessary to use them on any knee case. The arthroscope attached to the AVD does not occupy the already limited space or cause any difficulty in viewing from above during lateral release or medial imbrication procedures.

The Surgical Assistant should not be applied for any longer than one would a pneumatic tourniquet. It does have a potential tourniquet effect of 350 mm Hg. There have been no neurovascular complications with adherence to the limited application time.

I had two incidences of a ruptured tibial collateral ligament in my early experience with the Surgical Assistant prototype (1978). Both patients were over 70 years of age, and both were treated with splint immobilization. These injuries healed without laxity. Since that time I have been more cautious in applying valgus stress in older patients.

In discussions with other surgeons about the use of this instrument, I learned that most apply far less pressure to the extremity than I do. This is a result of lack of experience and confidence. It takes time and experience to develop the feel and yet not push so hard as to injure ligamentous structures. Actually, the ligamentous structures are more likely to be torn or injured by quick stress rather than a continuous, slow, gentle pressure.

The Surgical Assistant allows for 1 or 2 mm greater opening of the knee. This is important in visualization of the posterior extremes from the anterior portals.

The mechanical Surgical Assistant does not move or become fatigued. Operating room personnel may appreciate this type of device more than the surgeon; it avoids the tiring job of holding the thigh.

Foam insert

The closed-cell foam inserts are washable and have excellent cleansability (see Fig. 4-17, *B* and *C*). Their durability has been proved to exceed more than 350 cases before deformation of the foam. They are not steam autoclavable; they enlarge and deform if they are subject to high temperatures. Some compression of the foam is possible, but it does not deform enough to interfere with its function.

The first application into the frame is critical for the foam insert. It should sit absolutely squarely in the metal brackets, and the crossbar should be perfectly centered as the compression is applied. Once the first compression is applied to the closed-cell foam, it will conform to the metallic frame and establish a memory. This prevents the foam from sliding one way or the other. If it is applied eccentrically, the foam insert will tend to slide out of the frame; this is why exact positioning is important. Minimal crossbar rotation can ensure exact centering during compression.

INFLOW-OUTFLOW SYSTEM

The fluid reservoir should be 6 liters of saline suspended at least 1 meter above the patient (Fig. 4-18, *A*). The plastic bag container permits manual squeezing of the bag for increased pressure. Rigid bottles or containers do not have the same advantage.

A weighted IV pole or other well-secured apparatus is necessary for safety with elevated reservoir (Fig. 4-18, *B*).

The inflow tubing is sterile and Y shaped to control separate flows. It is now available in 8-foot lengths. The longer tubing allows higher placement and displacement of the reservoir from the surgical field.

The inflow cannula is 4.2 mm inside diameter (Fig. 4-18, *C*). Two small holes at the end provide flow when the end of the cannula is unintentionally against the far wall of the joint. The cannulas with holes are fine for the knee joint, but not the other joints. The lack of space in other joints may back the cannula out of the joint. If so, extrasynovial leakage may occur through small side holes. I use cannulas without holes for joints other than the knee. There is a small adaptor for inflow tubing to the cannula to provide secure fit. Alternately, the inflow can be on the arthroscope. To facilitate placement of the tube, a small adaptor acts as an interface with the arthroscope spigot. Direct attachment of the tube to the arthroscope is not tight and results in leakage.

The suction outflow tubing attaches to the arthroscope during the diagnostic phase and to the motorized instruments during the operative phase. On occasion the suction tubing is attached directly to the cannula of the arthroscope to remove hemarthrosis or in knees with large loose bodies.

The outflow is via the arthroscope during the diagnostic phase and during surgery on activated motorized instrumentation (Fig. 4-19, *A*). Otherwise, arthroscopy is performed without continuous flow (see Chapter 6).

The suction tube connects to the collection bottle (Fig. 4-19, *B*). This is a

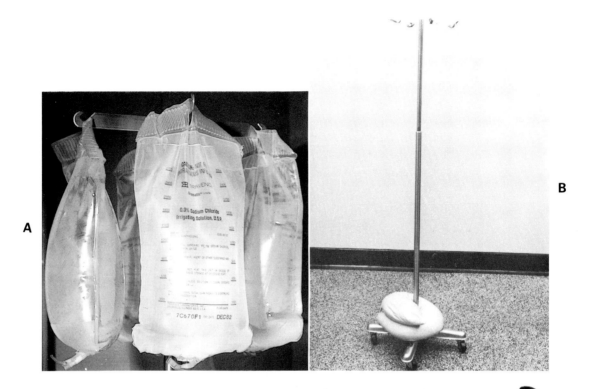

FIG. 4-18. Inflow system.

A Six liters of fluid suspended 1 meter above patient.

B Weighted IV pole secured with sandbag.

C Inflow cannulas, obturators, and tubing adaptor.

D Inflow adaptor on arthroscope permits direct attachment to arthroscope via Y-tubing.

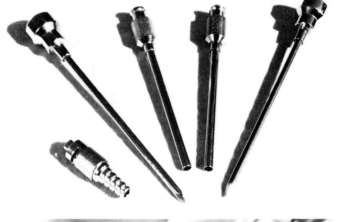

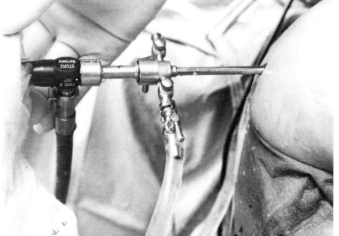

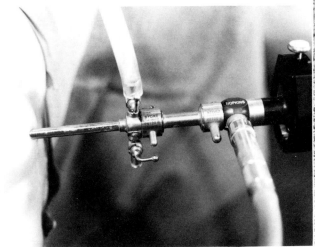

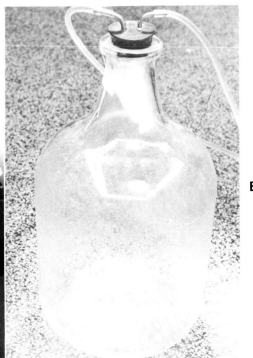

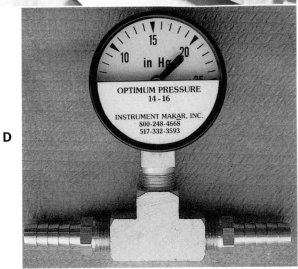

FIG. 4-19. Outflow system.

A Outflow on arthroscope during diagnostic phase.

B Large collection bottle accommodates even longest procedure and abundant fluid use. Collection bag is placed in top of suction bottle; thus decanting of all fluid is not necessary at end of procedure.

C Suction tube showing pieces of debrided articular material being removed from joint.

D Suction gauge placed in line near operative field.

large glass reservoir. A small cotton collection bag avoids the necessity of straining the entire collection of fluid for a specimen. The suction may be central or generated by machine in the operating room. Ingham Medical Center has a central system. It has been measured as 14 to 16 inches of mercury (40 cm Hg) in-line pressure. The Dyonics motorized instrumentation was calibrated on this pressure.

The suction pressure should be calibrated to a specific motorized system. The revolutions per minute, window size, and tubing diameter affect efficiency. If the motorized instruments used are other than Dyonics, the instruction manual should be checked for calibration.

The pressure is measured in-line as opposed to end-on (see Fig. 3-14). The end-on gives a closed-system measurement and an unrealistic peak pressure measurement results. The in-line pressure measures flow during actual conditions. A simple gauge is available for this calculation (Fig. 4-19, *D*).

Variations in pressure can be created by the second assistant clamping the outflow tube with intermittent manual pressure on the inflow reservoir. I have not seen a need for inflow pumps. If mechanical pressure is used, the intraarticular pressure should be monitored for safety. Some cases of compartment syndrome have occurred with mechanical pressure delivery of fluids.

CANNULA SYSTEM

The arthroscopic surgical system outlined in this textbook is predicated on the use of cannulas (see Fig. 4-18, *C*). The cannula system ensures joint penetration, not only initially but subsequently. It minimizes trauma with a single passage through the tissues. As much as possible, joint entries are made through the cannula to avoid any further trauma with probing, pushing, or channelization.

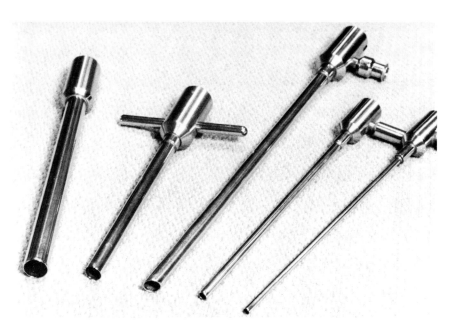

FIG. 4-20. Large operative cannulas for loose body removal. Cannulas vary in size from 8 mm (*left*) to 2 mm (*right*) OD. The latter holds a 1.7 mm Needlescope.

By design, the knife blades as well as the Dyonics ASS fit in and out through the cannula system. If there is any fracture of a blade, the cannula can be placed over the handle and the blade can be immediately removed. The cannula system may be interchangeable with the arthroscope cannula system.

There are two sizes of Dyonics cannulas: one accompanies the IASS, and the other accommodates the Arthroplasty System instrumentation. Each operative cannula comes with a sharp trochar and semisharp obturator. The sharp trochar is for skin and fascial penetration. The semisharp obturator is for joint entry. The appropriate size cannula is used depending on the surgical system to be employed.

The original calibration for the IASS was made with a 4.5 mm ID cannula. I routinely use this cannula to start cases by superomedial portal for inflow.

A cannula and obturator accompany the Ligamentous and Capsular Repair (LCR) system (see Fig. 4-51). This was intended for delivery of various metallic staples but can also be used for evacuation of loose bodies or debris. It is too large in diameter (1.3 cm OD) to place instruments and maintain joint distention.

Larger obturators and cannulas, up to 1 cm in size, are useful in removal of large loose bodies or multiple loose bodies of osteochondromatosis (Fig. 4-20).

The cannula system (2.7 mm OD) that accompanies the Needlescope may be used as auxiliary inflow in tight or isolated compartments for maximizing flow with motorized instrumentation.

Switching sticks

Switching sticks facilitate the interchange of cannulas of different sizes or lengths (Fig. 4-21) while securing position and avoiding further channelization or tissue trauma. Switching sticks are nothing more than two 9-inch rods, 4.0

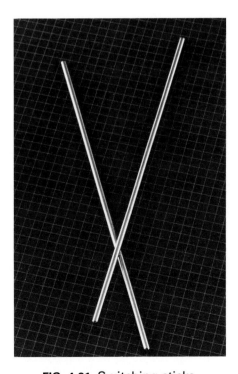

FIG. 4-21. Switching sticks.

mm OD. When the operative cannula is in one position and the arthroscope is in another, the instrumentation can be removed from the cannula and the switching stick inserted (see Fig. 6-87). The arthroscope is removed from its cannula system, which is a different shape, size, and length. A switching stick is placed in arthroscope cannula. The two switching sticks remain in the knee, looking very much like chopsticks. The cannulas are interchanged to their new positions over the switching sticks. The switching sticks are removed and replaced with the arthroscope and the instrument.

Wissinger rod

In securing the surgical exposure, especially in the shoulder or the elbow joints, I had previously visualized from one side of the joint and then by trial and error placed a No. 18 spinal needle from the opposite side of the joint. After entering the joint I attempted to place a cannula along the same course. This was not always an easy maneuver.

Dr. H. Andrew Wissinger, during a visit with me in East Lansing, Michigan, observed the shortcomings of this method. He recommended that the opposite portal be established from inside with a rod (Fig. 4-22).

The arthroscope and the cannula are placed against the desired point of entry on the far wall of the joint. The cannula is held in place and the scope

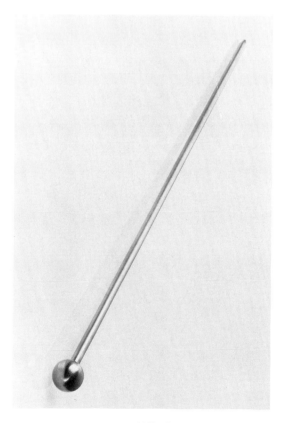

FIG. 4-22. Wissinger rod.

removed. A long obturator, the Wissinger rod, is placed down the arthroscope cannula and out in a retrograde fashion under the skin. The skin is incised. An operating cannula is placed over the rod and into the joint. The rod is removed, and the scope is replaced in its cannula. The instrument is then placed in the cannula. Proper opposite-side cannula position is thus facilitated. This method is used in the shoulder and elbow. The knee is not suitable anatomically for use of the Wissinger rod, and it is not necessary.

PALPATION INSTRUMENTS
No. 18 spinal needle

The instrument most commonly used to establish proper joint entry is the No. 18 spinal needle (Fig. 4-23, *A*). A 3-inch needle is used for the knee, elbow, and shoulder joints, and a 6-inch needle is used in the hip. X-ray control is necessary in the hip to determine location in deep tissues.

With minimal tissue disruption, the spinal needle locates a position on the skin for proper entry into the joint. The spinal needle can then be used for intraarticular palpation of the anticipated operative sites.

The No. 18 spinal needle can be the "third hand" in the joint. With both the arthroscope and instrument in a confined space, the spinal needle, if properly placed transcutaneously, can hold tissue up, down, out of the way, or in place without obstructing view or surgical manipulation. It is most useful in holding ends of anterior cruciate ligament out of the way during femoral notch preparation.

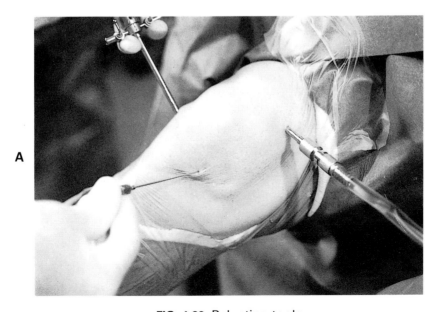

FIG. 4-23. Palpation tools.

A No. 18 spinal needle.
Continued.

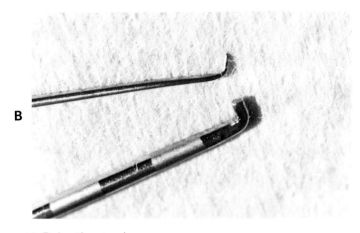

FIG. 4-23, cont'd. Palpation tools.

B Probes. Larger probe is Oretorp model, and smaller is special probe for arthroscopic surgery.

Probes

I prefer a probe without a fixed handle (Fig. 4-23, *B*). This allows passage through cannulas, so necessary in posterior compartments of the knee and at all times in joints other than the knee. The handle size is sufficient for holding. The pencil shape emphasizes fine tactile fingertip control. Introduction by cannula reduces tissue trauma. After entry, the cannula is removed from the probe to eliminate joint leakage. The cannula is then placed on the instrument table.

The probes can be either rigid or semimalleable. The rigid type is most commonly used. There may be a need for a semimalleable probe to reach certain areas not directly in line with the entry portal.

Two sizes of probes are necessary. The larger (2 mm) probe is most commonly used in the knee, and the smaller (1 mm) is used in the ankle joint or in small children.

Anodized black probes provide excellent visual contrast, especially if silver-metallic instruments are also in the visual field. Millimeter markings on the probe assist in estimation of anatomical or lesion size. The inflow cannula is convenient for palpation of the patellofemoral and suprapatellar areas (see Fig. 6-64).

A blunt obturator, with its larger size, may be best suited for palpation and manipulation of large defects or soft areas of articular cartilage (see Fig. 4-18, *C*).

GRASPING INSTRUMENTS
Miniature forceps

A miniature forceps can be placed through a 2 mm OD cannula, or even transcutaneously through a small puncture wound for biopsy of synovial membrane or articular cartilage (Fig. 4-24). It is possible to obtain a synovial specimen with the patient under local anesthesia using the sense of palpation alone; however, direct visualization is surer. The specimens are of adequate size for histological evaluation.

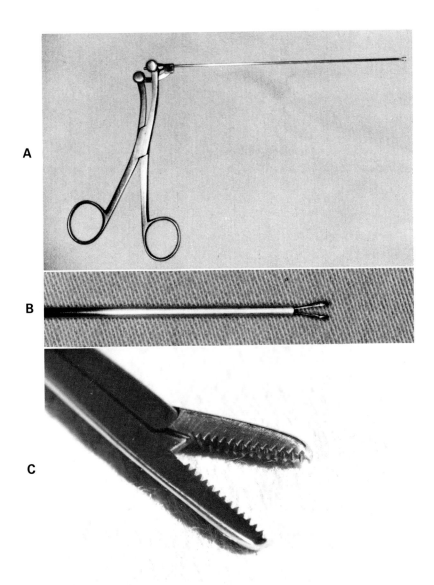

FIG. 4-24. Grasping forceps.

A Small biopsy forceps can be placed through 2 mm diameter cannula of Needle-scope. Biopsy can be done by a separate puncture under direct vision or blindly through existing puncture.

B Biting end of miniature biopsy forceps.

C Meniscal grabber.

Continued.

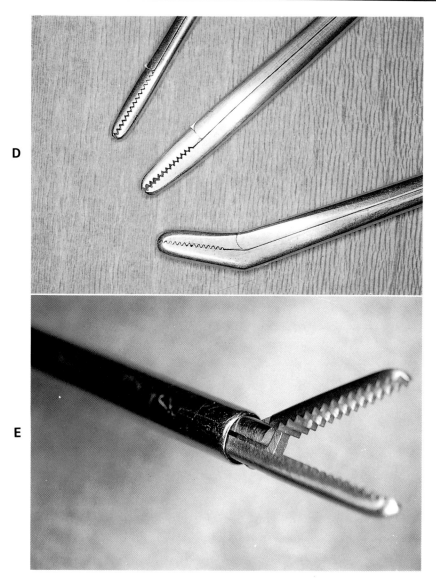

FIG. 4-24, cont'd. Grasping forceps.

D Various shapes and sizes.
E Small size passes through cannula.

The 2 mm forceps is used for intraarticular manipulation of suture for meniscal repair or grafting (see Fig. 4-50, *E*). It may be used as an adjunct in shoulder repair for pulling up glenohumeral ligaments for internal fixation. The superior approach through the supraspinatus muscle gives the proper approach.

Meniscal grasper

Kocher clamps were originally used as meniscus graspers. However, they tended to cut through the meniscus, and their size and shape was such that they caused injury to the articular cartilage.

Subsequently, a Schlissinger-type clamp was adapted from the neurosurgical instrumentation for arthroscopic surgery (Fig. 4-24, *C*). Two sizes are avail-

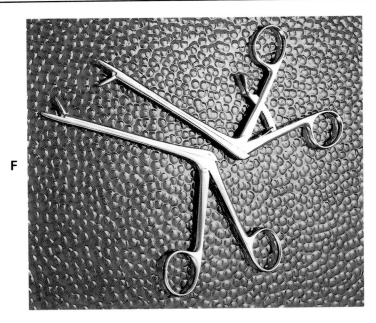

FIG. 4-24, cont'd

F Two styles: with and without rachet.

able: 3.1 × 5.5 mm and 3.3 × 3.5 mm. The larger is for routine grasping of meniscus or small, soft loose bodies. The smaller is for pieces in small spaces, that is, the posterior horn in a tight knee. Because of its size, forceful grasping of hard or large pieces will cause instrument breakage. This is especially so if rotation, angulation, and forceful traction are applied.

Breakage potential is less with the larger grasper. Breakage occurs at the pin, causing the grip to release. It is rare for the jaw of the grasper to fracture.

Two models are available, with and without a ratchet holding device (Fig. 4-24, *F*). I prefer the control and release of the plain model. In some cases, the security of grasping with the ratchet model may be an advantage.

A miniature Kocher-type clamp may be beneficial in tight areas with tenacious tissue (Fig. 4-25).

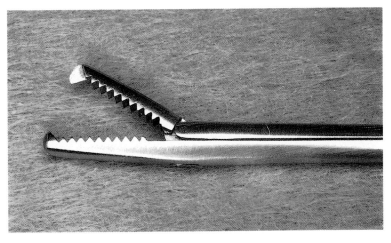

FIG. 4-25. Miniature Kocher-type clamp.

Loose body grasper

To accommodate the size of various loose bodies or foreign objects, pituitary forceps were modified with reverse teeth on the maxillary side and a cutout on the mandibular portion (Fig. 4-26). The reverse teeth reduce the chance of pinching the loose body out of the mechanism while grasping (the so-called watermelon-seed effect). The cutout on the mandibular jaw accommodates the configuration of the object. Because of its appearance and the popularity of the movie of the same name, the manufacturer chose to market this instrument under the name of Jaws.

There are two model sizes: 6.5 × 3.5 mm and 4.0 × 3.2 mm. The larger must be placed transcutaneously. The smaller has the advantage of being able to pass through the IASS cannula system; it is useful for multiple small objects. The small grasper is particularly effective within the posteromedial and lateral compartments of the knee or in other joints when cannula passage is mandatory.

A **B**

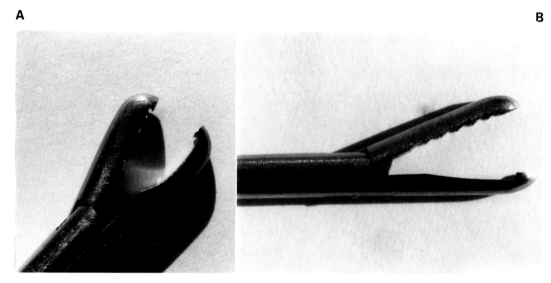

FIG. 4-26. Loose body graspers.

A Jaws modified pituitary forceps is excellent for removing loose bodies of rather large size, even with patient under local anesthesia. It is useful for grasping fragments of menisci that must be excised when patient requires general anesthesia.

B Reverse-tooth Jaws modified pituitary forceps. Notice reversed superior teeth, which guard against slippage of loose body. Scooped-out inferior portion of forceps holds oval-shaped foreign body. Jaws Jr., a smaller instrument, passes through an Intra-articular Shaver System cannula.

RETRIEVING INSTRUMENT
Golden Retriever

The Golden Retriever is a metallic tube (4.2 mm OD) with a powerful miniature magnet in one end (Fig. 4-27). It functions with both applied suction forces and magnetic power. It is anodized gold for rapid visual identification in an environment of silver instruments.

The Golden Retriever will be effective only if the broken instrument fragment has magnetic properties. This is why magnetic instruments are necessary in arthroscopic surgery.

The force of flow created by suction will mobilize a fragment and draw it into magnetic field. I have observed retrieval of pieces located out of sight in the remote recesses of the joint.

The suction tube applied to the end is purposely designed for a loose fit. If an adaptor is used to maximize suction, soft tissue often is drawn in between fragments and the magnet, interfering with attachment and retrieval. It was by design that the Golden Retriever cannot deliver suction as powerful as it would seem to be able to. In fact the suction should be removed the instant the metallic piece is close to the end of the tube to assure good contact without interposition of tissue.

The final retrieval of the fragment is accomplished by direct visualization (see Fig. 6-86). An IASS cannula is placed over the Golden Retriever. Under direct visualization, the fragment and Golden Retriever are removed through the IASS cannula system. The cannula is removed last.

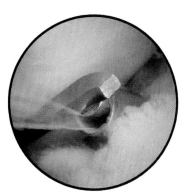

FIG. 4-27. Golden Retriever, a magnetized sucker for retrieval of magnetic, metallic loose fragments.

The surgeon absolutely should not retrieve a metallic fragment transcutaneously with any type of magnet, because the fragment could fall off outside the joint yet remain in the tissues, complicating removal.

CUTTING INSTRUMENTS
Knife blades

The knife blade has always been the traditional surgical means of tissue resection, and the same is so in arthroscopic surgery. However, the small confines of the arthroscopic environment necessitated the development of special sizes and shapes of knife blades (Figs. 4-28 to 4-30).

Originally I used the available disposable knife blades. These particular blades had a high incidence of fracture, especially along the stress risers of the numbers stamped on the blade. The use of these blades resulted in the conception and development of the Golden Retriever.

There was a need for sharp knife blades specifically designed for arthroscopic surgery. Obtaining them was not an easy matter. The market demand was not great enough in 1977 to attract the interest of manufacturers.

It became necessary to develop and produce blades specifically for arthroscopic surgery outside of the existing industry. My serendipitous acquaintance with a precision grinder, Mr. Ted Hill, resulted in the production of a series of knife blades specifically designed for arthroscopic surgery. Virtually all manufacturers have copied these designs.

An arthroscopic knife blade must be sharp and breakage resistant and have magnetic properties. The configuration of the cutting edge and shaft must be such that adjacent tissues are protected. The transition from cutting edge to shaft must be smooth to allow for gliding motion through capsular tissues. The knife must be deliverable by a cannula system; any knife blade placed blindly may cause tissue trauma. With separate passages, injury to the articular cartilage may occur. By use of a cannula, the blade is protected until it comes into view at the end of the cannula, the site of resection.

The Oretorp retractable blade provides a similar safety factor, but the blade is breakable. The shaft-blade junction is abrupt, which results in bumping or catching on tissues.

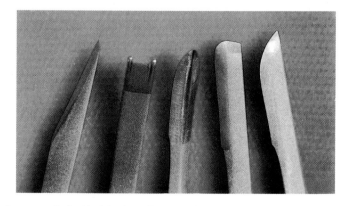

FIG. 4-28. Arthroscopic knife blades. From left to right 711, 747, 761, 764, and 767.

The first knife blades developed to meet arthroscopic specifications had the shapes of traditional blades. They were designated Instrument Makar (IM) blades 711, 747, 764, and 767 (see Fig. 4-28). The regular set blades are 3.4 mm in diameter and 23 mm long.

The IM 711 blade is used for cutting of skin and subcutaneous tissue for various portals. It may also be used for sectioning plica or fibrous bands.

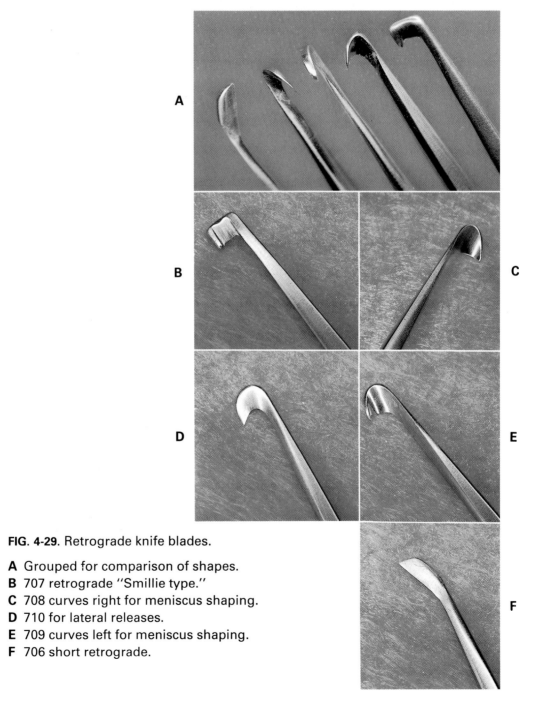

FIG. 4-29. Retrograde knife blades.

A Grouped for comparison of shapes.
B 707 retrograde "Smillie type."
C 708 curves right for meniscus shaping.
D 710 for lateral releases.
E 709 curves left for meniscus shaping.
F 706 short retrograde.

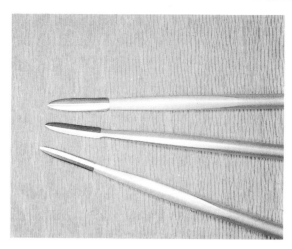

FIG. 4-30. Various sizes of 761 blades. Small sizes (mini 761s) are necessary for tight knees.

The IM 764 blade is used for meniscus cutting, especially of the posterior horn in a tight knee that will not accommodate the shape of a curved blade.

The IM 767 blade was used originally for lateral release. The technique was performed with both cutting and viewing from the medial side. With the retrograde method, the IM 710 blade has replaced the IM 767 for lateral release and medial imbrication procedures.

The IM 747 blade is a miniature Smillie-type blade with a slight curve that follows the condylar curve to the posterior meniscus horn. It has a protective guide on each side of the cutting edge.

None of the existing knives had the proper configuration for most arthroscopic meniscal resections, especially in the posterior horn. The convex surface of the femur is in the opposite plane of the meniscus incision. As a result, I developed a blade with a curvature that allowed passage past the condyle. It is semi-pointed and sharp at the tip, and there are cutting edges on both sides.

Once it is past the condyle, the tip is inserted into the meniscus (Fig. 11-28). The blade is rotated over 180 degrees. The tip points downward, as does the concave side. Cutting is performed in an oblique plane to preserve the triangular shape of the meniscus. The curvature of the blade permits transitional shaping of the posterior and anterior margins of resection.

Dr. Robert Hunter, during a visit from Minneapolis, named this the "banana blade." As the popularity of this knife grew, most companies advertised a banana blade. To date, none of the replicas have the sharpness, contours, or dimensions of the original. It is truly an arthroscopic surgical utility knife. It is called the 761 blade.

There were many requests for a retrograde blade set, but I did not see a need for it. However, after receiving a request from Dr. Richard Caspari of Richmond, Virginia, we designed five different retrograde blades of various sizes and shapes. My associates and I also used the blades and were surprised at their value. The 710 blade led to the retrograde method of lateral release. The diameter of the retrograde blades is 4.1 mm, and they are 23 mm in length.

The **706** is an inclined retrograde blade that is of limited usefulness (see Fig. 4-29, *F*). Other blades can perform the same functions it does. An occasional anterior horn tear has exactly the same configuration as this blade, making it the obvious choice.

The **707** is a reverse Smillie-type blade that permits retrograde cutting action yet has protective edges (see Fig. 4-29, *B*). It is used for the anterior horn of bucket-handle tears.

The **708** is a retrograde right-handed blade that has the point facing left and concave surface up (see Fig. 4-29, *C*). It is used to shape anterior horns. It is also good for extreme posterior compartment meniscal stumps when used with cannula protection to limit length of cutting stroke. It is also useful in shaping diskoid menisci.

The **709** is the mirror image of the 708 and has the same purpose. It has different cutting configurations for proper meniscus beveling in a given situation (see Fig. 4-29, *E*).

The **710** blade is a retrograde, biconcaved cutting surface that is sharp on the point (see Fig. 4-29, *D*). It is an integral part of lateral release and medial imbrication techniques. It is useful in section of adhesions and in quadricepsplasty.

Miniature knives

Because some knees are so tight, rotational cutting was not possible with the regular 761 blade (see Fig. 4-30). I designed two smaller blades of similar configuration. The shaft is the same 3.4 mm OD, but the tips are small enough for any posterior cutting without injury to the femoral or tibial condyle. They are used with the miniature grasper and 2.7 mm basket forceps in the tightest knees.

Because these blades are reusable, care must be taken in their handling during and between cases. The commonly used 761 and 710 blades are part of the routine set-up. They are held in separate slots in the plastic knife holder for protection. They are disinfected by cold methods between cases to reduce damage caused by jostling with other instruments in the autoclave. The less frequently used knives are individually wrapped and sterilized and held out of set-up. On request, they are unwrapped, used, and resterilized. With this method, sharpness and long blade life is assured. Each reusable blade is good for about 30 uses. Single-case use is a result of abuse of the edges.

Disposable blades

Since the time the original arthroscopic blades were designed, many have been adapted to disposable blades. The stress riser of the stamped number has been moved proximally. The objectionable abrupt junction between the handle and the blade itself was tapered with plastic. Occasional fracture of the plastic shafts has been reported, and retrieval of the fragments may be impeded by the nonmagnetic property of the plastic.

The main advantage of a disposable blade is its single-time use and sharpness. Per case, its actual cost is greater than the reusable blade.

The disadvantages of the disposable blades are their flatness and flexibility, which do not allow the meniscal penetration and the rotation that are so necessary in posterior compartment surgery. These blades are limited to cutting similar to that done with other flat blade configurations. They do not offer any specific arthroscopic surgical advantages. This is especially so of the disposable "banana blade."

Knife handles

The knife blade systems I recommend do not have fixed handles (Fig. 4-31). The rod shapes allow for the important cannula-delivery system. For the surgeon who desires to have a better grip for precision or power, knife handles can be attached. After the knife blades are passed through the cannula, the cannula is removed and a handle placed over the blade. With the large end down, a power grip can be achieved; with the small end down, a precision grip is possible. A lever with cam action provides locking. When cutting is complete, the cam action is released and the handle put back on the table. The cannula is passed over the knife blade and the knife blade removed. This method gives the surgeon the best of both worlds, power and precision. Handles are available for regular and retrograde blades.

Basket forceps

Basket forceps for arthroscopy have undergone a considerable evolutionary process (Fig. 4-32). They were the initial cutting instrument, borrowed from other endoscopic disciplines, to be used for resection of meniscal flaps or synovial plica. They have even been used in a rather primitive way for debridement of articular surfaces.

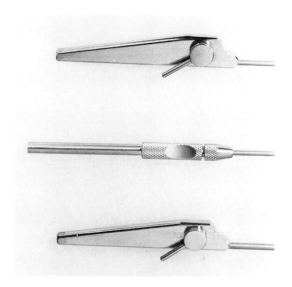

FIG. 4-31. Knife blade handles.

Because of its disadvantages the basket forceps has a lesser role in arthroscopy today. It must be passed without a cannula, and multiple passes injure the joint. Small fragments are left to obscure view or become free within the joint. The resection line is perpendicular, which fails to reproduce the normal triangular configuration of the meniscus. A knife and motorized instruments will do most jobs better, more cleanly, and faster than basket forceps. Nevertheless, there is a place for them in selected instances.

Basket forceps designs have advanced to create stronger, smaller instruments. They come in a multitude of shapes, sizes, angles, ups, downs, and arounds. Recently a forceps was introduced that incorporates suction. I believe most surgeons have complicated their surgical set-up enough with all the options available. The following are the features of basket forceps I have found useful. They should be small in size. The edges must be smooth and have no protruding parts. They must be strong and durable so they will cut well. A few properly selected basket forceps will do all jobs. I believe the basket forceps meets a perceived rather than a real need.

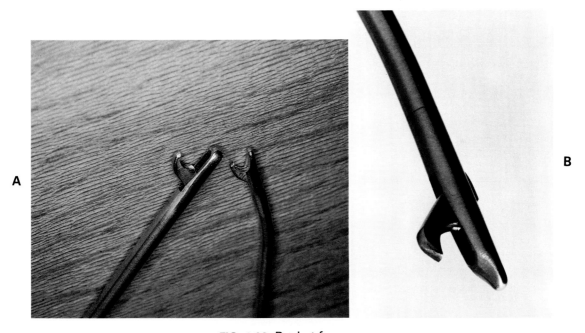

A

B

FIG. 4-32. Basket forceps.

A Curved and straight.
B Snowplow nose.

Variable axis system

The variable axis system provides various sizes and shapes of basket forceps and cutting instrumentation (Fig. 4-33, *A*). It allows cutting both right and left at various angles and with various sizes, without the added expense of having multiple handles. Cutting devices are interchangeable. The variable axis system also facilitates resharpening, because only the cutting devices need to be sent for maintenance.

I use two handles, each with most commonly used cutting shafts: the 2.7 mm angled and 3.5 mm with snowplow nose (see Fig. 4-33, *A*). Some may choose to routinely mount scissors; as a rule, I use basket forceps instead of scissors.

2.7 mm up-angle shaft, straight jaws

The 2.7 mm angled forceps has a contour that conforms to femoral condyle. (see Fig. 4-32). It reaches the posterior horn. It is small enough not to obstruct view and to selectively remove the upper or lower lip of a horizontal cleft tear. To my knowledge, George Shutt introduced this style, which is now marketed by many companies.

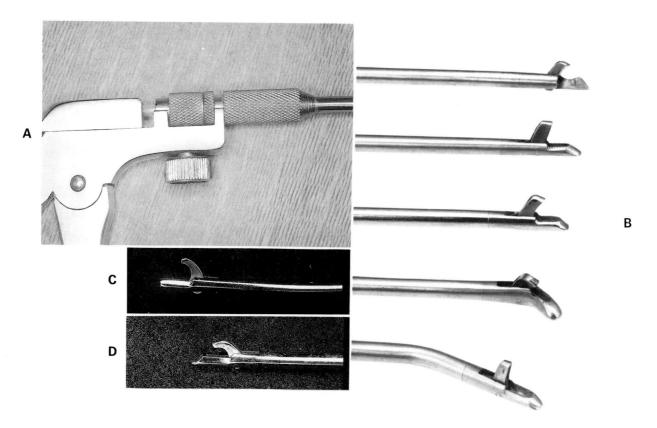

FIG. 4-33. Variable axis hand instrument system.

A Removable blade at handle.
B Various shapes, scissors, straight jaw, arc jaw, curved tip, curved shaft.
C Up-curved shaft, 2.7 mm, regular tip.
D Straight basket forceps, 2.7 mm, snowplow tip.

3.5 mm straight shaft, straight jaws

The 3.5 mm forceps is small enough to be used in most joints yet large enough to effect a meaningful bite (Fig. 4-34). It is especially useful if it is designed with a scooped nose to elevate the edge of the meniscus.

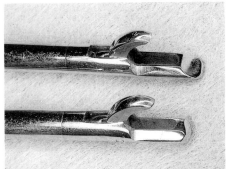

FIG. 4-34. 3.5 mm straight shaft, straight jaws.

5 mm straight shaft, 90-degree offset jaw

The right-angle punch has solved a problem in some people's hands, especially when used at the anterior horns of the meniscus (Fig. 4-35). Other basket forceps will not reach this area. The right-angle punch is easily controlled and visualized, effective, and sturdy.

A

FIG. 4-35. Straight shaft, 90-degree offset jaw.

A Close-up of 90-degree offset.
B Arthroscopic view of 90-degree offset on anterior horn of lateral meniscus.
C Jaws closed for cutting.
D Bite completed.

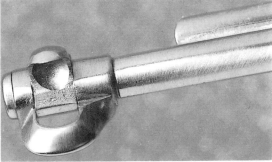

B
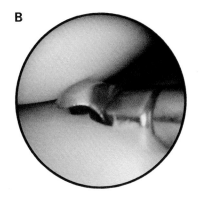

C
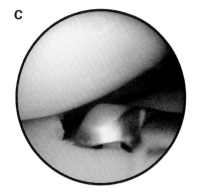

D
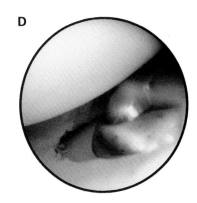

Other shapes and sizes

I have found little use for a greater variety of angles and shapes. It is expensive and unnecessary to have a shape and an angle for each and every bite. Surgical technique compensates for multiple-shaped tools, and a great variety of tools is not a substitute for good surgical technique.

Scissors

I have used a variety of scissors. Generally the durable scissors is too large, and others are too fragile. Until the variable axis scissors were available, I had not used scissors of any type beyond the trial stage. The variable axis scissors have proved to be both effective and durable (see Fig. 4-33, *B*). Their size and shape allow access to a variety of positions in the joint. They are sharp enough that the piece can be grasped and cut without a second instrument used to apply tension. No other scissors has this capability.

Curettes

Curettes are available in various sizes and shapes. The looped ones are particularly useful (Fig. 4-36, *A*). They are used to trim the edges of craters of articular cartilage. I use a standard 3 mm curette for biopsies (Fig. 4-36, *B*). An angled 3 mm curette has additionally been used as a probe in developing a space between the anterior cruciate pedicle and posterior cruciate ligament for semitendinosus graft.

Motorized drill and saw

Hand drills have traditionally consisted of a simple brace-and-bit system. I presently favor the Dyonics battery-powered motorized system. It is lightweight

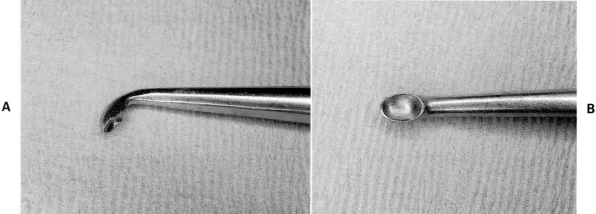

FIG. 4-36. Curettes.

A Angled curette.
B Regular curette.

and allows for Kirschner wire insertion and use of larger ($\frac{5}{16}$-inch) drill bits with good control and power. It is compact and easily maintained. There also is easy conversion to the oscillating saw system for combined procedures, such as osteotomy or tibial tubercle transplantation (Fig. 4-37).

Placement jigs

The advent of transcutaneous arthroscopically monitored anterior cruciate ligament grafting required proper insertion sites. Transcutaneous osseous drilling for surgical access to repair and placement sites demanded an instrument that could accurately and safely facilitate proper placement.

The simplest, most effective, and least expensive instrument for this purpose is Instrument Makar's Bow and Arrow (Fig. 4-38). The "bow" provides an arc for variable positioning. The "arrow" is not sharp and is designed for placement and removal through the arthroscope. The top of the arrow extends past the entry line to allow retraction of tissues for exposure and to prevent drilling past the tip (Fig. 4-38, C). Slight deviations in Kirschner wire direction may occur, but this system protects against missing the mark or passing-by out of sight. After the position of entry is established in the joint, the drill pin guide is placed at the other end of the bow. The arrow is designed so that the Kirschner wire will contact the cross-mark proximal to the tip. In other systems, the Kirschner wire meets the jig at a small tip. The sharp point of the drill guide is tapped into the bone to secure fixation (Fig. 4-38, D). The apparatus is tightened under tension. It still is necessary to hold the bow position, because no sharp point pene-

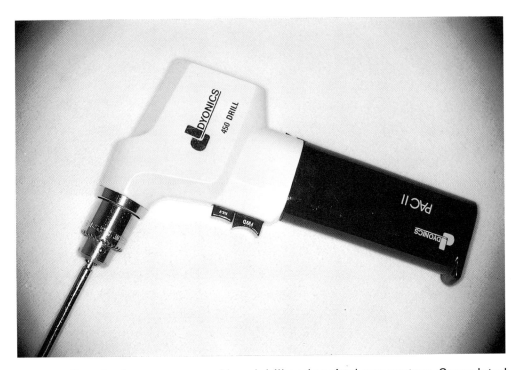

FIG. 4-37. Dyonics battery-powered hand drill and sagittal saw system. Cannulated drill is in place.

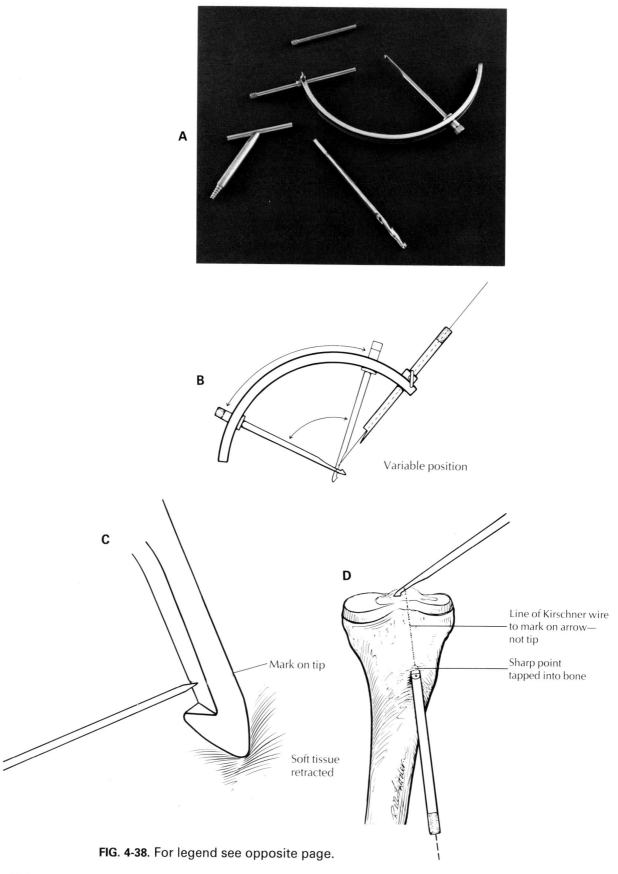

A

B

Variable position

C

Mark on tip

Soft tissue
retracted

D

Line of Kirschner wire
to mark on arrow—
not tip

Sharp point
tapped into bone

FIG. 4-38. For legend see opposite page.

trates the surface. The blunt point eliminates the chance of joint injury with placement. The Kirschner wire is placed through the drill guide until it is seen in the joint. The apparatus is then removed; the arrow first and then the bow and pin guide, leaving only the Kirschner wire. After proper placement is confirmed, a cannulated drill is placed over the Kirschner wire and the drill hole is completed (see Fig. 12-55). It may be used for either femoral or tibial graft insertion sites or for bone grafts in osteochondritis dissecans.

Other systems are available, including a geometrical system designed by Dr. James Fox of Thousand Oaks, California. This system, marketed by Dyonics, is based on the same arc principle; it is larger in construction and higher in price.

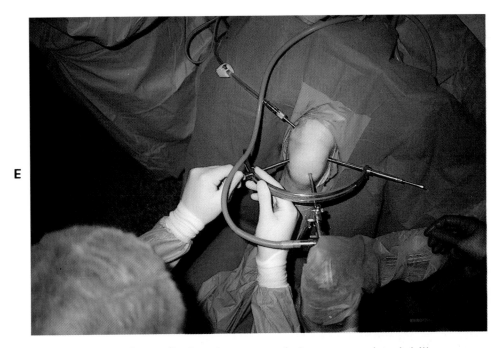

FIG. 4-38. Bow and Arrow jig for placement of pins or cannulated drills.

A Photograph of instruments.
B Variable positions of arrow on bow keeping Kirschner wire always at same point.
C Close-up of arrow tip shows line of contact not at tip. This protects from pass-bys.
D Arrow in place. Pin guide tapped into bone and ready for Kirschner wire delivery.
E Clinical use of Bow and Arrow jig.

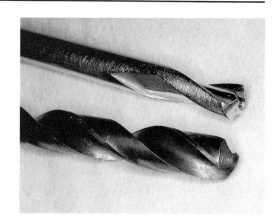

FIG. **4-39**. Drill bits; various sizes. Cannulated and solid shaft.

Drill bits

Various drill bit sizes are selected on the basis of operative requirements. Short-fluted drills are necessary for intraarticular work to avoid injury to adjacent tissues. A 1 mm diameter drill bit or even a Kirschner wire is used for drilling in osteochondritis dissecans. A drill bit of ⁵⁄₁₆-inch diameter is used for holes to secure anterior cruciate ligament grafts. Cannulated drill bits can be placed over preliminarily placed Kirschner wires. Specialized drill bits (Fig. 4-39) are used with cannulated screw sets and the Bow and Arrow system.

Tendon stripper

A tendon stripper was designed by Dr. Paul Brand for removing palmaris longus or plantaris tendon for hand surgical procedures. A shortened version (12 inches) provides a means of removing semitendinosus tendon for knee ligament repairs (Fig. 4-40).

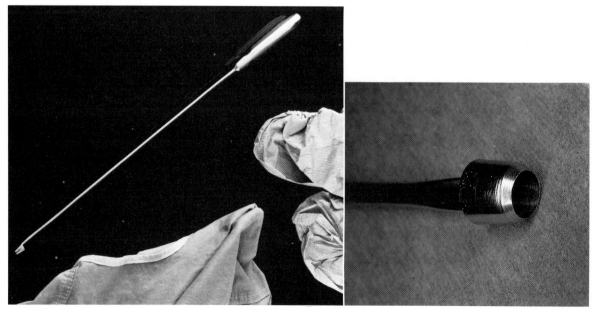

FIG. **4-40**. Tendon stripper.

Arthroscopic motorized instrumentation

Simultaneous resection and removal of tissue is best accomplished by motorized instrumentation. In 1975, in conjunction with engineers from Dyonics Corporation, a battery-powered electric motor–driven, rotating-cutting-suction device was developed. The first prototype consisted of two tubes, one inside the other and each with a terminal window. Another prototype with a side window "resected" the fuzz from a submerged peach in a laboratory environment. Suction carried the material away from the resection site.

The first case experience was with a battery-powered, hand-activated model (see Fig. 1-5). It worked, but the level of attention necessary to manipulate the instrument and compress the activator switch with the same hand resulted in fatigue. We then switched to the foot pedal as the means of activation and added a larger, more powerful motor.

A single-head cutting device and drain case attached to the motor by a threaded coupling. The single cutting head was bullet shaped for safety and strength, and the window was recessed from the tip. The initial model had serrated edges to the window by the manufacturer's initiative. This was removed later because of inadvertant articular scraping. This instrument became known as the Dyonics Intra-articular Shaver (Fig. 4-41) and was introduced commercially in December, 1976. Subsequently the drain case became a separate structure, permitting interchangeability of various cutting heads.

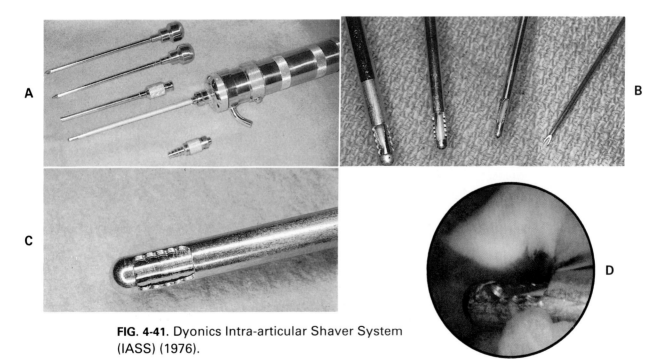

FIG. 4-41. Dyonics Intra-articular Shaver System (IASS) (1976).

A Motor, drive shaft, and cannula system.
B Various cutting heads with No. 18 spinal needle to right for reference.
C Close-up of original shaver head.
D Arthroscopic view of original shaver cutting synovium.

Continued.

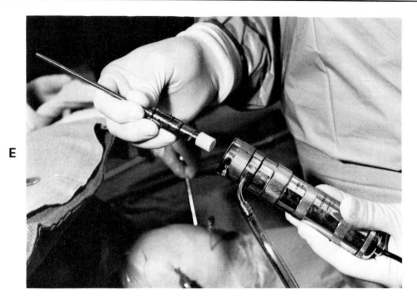

FIG. 4-41, cont'd

E Intra-articular Shaver System has quick release from the crankcase to accommodate interchangeable heads. Instruments are manufactured by Dyonics, Inc., Andover, Mass.

The second development in motorized instrumentation occurred in 1981 with the introduction of the Dyonics Arthroplasty System (Fig. 4-42). The model offered a larger motor with greater torque and more revolutions per minute. It facilitated synovectomy and osseous debridement as in abrasion arthroplasty. Various head sizes and configurations have since been developed.

In 1985 Dyonics introduced the third-generation motor for its system. It is called the Advanced Arthroscopic Surgical System (AASS) Model 85 (Fig. 4-43).

With this advance came a lighter, smaller, and more powerful motor. In addition, a single power source permits running both the IASS and Arthroplasty System as well as a miniaturized small joint system. The various interchangeable drain cases electronically select the proper central voltage for the drive system. Variable speed controls are available within a functional range for each system. The system eliminates the rotating side arm suction spigot of the previous drain case, resulting in less obstruction adjacent to the surgical site. The direct-line outflow to the rear of the instrument eliminates clogging and facilitates cleaning and maintenance. In accordance with the Dyonics Corporation's philosophy, this model does not antiquate existing products but does represent a significant technical advancement.

The small joint set extends the usefulness of the AASS to the elbow, ankle, wrist and finger joints (Fig. 4-44).

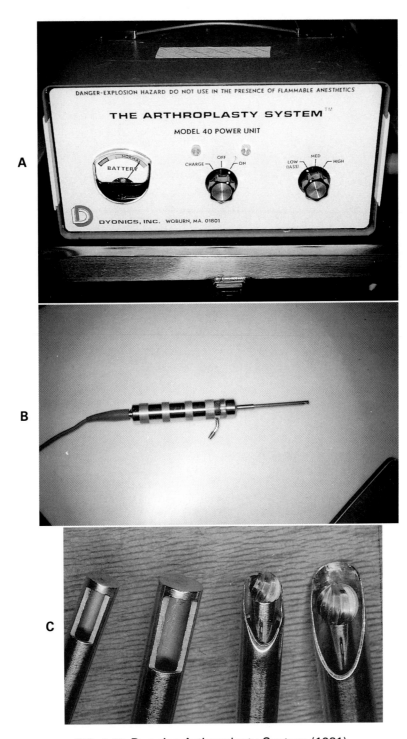

FIG. 4-42. Dyonics Arthroplasty System (1981).

A Battery power source.
B Motor was larger than that of IASS.
C Original synovial and abrading cutting heads.

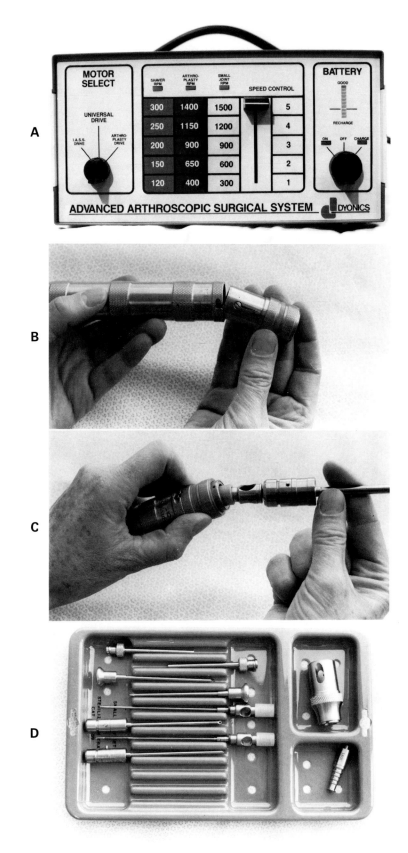

FIG. 4-43. Advanced Arthroscopic Surgical System (AASS) Model 85. **A,** Power source. **B,** Universal motor drive. **C,** Drain cases for various cutting heads electronically adjust rpm. **D,** Various cutting heads and adaptors.

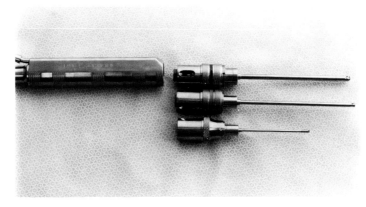

FIG. 4-44. Small joint accessory of AASS. Motor, drain case, and small cutting heads.

Cutting effectiveness

The surgeon often perceives that cutting effectiveness is related to fast rpm and sharp edges. Both ideas are wrong. The common perception is that faster is better. This is not always true. A variable-speed instrument is optimal.

The original IASS had below 100 rpm in a liquid medium. Gradually, as improvements in metallurgy developed, speed was increased above 100 rpm.

In general, the harder the tissue to be cut, the slower the rpm requirements; that is, there must be a time long enough with the window open for the material to enter. The reverse is true for soft pliable tissue, such as synovium. Over 1,000 rpm is required to avoid deep, unregulated resections. Faster speeds are required for resection of bone. Speed affects efficiency, but only when matched to tissue type.

The Dyonics system has a built-in stall mechanism for safety purposes. The calibrated stall avoids unnecessarily deep resection and provides a mechanism of control for surgeons at all levels of experience.

The cutting edges of the shaver and trimmer are ragged on microscopic inspection, like conventional scissors. The cutter has matched-angle sharp edges. Disposable cutting heads are a perceived need. I used my last cutter for 6 months and 300 cases. Even an abused cutter will cut bone or the end of the arthroscope if the window is open long enough for entry.

It should be pointed out that faster speeds, greater power (torque), and sharp blades alone do not make a faster operation. The surgeon's manipulation skill determines effectiveness.

There must be a balance of rpm, torque, flow, and cutting head selection for tissue type and surgical manipulation (see Chapter 6).

Various cutting attachments

IASS (Intra-articular Shaver System)

Shaver (3.0 and 4.5 mm) (Fig. 4-45, *A*). The bullet-nosed shaver head is commercially available but rarely used, because it is less effective at cutting than more recent configurations.

Cutter (3.5, 4.5, and 5.5 mm) (Fig. 4-45, *B*). The keyhole-shaped cutter was developed in 1978. This unique design provided a means of end and side cutting. Resection of tough meniscal tissue is possible. Resection of distally based flaps of articular cartilage and fibrous adhesions, even plica, are among its capabilities. The cutter will cut bone but is not intended for that purpose; therefore care must be taken not to injure normal articular cartilage.

Trimmer (3.5 and 4.5 mm) (Fig. 4-45, *C*). The trimmer was the first modification of the shaver head. It placed the window closer to the end of the tube. This provided more effective cutting with tipping-in of the end into the lesion. It was designed for debridement of degenerative articular cartilage and was used for synovectomy before the Arthroplasty System was developed.

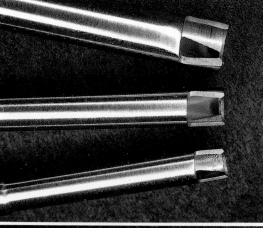
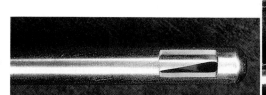
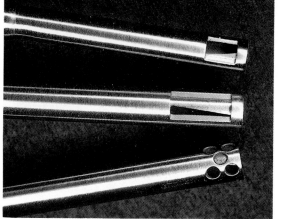

FIG. 4-45. Various cutting heads (AASS).

A Shaver, 4.5 mm.
B Cutters 3.5, 4.5, and 5.5 mm.
C *Top*, trimmers 3.5, 4.5 mm. *Bottom*, whisker 4.5 mm.

Whisker (4.5 mm) (see Fig. 4-45, *C*). The whisker was developed while trying to place a secondary portal opposite a prototype trimmer to enhance flow and avoid clogging. The problem was solved in another way on the trimmer head, but smaller material was observed to enter and be cut in the 1 mm hole.

A second design with several holes resulted in the whisker. This cutting head is more effective when attached to the Arthroplasty System with its faster speeds. It is used for small fragmentation.

Drill chuck and cannula (Fig. 4-45, *D*). The desire to drill small access holes in osteochondritic lesions resulted in adaptation of the Jacobs drill chuck to the IASS. A cannula with obturators allows transcutaneous access without tying up tissue. It also comes with the Arthroplasty System. The greater torque and higher speed of this system are advantageous.

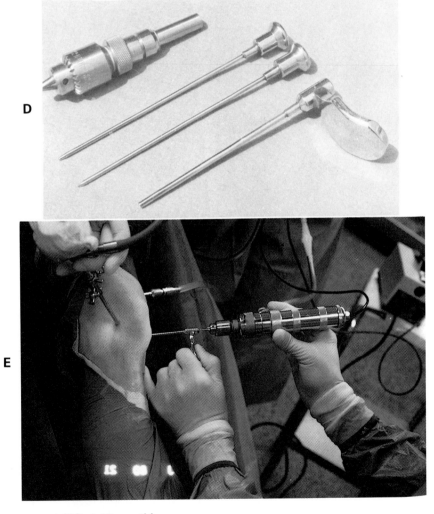

FIG. 4-45, cont'd

D Drill chuck and cannula.
E Clinical use of motorized drill chuck for pin position.

ARTHROPLASTY SYSTEM

Drill chuck and cannula. (Same design as IASS but couples to AAS.)

Regular synovial resector (4.5 and 5.5 mm) (Fig. 4-46). The trimmer design was adapted to the larger, faster system and is effective for synovectomy. It is more easily controlled and less aggressive than the full-radius model. It is safer when used adjacent to normal articular cartilage. It is effective on soft degenerative articular lesions.

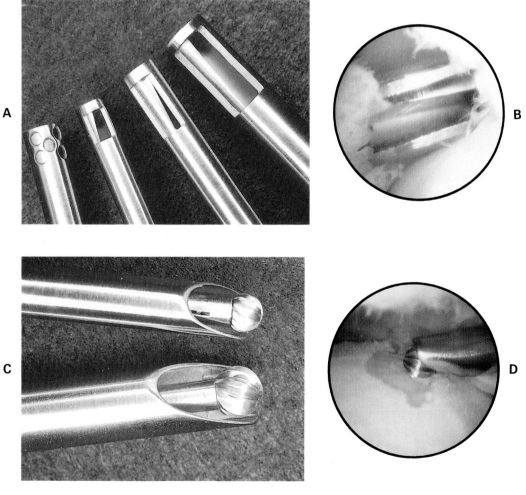

FIG. 4-46. Arthroplasty System

A Synovial resectors, regular shape.
B Arthroscopic view of synovial resector.
C Abraders in two sizes.
D Arthroscopic view of abrader.

Full-radius synovectomy blade (3.5 and 5.5 mm) (Fig. 4-47). Dr. Thomas Rosenberg introduced this design to Dyonics. It greatly enhanced the efficiency and aggressiveness for synovectomy. The head configuration permits cutting on the end as well as the side. It will cut normal articular cartilage, even cancellous bone. Therefore care must be taken even by an experienced arthroscopic surgeon.

Full-radius whisker blade (3.5 and 5.5 mm)(Fig. 4-47, *B*). This cutting head is best suited for faster speeds. It is especially well suited for removal of fine furry articular cartilage. It serves well as a final clean-up instrument, and it is particularly well suited for synovectomy of villae. It will spare the basement membrane and capsule. The removal of small metallic fragments without cutting other tissue is facilitated by the whisker.

The 3.5 mm is the instrument head of choice for small joint synovectomy. The smaller holes prevent decompression and joint collapse in small reservoir joints, that is, the elbow and ankle. It will not cut out of capsule, thereby protecting adjacent neurovascular structures.

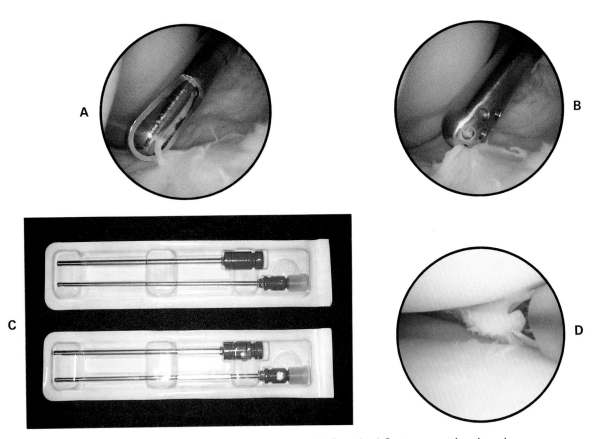

FIG. 4-47. Advanced Arthroscopic Surgical System cutting heads.

A Full-radius synovial resector.
B Synovial whisker.
C Disposable blades.
D Disposable cutter resecting meniscus.

Abrader (4.5 and 5.5 mm) (Fig. 4-46, *C*). This cutting head was designed to facilitate superficial debridement (1 to 2 mm) of exposed bony surfaces. It also serves to resect osteophytes and prepares bony sites for attachments necessary for arthroscopically monitored anterior cruciate ligament repair or grafting.

The 4.5 mm abrader passes through the cannula system. It is most useful when portals of shoulder joints are·interchanged, when a cannula approach is essential. The 5.5 mm abrader is more aggressive and effective. It is favored in the knee for abrasion, resection of osteophytes, and graft site preparation. Its size precludes cannula insertion. Careful transcutaneous placement is facilitated by pressure with gentle rotation.

Both abraders have a retractable shaft on the cutting burr (for pistoning) to avoid inadvertent deep cutting if excessive pressure is applied.

REPAIR AND RECONSTRUCTION INSTRUMENTS
Needles

Traditional surgical repairs are performed with needles. Transcutaneous suturing can be done arthroscopically. Repairs typically accomplished this way include meniscus tears and grafts and medial capsular imbrication procedures for patellar malalignment.

The No. 18 spinal needle is used to determine instrument placement site. It is also used for palpation and for holding intraarticular structures out of the way or in place as desired (Fig. 4-48, *A*). It occupies minimal space and does not obstruct viewing.

Free-hand surgical repairs for medial imbrication employ a curved cutting needle: the Anchor brand King ⅜-inch circle 1841-3¾-D (Fig. 4-48, *C*). The length and curve are sufficient to span the medial imbrication site. The same needle has been employed for meniscal repair.

A shorter curved needle has been used for transcutaneous tibial collateral ligament repair (see Fig. 14-48, *B*).

The smaller needle, ½-circle 1824-9D has been used for open meniscal and anterior cruciate ligament suturing (Fig. 4-48, *D*).

The straight Keith abdominal needle (1827 27-18D) is suitable for meniscus repair (Fig. 4-48, *E*). It also fits the straight Meniscus Mender.

Meniscus Mender

A variety of instruments exist for repair of meniscal tissue. They all are based on a similar principle, that of delivering a suture from inside to out. They are available in both straight and curved styles, both single and double barrel. This group of instruments has limitations for repairing posterior horn lesions; even the curved delivery systems have been the subject of reports of neurovascular injury or nerve entrapment.

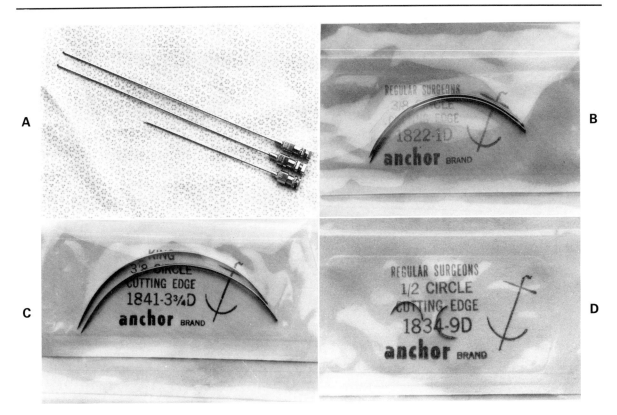

FIG. 4-48. Needles.

A No. 18 spinal needles in various lengths. Short for knee, longer for hip.
B 3/8-inch, 1822-ID circle for transcutaneous suturing.
C 3/8-inch 1841 3-3/4 for medial imbrication
D Smaller needle for transcutaneous ACL suturing

I designed a very safe, simple, single- and double-barrel system, the Meniscus Mender (Fig. 4-49). The needles are long enough to exit skin and still be visualized inside the knee. The delivery mechanism assures that 1 cm of needle remains visible in the knee, even if it is not identified from the outside. This prevents loss of the needle. When improperly placed or broken, the needle is magnetically retrievable.

The size of the delivery system barrels precludes extreme posterior approaches, thus avoiding neurovascular accidents. The size also permits a large needle, which reduces the chances of deformation, maltracking, or breakage. The design adheres to the adage, "Do no harm." The joint can always be opened for meniscal repair.

The single-barrel system provides for variability in site and width of suture placement (Fig. 4-49, *B*). The double-barrel model provides for single suture delivery simultaneously on two needles. This advantage is weighed against set distance between suture sites. Both systems use standard Keith needles and are musket- or retrograde-loaded.

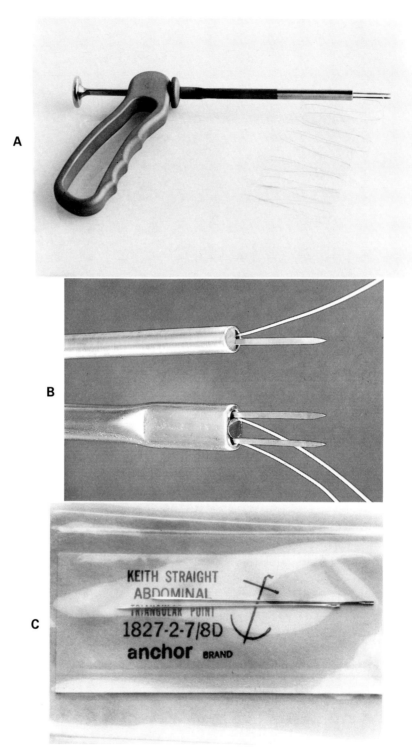

FIG. 4-49. Meniscus Mender I.

A Hand instrument for Keith needle delivery.
B Close-up of single barrel and double barrel.
C Keith needle.

Meniscus Mender II

Recently I have abandoned the inside-out technique for safer, faster, more flexible insertion methods using No. 18 spinal needles placed from the outside in. Modifications of various curvatures permit posterior repairs and capsular security.

I have employed a set of No. 18 spinal needles, a miniature self-spreading cable loop on metal stylet, and a miniature suture-holding forceps (Fig. 4-50).

The specifics of this technique are described in Chapter 11.

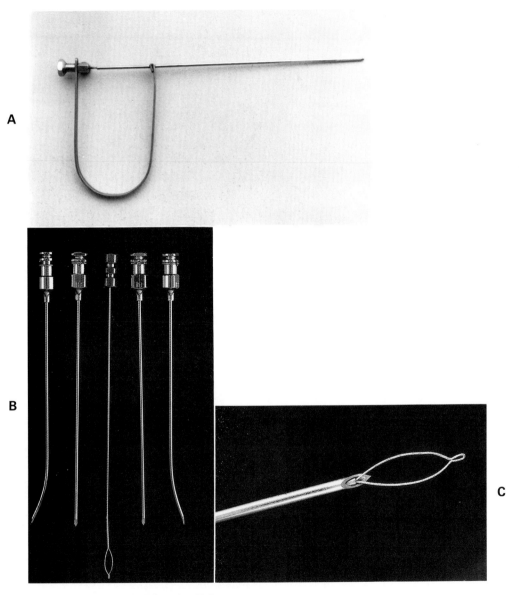

FIG. 4-50. Meniscus Mender II System.

A Hand instrument; suture grasper.
B Special curved needles with IM loop.
C Close-up of IM loop exiting No. 18 spinal needle.

The ligamentous and capsular repair (LCR) system

The LCR system was designed for arthroscopic reattachment of the torn anterior cruciate ligament (Fig. 4-51). It has been used to reattach the posterior cruciate ligament, reattach the medial retinaculum to the patella in dislocation, and in shoulder surgery to repair glenohumeral ligaments. Even biceps (long head) tendon stabilization has been performed arthroscopically.

The system consists of a cannula, an interlocking obturator, a driver-extractor and various sizes of staples (Fig. 4-51, B and C). The cannula is large enough to deliver any of the staples. After the staple is placed intraarticularly, the cannula is withdrawn and secured to the driver-extractor by a rotation and locking-screw mechanism. This avoids sliding of the cannula during impaction-extraction.

The driver-extractor has a built-in sliding hammer. This permits the surgeon to watch the staple placement on the television screen instead of watching the end of the driver, as with a separate mallet. To better control force, the built-in hammer avoids side or missed hits. Extraction is immediately available by reversing the directional force of the sliding hammer. There are threads at the distal end for staple attachment.

The staples are round for cannula insertion. They come in two styles (see Fig. 4-51, A) and diameters, 5.5 and 6.7 mm. The limbs have reverse-angled

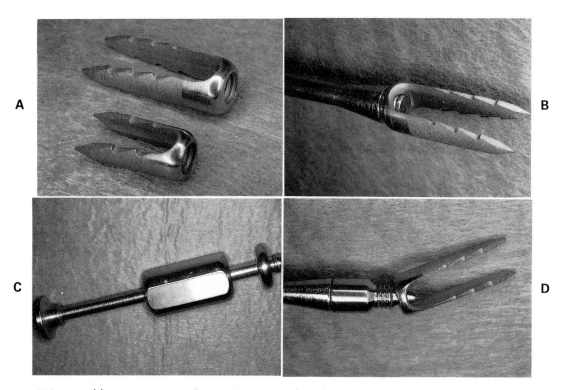

FIG. 4-51. Ligamentous and capsular repair (LCR) system

A Close-up of staples.
B Staple on driver-extractor.
C Close-up of cannula attached to driver and sliding hammer.
D Bullet-nose extractor tip.

teeth for securing to bone. The smaller staples are used in children and small adults; the larger staples are more commonly placed.

Recently the head has been rounded and reduced in size. This avoids compression on an anterior cruciate ligament pedicle graft with knee extension or protrusion on the glenoid.

The head and hips of the staples are shiny, and the legs are frosted. These landmarks allow the surgeon to gauge depth of insertion so that the limbs of the staples are adequately embedded in bone with space remaining in the crotch of the staple to house tissue. Otherwise, the gauging of depth would be inaccurate and complete insertion would cut through tissue held by the staple.

By design, the staples are malleable. This ensures direct placement without stressing the metal. Any rotational or angular stress applied to gain placement or to make something fit will fail. Placement must be into cancellous bone and along a direct line of impaction. Both compression and deviation of the staple limbs have been observed, because the metal conforms to rather than breaks through bone. In either event, no technical or clinical problem occurred with minor deformation of the staples. Subsequent extraction has not been a problem.

Major deformation, up to 90 degrees of angulation and 180 degrees of rotation of a limb of the staple, has not resulted in breakage. I am aware of two cases of fracture of the staple with more angulation and 180 degrees of rotation with continued impaction (hammering).

The metal has magnetic properties to facilitate retrieval if necessary, either broken or en toto. The metal is noncorrosive (Fig. 4-52).

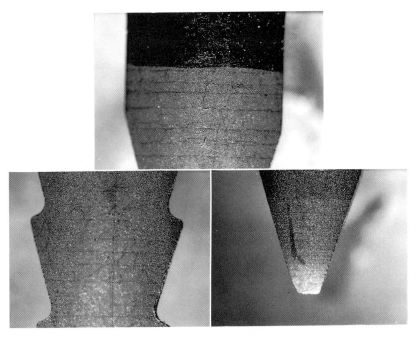

FIG. 4-52. Close-ups of IM staple implanted over 1 year earlier. No corrosion.

Routine extraction is facilitated by a softer metal, bullet-nosed staple remover (see Fig. 4-51, *D*). The shape allows the softer metal tip to enter and secure the staple to the extractor. The bullet-nosed staple remover is self-centering, even if the longitudinal axes of the extractor and staple are not aligned. It was not intended for insertion or implantation.

Cannulated screw sets

Transcutaneous arthroscopically monitored reduction-internal fixation of bone fragments is technically challenging (Fig. 4-53).

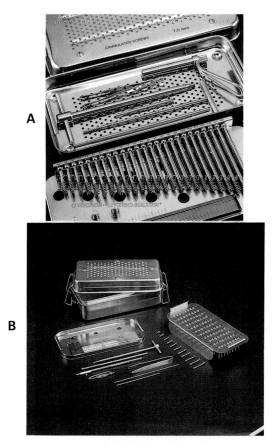

FIG. 4-53. Cannulated screw set.

A Large size for tibial plateau fractures.
B Small set for osteochondritis dessicans.

A cannulated screw set facilitates this type of surgical procedure. The fragments are reduced, and the guide pin holds the reduction (Fig. 4-54). This pin maintains reduction during drilling, tapping, and screw fixation. After reduction and internal fixation the guide pin is removed.

Gradations in size and length are available: large, 40 to 130 mm in 5 mm gradations; and miniature, 10 to 30 mm in 2 mm gradations.

Washers are available for a compression effect.

Large cannulated screw sets are used in femoral and tibial condylar fractures. The miniature set is used for osteochondritis dissecans.

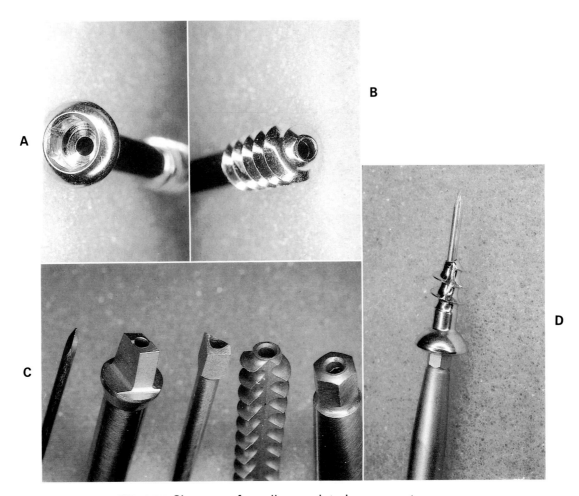

FIG. 4-54. Close-up of small cannulated screw system.

A Head of screw.
B End of screw with cancellous threads.
C *Left to right:* guide pin, countersink, drill, tap, screwdriver.
D Screw on screwdriver over guide pin.

ORGANIZATION OF INSTRUMENTATION

The organization of arthroscopic instrumentation can be considered along with the general groupings; that is, image transmission; probing; cutting, hand and motorized; and repair. Choices in each category will fit the existing budget and the surgeon's training, surgical system, and technical dexterity.

After instrumentation is procured, organization should include preoperative, operative, and postoperative placement and care. Instruments should be assigned the same place, pattern, and alignment for each case. This avoids unnecessary searches and delays. Organization maps will help different personnel participate properly (see Chapter 3).

CARE OF INSTRUMENTATION

Arthroscopic instruments are expensive, and they are more fragile than standard orthopedic instruments (Fig. 4-55). Proper care of instruments must be observed at all times. Besides obvious breakage related to dropping or excessive bending, injury can occur during clean-up, take-down, scrubbing, sorting, and packaging. Continuous educational efforts must be made to minimize breakage and maximize efficiency. The entire staff must take an interest, but the leadership must be by the surgeon's example.

It seems highly unlikely that a person who was not interested in arthroscopic surgery or a person on a rotational basis could take the kind of care of the arthroscopic surgical instruments, the video equipment, the suction and flows, and so on, that is necessary for this type of work.

If there is no one assigned to this activity at an institution, the surgeon can anticipate the care of the instruments to be unsuccessful. The cost of either repairing or replacing surgical instrumentation will be exceedingly high and unnecessary. It would be worth that dollar savings to have a team or an interested person to care for the instrumentation. I own my instruments, and only one person cares for them interoperatively and stores them between surgical dates.

STERILIZATION AND DISINFECTION

All metallic instrumentation may be steam autoclaved, as may as most light guides. Arthroscopes deteriorate with steam autoclaving, even the ones that are advertised as being autoclaveable. It shortens the life of the scope by deterioration of the lens sealants. Ethylene oxide gas sterilization is preferred. As a practical matter, disinfection by cold soaking in activated glutaraldehyde is clinically safer (See Chapter 3).

Cold soaking is also used for motors to avoid the time necessary for the motor cool down for comfortable handling after autoclaving. Hand-held television cameras are treated in the same manner or covered with sterile plastic. Knife blades are soaked in plastic containers to minimize handling injury, although they can be steam autoclaved.

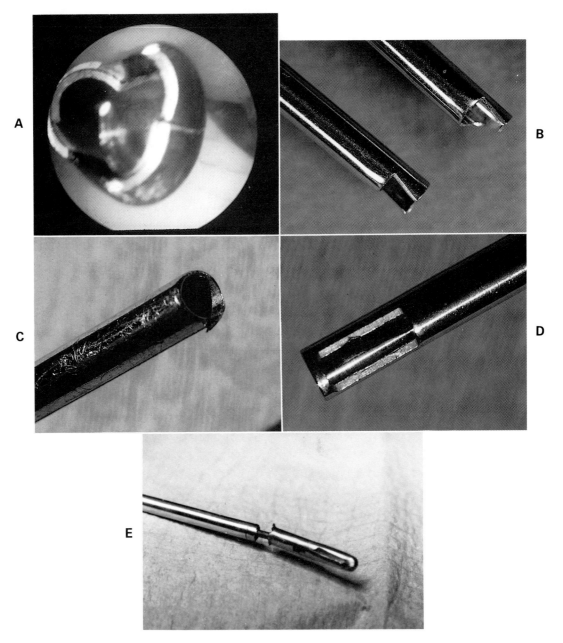

FIG. 4-55. Instrument breakage.

A Broken cutter tip in early model.
B Fragment broken off inner rotating tube.
C Metal cut off tip of arthroscope cannula.
D Synovial resector with notch in edge after cutting cannula shown in **C**.
E Broken forceps.

VARIOUS ENERGY SOURCES
High-speed motor

The Midas Rex arthroscopic motorized instrumentation is a high-speed cutting device with a speed greater than 10,000 rpm. It was adapted from air-powered instrumentation for cement and bone resection. I have used it only in the laboratory. It is my opinion that the size, shape, contour, and concept were not, at the time of my observation, acceptable for the field of arthroscopic surgery.

I have also had an opportunity to watch videotapes of clinical cases performed with the Midas Rex. It was my opinion that the frequency of intraarticular cartilage injury depicted in those videotapes would not be acceptable in clinical practice. In its developmental state, it cannot be recommended for clinical use.

Recently Acufux introduced a high-speed auger and cutting design in conjunction with Dr. Richard Caspari. Dyonics offers a similar high-speed cutter called Turbo. The design and speed are aggressive in cutting meniscus or other tissue it touches as well. Clogging has been a problem. Turbulence may cause a momentary loss of visualization of the resection site. Control of resection requires a careful hand.

The introduction of these high-powered, aggressive meniscal resectors comes at a time in which emphasis is on preservation of tissue and meniscus repair.

Electrothermal

Electrothermal instrumentation was developed in response to cases of hemarthrosis following a certain technique of lateral release. Lateral release techniques employed a posterior incision near the lateral intermuscular septum in an area of maximum vessel size. More bleeding occurred than if the procedure were done as I have outlined in this textbook (see Chapter 10).

At any rate, bleeding is still a problem and hemostasis is a basic surgical principle. In my opinion the electrothermal method offers one major advantage, the opportunity to achieve hemostasis by electrocoagulation. However, I believe this advantage is outweighed by the disadvantages. These involve the cost ($3,500), the single use of the system, the slower technique as compared to cutting with a knife blade, and the requirement of sterile water rather than saline as a medium. The disadvantage of the sterile water is that it has the postoperative potential, if it dissects into the thigh area, to cause considerable discomfort. Postoperative pain has resulted in anklyosis after this lateral release technique. McGinty has used CO_2 medium.

The instrument is in the developmental stage for resection of menisci. I believe laboratory and clinical studies should demonstrate containment of the energy source at the end and avoidance of injury to the adjacent articular tissues. It is not sufficient to resect the meniscus and demonstrate that the articular cartilage is not injured at a particular time. The energy source is not unidirectional but in a form that looks very much like the mushroom of an explosion around the end of the tip. It is not limited just to the tip or directed away from the tip. The articular cartilage, being a tissue of low metabolism, does not respond to contusion or laceration for up to 1 year. Studies should involve histological studies in the laboratory and second-look arthroscopy clinically to prove the safety of electrothermal instrumentation.

My last objection is that most of these procedures can be done more effectively and with less risk by mechanical methods.

Laser

Drs. Terry Whipple and Dick Caspari have done considerable animal studies with lasers. They have demonstrated the tissue response as well as many technical difficulties. The least of these is loss of the sense of palpation, which is so vital to a surgeon, as well as the sense of direction or depth of the energy cut. Smoke or debris has to be washed out separately.

My discussion with Dr. James Smith of Seattle, the only person to my knowledge who has done human work with lasers, indicates that the procedure is laborious; approximately 1½ hours are required for procedures that otherwise take a few minutes. Laser arthroscopic surgery is still in the early developmental stage as of this writing, and it is certainly experimental for human use. Smith recently placed a moratorium on his series to await adequate follow-up.

Cryosurgery

Cryosurgery has not been of practical value in resecting tissue or effecting hemostasis.

REFERENCES

1. Crow, S., et al.: Disinfection or sterilization? Four views on arthroscopes, AORN J. **37**:854, 862, 1983.
2. Johnson, L.L.: Needlescope. In American Academy of Orthopaedic Surgeons Symposium on arthroscopy and arthrography of the knee, St. Louis, 1978, The C.V. Mosby Co.
3. Johnson, L.L., et al.: Cold sterilization method for arthroscopes using activated dialdehyde, Orthop. Rev. **6**:75, 1977.
4. Johnson, L.L., et al.: Two percent glutaraldehyde: a disinfectant in arthroscopy and arthroscopic surgery, J. Bone Joint Surg. **64A**:237, 1982.
5. McGinty, J.A.: personal communication, 1983.
6. Prescott, R.: Optical principles of endoscopy. J. Med. Primatol. **5**:133, 1976.
7. Prescott, R.: Optical design and care of the endoscope. In American Academy of Orthopaedic Surgeons Symposium on arthroscopy and arthrography of the knee, St. Louis, 1978, The C.V. Mosby Co.
8. Smith, J.A.: Personal communication, 1983.
9. Stearns, C.M.: Preparation of arthroscopic instrumentation: the sterilization vs. disinfection controversy, Orthop. Nurs. **2**:38, 1983.
10. Takagi, K.: The classic arthroscope (from J. Jap. Orthop. Asoc. 1939), Clin. Orthop. **167**:6 1982.
11. Whipple, T.L., Caspari, R.B., and Myers, J.F.: Arthroscopic laser meniscectomy in a gas medium, Arthroscopy **1**:2-7, 1985.

Documentation

Documentation is an important and integral dimension of arthroscopic surgery. The diagnostic observations are detailed because of the thoroughness of the examination and the magnification factor. The operative work is exacting, with many precise maneuvers. Recall of details would be incomplete and of little value.

A description of the surgical findings and procedure should be documented immediately after every arthroscopic procedure. Experience has shown that any lapse of time between the end of a procedure and documentation of the findings (i.e., for the performance of another arthroscopic examination) results in diminished recall. Therefore a dictated or computer-generated operative report should be completed immediately following the procedure, before telephone calls, before patient discharge, and before extraneous conversation.

Often there is a planned interval between the diagnostic arthroscopic evaluation and the time of definitive surgery, and some details can be forgotten. It is important to record not only the findings but also the recommendation for the future surgical plan. This way the report will be available at the time of the anticipated surgical intervention, which is especially important if the surgery is to be performed by someone other than the diagnostic arthroscopist.

HANDWRITTEN CHART NOTES

The patient's hospital chart should indicate that the patient has had an operation and by what means, by what surgeon, assistants, and anesthesiologist, and by what type of anesthetic. The main features should be handwritten in the hospital record for immediate reference by the nursing staff and/or by others in case of emergency. It should include the date, the postoperative diagnosis, and the patient's health status at the conclusion of the procedure. It can also be helpful to include some information in the patient's office or clinic record in case of lost dictation.

DICTATED NARRATIVE

The dictated narrative entered on the patient's record should include a medical history and the findings at physical examination. Prearthroscopic and postarthroscopic diagnoses are documented (see box on pp. 248-249). The procedure should always be recorded in a routine manner regardless of how it may have been accomplished technically. The different compartments of the knee joint should always be dictated in the same order and separated into paragraphs. It is also important to mention the approach used in entering each compartments (e.g., "Transcondylar posteromedial through the utility approach" or "transcutaneous posteromedial approach"). If a compartment is not inspected, this should be indicated.

Patellar and suprapatellar pouch findings are usually recorded first because this area is examined first. In patients with tight, fat, or scarred knees, complete inspection under the patella may not be possible from the initial anteromedial puncture, and the area will need to be inspected later by a suprapatellar portal. Still, the findings in this area are recorded first on the dictated narrative.

The next paragraph usually describes the anterolateral compartment, its meniscal tissue, and its articular surfaces.

Findings in the intercondylar notch are described in the next paragraph, including the status of the fat pad and the ligamentum mucosa. The results of inspection of the anterior and posterior cruciate ligaments should be described and the presence or absence of loose bodies and osteophytes recorded.

Documentation of the anteromedial compartment should include the findings of the articular surface and the meniscal tissue examination.

Findings in the posteromedial compartment include those of the articular surface and the meniscus, as well as the presence of loose bodies or synovitis. The status of the posterior cruciate ligament can be described. A Baker's cyst may also have been seen.

Recorded findings of the posterolateral compartment should include the sta-

EXAMPLE OF DICTATED NARRATIVE: DIAGNOSTIC ARTHROSCOPY

The patient is a 28-year-old white man who has had previous medial and lateral meniscectomies, with attenuation of the anterior cruciate ligament. He has catching and pain on the outer aspect of the right knee in spite of lateral meniscectomy. Arthrography does not show any specific abnormality.

Physical examination shows a stable patella and a relatively stable knee, with moderate evidence of anterior cruciate laxity demonstrated by positive lateral pivot shift, Lachman test, and neutral Slocum test. There is some crepitus over the lateral joint line in the lateral femoral condyle, but no acute tenderness, heat, or effusion.

Clinical diagnosis

Status postoperative medial and lateral meniscectomies, right knee: tear in anterior cruciate ligament. Moderate instability.

Preoperative diagnosis

Status postoperative medial and lateral meniscectomies: tear in anterior cruciate ligament; degenerative arthritis in lateral compartment.

Postoperative diagnosis

1. Posterior horn remnant of lateral meniscus
2. Degenerative arthritis, moderately severe, in lateral femoral condyle
3. Status postoperative medial meniscectomy
4. Attenuated anterior cruciate ligament

Procedure

The patient was placed on a regular table. A tourniquet was placed high on the right thigh. The entire right knee was prepared with Betadine and sterilely draped to expose the area.

Plain lidocaine 1% was injected into the infrapatellar fat pad and the infrapatellar branch of the saphenous nerve. A sharp and then a blunt trocar were placed in the joint, and the joint was distended with saline.

The undersurface of the patella was seen and found to be smooth. There is mild synovitis of the joint. Minimal stardusting was vacuumed out of the joint.

The lateral compartment shows diffuse degenerative articular changes, chunky and fibrillar in nature.

The lateral meniscus is rather prominent near the area of the posterior horn and showed some adjacent tibial condylar fibrillation.

The intercondylar notch shows an attenuated anterior cruciate ligament off femur, attached to posterior cruciate.

The medial compartment shows a small regenerated meniscus and no articular injury.

EXAMPLE OF DICTATED NARRATIVE: DIAGNOSTIC ARTHROSCOPY—cont'd

A separate posteromedial puncture shows only a minimal remnant of the posterior meniscus, with no separation.

A separate posterolateral puncture shows a rather large posterior lateral meniscus. The meniscus was palpated and popped back and forth. The patient feels that this duplicates his symptoms of instability in the lateral joint line.

The fluid and equipment were removed. A sterile dressing was applied, and the patient was taken to the recovery room in good condition.

Recommendations

I would recommend that the posterior horn of the lateral meniscus be removed. Some shaving of the lateral femoral condyle might be in order. Reconstructive surgery is indicated for the ACL. The patient should be told that the prognosis is not good because of the presence of degenerative lateral compartment disease.

---

tus of the synovium, any loose bodies, and the meniscus, its attachments, the popliteus tendon, and articular surfaces.

When looking down either the medial and lateral gutters for the presence of loose bodies, a check can be made of the meniscal attachments. Attention can also be given to the plicae, and these findings should be recorded.

Technical problems should be documented as should the completeness of the examination. The mechanical tightness inherent in the knee or any difficulty encountered in visualizing a particular part are important dimensions to identify. Areas that were not visualized should be reported as such and should not be considered a failure of the technique. A physical limitation to visualization may exist and would be important to report.

The narrative is finished with recommendations.

WORKSHEETS AND DIAGRAMS

For patients undergoing a diagnostic arthroscopy performed for another orthopedic surgeon, the use of a worksheet can be helpful (Fig. 5-1). The top copy provides a record that can be placed in an envelope and accompany the patient on his return visit to the referring physician, eliminating delays in communication. Often the typewritten copy is not available when the patient returns to the referring physician's office. This method provides the physician with the information needed to have an intelligent discussion with the patient. The undersheet is a copy of NCR paper that becomes a part of the office or clinic chart.

Diagrams, charts, or drawings can be helpful, especially early in the arthroscopic experience (Fig. 5-2). Familiarity with arthroscopic descriptions can diminish the need for diagrams. Diagrams can be either drawn freehand, premade, or borrowed from someone else. Filling in blanks speeds documentation. More definite illustration of findings can be added, including the findings from the posteromedial and posterolateral compartments.

Arthroscopy: dictated report to follow

Name _____   Office # _____   Date _____

Referring doctor _____   Age _____ Race _____ Sex _____

R   L   Hip   Knee   Ankle   Shoulder   Elbow   Wrist   Finger

Onset: _____   How: _____   When: _____   Where: _____

Complaints	Site	Physical exam		X-ray
Pain	Antero	Normal	Warm	Normal
Crepitus		Obese	Patellar	Narrowing
Catching	Medial	ROM	Pain	Osteochondritis
Locking		Incision	Crepitus	Patellar defect
Swelling	Lateral	Instability	Instability	Loose body
Heat		Tibia vara	Dislocation	Calcification
Instability	Postero	Genu valgum	Pain w/ push	Fracture
Giving out		Tender	Pain w/ contr.	Arthrogram
Popping	Patellar	Swollen		
Numbness		Positive McMurray		

Surgery: _____

Anesthesia: Local   General   Spinal   IV regional   Apprehensive   Relaxed
_____

Pre-op DX _____

Post-op DX _____

Findings:
Patella _____

Suprapatellar pouch _____

A-L _____

ICN _____

A-M _____

P-M _____

P-L _____

Alternate
puncture _____

Therapeutic: Loose bodies   Lavage   Forceps   Removal   Section plica   Biopsy
                Intraarticular shaving   Patella   Condyles   Meniscectomy
Recommendations: _____

Lanny L. Johnson, M.D.

FIG. 5-1. Worksheet is filled out with ballpoint pen and taken by patient back to referring physician. This is NCR paper, which provides copy for our records.

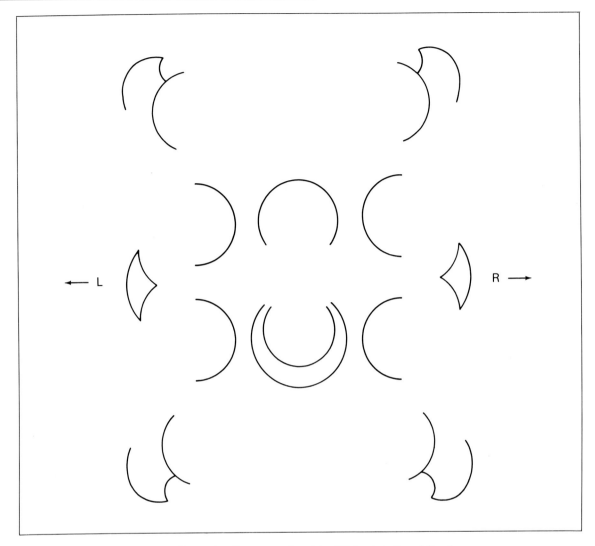

FIG. 5-2. Sample diagram sheet to fill in details of findings

COMPUTERIZED RECORD
The computer as a surgical instrument

In my practice lifetime of 19 years, the demands on the physician to collect, record, and retrieve information have grown enormously. Years ago, a handwritten note in either the office record or the hospital chart would suffice if it identified the patient's diagnosis and treatment. The increasing requirements for hospital accreditation stipulate history and physical examination documentation on admission. Governmentally instituted regulations require signed discharge summary on diagnosis-related groups (DRGs) within 24 hours of discharge. The hospital's and physician's payment depend on compliance with these regulations. There are increasing documentation requirements in the face of increasing time constraints. It almost seems that the last reason for medical record information is its value in patient care.

The medicolegal climate necessitates the keeping of complete and accurate records that support the standards of patient care.

After the events of hospitalization and/or surgery the patient needs information for insurance forms, legal inquiries, and workmen's compensation applications along with letters to referring physicians or consultants.

Many surgeons use their weekends for paperwork; this is a nonproductive and "not-for-profit" enterprise.

The proper use of a computer can greatly reduce the surgeon's expenditures of time and effort in responding to informational requests. It also affords the opportunity to maintain impeccable records for legal purposes.

The computer's capacity for single input and multiorganizational delivery makes internal auditing possible. The opportunity to study one's own experience by case retrieval and to learn of one's own diagnostic tendencies can only improve skills. Just as diagnostic arthroscopy provides more accurate diagnosis and directs the surgical plan, the properly designed computer program can assist the surgeon in diagnostic accuracy preoperatively. With the proper informational base, the surgeon can recall his or her own results on a given diagnosis with conservative or surgical treatment. This way the surgeon may better advise patients on complications, time off work, and prognosis.

An informational system combined with other physicians forms a data base for the surgeon to compare his or her diagnosis with those of others given the same information.

After the clinical impression, the available medical literature on the same topic may be reviewed on the computer screen.

The computer is limited to providing and collating information. It allows the surgeon time to effectively educate himself or herself and the patient concerning the problem and treatment choices.

To date surgical technique remains a skill that depends on the intelligence and eye-hand coordination of the physician. I envision the computer assisting with intraoperative decision making in the future. A computer inquiry is based on a patient's age, sex, diagnosis, and specific surgical findings. To date this has been a matter of surgeon recall, experience, and training applied to the problem at hand. A printout of possible choices including standard deviations becomes immediately available.

The prospects for this type of technology to be integrated into medical practice are so exciting to me that in 1980 I started to develop a patient management software program for arthroscopic surgery.

Patient history, physical examination, x-ray, clinical impression, arthroscopic surgical report, and follow-up evaluation programs along with research protocol for the knee joint were developed. A similar program is underway for the shoulder.

The software program was first worked out on paper forms; therefore revision has been the name of the game. The objective was to make it easier, not more difficult, to manage this patient information. Integration with existing business packages was a second priority. The following dimensions are operational.

Patient history form (Fig. 5-3)

The patient history form is sent to the patient on scheduling of the initial office appointment and completed before the interviews in the physician's office. This allows the patient time for recall, accuracy, and completeness. The physician then reviews the form and makes inquiries, deletions, or additions.

The form is ready for computer input following a menu system by the office staff.

A typed narrative is available on command. The information is stored for future reports and for research purposes.

Physical examination form (Fig. 5-4)

The physical examination form is completed on the initial examination. It ensures completeness based on filling in blanks. Except for the specific measurements, most of the form is completed after performance of the examination. The recording of measurements at the time avoids errors of memory. A routine of always measuring and recording the patient's right side first avoids any confusion introduced by which limb is affected or the position of the patient during the examination.

Information is stored for narrative reports or research purposes.

X-ray form (Fig. 5-5)

The x-ray form is more comprehensive than might be practical for use in daily practice. The data are listed in order of frequency, with the most common factors appearing first. Its comprehensiveness is useful for research purposes. If the x-ray film is saved, specific parameters can be entered at the time of research and then subjected to computer analysis.

A computer-generated narrative is available.

Clinical impression

A clinical impression is formulated based on the information given. It usually precedes any clinical laboratory tests. The term is not to be confused with nor does it imply a pathological diagnosis. The pathological diagnosis would be established after definitive tests, after time for clinical observation, or after arthroscopic observation.

Arthroscopic surgical report (Fig. 5-6)

The crux of the entire system is the arthroscopic surgical report. This document records the pathological diagnosis and the surgical treatment. The postoperative management and prognosis are included. From this document, coupled with the previous records, all future recall, correspondence, and letters to referring physicians, both the patient's and the insurance company's may be generated.

The ability to provide a same-day discharge summary and a copy of the report is now within the capacity of the computer system.

For medicolegal and institutional reasons it is important to recognize that this method, although it is computer synthesized, is a more complete and individ-

Text continued on p. 288.

SEQUENCE NO.

FORM #1

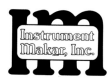

PATIENT INFORMATION QUESTIONNAIRE: KNEE

PURPOSE

By having you finish this form we are able to obtain maximum patient input which contributes to the completeness of your medical records. This form must be filled out for proper reports.

Please do not attach materials or letters as an alternative to completing this form.

INSTRUCTIONS

Please fill out the following questionnaire to the best of your ability, answering each question as it applies to you TODAY. Complete this form for the problematic knee. If both knees are a problem, then a similar form needs to be completed for the **second knee**. If you have any questions about items in this questionnaire, please check with the receptionist. We will be happy to assist you.

ATTACH COPIES OF DOCTOR'S, HOSPITAL'S, X-RAY OR SURGICAL REPORTS IF AVAILABLE.

1. PATIENT NAME: _____   2. PATIENT #: _____
   (LAST)   (FIRST)   (MIDDLE INITIAL)

3. DATE: _____/_____/_____
         MO   DAY   YR

PROBLEM #: _____   SURGEON'S COMMENTS: _____

PROBLEM#: If this is the patient's first office visit, the patient's problem # is 1. If the patient returns for the same problem, the problem should be assigned the original problem #.

FOR PHYSICIAN'S USE ONLY: If the patient is seen for an entgirely new problem, one in the same joint or in a different joint, then the problem # is 2. Each new problem the patient is seen for must be given a sequential problem #.

FIG. 5-3

A Patient information questionnaire.

PATIENT INFORMATION QUESTIONNAIRE: KNEE

4. Street address: _____

5. City: _____   6. State: _____   7. Zip code: _____

8. Country: _____

9. Age: _____   10. Sex: M ☐ F ☐   11. Height: _____   12. Weight: _____

13. Date of birth: Month _____   Day _____   Year _____

14. Social Security Number: _____

15. Home telephone:(_____)_____   16. Work telephone:(_____)_____

17. Telephone number where you can be reached during the day: (_____)_____

18. Medicaid #:_____   19. Medicare #:_____
                (5 NUMBERS)   (3 GROUPS OF 4 NUMBERS)

    BLUE CROSS/BLUE SHIELD:

20. Group #: _____   21. Service Code: _____
             (5 NUMBERS)   (3 GROUPS OF 4 NUMBERS)

22. Contract #: _____   23. B.C. Plan Code: _____
               (9 NUMBERS)   (4 NUMBERS)

24. Other Insurance: name _____

25. Other Insurance: policy number _____

26. Responsible party and/or subscriber's name:_____

27. Employment: 1. sedentary   2. physical

28. Is this a Worker's Compensation case?   1. yes   2. no   3. company _____

29. Is this a legal or third person liability case?   1. yes   2. no

A

---

41. Which joint are you having problems with?
    1) right knee
    2) left knee

42. If your knee is bothering you, please measure the distance around each knee in centimeters (2.54 cm. to the inch) and fill in the spaces provided: 1) right _____   2) left _____

43. MY MAJOR COMPLAINT is (please circle just ONE):
    1. pain
    2. aching—sore
    3. swelling
    4. grinding
    5. loss of motion
    6. giving out
    7. locking
    8. loss of work
    9. loss of activities
    10. other (please explain) _____

FIG. 5-3, cont'd

A Patient information questionnaire.

Continued.

Patient Information Questionnaire: Knee (continued) 3

44. ONSET OF THE PROBLEM: please circle those that apply and enter the date or duration of the problem if it is known—
    1) gradually, since _____
    2) suddenly, on _____
    3) vehicle accident, on _____
    4) injury, on _____
    5) injury while playing sports, on _____
    6) injury at work, on _____
    7) don't know

(If you are experiencing PAIN, please answer this section. If not, please skip to question 60.)

PHYSICIAN'S NOTES

50. LOCATION OF PAIN: please circle those that apply—
    1) front   5) kneecap
    2) back   6) all over
    3) inner side   7) deep inside
    4) outer side

51. MECHANISM OF INJURY (Details of Problem):

52. FREQUENCY OF PAIN: please circle those that apply—
    1) none
    2) occasionally
    3) constantly
    4) recent onset
    5) with activity
    6) even when resting

53. TIME OF DAY WHEN PAIN OCCURS: please circle those that apply—
    1) morning
    2) all day
    3) end of the day
    4) interrupts my sleep

A

54. PAIN MADE WORSE WHEN: please circle those that apply—
    1) sitting
    2) standing
    3) walking
    4) getting up to walk
    5) running
    6) physical therapy
    7) after exercise

55. PAIN RELIEVED BY: please circle those that apply—
    1) nothing
    2) rest
    3) activity
    4) medicine—if so, what kind? _____
    5) physical therapy—heat or cold application
    6) moving the knee

60. SWELLING OF THE AFFECTED AREA: please circle those that apply—
    1) none ever
    2) originally, but not since
    3) doesn't go away—swelling is constant
    4) frequently
    5) after giving out or buckling
    6) only after exercise or use of the joint

FIG. 5-3, cont'd

A Patient information questionnaire.

61. GRATING OR GRINDING NOISES OR SENSATIONS IN THE JOINT: please circle those that apply—
 1) none
 2) feel with my hand
 3) getting up from a chair
 4) noticeable when climbing stairs
 5) noticeable when walking
 6) only when doing deep knee bend

62. LOCKING JOINT (JOINT STICKS): please circle those that apply—
 1) never
 2) at first, but not now
 3) frequently or occasionally
 4) just started
 5) constantly or continually

63. WHEN KNEE GIVES OUT OR BUCKLES: please circle those that apply—
 1) this does not apply to me
 2) at time of original injury
 3) at present time
 4) often
 5) while walking
 6) while climbing stairs
 7) while pivoting on the leg

64. WHERE KNEE GIVES OUT OR BUCKLES: please circle those that apply—
 1) this does not apply to me
 2) knee cap area
 3) knee shifts (entire)
 4) deep inside the knee

70. STIFFNESS OF THE JOINT: please circle those that apply—
 1) none
 2) always
 3) after activity
 4) in the morning
 5) end of day

75. RANGE OF MOTION IN THE JOINT: please circle those that apply—
 1) same as ever
 2) unable to fully straighten the joint
 3) unable to fully bend or flex the joint

76. MOBILITY OF THE JOINT: please circle those that apply—
 1) able to walk normally
 2) able to walk with a limp
 3) unable to walk
 4) able to run normally
 5) unable to run
 6) able to use affected joint (other than knee) as usual
 7) unable to use affected joint (other than knee) as usual

PHYSICIAN'S NOTES

A

FIG. 5-3, cont'd

A Patient information questionnaire.

Continued.

Patient Information Questionnaire: Knee (continued)   5

80. ALIGNMENT OF THE KNEE: please circle those that apply—
     1) straight
     2) bowlegged
     3) knock-kneed
     4) becoming more bowlegged
     5) becoming more knock-kneed
     6) no change in alignment

81. MAXIMUM DISTANCE ABLE TO WALK (without knee symptoms):
     1. 1/8 mile
     2. 1/4 mile
     3. 1/2 mile
     4. 3/4 mile
     5. 1 mile
     6. no limit

82. ACTIVITIES UNABLE TO DO BECAUSE OF AFFECTED JOINT:
     please circle those that apply—
     1) none
     2) work at my job—how long off work? _____ months
     3) housework
     4) shopping
     5) recreation activities I enjoy
     6) participate in competitive sports

83. AIDS TO WALKING CURRENTLY IN USE:
     please circle those that apply—
     1) none
     2) cane
     3) crutches
     4) walker
     5) wheelchair
     6) brace

PHYSICIAN'S NOTES

A

FOR THIS CONDITION:

90. Were you treated by a family physician?   3. Name: _____
     1. Diagnosis: _____   4. Address: _____
     2. Treatment: _____   _____

91. Were you treated by an orthopedic surgeon?   3. Name: _____
     1. Diagnosis: _____   4. Address: _____
     2. Treatment: _____   _____

92. Were you treated at an emergency room?   3. Hospital: _____
     1. Diagnosis: _____   4. Address: _____
     2. Treatment: _____   _____

93. What physician referred you to us?
     1. Name: _____
     2. Address: _____

FIG. 5-3, cont'd

A Patient information questionnaire.

---

100. Did you have **X-RAYS** taken?
    1. NONE
    2. yes
        FIRST SET
        3) where: _____
        4) when: _____
        5) results: _____
        SECOND SET
        6) where: _____
        7) when: _____
        8) results: _____

101. Did you have an **ARTHROGRAM** (dye test)?
    1. NONE
    2. yes
        FIRST
        3) where: _____
        4) when: _____
        5) results: _____
        SECOND
        6) where: _____
        7) when: _____
        8) results: _____

105. Did you have an **ARTHROSCOPY or ARTHROSCOPIC SURGERY** performed (looking into the joint)?
    1. NONE
    2. yes
        FIRST
        3) where: _____
        4) when: _____
        5) by whom: _____
        6) results: _____
        SECOND
        7) where: _____
        8) when: _____
        9) by whom: _____
        10) results: _____

A

FIG. 5-3, cont'd

A Patient information questionnaire.   *Continued.*

Patient Information Questionnaire: Knee (continued)   7

106. Did you have **OPEN SURGERY** on the joint?
    1. NONE
    2. yes
      FIRST
        3) where: _____
        4) when: _____
        5) why: _____
        6) by whom: _____
        7) results: _____
      SECOND
        8) where: _____
        9) when: _____
       10) why: _____
       11) by whom: _____
       12) results: _____

REVIEW OF SYMPTOMS
115. Do you have any of the following medical problems?
    Please circle those that apply.   OTHER PROBLEMS: please describe problem and symptoms
      1) heart disease   _____
      2) high blood pressure   _____
      3) diabetes   _____
      4) lung disease   _____
      5) rheumatoid arthritis   _____
      6) other form of arthritis   _____
      7) inherited disease   _____
      8) gout   _____
      9) stomach ulcer   _____
     10) bleeding tendency   _____
     11) circulation problems in affected leg   _____

116. Have you been under doctor's care in the past two years?
    1. NONE
    2. yes
      3) by whom: _____
      4) where: _____
      5) why: _____

117. Please list the medications you are currently taking and the dosage of each in the space below:
    1)_____   3)_____
    2)_____   4)_____

A

FIG. 5-3, cont'd

A Patient information questionnaire.

8

118. Have you taken any of the following MEDICATIONS
within the **past 6 months**?
   1) cortisone (pills) (shots) (shots in joint)
   2) high blood pressure pills
   3) water pills
   4) heart medicine
   5) insulin

119. Please list **all** known ALLERGIES:

_____

_____

_____

_____

120. Please list any major surgeries which you may have had (along with any complications that may have
occurred) in the space below:

Surgeries	Complications
1)_____	1)_____
2)_____	2)_____
3)_____	3)_____

121. Please rate your overall level of physical health (please circle just ONE):
   1. excellent
   2. very good
   3. good
   4. fair
   5. poor

A

CERTIFICATION OF AUTHENTICITY

I hereby certify that the above information is true and correct within the best of my ability.

Signed: _____

Date: _____

DID YOU SKIP ANY PAGES?

**Check to see that you didn't skip any pages. If you failed to answer important questions or
skipped a page by mistake, we will return this questionnaire to you for completion.**

DOCTOR'S SIGNATURE _____

FIG. 5-3, cont'd

A Patient information questionnaire.

Continued.

B

PATIENT INFORMATION QUESTIONNAIRE: KNEE

4. Street address: _4631 WOODRIDGE_

5. City: _BATTLE CREEK_   6. State: _MI_   7. Zip code: _49017_

8. Country: _USA_

9. Age: _51_   10. Sex: M ☐ F ☒   11. Height: _5'7"_   12. Weight: _179_

13. Date of birth: Month _5_ Day _4_ Year _34_

14. Social Security Number: _____

15. Home telephone: (_616_) _583 - 9631_   16. Work telephone: (____) _____

17. Telephone number where you can be reached during the day: (____) _____

18. Medicaid #: _____   19. Medicare #: _____
                    (5 NUMBERS)   (3 GROUPS OF 4 NUMBERS)

BLUE CROSS/BLUE SHIELD:

20. Group #: _____   21. Service Code: _____
                (5 NUMBERS)   (3 GROUPS OF 4 NUMBERS)

22. Contract #: _____   23. B.C. Plan Code: _____
                (9 NUMBERS)   (4 NUMBERS)

24. Other Insurance: name _TRAVELERS INSURANCE_

25. Other Insurance: policy number _XY 105 - LA2_

26. Responsible party and/or subscriber's name: _SAMUEL SAMPLE_

27. Employment: (1.) sedentary   2. physical

28. Is this a Worker's Compensation case?   1. yes   (2.) no   3. company _____

29. Is this a legal or third person liability case?   1. yes   (2.) no

---

41. Which joint are you having problems with?
    1) right knee
    (2) left knee

42. If your knee is bothering you, please measure the distance around each knee in centimeters (2.54 cm. to the inch) and fill in the spaces provided: 1) right _16_   2) left _17¾_

43. MY MAJOR COMPLAINT is (please circle just ONE):
    (1.) pain
    (2.) aching—sore
    3. swelling
    (4.) grinding
    5. loss of motion
    (6.) giving out
    7. locking
    8. loss of work
    (9.) loss of activities
    10. other (please explain) _____

FIG. 5-3, cont'd

B Example completed patient information questionnaire.

Patient Information Questionnaire: Knee (continued)   3

44. ONSET OF THE PROBLEM: please circle those that apply and
    enter the date or duration of the problem if it is known—
        1) gradually, since _____
        2) suddenly, on _____
        3) vehicle accident, on _____
        (4) injury, on __7- 12 -84_____
        5) injury while playing sports, on _____
        6) injury at work, on _____
        7) don't know

    (If you are experiencing PAIN, please answer this section. If not,
    please skip to question 60.)

50. LOCATION OF PAIN: please circle those that apply—
        1) front   (5) kneecap
        2) back   6) all over
        (3) inner side   7) deep inside
        4) outer side

52. FREQUENCY OF PAIN: please circle those that apply—
        1) none
        2) occasionally
        3) constantly
        4) recent onset
        (5) with activity
        6) even when resting

53. TIME OF DAY WHEN PAIN OCCURS:
    please circle those that apply—
        1) morning
        (2) all day
        3) end of the day
        4) interrupts my sleep

54. PAIN MADE WORSE WHEN: please circle those that apply—
        1) sitting
        (2) standing
        (3) walking
        (4) getting up to walk
        5) running
        (6) physical therapy
        7) after exercise

55. PAIN RELIEVED BY: please circle those that apply—
        1) nothing
        (2) rest
        3) activity
        (4) medicine—if so, what kind? _TYLENOL_____
        5) physical therapy—heat or cold application
        6) moving the knee

60. SWELLING OF THE AFFECTED AREA:
    please circle those that apply—
        1) none ever
        2) originally, but not since
        (3) doesn't go away—swelling is constant
        4) frequently
        5) after giving out or buckling
        6) only after exercise or use of the joint

PHYSICIAN'S NOTES

51 MECHANISM OF INJURY
   (Details of Problem):

FIG. 5-3, cont'd

B Example completed patient information questionnaire.   *Continued.*

Arthroscopic surgery: principles and practice

B

61. GRATING OR GRINDING NOISES OR SENSATIONS IN THE
    JOINT: please circle those that apply—
    1) none
    2) feel with my hand
    3) getting up from a chair
    4) noticeable when climbing stairs
    5) noticeable when walking
    6) only when doing deep knee bend

62. LOCKING JOINT (JOINT STICKS):
    please circle those that apply—
    1) never
    2) at first, but not now
    3) frequently or occasionally
    4) just started
    5) constantly or continually

63. WHEN KNEE GIVES OUT OR BUCKLES:
    please circle those that apply—
    1) this does not apply to me
    2) at time of original injury
    3) at present time
    4) often
    5) while walking
    6) while climbing stairs
    7) while pivoting on the leg

64. WHERE KNEE GIVES OUT OR BUCKLES:
    please circle those that apply—
    1) this does not apply to me
    2) knee cap area
    3) knee shifts (entire)
    4) deep inside the knee

70. STIFFNESS OF THE JOINT:
    please circle those that apply—
    1) none
    2) always
    3) after activity
    4) in the morning
    5) end of day

75. RANGE OF MOTION IN THE JOINT:
    please circle those that apply—
    1) same as ever
    2) unable to fully straighten the joint
    3) unable to fully bend or flex the joint

76. MOBILITY OF THE JOINT: please circle those that apply—
    1) able to walk normally
    2) able to walk with a limp
    3) unable to walk
    4) able to run normally
    5) unable to run
    6) able to use affected joint (other than knee) as usual
    7) unable to use affected joint (other than knee) as usual

PHYSICIAN'S NOTES

FIG. 5-3, cont'd

B Example completed patient information questionnaire.

Patient Information Questionnaire: Knee (continued)   5

80. ALIGNMENT OF THE KNEE: please circle those that apply—
    1) straight
    2) bowlegged
    3) knock-kneed
    4) becoming more bowlegged
    5) becoming more knock-kneed
    6) no change in alignment

81. MAXIMUM DISTANCE ABLE TO WALK (without knee symptoms):
    1. 1/8 mile
    2. 1/4 mile
    3. 1/2 mile
    4. 3/4 mile
    5. 1 mile
    6. no limit

82. ACTIVITIES UNABLE TO DO BECAUSE OF AFFECTED JOINT:
    please circle those that apply—
    1) none
    2) work at my job—how long off work? _____ months
    3) housework
    4) shopping
    5) recreation activities I enjoy
    6) participate in competitive sports

83. AIDS TO WALKING CURRENTLY IN USE:
    please circle those that apply—
    1) none
    2) cane
    3) crutches
    4) walker
    5) wheelchair
    6) brace

PHYSICIAN'S NOTES

B

FOR THIS CONDITION:

90. Were you treated by a family physician?
    1. Diagnosis: _____
    2. Treatment: _____
    3. Name: _____
    4. Address: _____
    _____

91. Were you treated by an orthopedic surgeon?
    1. Diagnosis: _____
    2. Treatment: _____
    3. Name: _____
    4. Address: _____
    _____

92. Were you treated at an emergency room?
    1. Diagnosis: _____
    2. Treatment: _____
    3. Hospital: _____
    4. Address: _____
    _____

93. What physician referred you to us?
    1. Name: _____
    2. Address: _____

FIG. 5-3, cont'd

B Example completed patient information questionnaire.   *Continued.*

Re: Susan Sample 12345
4631 Woodridge
Battle Creek, MI 49017
USA
DOB: 05/04/1934
Worker's Compensation: No
Liability case: No

This 51-year-old female was evaluated on March 15, 1985.

Her chief complaints were pain, aching, and soreness, grinding, giving out, as well as loss of activities due to the left knee. The problem started from an injury on 07/12/84.

She complained of knee pain on the inner side and in the kneecap area. The pain occurs with activity and throughout the day. The pain is made worse when standing, walking, getting up to walk, as well as during physical therapy and is relieved by rest as well as Tylenol.

There was constant swelling.

Grating or grinding noises or sensations in the joint occur when getting up from a chair, climbing stairs, when walking, as well as being felt with the hand.

There was locking of the joint frequently or occasionally. Her knee gave out or buckled at the time of the original injury. Her knee gives out or buckles in the kneecap area as well as deep inside the knee.

Stiffness in her joint is present after activity and at the end of the day. The range of motion in the joint is the same as ever. In regards to her mobility, she is able to walk but with a limp and unable to run.

The alignment of her knee is becoming more knock-kneed.

C

FIG. 5-3, cont'd

C Example dictated narrative based on completed questionnaire. See correlations in shaded areas.

PHYSICAL EXAM: KNEE

SEQUENCE NO

FORM #2

1. _____
   Last   First   Middle

2. _____
   Chart #

3. _____
   Physician

4. _____
   Physician #

5. _____
   Month   Day   Year

6. PROBLEMATIC JOINT
   1. RIGHT KNEE   2. LEFT KNEE

7. OPPOSITE KNEE
   1. Asymptomatic   1. Normal exam
   2. symptomatic   2. abnormal exam

10. GETTING UP FROM CHAIR   1) NORMAL
    2) slow
    3) good leg first
    4) arm help

11. GAIT   1) NORMAL
    2) limps
    3) straight leg
    4) bent knee
    5) support _____

15. ALIGNMENT (SUPINE)

	RIGHT	LEFT
VALGUS	1._____	1._____
Q angle	2._____	2._____
varus	3._____	3._____
pseudoopening	4. (+) (−)	4. (+) (−)

16. (Full) RANGE OF MOTION (Limited)

	RIGHT	LEFT
Active Extension	1._____	1._____
Active Flexion	2._____	2._____
Heel from buttock	3._____cm	3._____cm
Passive Extension	4._____	4._____
Passive Flexion	5._____	5._____
Heel from buttock	6._____cm	6._____cm

17. CIRCUMFERENCE

	RIGHT	LEFT
Thigh	1._____cm	1._____cm
Knee	2._____cm	2._____cm
Calf	3._____cm	3._____cm

20. APPEARANCE

Skin	1) Normal	2) Abnormal	How:_____
Color	1) Normal	2) Abnormal	How:_____
Temperature	1) Normal (cool)	2) Abnormal	How:_____
Texture	1) Normal	2) Abnormal	How:_____

21. SKIN INCISIONS   1) NONE   2) Present
    1. arthroscopic   1. single   1. healed   1. tender
    2. open   2. multiple   2. healing   2. swollen
    3. varicose vein surgery   3. open   3. reddened
                                     4. draining

22. SITE OF INCISIONS   LENGTH:
    1. anterior   1. medial   1. longitudinal   1. _____cm
    2. posterior   2. lateral   2. transverse   2. _____cm

FIG. 5-4. Physical examination form.   *Continued.*

25. JOINT EFFUSION   1) NONE
     2. mild   3. moderate   4. maximal

26. TENDERNESS   1) NONE   2) Present
     1. anterior   1. joint line   1. _____ ligament
     2. posterior   2. suprapatellar   2. _____ tendon
     3. medial   3. patella   3. _____ nerve
     4. lateral   4. parapatellar   4. _____ muscle
                5. femur
                6. tibia
                7. tibial tubercle
                8. fibula

30. COMPARTMENTS ASSESSMENT   1) NORMAL   2) Abnormal
     1. crepitus   1. medial   1. compartment   1. meniscal
     2. catching   2. lateral   2. articular cartilage
     3. popping   3. synovial
                                         4. extra articular

31. PATELLOFEMORAL ASSESSMENT   1) NORMAL   2) Abnormal
     1. crepitus   1. patellar   1. pain w/compression   1. lateral tilt   1. subluxable
     2. catching   2. trochlear   2. pain w/distal push   2. J-sign   2. dislocatable
     3. popping   3. synovial   3. grimace w/lateral push
     4. extra articular

35. MANIPULATION   1) NORMAL   2) Abnormal
     1. McMurray test _____
     2. Appley test _____
     3. Other _____

36. BURSAE   1) NORMAL   2) Present
     1. Prepatellar
     2. pes anserina
     3. semimembranous
     4. Baker's cyst

37. MASS   1) NONE
     1. cystic   1. anterior   1. meniscus
     2. solid   2. posterior   2. _____
                3. medial
                4. lateral

40. LIGAMENTOUS STABILITY   1) NORMAL   2) Abnormal
SPECIFIC INSTABILITY:

ANTERIOR	MAGNITUDE	POSTERIOR	MAGNITUDE
1. Lachman	(+) (−) ____	8. Rotary Posteromedial	(+) (−) ____
2. Pivot Shift	(+) (−) ____	9. Neutral Posterior	(+) (−) ____
3. Antermedial Slocum	(+) (−) ____	10. Rotary Posterolateral	(+) (−) ____
4. Neutral Slocum	(+) (−) ____	11. Reverse Pivot	(+) (−) ____
5. Anterolateral Slocum	(+) (−) ____		
DIRECT MEDIAL		DIRECT LATERAL	
6. Extension	(+) (−) ____	12. Extension	(+) (−) ____
7. 15-30° Flexion	(+) (−) ____	13. 15-30° Flexion	(+) (−) ____
		14. Pseudoopening	(+) (−) ____
		15. Other _____	(+) (−) ____

FIG. 5-4, cont'd. Physical examination form.

45. COMPARISON MEASUREMENTS

	RIGHT		LEFT	
Position ___° 1. ____	2. ____ lbs. ___ mm ___ mm ___ mm	4. ____ lbs. ___ mm ___ mm ___ mm	6. ____ lbs. ___ mm ___ mm ___ mm	8. ____ lbs. ___ mm ___ mm ___ mm
	Avg. 3. ____	Avg. 5. ____	Avg. 7. ____	Avg. 9. ____
Position ___° 1. ____	2. ____ lbs. ___ mm ___ mm ___ mm	4. ____ lbs. ___ mm ___ mm ___ mm	6. ____ lbs. ___ mm ___ mm ___ mm	8. ____ lbs. ___ mm ___ mm ___ mm
	Avg. 3. ____	Avg. 5. ____	Avg. 7. ____	Avg. 9. ____
Position ___° 1. ____	2. ____ lbs. ___ mm ___ mm ___ mm	4. ____ lbs. ___ mm ___ mm ___ mm	6. ____ lbs. ___ mm ___ mm ___ mm	8. ____ lbs. ___ mm ___ mm ___ mm
	Avg. 3. ____	Avg. 5. ____	Avg. 7. ____	Avg. 9. ____
Position ___° 1. ____	2. ____ lbs. ___ mm ___ mm ___ mm	4. ____ lbs. ___ mm ___ mm ___ mm	6. ____ lbs. ___ mm ___ mm ___ mm	8. ____ lbs. ___ mm ___ mm ___ mm
	Avg. 3. ____	Avg. 5. ____	Avg. 7. ____	Avg. 9. ____

50. POSTERIOR KNEE   1) NORMAL   2) Abnormal
    1. tender   1. mass
    2. swollen   2. Baker's cyst

51. HAMSTRINGS   1) NORMAL   2) Abnormal
    1. tight
    2. weak

52. CALF   1) NORMAL   2) Abnormal
    1. swollen
    2. painful
    3. positive Homan's sign

53. HEELCORDS   1) NORMAL   2) Abnormal
    1. tight
    2. tender

60. MUSCLE STRENGTH   1) NORMAL
    1. knee   1. extension   1. normal   1. VMO R (+) (−)
    2. hip   2. flexion   2. abnormal   2. VMO L (+) (−)
           3. abduction
           4. adduction

61. NEUROLOGICAL   1) NORMAL   2) Positive _____

62. CIRCULATION   1) NORMAL   2) Abnormal
    1. diminished   1. popliteal   1. varicose veins
    2. absent   2. P. T.
           3. D. P.

FIG. 5-4, cont'd. Physical examination form.   *Continued.*

70. AMPUTATION   1) NONE   2) B. K.   3) A. K.

71. PATIENT COOPERATION
    1) Good
    2) Failed to Relax
    3) Failed to Cooperate

72. CLINICAL IMPRESSION _____

Signature _____

FIG. 5-4, cont'd. Physical examination form.

X-RAY EVALUATION FORM: KNEE

SEQUENCE NO

FORM #3

1. _____
   Last   First   Middle

2. _____
   Chart #

3. _____
   Doctor

4. _____
   Physician #

5. _____
   Month   Day   Year

6. 1. Our office
   2. Other facility _____

7. PROBLEMATIC JOINT
   1. RIGHT KNEE   2. LEFT KNEE

8. Plain FILMS Projections

	Here	Where	Date
AP supine			
Standing AP 0°			
45° flexion			
Lateral 30°			
contraction-extension			
Tunnel			
Oblique			
Merchant 45°			
_____ °			

9. X-RAY DESCRIPTION   1. NO ABNORMALITIES

   1. Degenerative changes
   1. Joint space narrowing
   3. Osteophyte formation
   4. Loose body
   5. Osteochondritis
   6. Osgood-Schlatter
   7. Calcification

   1. anterior
   2. posterior
   3. medial
   4. lateral
   5. superior
   6. distal
   7. intercondylar

   1. compartment
   2. femur
   3. tibia
   4. patella
   5. vessels
   6. soft tissues

   1. varus position _____ °
   2. valgus position _____ °

10. X-RAY Interpretation:
   _____

PATELLA:

20. MERCHANT VIEW   1) NORMAL   2) Abnormal
   1. 20°   1. Lateral Position   7. Degenerative Changes
   2. 30°   2. Lateral Overhang
   3. 45°   3. Lateral Facet Sclerosis
   4. 60°   4. Medial Bone Avulsion
   5. 90°   5. Fracture
                 6. Dislocation

21. LATERAL VIEW   1) NORMAL   2) Abnormal
   1. Scalloping
   2. Sclerosis
   3. Osteochondritis Dissecans
   4. Bi Tri Partite
   5. Degenerative Changes

FIG. 5-5. X-ray form.   *Continued.*

22. POSITION   1) NORMAL   2) high   3) low

                                      Extension-Contraction view

    P/T Ratio _____ / _____ = _____   RT_____mm   LF_____mm

25. MEASUREMENTS

	RIGHT	LEFT
Lateral offset	1._____mm	1._____mm
Angles		
Parallel	2._____mm	2._____mm
Apex Medial	3._____mm	3._____mm
Apex Lateral	4._____mm	4._____mm
Patellofemoral Space		
Medial	5._____mm	5._____mm
Apex	6._____mm	6._____mm
Lateral	7._____mm	7._____mm

26. PATELLAR offset _____mm

27. PATELLOFEMORAL ANGLES
    1. parallel
    2. apex medial _____mm
    3. apex lateral _____mm

28. PATELLOFEMORAL MEASURED SPACE
    1. medial _____mm
    2. apex _____mm
    3. lateral _____mm

35. FOREIGN BODY OR SURGICAL IMPLANT

1. femur	1. screw
2. tibia	2. staple
3. fibula	3. nail
4. patella	4. plate
5. soft tissues	5. wire

45. FRACTURE

1. recent	1. open	1. femur	1. simple	1. transverse
2. previous	2. closed	2. tibia	2. comminuted	2. oblique
		3. fibula		3. spiral
		4. patella		4. butterfly

1. united	1. acceptable Position
2. delayed Union	2. displacement
3. malunion	3. angulation
	4. articular offset

60.

Type	Date	Normal	Abnormal	How?	By report	By review
Arthrogram						
Tomogram						
Bone Scan						
CAT Scan						

Signature _____

FIG. 5-5, cont'd. X-ray form.

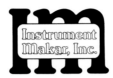

SEQUENCE NO

FORM #5

DIAGNOSTIC AND OPERATIVE
ARTHROSCOPIC SURGERY FORM: KNEE

INSTRUCTIONS

— CIRCLE words which best describe your observation.

— For questions where multiple sentences will be generated:
    1. Use dark ink to denote the primary observation and connect the circles with lines.
    2. Use red ink to denote a secondary observation and connect the circles with lines.

— X-out errors.

— IN BILATERAL CASES - USE TWO FORMS.

— N/V: Abbreviation for "Not Visualized."

— If elaboration is necessary use question #182.

1. NAME:_____ 2. HOSPITAL #:_____
          (LAST)   (FIRST)   (MIDDLE INITIAL)

3. PATIENT #:_____ 4. SURGERY DATE:____/____/____ 5. JOINT OPERATED ON: 1. Right 2. Left
                                   MO   DAY   YR

PROBLEM #:_____ SURGEON'S COMMENT:_____

PROBLEM #:   If this is the patient's first office visit, the patient's problem # is 1. If the patient returns for the same problem, the problem should be assigned the original problem #.
If the patient is seen for an entirely new problem, one in the same joint or in a different joint, then the problem # is 2.
Each new problem the patient is seen for must be given a sequencial problem #.

FIG. 5-6. Arthroscopic surgical form.   *Continued.*

DIAGNOSTIC AND OPERATIVE ARTHROSCOPIC SURGERY FORM: KNEE

6. Patient Status;   1. inpatient admitted: _____/_____/_____   2. outpatient   3. admitted following surgery
MO   DAY   YR

7. Name of Surgeon: _____   8. Surgeon #:_____

9. 1st Assistant: _____

10. 2nd Assistant: _____

11. Anesthesiologist: _____

12. Type of Anesthetic: 1. general   2. endotracheal   3. spinal   4. epidural   5. local   6. block

    7. aborted - reason_____

13. Patient Position: 1. supine   2. prone   3. (R) (L) lateral decubitus

14. Type of Table: 1. regular   2. fracture

15. Past Surgical History—OPEN (on involved knee):

    1) arthrotomy   _____   4) ligament repair   _____   7) synovectomy   _____

    2) meniscectomy   _____   5) osteotomy   _____   8) _____   9) _____

    3) patellar alignment   _____   6) total knee   _____

16. Past Surgical History—DIAGNOSTIC ARTHROSCOPY: How Many:_____   Last Dx:_____

17. Past Surgical History—ARTHROSCOPIC SURGERY (on involved knee):

    1) meniscectomy   _____   3) abrasion arthroplasty   _____   5) ligament repair   _____

    2) condylar shave   _____   4) patellar alignment   _____   6) _____   7) _____

18. PRIMARY SYMPTOM LOCATION: 1. NONE   2. generalized   3. localized

				Nature of Lesions:	
1. suprapatellar	1. anterior	1. femur	1. meniscal	1. loose body
2. patellar	2. medial	2. joint line	2. condylar	2. osteophyte
3. patellofemoral	3. lateral	3. collateral ligament	3. synovial	3. Baker's cyst
4. patellar tendon	4. posterior	4. cruciate ligament	4. ankylosis	4. cyst
5. tibial tubercle		5. tibia	5. instability	5. pes ancerina
			6. position	6. fracture

19. LOCATION OF SIGNS: 1. NONE   2. generalized   3. localized

				Nature of Lesions:	
1. suprapatellar	1. anterior	1. femur	1. meniscal	1. loose body
2. patellar	2. medial	2. joint line	2. condylar	2. osteophyte
3. patellofemoral	3. lateral	3. collateral ligament	3. synovial	3. Baker's cyst
4. patellar tendon	4. posterior	4. cruciate ligament	4. ankylosis	4. cyst
5. tibial tubercle		5. tibia	5. instability	5. pes ancerina
			6. position	6. fracture

FIG. 5-6, cont'd. Arthroscopic surgical form.

EXAM UNDER ANESTHESIA

30. RANGE OF MOTION:

		R	L
1. full	extension	1. _____ °	1. _____ °
2. limited	flexion	2. _____ °	2. _____ °
3. locked	heel-buttock	3. _____cm	3. _____cm

31. PATELLAR STABILITY:

1. NORMAL   1. in extension
2. unstable   2. at 45° flexion

32. LIGAMENTOUS STABILITY: 1) NORMAL   2) abnormal

ANTERIOR:
1. Lachman   (+) (−) _____
2. Pivot Shift   (+) (−) _____
3. Anteromedial Slocum   (+) (−) _____
4. Neutral Slocum   (+) (−) _____
5. Anterolateral Slocum   (+) (−) _____

POSTERIOR:
8. Rotary Posteromedial   (+) (−) _____
9. Neutral Posterior   (+) (−) _____
10. Rotary Posterolateral (+) (−) _____
11. Reverse Pivot   (+) (−) _____

DIRECT MEDIAL:
6. Extension   (+) (−) _____
7. 15-30° Flexion   (+) (−) _____

DIRECT LATERAL:
12. Extension   (+) (−) _____
13. 15-30° Flexion   (+) (−) _____
14. Pseudo opening   (+) (−) _____
15. Other_____   (+) (−) _____

33. COMPARISON MEASUREMENTS:

	RIGHT		LEFT	
Position ° 1. _____	2. _____lbs. mm mm mm	4. _____lbs. mm mm mm	6. _____lbs. mm mm mm	8. _____lbs. mm mm mm
	Avg. 3. _____	Avg. 5. _____	Avg. 7. _____	Avg. 9. _____
Position ° 1. _____	2. _____lbs. mm mm mm	4. _____lbs. mm mm mm	6. _____lbs. mm mm mm	8. _____lbs. mm mm mm
	Avg. 3. _____	Avg. 5. _____	Avg. 7. _____	Avg. 9. _____
Position ° 1. _____	2. _____lbs. mm mm mm	4. _____lbs. mm mm mm	6. _____lbs. mm mm mm	8. _____lbs. mm mm mm
	Avg. 3. _____	Avg. 5. _____	Avg. 7. _____	Avg. 9. _____
Position ° 1. _____	2. _____lbs. mm mm mm	4. _____lbs. mm mm mm	6. _____lbs. mm mm mm	8. _____lbs. mm mm mm
	Avg. 3. _____	Avg. 5. _____	Avg. 7. _____	Avg. 9. _____

FIG. 5-6, cont'd. Arthroscopic surgical form.   *Continued.*

4   **Diagnostic and Operative Arthroscopic Surgery Form: Knee (continued)**

(Please designate GENERAL GROUPING and LOCATION — PRINT CLEARLY)

40. PRE-OP DIAGNOSIS: _____

41. POST-OP DIAGNOSIS: 1. Same
2. None made

3. Additional _____

4. Different _____

DIAGNOSTIC ARTHROSCOPY

45. SKIN PREPARATION: 1. Betadine   1. scrub
2. Phisohex   2. paint
3. other_____   3. minutes_____

46. TOURNIQUET: 1. no   2. yes, at_____mm. Hg.

47. THIGH HOLDER: 1. no   2. yes, (below, over, above) the tourniquet

48. INITIAL INFLOW SITE:
1. cannula   1. superior   1. medial
2. scope   2. inferior   2. lateral
3. posterior

49. JOINT FLUID: 1. NORMAL   2. abnormal
1. minimal   1. yellow   1. mucinous   1. cultured
2. moderate   2. serosanguinous 2. purulent   2. laboratory analysis
3. massive   3. bloody   3. snowy (loose bodies)
4. brown

50. MEDIUM FOR ARTHROSCOPY:
1) saline   3) air   5) CO_2 7) Other_____
2) sterile water 4) N_2 6) Ringer's Lactate

51. PRESSURE ON INFLOW:
1. gravity   1. intermittent   pressure: flow:
2. manual   2. variable   _____Hg   _____cc/min.
3. mechanical

55. LOOSE BODIES: 1. NONE   2. N/V   3. Present (number_____)
1. small   1. dispersed   1. anterior   1. suprapatellar   1. cartilage
2. medium   2. in joint   2. posterior   2. intercondylar   2. meniscal
3. large   3. extrasynovial 3. medial   3. gutter   3. bony
4. combination 4. synovial attached 4. lateral   4. Baker's cyst   4. foreign body_____
5. compartment   5. implant_____

56. SYNOVIAL REACTION: 1. NONE   2. N/V   3. Present
1. minimal   1. localized   1. degenerative   1. rheumatoid   1. pigmented villinodular
2. moderate   2. diffuse   2. inflammatory   2. fibrinoid   2. osteochondromatosis
3. excessive   3. to injury   3. gout   3. chondromatosis
4. from surgery   4. pseudogout
5. hemorrhagic   5. crystalline

FIG. 5-6, cont'd. Arthroscopic surgical form.

Diagnostic and Operative Arthroscopic Surgery Form: Knee (continued)   5

57. SUPRAPATELLAR PLICA: 1. NONE   2. N/V   3. present   4. pathologic
    1. fenestrated   1. medial
    2. surgically absent   2. lateral
    3. regrown
    4. enlarged

58. MEDIAL SHELF PLICA: 1. NONE   2. N/V   3. present   4. pathologic
    1. fenestrated   1. medial
    2. surgically absent   2. lateral
    3. regrown
    4. enlarged

59. FIBROTIC BAND: 1. NONE   2.N/V   3. Present
    1. single   1. anterior   1. suprapatellar
    2. multiple   2. posterior   2. intercondylar
    3. massive   3. medial   3. interosseuous
    4. compressive   4. lateral   4. gutter
                                          5. compartment

63. PATELLOFEMORAL JOINT POSITION, TRACKING AND SURFACE: 1) NORMAL   2) N/V   3) abnormal
        1. viewed above   2. viewed below   3. by probing

IF PATELLA WAS ABNORMAL, CONTINUE WITH QUESTION 64.
IF PATELLA WAS NORMAL, SKIP TO QUESTION 70.

---

64. PATELLAR POSITION AND TRACKING: 1. NORMAL   2. N/V   3. abnormal
    1. acute   1. alta   1. displacement
    2. chronic   2. medial   2. subluxation
    3. recurrent   3. lateral   3. dislocation
    4. congenital   4. baja   4. compression
    5. post surgical   5. position

65. PATELLAR SURFACE: 1. NORMAL   2. N/V   3. abnormal   4. post patellectomy

				Size:	Depth:
1. traumatic	1. healing	11. fissure(s)	1. anterior	1. ____cm.	1. superficial
2. degenerative	2. healed	12. crabmeat	2. posterior		2. 1/2 thickness
3. cortical	3. soft	13. furry	3. medial	by	3. to bone
depression	4. firm	14. granular	4. central	2. ____cm.	4. bone exposed
4. avulsion	5. hard	15. flap	5. lateral	3. measured	5. ____mm.
5. synovial	6. smooth	16. undermined	6. diffuse		6. measured
pannus	7. osteophyte	17. osteochondritis	7. proximal		
	8. rounded	dissecans	8. distal		
	9. blister	18. crystalline			
	10. bubble	19. osteonecrosis			

66. FEMORAL TROCHLEA: 1. NORMAL   2. N/V   3. abnormal

				Size:	Depth:
1. traumatic	1. healing	11. fissure(s)	1. anterior	1. ____cm.	1. superficial
2. degenerative	2. healed	12. crabmeat	2. posterior		2. 1/2 thickness
3. cortical	3. soft	13. furry	3. medial	by	3. to bone
depression	4. firm	14. granular	4. central	2. ____cm.	4. bone exposed
4. avulsion	5. hard	15. flap	5. lateral	3. measured	5. ____mm.
5. synovial	6. smooth	16. undermined	6. diffuse		6. measured
pannus	7. osteophyte	17. osteochondritis	7. proximal		
	8. rounded	dissecans	8. distal		
	9. blister	18. crystalline			
	10. bubble				

FIG. 5-6, cont'd. Arthroscopic surgical form.   *Continued.*

70. MEDIAL COMPARTMENT: 1. NORMAL   2. N/V   3. abnormal   4. loose bodies (defined in question 55.)
        1) by visualization   2) by probing

IF MEDIAL COMPARTMENT WAS ABNORMAL, CONTINUE WITH QUESTION 71.
IF MEDIAL COMPARTMENT WAS NORMAL, SKIP TO QUESTION 78.

---

71. MEDIAL FEMORAL CONDYLE: 1. NORMAL   2. N/V   3. abnormal

				Size:	Depth:
1. traumatic	1. healing	11. fissure(s)	1. anterior	1. _____cm.	1. superficial
2. degenerative	2. healed	12. crabmeat	2. posterior		2. 1/2 thickness
3. cortical	3. soft	13. furry	3. medial	by	3. to bone
depression	4. firm	14. granular	4. central	2. _____cm.	4. bone exposed
4. avulsion	5. hard	15. cobblestone	5. lateral	3. measured	5. _____mm.
	6. smooth	16. flap	6. diffuse		6. measured
	7. osteophyte	17. osteochondritis			
	8. chondronecrosis	dissecans			
	9. blister	18. crystalline			
	10. bubble	19. osteonecrosis			

72. MEDIAL TIBIAL CONDYLE: 1. NORMAL   2. N/V   3. abnormal

				Size:	Depth:
1. traumatic	1. healing	11. fissure(s)	1. anterior	1. _____cm.	1. superficial
2. degenerative	2. healed	12. crabmeat	2. posterior		2. 1/2 thickness
3. cortical	3. soft	13. furry	3. medial	by	3. to bone
depression	4. firm	14. granular	4. central	2. _____cm.	4. bone exposed
4. avulsion	5. hard	15. cobblestone	5. lateral	3. measured	5. _____mm.
	6. smooth	16. flap	6. diffuse		6. measured
	7. osteophyte	17. osteochondritis			
	8. chondronecrosis	dissecans			
	9. blister	18. crystalline			
	10. bubble	19. osteonecrosis			

73. MEDIAL MENISCUS: 1. NORMAL   2. N/V   3. abnormal

1. traumatic	1. torn	1. reduced	1. above meniscus	1. flap	1. anterior
2. degenerative	2. fringe degeneration	2. displaced	2. under meniscus	2. longitudinal	2. medial
3. scarred	pathologically absent	3. reducible	3. posterior	3. radial	3. posterior
4. healed	3. total	4. displaceable	4. medial	4. horizontal	4. superior
	4. partial		5. notch	5. oblique	surface
	surgically absent	1. single		6. complex	5. interstitial
	5. total	2. double		7. cystic	6. undersurface
	6. partial	3. triple		8. discoid	7. periphery
	7. retained posterior horn			9. compression	8. middle
	8. crystalline			10. bucket handle	9. inner edge
					10. meniscotibial
					ligament

74. MEDIAL GUTTER: 1. NORMAL   2. N/V   3. abnormal
        1. fibrous adhesion   2. fenistrated plica   3. loose bodies   4. osteophyte   5. synovitis   6. tear-TCL
        7. tear-patellar retinaculum

FIG. 5-6, cont'd. Arthroscopic surgical form.

75. POSTEROMEDIAL COMPARTMENT: 1. NORMAL   2. N/V   3. abnormal   4. confirmed anterior findings
    Approach: Lesions not otherwise seen:
        1. transcondylar   1. meniscal tear
        2. transcutaneous   2. loose bodies
                                            3. synovitis
                                            4. torn posterior cruciate
                                            5. Baker's cyst
                                            6. blood clot

78. INTERCONDYLAR NOTCH AREA: 1. NORMAL   2. N/V   3. abnormal
                1) by visualization   2) by probing

IF INTERCONDYLAR NOTCH WAS ABNORMAL, CONTINUE WITH QUESTION 79.
IF INTERCONDYLAR NOTCH WAS NORMAL, SKIP TO QUESTION 85.

---

79. OBSERVATION OF SPACE: 1. NORMAL
      2) loose body   3) osteophyte-femoral notch   4) osteophyte-tibia   5) displaced medial meniscus
      6) displaced lateral meniscus   7) synovitis   8) fibrosis

80. MEMBRANEOUS LIGAMENT: 1. INTACT
      2) absent   3) imperforate   4) accessory bands   5) hemorrhagic   6) regenerated

81. ANTERIOR CRUCIATE LIGAMENT: 1. NORMAL   2. N/V   3. abnormal
    1. torn-complete   1. femur   1. anterormedial   1. acute/red
    2. torn-partial   2. midsubstance   2. intermediate   2. chronic/yellow-white
    3. torn-interstitial   3. tibia   3. posterolateral   3. enlarged tibial spine
                    4. with bone

    4. attached to P.C.
    5. healing   Separate Bands: Drawer sign-45° flexion   Post-op Repair:
    6. healed   how many_____   greater than 5mm in . . .   1. primary
    7. absent   1. neutral   2. pedicle
                                     2. medial rotation   3. graft_____
                                     3. lateral rotation   4. staple
                                                          5. suture

82. POSTERIOR CRUCIATE LIGAMENT: 1. NORMAL   2. N/V   3. abnormal
    1. torn-partial   1. femur   1. acute/red
    2. torn-complete   2. midsubstance   2. chronic/yellow-white
    3. interstitial   3. tibia   3. post-op repair
    4. absent   4. with bone

85. LATERAL COMPARTMENT: 1. NORMAL   2. N/V   3. abnormal   4. loose bodies (see question 55.)
                1) by visualization   2) by probing

IF LATERAL COMPARTMENT IS ABNORMAL, CONTINUE WITH QUESTION 86.
IF LATERAL COMPARTMENT IS NORMAL, SKIP TO QUESTION 95.

FIG. 5-6, cont'd. Arthroscopic surgical form.   *Continued.*

8   **Diagnostic and Operative Arthroscopic Surgery Form: Knee (continued)**

86. LATERAL FEMORAL CONDYLE: 1. NORMAL   2. N/V   3. abnormal

				Size:	Depth:
1. traumatic	1. healing	11. fissure(s)	1. anterior	1. _____cm.	1. superficial
2. degenerative	2. healed	12. crabmeat	2. posterior	by	2. 1/2 thickness
3. cortical	3. soft	13. furry	3. medial		3. to bone
depression	4. firm	14. granular	4. central	2. _____cm.	4. bone exposed
4. avulsion	5. hard	15. fracture	5. lateral	3. measured	5. _____mm.
	6. smooth	16. osteochondritis	6. diffuse		6. measured
	7. osteophyte	dissecans			
	8. chondronecrosis	17. crystalline			
	9. blister	18. osteonecrosis			
	10. bubble				

87. LATERAL TIBIAL CONDYLE: 1. NORMAL   2. N/V   3. abnormal

				Size:	Depth:
1. traumatic	1. healing	11. fissure(s)	1. anterior	1. _____cm.	1. superficial
2. degenerative	2. healed	12. crabmeat	2. posterior	by	2. 1/2 thickness
3. cortical	3. soft	13. furry	3. medial		3. to bone
depression	4. firm	14. granular	4. central	2. _____cm.	4. bone exposed
4. avulsion	5. hard	15. fracture	5. lateral	3. measured	5. _____mm.
	6. smooth	16. osteochondritis	6. diffuse		6. measured
	7. osteophyte	dissecans			
	8. chondronecrosis	17. crystalline			
	9. blister	18. osteonecrosis			
	10. bubble				

88. LATERAL MENISCUS: 1. NORMAL   2. N/V   3. abnormal

1. traumatic	1. torn	1. reduced	1. above meniscus	1. flap	1. anterior
2. degenerative	2. fringe degeneration	2. displaced	2. under meniscus	2. longitudinal	2. medial
3. scarred	pathologically absent	3. reducible	3. posterior	3. radial	3. posterior
4. healed	3. total	4. displaceable	4. medial	4. horizontal	4. superior
	4. partial		5. notch	5. oblique	surface
	surgically absent	1. single		6. complex	5. interstitial
	5. total	2. double		7. cystic	6. undersurface
	6. partial	3. triple		8. discoid	7. periphery
	7. retained posterior horn			9. compression	8. middle
	8. crystalline			10. bucket handle	9. inner edge
					10. meniscotibial ligament

89. POPLITEAL TENDON AND SHEATH: 1. NORMAL   2. N/V   3. abnormal

Tendon:	Meniscal attachments:		Lesions not otherwise seen:
1. intact	Superior:	Inferior:	1. loose bodies
2. torn	1. intact	1. intact	2. osteophytes
3. absent	2. torn	2. torn	3. synovitis

90. LATERAL GUTTER: 1. NORMAL   2. N/V   3. abnormal
    1) fibrous adhesion   2) plica   3) loose bodies   4) osteophyte   5) synovitis

91. POSTEROLATERAL COMPARTMENT: 1. NORMAL   2. N/V   3. abnormal   4. confirmed anterior findings

Approach:	Lesions not otherwise seen:
1. transcondylar	1. mensical tear
2. transcutaneous	2. loose bodies
	3. synovitis
	4. blood clot

FIG. 5-6, cont'd. Arthroscopic surgical form.

Diagnostic and Operative Arthroscopic Surgery Form: Knee (continued) 9

95. SURGERY PERFORMED: 1. YES   2. no   3. not indicated   4. deferred

IF ARTHROSCOPIC SURGERY WAS PERFORMED, CONTINUED WITH QUESTION 96.
IF OPEN SURGERY WAS PERFORMED, SKIP TO QUESTION 136.
IF NO SURGERY WAS PERFORMED, SKIP TO QUESTION 151.

OPERATIVE ARTHROSCOPY

96. SURGICAL APPROACH:

				Procedure:
1. transcutaneous	1. femur	1. anterior	1. television monitoring	1. resection
2. transosseous	2. tibia	2. posterior	2. direct viewing	2. alignment
		3. medial	3. x-ray control	3. repair
1. single		4. lateral	4. image intensification	4. position
2. multiple		5. proximal		5. removal
		6. distal		

98. THERAPEUTIC LAVAGE: 1. ALL compartments
    2) anterior compartments   3) posteromedial   4) posterolateral   5) Baker's cyst

99. LOOSE BODY REMOVAL:

Compartment:	Tissue Type:	Method:
1. all	1. cartilage	1. lavage
2. suprapatellar	2. meniscus	2. forceps
3. anterior	3. bone	3. motorized instruments
4. posterior	4. other_____	4. suction-magnet
5. medial	5. implant_____	5. other_____
6. lateral		
7. intercondylar notch		
8. Baker's cyst		

102. SYNOVECTOMY:

1. localized	1. all compartment	1. suprapatellar plica
2. generalized	2. suprapatellar	2. medial shelf plica
3. adhesiolysis	3. anterior	3. membraneous ligament
4. _____bursa	4. posterior	4. fat pad
	5. medial	5. anomalous band
	6. lateral	6. Baker's cyst
		7. gutter
		8. popliteus sheath
		9. parapatellar synovitis
		10. pathological lesion

103. CHONDROPLASTY:

1. superficial	1. all compartments	1. distal	1. patellar
2. 1/2 thickness	2. medial	2. proximal	2. trochlea
3. to exposed bone	3. central	3. anterior	3. femur
	4. lateral	4. posterior	4. tibia
	5. entire surface		5. intercondylar notch

104. ABRASION ARTHROPLASTY:

1. small (1/3 surface)	1. all compartments	1. distal	1. patellar
2. moderate (2/3 surface)	2. medial	2. proximal	2. trochlea
3. large (entire)	3. central	3. anterior	3. femur
	4. lateral	4. posterior	4. tibia
	5. entire surface		5. intercondylar notch

FIG. 5-6, cont'd. Arthroscopic surgical form. *Continued.*

10   **Diagnostic and Operative Arthroscopic Surgery Form: Knee (continued)**

105. OSTEOPHYTE REMOVAL:
     1. small   1. all compartments   1. superior   1. patellar (facetectomy)
     2. medium   2. medial   2. anterior   2. intercondylar notch
     3. large   3. central   3. posterior   3. femur
                           4. lateral   4. distal   4. tibia
                                                   5. proximal

106. OSTEOCHONDRITIS DISSECANS:
     1. drilled   1. base   1. internal fixation-screw(s)
     2. debrided   2. fragment   2. internal fixation-wire(s)
                                                   3. graft_____

107. DRILLING CHONDROPLASTY:
     1. anterior   1. patella
     2. posterior   2. trochlea
     3. medial   3. femur
     4. central   4. tibia
     5. lateral
     6. distal
     7. proximal

110. CAPSULAR RELEASE:
     1. medial   3. superior   5. posterior
     2. lateral   4. anterior   6. quadriceps plasty

111. CAPSULE REPAIR:
     1. short (1cm)   1. anterior   1. medial
     2. long   2. posterior   2. lateral

112. PATELLAR REALIGNMENT:
     1. arthroscopic   4. medial imbrication   7. patellar tendon advancement
     2. combined with open surgery   5. fixation with suture   8. patellar tendon recession
     3. lateral release   6. fixation with metal implant

115. MEDIAL MENISCUS Rx: 1.(Narrative)
     1. subtotal   1. resection   1. free graft   1. suture_____
     2. total   2. repair   2. pedicle graft   2. instrumentation_____
                           3. reshaping   3. allograft
                                                   4. other_____
                                                   5. donor_____

     1. anterior   1. inner rim
     2. middle   2. central
     3. posterior   3. outer
                           4. entire

116. LATERAL MENISCUS Rx: 1. (Narrative)
     1. subtotal   1. resection   1. free graft   1. suture_____
     2. total   2. repair   2. pedicle graft   2. instrumentation_____
                           3. reshaping   3. allograft
                                                   4. other_____
                                                   5. donor_____

     1. anterior   1. inner rim
     2. middle   2. central
     3. posterior   3. outer
                           4. entire

FIG. 5-6, cont'd. Arthroscopic surgical form.

Diagnostic and Operative Arthroscopic Surgery Form: Knee (continued) 11

120. ANTERIOR CRUCIATE:
    1. partial
    2. total

    1) Narrative
        1. primary
        2. delayed primary
        3. secondary
        4. reconstruction

    Fixation:
        1. femur
        2. tibia

    Notch Preparation:
        1. synovectomy
        2. osteoplasty
        3. drill hole

    Site:
        1. intra-articular
        2. extra-articular
        3. femur
        4. tibia

    Method:
        1. staple
        2. screw
        3. sutures

    Augmentation:
        1. pedicle
        2. meniscus
        3. graft_____

121. POSTERIOR CRUCIATE:
    1. partial
    2. total

    1) Narrative
        1. primary
        2. delayed primary
        3. secondary
        4. reconstruction

    Fixation:
        1. femur
        2. tibia

    Notch Preparation:
        1. synovectomy
        2. osteoplasty
        3. drill hole

    Site:
        1. intra-articular
        2. extra-articular
        3. femur
        4. tibia

    Method:
        1. staple
        2. screw
        3. sutures

    Augmentation:
        1. pedicle
        2. meniscus
        3. graft_____

122. TIBIAL COLLATERAL:

    1. primary repair
    2. delayed primary
    3. secondary repair
    4. reconstructed

    1. staple
    2. screw
    3. suture

    Augmentation:
        1. graft_____
        2. other_____

123. LATERAL COLLATERAL:

    1. primary repair
    2. delayed primary
    3. secondary repair
    4. reconstructed

    1. staple
    2. screw
    3. suture

    Augmentation:
        1. graft_____
        2. other_____

125. ARTHROSCOPIC FRACTURE OPEN REDUCTION:
    1. displaced
    2. undisplaced
    3. avulsion

    1. patella
    2. femur
    3. tibia
    4. fibula

    Fixation:
        1. wire
        2. screw
        3. other_____

126. BIOPSY:
    1. intra articular
    2. extra articular

    1. synovial
    2. meniscal
    3. cartilage
    4. ligament

    1. anterior
    2. posterior
    3. medial
    4. lateral

    1. patella
    2. trochlea
    3. femur
    4. tibia

135. CUTTING INSTRUMENTS: 1) hand   2) motorized   3) electrocaudery   4) laser   5) cryosurgical

FIG. 5-6, cont'd. Arthroscopic surgical form.   *Continued.*

OPEN SURGERY

136. OPEN SURGERY PERFORMED: 1. yes   2. no (skip to question 151.)

137. INCISION:
Site: Purpose:
  1. combined   1. harvest_____graft
  2. anterior   2. insert_____graft
  3. posterior   3. transfer patellar tendon
  4. medial   4. repair
  5. central   5. other_____
  6. lateral
  7. transverse
  8. oblique

138. EXCISION:
  1. bursa   1. anterior
  2. scar   2. posterior
  3. neuroma   3. medial
  4. suture   4. lateral
  5. other_____

141. ARTHROTOMY:
Site: Purpose:
  1. anterior   1. loose body
  2. posterior   2. foreign body
  3. medial   3. meniscectomy (partial) (total)
  4. lateral   4. meniscal repair
                                              5. patellectomy
                                              6. other_____

142. OPEN RECONSTRUCTION REPAIR, ALIGNMENT, OR REALIGNMENT: 1) Narrative

1. reconstruction	1. anterior	1. patellar-retinaculum	1. ligament	1. imbrication	1. staple
2. repair	2. posterior	2. anterior cruciate	2. capsule	2. advancement	2. screw
3. alignment	3. medial	3. posterior cruciate	3. tendon	3. recession	3. suture
	4. central	4. quadriceps			
	5. lateral	5. patellar tendon			
		6. collateral			
		7. popliteus			

143. OSTEOTOMY: 1) Narrative
  1. varus producing   1. tibia
  2. valgus producing   2. femur
  3. elevation (Maquet)

150. WOUND CLOSURE:
  1) sponge count correct   5) closed in layers with_____
  2) all instruments accounted for   6) skin approximated with_____
  3) wound irrigated-debrided   7) sterile dressing applied
  4) hemostasis control with_____   8) packed open with dressing of_____

151. CLOSED REDUCTION OF FRACTURE: 1) tibia   2) femur   3) patella   4) fibula

152. MANIPULATION: Final range of motion   ext. ____°   Flex. ____°

FIG. 5-6, cont'd. Arthroscopic surgical form.

DOCUMENTATION

155. OPERATIVE TIME: _____(min.)   156. TOURNIQUET TIME _____(min.)   157. ANESTHESIA TIME _____(min.)

158. TELEVISION RECORDING DONE:
    1) continuous   1) inside   1) 1/2 inch Beta   1) teaching value
    2) edited   2) outside   2) 3/4 inch cassette   2) research value
                                             3) VHS
                                             4) disc

159. SLIDE PHOTOGRAPHY DONE:
    1) inside   1) teaching value   lesion_____
    2) outside   2) research value
                         3) for text book

160. MOVIE RECORDING DONE:
    1) inside   1) 16 mm.   1) teaching value   lesion_____
    2) outside   2) 35 mm.   2) research value

161. PHOTOGRAPHIC PRINTS DONE:
    1) inside   1) black & white   1) teaching value   lesion_____
    2) outside   2) color   2) research value

PATHOLOGY

165. GROSS SPECIMEN PHOTO TAKEN: 1) slide   2) video   3) movie   lesion_____

167. MICROSCOPIC SECTION REQUESTED:
    1) H & E   1) teaching value   lesion_____
    2) special stain   2) research value
    3) electron microscopy 3) textbook   slide #_____

FIG. 5-6, cont'd. Arthroscopic surgical form.   *Continued.*

14 **Diagnostic and Operative Arthroscopic Surgery Form: Knee (continued)**

POST OP MANAGEMENT

170. GENERAL STATEMENTS 1) ALL of following
    2) sterile dressing applied 5) tolerated procedure well
    3) tourniquet released 6) delivered to recovery room in good condition
    4) circulation returned immediately

171. IMMOBILIZATION: 1. NONE 2. splinted_____° 3. casted_____° 4. CPM-ROM ext._____° 5. flex._____°

172. PATIENT INSTRUCTION SHEET PROVIDED: 1. YES 2. no

173. MEDICATION PRESCRIPTION PROVIDED: 1) NO 2) Tylenol #_____ 3) Percodan 4) other_______________

175. AMBULATION:

Weight bearing:		For:	Then:	Duration:
1. full (FWB)	1. now	1. _____days	1. PWB	1. _____days
2. partial (PWB)		2. _____weeks	2. FWB	2. _____weeks
3. none (NWB)		3. _____months		3. _____months

180. RECOMMENDATIONS:
    Call for return appointment:

	In:	Off work:
1. our office	1. _____days	1. _____days
2. referring Dr. office	2. _____weeks	2. _____weeks
	3. _____months	3. _____months

182. COMMENTS / ELABORATION:____

184. TECHNICAL PROBLEMS:____

186. SPECIAL VIEWING OR SURGICAL APPROACHES____

FIG. 5-6, cont'd. Arthroscopic surgical form.

Diagnostic and Operative Arthroscopic Surgery Form: Knee (continued)   15

190. PROGNOSIS:
    1. excellent
    2. good
    3. fair
    4. poor
    5. medical condition not stationary

191. COPY OF REPORT TO: 1) Referring Physician   2) Patient   3) Company   4) Insurance Carrier

192. DRAWING (below):   1. YES   2. no

DRAWING

Signature _____

FIG. 5-6, cont'd. Arthroscopic surgical form.

ualized report than that produced by other means. I share others' objection to generalized computerized reports produced in "cookie-cutter" fashion. They are popular but reflect little specific information about the individual procedure beyond the patient's name and the date.

The arthroscopic surgical report form is filled out immediately after the procedure. Failure to do this or grouping cases together for reporting will convince the surgeon of the necessity to fill it out right away. Even dictating the case before filling out the form will point out many deletions in the dictation. The hand-checked forms serve as a back-up to electronic storage.

At first appearance, the number of choices on the form is overwhelming. There are thousands of individual choices and many times that number of combination. These choices were produced over 4 years of daily arthroscopic surgical practice and about 3,000 experiences. It would not be feasible for the surgeon to read each possible answer anymore than he or she could look at and identify each cell in the knee joint.

In practice the surgeon scans the knee arthroscopically, looking at millions of cells and picking out areas for closer attention. The surgeon observes the knee by compartment, by tissue type, and by structure. Pathological lesions are given more attention and observation. The arthroscopic surgical form is filled out in the same manner.

If the patellofemoral area is observed to be normal, then one circle is made at the beginning of that section and the surgeon moves on to the next paragraph. If the medial meniscus is torn then the compartment is abnormal, but the condyles are normal. The meniscus tear is characterized in the same logical sequence as it is observed arthroscopically.

With familiarity, completion of the arthroscopic surgical form takes only 2 minutes for the most simple case and 5 minutes for the most complex. In any case, both take less time than dictation alone. The completed forms are entered into a computer. A dictated narrative is produced with intelligent sentences and correct grammar no matter what responses of combinations are circled (Fig. 5-7). In addition, future reports, summaries, medicolegal work, and insurance forms are all reproduced with the push of a button. The bonus of the research dimension should change case reviews from a discouraging, painstaking event to one of curiosity, satisfaction, and expectation. Computer-generated referral letters may also be produced (Fig. 5-8).

Follow-up form

To facilitate patient case review and research, the follow-up patient information and evaluation form was designed. It encompasses and correlates with the patient information, physical examination, and x-ray forms. Complications, subsequent evaluations, and treatment are included.

This information is subjected to computer analysis and comparison evaluations for research purposes.

I trust that the reader recognizes the computer as an instrument that works in his or her hands like any other device in the treatment and management of the patient.

Text continued on p. 300

```
RE:        John Doe

CHART #:   67797

Date of operation:          February 26, 1986
Date of documentation:      February 26, 1986

Joint operated on:          Right knee

Patient status:             Inpatient

Surgeon:                    Gus Lowe, M.D.

Anesthesiologist:           Mary Smith, M.D.
Type of anesthesia:         General

PAST SURGICAL HISTORY:  The patient previously underwent the following open
surgical procedure(s):  a fractured patella on the involved knee.

SYMPTOM LOCATION:  The patient's symptoms were generalized in location and
the disease process was not specific in nature.  The disease process or
problem appears to be ankylosis.

LOCATION OF SIGNS:  The patient's physical signs were generalized in loca-
tion, and the disease process was not specific in nature.  The signs indi-
cate the problem was ankylosis.

EXAMINATION UNDER ANESTHESIA:  The range of motion of the right knee was
0 degrees extension and 75 degrees flexion.  There was a stable patella
and no ligamentous instability.  The alignment was straight.

PREOPERATIVE DIAGNOSIS:     Ankylosis

POSTOPERATIVE DIAGNOSIS:    (In addition to preoperative diagnosis)
                            Degenerative arthritis, patellofemoral; loose
                            body

A diagnostic arthroscopic procedure was performed.

Operative arthroscopic procedure(s) performed:
                                              Insurance codes
                    Therapeutic lavage          21217
                    Loose body removal          21217
                    Synovectomy                 21279
                    Chondroplasty               21332
                    Capsular release            i.c.

PREPARATION:  A satisfactory general anesthestic was administered by
Mary Smith, M.D.  The patient was placed in the supine position on a
regular table.  A tourniquet was placed high on the thigh and elevated
to 450 mm Hg.  The procedure was performed using a mechanical thigh-
holding device placed below the tourniquet and draped out of the
sterile area.  A Betadine skin preparation was performed.  The inflow
site was via a cannula placed superior and medial.  The joint fluid
was normal in amount, color, and consistency.  Saline solution was
used for joint distention.  The inflow was by gravity.
```

FIG. 5-7. Computerized synthesis of sample patient surgical reports.

Continued.

```
Knee Surgery Report for John Doe   (67797)   Page - 2

Operative findings:  The arthroscopy identified a loose body, which was
attached to the synovium in the anterior area.  The loose body was medium
in size and of bony material.  There was moderate diffuse reaction to
injury.  The suprapatellar plica was absent.  The medial shelf was not
present.  Fibrotic bands were present.  Multiple fibrotic bands were seen
in the suprapatellar compartment.

The patellofemoral area had pathological changes as visualized when
viewed from below as well as by probing.

The patellar surfaces were abnormal, demonstrating a diffuse traumatic
soft and crabmeat lesion; half-thickness in depth.  The patellofemoral
joint position and tracking were normal.

The femoral trochlear area was abnormal, demonstrating a degenerative firm
and furry lesion located central; half-thickness in depth.

The medial compartment and its contents were normal.

The medial femoral condylar surfaces were abnormal, demonstrating a
degenerative soft and furry lesion located central; superficial in depth.

The medial tibial condylar surfaces were normal.  The medial meniscus was
normal.  The medial-gutter was normal.

The posteromedial compartment and its contents were not visualized.

The intercondylar notch area and its contents were normal.

The lateral compartment was normal.

Arthroscopic surgery was performed.

The surgical approach was transcutaneous via multiple portals.  Television
monitoring was used to identify lesions.

A therapeutic lavage was performed in all compartments.

Bony material was removed from anterior compartment by forceps.  A
synovectomy was localized to the suprapatellar compartment.  A
synovectomy was performed in the medial and lateral compartments.
The synovectomy specifically excised the gutter linings.

A half-thickness chondroplasty was performed on the medial patellar
surface and femoral trochlea.

A capsular release was performed in the medial, lateral, and superior
area, effecting a quadricepsplasty.

The operative procedures were performed with hand and motorized
instrumentation.

An adequate resection was accomplished.
```

FIG. 5-7, cont'd. Computerized synthesis of sample patient surgical reports.

```
Knee Surgery Report for John Doe    (67797)    Page - 3

The knee was gently manipul.ted without incident to a final range of motion
with 0 degrees of extension and 145 degrees of flexion.

DOCUMENTATION:  Documentation monitored inside by continuous video in 1/2-
inch Beta format.  Documentation monitored outside by edited video in
3/4-inch cassette format.

POSTOPERATIVE MANAGEMENT:  The extremity was placed in a CPM machine with
ROM:  0 degrees extension to 145 degrees flexion.  A sterile dressing was
applied; the tourniquet was released; circulation returned immediately; the
patient tolerated the procedure well; and the patient was delivered to the
recovery room in good condition.

A patient instruction sheet was provided.  A prescription was written for
Tylenol No. 3.

Ambulation should be full weight bearing immediately.

Prognosis:  Good.




                                        Gus Lowe, M.D.


   Form sequence number:   3124

   Form type:   6
```


```
                              END OF REPORT
```

FIG. 5-7, cont'd. Computerized synthesis of sample patient surgical reports.

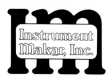

FOLLOW-UP QUESTIONNAIRE: KNEE

PURPOSE

By having you finish this form we are able to obtain maximum patient input which contributes to the completeness of our research. This form must be filled out for proper reports. Please do not attach materials and refer to them as an alternative to completing this questionnaire.

INSTRUCTIONS

Please fill out the following questionnaire to the best of your ability, answering each question as it applies to you TODAY. Complete this form for the knee you are having a problem with. If both knees are a problem, then a similar form needs to be completed for the **second knee**. If you have any questions about items in this questionnaire, please check with the receptionist. We will be happy to assist you.

1. PATIENT NAME: _____ 2. PATIENT #:_____
   (LAST)   (FIRST)   MIDDLE INITIAL)

3. DATE OF EXAMINATION:____/____/____ 4. KNEE EXAMINED: 1. right 2. left
   MO   DAY   YR

FOR PHYSICIAN'S USE ONLY

PROBLEM #: _____ SURGEON'S COMMENT: _____

PROBLEM #:   If this is a follow-up on the patient's first office visit, the patients' problem # is 1. If the patient returns again for the same problem, the problem should be assigned the original problem #.
If the patient is seen for an entirely new problem, one in the same joint or in a different joint, then the problem is # 2. Each new problem the patient is seen for must be given a sequencial problem #.

FIG. 5-8. Follow-up questionnaire.

PATIENT'S FOLLOW-UP QUESTIONNAIRE: KNEE

5.   PATIENT HAS PRESENT COMPLAINT: 1. NO   2. yes

6.   General description of arthroscopic surgical result: 1. improved   2. same   3. worse   4. N/A

IF PATIENT HAS PRESENT COMPLAINT, CONTINUE WITH QUESTION 7.
IF PATIENT HAS NO PRESENT COMPLAINT, SKIP TO QUESTION 21.

---

8.   FREQUENCY OF PAIN: please circle those that apply—
    1) NONE
    2) occasionally
    3) constantly
    4) with activity
    5) even when resting
    6) lately

9.   TIME OF DAY WHEN PAIN OCCURS: please circle those that apply—
    1) morning
    2) all day
    3) end of the day
    4) when asleep at night

10. PAIN MADE WORSE WHEN: please circle those that apply—
    1) sitting
    2) standing
    3) walking
    4) getting up to walk
    5) running
    6) physical therapy

11. PAIN RELIEVED BY: please circle those that apply—
    1) NOTHING
    2) rest
    3) activity
    4) medicine—if so what kind?_____
    5) physical therapy—heat or cold application
    6) moving the knee

12. STIFFNESS OF JOINT: please circle those that apply—
    1) NONE
    2) always
    3) after activity
    4) in morning
    5) end of day

15. SWELLING OF THE AFFECTED AREA: please circle those that apply—
    1) NONE EVER
    2) originally, abut not since
    3) doesn't go away—swelling is constant
    4) frequently
    5) after giving out or buckling
    6) only after exercise or use of the joint

16. SWELLING AFTER PLAYING SPORTS: please circle those that apply—
    1) NEVER
    2) originally, but not now
    3) OK at first, but recently
    4) intermittent with activity
    5) most of the time

PHYSICIAN'S NOTES

7.   MECHANISM OF INJURY

  (details of problem):

FIG. 5-8, cont'd. Follow-up questionnaire.   *Continued.*

25. GRATING OR GRINDING NOISES OR SENSATIONS IN THE JOINT:
   please circle those that apply—
   1) NONE
   2) feel with my hand
   3) getting up from a chair
   4) noticeable when climbing stairs
   5) noticeable when walking
   6) only when doing deep knee bend

36. WHEN KNEE GIVES OUT OR BUCKLES: please circle those that apply—
   1) this does not apply to me
   2) at time of original injury
   3) at present time
   4) often
   5) while walking
   6) while climbing stairs
   7) while pivoting on the leg

50. RANGE OF MOTION IN THE JOINT: please circle those that apply—
   1) SAME as ever
   2) unable to fully straighten the joint
   3) unable to fully band or flex the joint

51. MOBILITY OF THE JOINT: please circle those that apply—
   1) able to walk normally
   2) able to walk with a limp
   3) unable to walk
   4) able to run normally
   5) unable to run

   6) able to use affected joint as usual
   7) unable to use affected joint as usual

57. ALIGNMENT OF THE KNEE: please circle those that apply—
   1) STRAIGHT
   2) bowlegged
   3) knock-kneed
   4) becoming more bowlegged
   5) becoming more knock-kneed
   6) no change in alignment

58. ACTIVITIES:
   1) EQUAL PERFORMANCE at same sports as before
   2) same sports as before surgery, lower performance
   3) active, but with different sports
   4) significantly limited
   5) no sports possible now

59. Maximum distance patient is able to walk NOW (without symptoms):
   please circle one that applies—
   1) 1/8 mile
   2) 1/4 mile
   3) 1/2 mile
   4) 3/4 mile
   5) 1 mile
   6) no limit

62. ACTIVITIES UNABLE TO DO WITH AFFECTED JOINT:
   please circle all that apply—
   1) NONE
   2) work at my job—how long off work? _____
   3) housework
   4) shopping
   5) recreation activities I enjoy
   6) participate in competitive sports

PHYSICIAN'S NOTES

FIG. 5-8, cont'd. Follow-up questionnaire.

63. AIDS TO WALKING CURRENTLY IN USE:　please circle all that apply—
　　　　1) NONE
　　　　2) cane
　　　　3) crutches
　　　　4) walker
　　　　5) wheelchair
　　　　6) brace

65. SUBSEQUENT INJURY TO SAME JOINT:
　　　　1) NONE
　　　　2) yes
　　　　3) description:_____

70. SUBSEQUENT VISIT TO PHYSICIAN CONCERNING JOINT:
　　　　1) NONE
　　　　2) yes
　　　　3) physician:_____

75. SUBSEQUENT X-RAYS OF JOINT:
　　　　1) NONE
　　　　2) yes
　　　　3) when:_____
　　　　4) where:_____
　　　　5) result:_____

77. SUBSEQUENT TREATMENT BY PHYSICIAN: (please circle all that apply)
　　　　1) NONE
　　　　2) shots
　　　　3) medicine-pills
　　　　4) physical therapy
　　　　5) bracing
　　　　6) hospitalization

　　　　IF THE PATIENT HAS NOT HAD SUBSEQUENT TREATMENT, THEN THE PATIENT IS FINISHED WITH THIS FORM.
　　　　　　　　　　THE PHYSICIAN WILL COMPLETE THE REMAINDER.

85. SUBSEQUENT ARTHROSCOPIC SURGERY:
　　　　1) NONE
　　　　2) yes
　　　　　FIRST
　　　　　3) where:_____
　　　　　4) when:_____
　　　　　5) why:_____
　　　　　6) by whom:_____
　　　　　7) results:_____
　　　　　SECOND
　　　　　8) where:_____
　　　　　9) when:_____
　　　　　10) why:_____
　　　　　11) by whom:_____
　　　　　12) results:_____

FIG. 5-8, cont'd. Follow-up questionnaire.　　　　　　　　　*Continued.*

86. SUBSEQUENT OPEN SURGERY:
    1) NONE
    2) yes
        3) where:_____
        4) when:_____
        5) why:_____
        6) by whom:_____
        7) results:_____

90. COMPLICATIONS AFTER SURGERY:
    1) NONE
    2) yes, see below

92. COMPLICATION:
    1) Infection   8) Atelectasis
    2) Thrombophlebitis   9) Pneumonia
    3) Pulmonary Embolism   10) Urinary Retention
    4) Hemorrhage-Bleeding   11) Ileus
    5) Bleeding in Joint   12) Extremity Neurovascular Problem
    6) Effusion   13) Ligament Injury
    7) Fistula

THANK YOU. PLEASE STOP HERE AND RETURN

FOR DOCTOR'S USE ONLY.

PHYSICAL EXAMINATION: KNEE

110. Examining physician: _____   133. Physician #: _____

115. FOLLOW-UP METHOD: 1) questionnaire   2) telephone conversation   3) written letter   4) chart review
    5) specific follow-up evaluation   6) other follow-up evaluation

120. WERE FOLLOW-UP X-RAYS TAKEN: 1. yes   2. no

125. GETTING UP FROM CHAIR   1) NORMAL
    2) slow
    3) good leg first
    4) arm help

130. GAIT: 1) NORMAL
        2) limps
        3) straight leg
        4) bent knee
        5) support_____

135. ALIGNMENT (SUPINE)

	RIGHT	LEFT
VALGUS	_____	_____
Q angle	_____	_____
varus	_____	_____
pseudoopening	(+) (−)	(+) (−)

FIG. 5-8, cont'd. Follow-up questionnaire.

140. (Full) RANGE OF MOTION (Limited)

Active Extension   _____   _____
Active Flexion   _____   _____
Heel from buttock   _____cm   _____cm

Passive Extension   _____   _____
Passive Flexion   _____   _____
Heel from buttock   _____cm   _____cm

142. CIRCUMFERENCE

Thigh   _____cm   _____cm
Knee   _____cm   _____cm
Calf   _____cm   _____cm

144. APPEARANCE   Skin   1) Normal   2) Abnormal How:_____
                   Color   1) Normal   2) Abnormal How:_____
                   Temperature 1) Normal (cool) 2) Abnormal How:_____
                   Texture   1) Normal   2) Abnormal How:_____

146. SKIN INCISIONS   1) NONE   2) Present
     1. arthroscopic   1. single   1. healed   1. tender
     2. open   2. multiple   2. healing   2. swollen
     3. varicose vein surgery   3. open   3. reddened
                                       4. draining

148. SITE OF INCISIONS   LENGTH:
     1. anterior   1. medial   1. longitudinal   1. _____cm
     2. posterior   2. lateral   2. transverse   2. _____cm

150. JOINT EFFUSION   1) NONE
     2. mild   3. moderate   4. maximal

152. TENDERNESS   1) NONE   2) Present
     1. anterior   1. joint line   1. _____ ligament
     2. posterior   2. suprapatellar   2. _____ tendon
     3. medial   3. patella   3. _____ nerve
     4. lateral   4. parapatellar   4. _____ muscle
                     5. femur
                     6. tibia
                     7. tibial tubercle
                     8. fibula

154. COMPARTMENTS ASSESSMENT 1) NORMAL   2) Abnormal
     1. crepitus   1. medial   1. compartment   1. meniscal
     2. catching   2. lateral   2. articular cartilage
     3. popping   3. synovial
                                                       4. extra articular

156. PATELLOFEMORAL ASSESSMENT 1) NORMAL   2) Abnormal
     1. crepitus   1. patellar   1. pain w/compression   1. lateral tilt   1. subluxable
     2. catching   2. trochlear   2. pain w/distal push   2. J-sign   2. dislocatable
     3. popping   3. synovial   3. grimace w/lateral push
     4. extra articular

158. MANIPULATION   1) NORMAL   2) Abnormal
     1. McMurray test _____
     2. Appley test _____
     3. Other _____

FIG. 5-8, cont'd. Follow-up questionnaire.   *Continued.*

Follow-up Questionnaire: Knee (continued)

160. BURSAE   1) NORMAL   2) Present
   1. Prepatellar
   2. pes anserina
   3. semimembranous
   4. Baker's cyst

162. MASS   1) NONE
   1. cystic   1. anterior   1. meniscus
   2. solid   2. posterior   2. _____
                    3. medial
                    4. lateral

164. LIGAMENTOUS STABILITY 1) NORMAL   2) Abnormal
SPECIFIC INSTABILITY:

ANTERIOR	MAGNITUDE	POSTERIOR	MAGNITUDE
1. Lachman	(+) (−) ____	8. Rotary Posteromedial	(+) (−) ____
2. Pivot Shift	(+) (−) ____	9. Neutral Posterior	(+) (−) ____
3. Antermedial Slocum	(+) (−) ____	10. Rotary Posterolateral	(+) (−) __ __
4. Neutral Slocum	(+) (−) ____	11. Reverse pivot	(+) (−) ____
5. Anterolateral Slocum	(+) (−) ____		

DIRECT MEDIAL		DIRECT LATERAL	
6. Extension	(+) (−) ____	12. Extension	(+) (−) ____
7. 15-30° Flexion	(+) (−) ____	13. 15-30° Flexion	(+) (−) ____
		14. Pseudoopening	(+) (−) ____
		15. Other _____	(+) (−) ____

166. COMPARISON MEASUREMENTS

	RIGHT		LEFT	
Position	2. ____ lbs.	4. ____ lbs.	6. ____ lbs.	8. ____ lbs.
	mm	mm	mm	mm
1. ____	mm	mm	mm	mm
	mm	mm	mm	mm
	Avg. 3. ____	Avg. 5. ____	Avg. 7. ____	Avg. 9. ____

	RIGHT		LEFT	
Position	2. ____ lbs.	4. ____ lbs.	6. ____ lbs.	8. ____ lbs.
	mm	mm	mm	mm
1. ____	mm	mm	mm	mm
	mm	mm	mm	mm
	Avg. 3. ____	Avg. 5. ____	Avg. 7. ____	Avg. 9. ____

	RIGHT		LEFT	
Position	2. ____ lbs.	4. ____ lbs.	6. ____ lbs.	8. ____ lbs.
	mm	mm	mm	mm
1. ____	mm	mm	mm	mm
	mm	mm	mm	mm
	Avg. 3. ____	Avg. 5. ____	Avg. 7. ____	Avg. 9. ____

	RIGHT		LEFT	
Position	2. ____ lbs.	4. ____ lbs.	6. ____ lbs.	8. ____ lbs.
	mm	mm	mm	mm
1. ____	mm	mm	mm	mm
	mm	mm	mm	mm
	Avg. 3. ____	Avg. 5. ____	Avg. 7. ____	Avg. 9. ____

168. POSTERIOR KNEE   1) NORMAL   2) Abnormal
   1. tender   1. mass
   2. swollen   2. Baker's cyst

170. HAMSTRINGS   1) NORMAL   2) Abnormal
   1. tight
   2. weak

FIG. 5-8, cont'd. Follow-up questionnaire.

298

172. CALF   1) NORMAL   2) Abnormal
     1. swollen
     2. painful
     3. positive Homan's sign

174. HEELCORDS   1) NORMAL   2) Abnormal
     1. tight
     2. tender

176. MUSCLE STRENGTH   1) NORMAL
     1. knee   1. extension   1. normal   1. VMO R (+) (−)
     2. hip   2. flexion   2. abnormal   2. VMO L (+) (−)
                    3. abduction
                    4. adduction

178. NEUROLOGICAL   1) NORMAL   2) Positive _____

180. CIRCULATION   1) NORMAL   2) Abnormal
     1. diminished   1. popliteal   1. varicose veins
     2. absent   2. P. T.
                     3. D. P.

182. AMPUTATION   1) NONE   2) B. K.   3) A. K.

184. PATIENT COOPERATION
     1. Good
     2. Failed to Relax
     3. Failed to Cooperate

Signature _____

FIG. 5-8, cont'd. Follow-up questionnaire.   *Continued.*

Computer glossary

I have included a simple computer glossary for both the reader's reference and my own. The use of computers in the practice of arthroscopic surgery will expand; therefore a glossary seems appropriate.

Acoustic coupler:	A type of modem that allows one computer to communicate with another computer or with a terminal device via telephone. The handset of the telephone is placed into this unit.
Applications software:	A software program that performs a specific user-oriented task, such as ration balancing or payroll. Applications software can either be purchased as a package or be custom designed by a programmer.
Backup:	The copying of one or more files onto a storage medium for safekeeping in case the original is damaged or lost.
Basic:	(*B*eginner's *A*ll-Purpose *S*ymbolic *I*nstruction *C*ode) A programming language designed to be easy to learn and use.
Batch processing:	A system for processing groups of similar tasks at the same time on the same machine.
Baud:	A measurement of communication speeds between devices; generally means bits transferred per second. The number is divided by 10 to arrive at the characters per second.
Binary code:	A code where 0 (zero) and 1 (one) are the only characters that can be used. Numbers are represented in powers of 2.
Bit:	A contraction of "binary digit", either a 0 or a 1, which represents a two-way choice; the smallest unit of information that the computer recognizes. A bit is equivalent to the presence or absence of an electrical pulse (0 or 1). Bits are usually grouped in nibbles (4 bits), bytes (8 bits), or larger units.
Boot:	To bring a computer system up by loading a program from external storage.
Buffer:	Temporary storage for data in a computer's memory. Compensates for differences in speeds of processors and peripheral devices such as storage units, terminals, and printers.
Bug:	A programming error that causes a malfunction or stoppage of a program.
Byte:	A group of bits (usually 8). A byte can be used to represent one character (number or letter) of information, all or part of binary numbers, and machine language instructions.
Chip:	A thin semiconductor wafer on which electronic components are deposited in the form of integrated circuits.

COBOL: (*Co*mmon *Bu*siness *O*riented *L*anguage) A high-level programming language.

Code: A set of expressions generated by a programmer or by the computer to construct programs.

Compile: The process whereby a program written in a programming language is changed to a machine language.

Compiler: A program that transfers program language to machine language.

Computer: A general-purpose electrical system designed for the manipulation of information. Incorporating a central processing unit (CPU), memory, input/output (I/O) facilities, power supply, and cabinet.

Concurrent processing: Efficient use of the computer system whereby the instructions for processing two or more jobs are alternated in such a way that the jobs have the appearance of being processed at the same time.

Console: Typically the input station designated as the computer operator's station.

Copy-protect: A method to prevent copying over information already recorded on a diskette or other storage medium.

Configuration: The design of a computer system.

CP/M: (*C*ontrol *P*rogram/*M*onitor) An operating system for microcomputers, developed by Digital Research Corp., and used on many 8-bit microcomputers.

CPU: (*C*entral *P*rocessing *U*nit) The housing of the computer's main processor (see *Processor*) and main memory (see *RAM*). The work or execution is performed here.

CRT: (*C*athode *R*ay *T*ube) The television tube used to display pictures or characters. Also, the computer terminal made from a CRT. See *VDT*.

Cursor: An electronically generated symbol that appears on the display screen to tell the operator where the next character will appear.

Custom software: Computer programs prepared for a specific purpose. Contrast with *Packaged software,* in which the programs are written in advance, usually for general purposes.

Daisy-wheel printer: Letter-quality impact printer in which the characters reside on the outside edge of a wheel.

Data: The information available for processing by an application program.

Data base: A collection of stored information available for processing.

Data base management system: A software application tool useful in storing, retrieving, modifying and querying information in a data base.

Data communications: Process of transmission of data from one location to another, between two computers; or between a computer and a remote terminal.

Data entry: Transcription or original entry of data from a source documents to the application program.

Data file: A set of related data records that follow a specific order.

Data processing: The actual execution of operations outlined by the application program on the data.

Data processing system: Network of hardware and software necessary to allow input, throughput, and output.

Debugging: The process whereby the programmer and/or computer detect, locate, and correct mistakes or malfunctions

Device: An expression used for components of hardware in a computer system.

Density: A term used to describe the distance between magnetic information on tapes or floppy disks. Higher density means greater information storage capability.

Direct connect modem: In contrast to an acoustic modem, a direct connect modem is hard-wired directly to the data transmission line.

Directory: The index of programs that tracks the program location on the storage device catalog.

Disk: A circular plate with magnetic material on both sides. This plate rotates for the storage and retrieval of data by one or more "heads," which transfer the information to and from the computer. The computer-readable information may be placed on a floppy or a rigid (hard) disk, and may have information on one or both sides. Also known as diskette or disc.

Diskette: A flexible disk that is inexpensive and very portable.

DOS: (*Disk Operating System*) The program responsible for the housekeeping and communications between the disk storage device and the computer. The DOS is also usually responsible for communications between the computer and peripheral units.

Dot matrix printer: A printing device that prints characters constructed from a pattern of dots selected from a fixed matrix.

Downtime: The period during which a computer is not operating.

Editing: The changing or modifying programs, data, or documents.

Editor: A program that manipulates text information and allows the user to make corrections, additions, deletions, and other changes.

Erase: Overwriting or clearing of information from its storage medium.

External storage: The storage of programs and information that would otherwise be lost if the computer were turned off; for example, tapes and disks. Also known as *mass storage.*

Field: A subset of a record, a specific area for a particular type of data.

File: A collection of related records stored as a unit.

Flowchart: A symbolic representation of all steps in processes with the purpose of problem definition, analysis, and solution. Used extensively in program documentation.

Firmware: Built-in programs. These programs are permanently stored on components of the hardware and typically cannot be erased or modified.

Flexible disk: Also called floppy disk. A magnetic storage medium made up of a flat, bendable plastic disk.

Format: The layout, design, and specifications of a printed document, including type size and style, margins, headings, and so on.

FORTRAN: (*For*mula *trans*lation) A programming language typically used in scientific applications.

Function keys: Additional keys on a keyboard that are used to perform operations definable by the user or program.

Graphics: The presentation of information pictorially rather than alphanumerically.

Hard copy: A paper printout. ("Hard" in that it can actually be held, as opposed to copy that can only be read on a screen.)

Hardware: The physical components of a computer system, that is, the mechanical and electronic equipment.

Head: The device that reads, writes, and erases data on a magnetic storage medium.

Indexed file: A method of file organization in which record keys and disk locations are stored in an index. This allows direct access to individual records.

Input: (1) The data that is entered into programs. (2) The act of entering data into a computer. (3) The data used by programs and subroutines to produce output.

Input device: Any machine that allows entering of commands or information into the computer. An input device could be a keyboard, tape drive, disk drive, microphone, light pen, digitizer, or electronic sensor.

Input/Output (I/O):	The process or equipment used in the computer system for communication.
Inquiry:	A request for information that is available in storage or that can be made available through processing of the available information.
Intelligent terminal:	(Smart terminal) A terminal that has some data processing capability or local computing capacity.
Interactive:	A program or computer that communicates with the user or another computer.
Interface:	The juncture at which two computer components (hardware and/or software) meet and interact with each other. Also used to apply to human-machine interaction.
K:	Computer shorthand for the quantity 1,024. The term is usually used to measure computer storage capacity and transfer rates.
LAN:	Local Area Network
Mainframe:	The largest of computers. With an expansive internal memory and fast processing time, costs range into the millions of dollars.
Memory:	The section of the computer in which instructions and data are stored. Each item in memory has a unique address that the CPU can use to retrieve information.
Microcomputer:	A small but complete microprocessor-based computer system, including CPU, memory, I/O interfaces, and power supply.
Microprocessor:	LSI implementation of a complete process or (ALU and control unit) on a single chip.
Minicomputer:	A small computer, intermediate in size between a microcomputer and a mainframe computer.
Modem:	(*Mod*ulator-*Dem*odulator) A device that transforms a computer's electrical pulses into audible tones for transmission over telephone line to another computer. A modem also receives incoming tones and transforms them into electrical signals that can be processed and stored by the computer. See *Acoustic Coupler* and *Direct Connect Modem.*
On-Line:	The time spent accessing, retrieving, or storing information on the computer.
Operating system:	A collection of programs for operating the computer. Operating systems perform housekeeping tasks such as input/output between the computer and peripheral systems and accept and interpret information from the keyboard.
Output:	Any processed information coming out of a computer via any medium (print, CRT, etc.) or the act of transferring information to these media.

Output device: A machine that transfers programs or information from the computer to some other medium. Examples of output devices include tape, disk, and bubble memory drives; computer printers, typewriters, and plotters; the computer picture screen (video display); robots; and sound synthesis devices that enable the computer to talk and/or play music.

Overhead: The amount of the computer's memory required to organize the operation of the system.

Packaged software: A program designed to be marketed for general use, unadapted to any particular installation.

Parallel: In communications, the method of sending an entire character or word at a time over a series of computer lines rather than breaking them up into their component elements. Parallel communication between the computer and printers is generally faster. Contrast with *Serial.*

Peripheral: A device attached to a computer (for example, the CRT or printer.)

Program: A sequence of instructions directing a computer to perform a particular function; a statement of an algorithm in a programming language.

Plug-compatible: Two devices that can work together without a separate interface device.

RAM: (*R*andom *A*ccess *M*emory) RAM serves as a computer's scratch pad. Information is usually transferred into RAM from permanent storage.

Record: A collection of data stored on a diskette or other medium that may be recalled as one unit. Records may be of either fixed or variable length. One or more records usually make up a data file.

Real time: Refers to events as they actually happen (in comparison to computer time, which is measured in millionths of a second).

Resolution: The quality of the image on the CRT, as influenced by the number of pixels on the screen, described by rows and columns. The greater the number of pixels, the higher the resolution. Typical values range from 128 × 128 to 1024 × 1024.

Response time: The time required for the system to respond to the user's request or accept the user's inputs.

ROM: (*R*ead *O*nly *M*emory) Memory containing fixed data or instructions that are permanently loaded during the manufacturing process. A computer can use the data in ROM but cannot change it.

Sequential access: A storage method (such as a magnetic tape) by which data can only be reached or retrieved by passing through all intermediate locations between the current one and the desired one.

Serial: The handling of data one item after another. In communications, a serial transmission breaks each character into its component bits and sends these bits one at a time to a receiving device, where they are reassembled.

Software: A general term for computer programs and documentation involved in the operation of the computer.

Source code: The readable computer commands written in a programming language. It requires an interpreter or compiler. It is sometimes referred to as a source program.

Storage: The general term for any device that is capable of holding data for later retrieval.

Tape: Inexpensive mass storage medium. Must be accessed sequentially.

Teletext: Textual information transmitted to people's homes via their television set. Information is usually maintained and updated on a computer.

Terminal: A keyboard with a CRT and/or printer that can be connected to a computer.

Time-sharing: A method of sharing the resources of the computer between several users so that several people can appear to be running different computer tasks simultaneously.

Tractor feed: An attachment used to move paper through a printer. The roller that moves the paper has sprockets on each end, which fit into the fan-folded paper's matching pattern of holes.

UNIX: A computer operating system originally developed by Bell Laboratories for its internal use. One of the primary objectives of UNIX is to allow the same computer programs to run on a diverse range (i.e., different manufacturers) of computers.

Utility program: A program used to assist in the operation of the computer, for example, a sorting routine, a printout program, or a file conversion program. Generally these programs perform housekeeping functions and have little relationship to the actual processing of the data.

VDT: (*Video Display Terminal*) A CRT with keyboard.

Word: A datum or the set of characters that occupies one storage location. In microcomputing, the terms *character, word,* and *byte* are interchangeable. In most minicomputers, a word is equal to two bytes.

Word processor: A text-editing system for electronically writing, formatting, and storing letters, reports, and manuscripts before printing.

STILL PHOTOGRAPHY

Photography is a function of light producing an image on photographic film. In arthroscopy the variables are the amount of light that can be thrown on an object, the amount that can be absorbed by the object, and the subsequent amount that will reflect back through the lens of the arthroscope to the camera. Therefore a powerful light source is necessary.

Factors

Light source

Most light sources are adequate for direct arthroscopic viewing regardless of scope size or quality. For small-scope photography, a powerful light source is required. A source with a 150-watt tungsten bulb will produce a dull, dark, yellow picture with the best of the large arthroscopes.

The serious arthroscopist requires a powerful light source for all photographic needs. The 300-watt Dyonics models 500 and 510 have been used for years. They are comparable to xenon and recent metalic halogen systems when compared by video documentation.

Scope size

The diameter of the arthroscope as well as the number of light bundles going down it affect the amount of light that can be thrown on the object. The more light bundles going down the arthroscope, the more light. The smaller diameter of the arthroscopic lens, the smaller the amount of light that can be transmitted back through the arthroscope to the film. Smaller arthroscopes have less photographic capacity, not necessarily because of their quality but because of their ability to transmit a quantity of light. An excellent photograph is less likely to be obtained with a 1.7 mm diameter Needlescope than with a 5 or 6.5 mm arthroscope.

At present most arthroscopes in the 5 to 6.5 mm diameter range will produce excellent photographic images, given the same quality and quantity of light.

Light guides

Another variable in photographic quality is the transmission of light along the fiberglass bundles. If there is breakage of the bundles, which occurs with time, or corrosion over the end of the bundles, light transmission will diminish.

Light bulbs

Light bulbs lose their power and effectiveness over time. As the materials in the light bulb break down the light will become diminished to a rather significant degree. The bulb will still illuminate but the effective light will be greatly compromised, too much so to use for documentation. Often this reduction in illumination is not recognized on direct viewing. Thus to produce excellent photographic work and bright video images, frequent bulb inspection and replacement are essential.

35 mm still photography

Everyone who embarks on the practice of arthroscopy desires to produce photographic documentation.[4] A particular slide may at first be of interest to the arthroscopist and the patient but with time brings only a "ho-hum" reaction, even from the arthroscopist.

Unless extreme care is exercised in taking the photographs, identifying the slides, and placing the documentation in the chart before too much time goes by, matching an individual slide to a given patient can be virtually impossible. For most orthopedic surgeons slide photography is not a practical recording method, except for rare cases or medicolegal claims, or when the surgeon is establishing a slide file for teaching, research, and/or publication purposes.

Slide photography has some limitations because of the number of frames on any given roll of film. By the time the film has been developed the surgeon may have forgotten much about the patient and the procedure. Unless one is compulsive about record keeping, (i.e., identifying film as to exact patient, date, compartment, and findings) few slides may be of any recognizable value. Also, with hundreds of slides on a variety of patients, many duplications can occur. I have overcome some of these problems by using the Olympus OM System with a Databack II unit. This allows the recording of the patient's last initial and the date of the procedure on the photograph. When properly used, this method can assist with slide identification (Fig. 5-9).

Camera and adaptor

Currently I use the 35 mm Olympus OM 1 single-lens reflex camera for arthroscopic photography. The use of a motor drive eliminates hand manipulations and facilitates sequential filming (Fig. 5-9, *A*). The Olympus OM system provides a power winder that can deliver 3 shots per second. The winder facilitates the taking of serial photographs during surgical procedures. I have seen

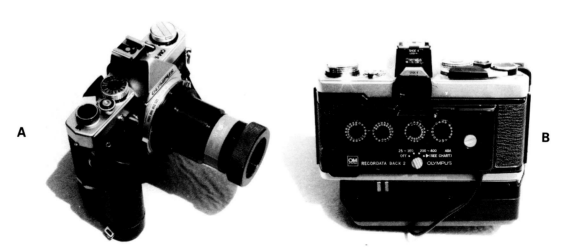

A   B

FIG. 5-9. 35 mm slide photographic camera.

A Motor drive and direct scope attachment with single lens.
B Databack 2 for Olympus system.

no need for a faster automatic winder (which can deliver a speed of 5 shots per second).

The adaptor should be a high-quality, hand-picked lens with multiple coatings to provide an ideal picture. It should be calibrated so that the circular image comfortably fills the slide frame for viewing (see Fig. 11-16,A).

There also should be an easily removable yet secure arthroscopic ocular attachment. Adequate length between the camera and the arthroscope ensures sterility, but it should not be so long as to form a great lever arm. These attachments are available for both the Nikkon F and Olympus OM systems.

Some endoscopists favor a pinch-type adaptor that hooks onto the end of a conventional lens system. This can produce a larger image on the film; however, because of the multiple lenses the image must traverse, there is less clarity and brightness. In addition, the pinch-type adaptor is easily disengaged during manipulation.

Film

I favor Kodak Ektachrome ASA 400 film. This is used with the Dyonics Model 510 light source, which generates illumination in the 550 K range, to allow direct-attachment, available-light photography to be performed without connecting any apparatus. With a Storz (4 mm) rod lens scope, most slides are shot at a speed of $\frac{1}{15}$ or $\frac{1}{30}$ second, depending on the object's color or brightness. (Table 5-1).

A faster speed is used on the brighter femoral condyles ($\frac{1}{60}$ second). A slower speed ($\frac{1}{4}$ second) is used for photographs across the suprapatellar pouch. Considerable light is absorbed in the large space.

When the smaller Needlescope is used, it is necessary to shoot at speeds of between $\frac{1}{4}$ and $\frac{1}{8}$ second.

It should be mentioned that this direct-attaching, single-lens system removes consideration for f-stops and through-the-lens metering. By trial and error, the surgeon can develop a simple system that is reproducible in virtually every knee.

Kodak Kodachrome ASA 64 film is used with the Storz flash generator. This produces the best and most consistent endoscopic photograph. The disadvantage is the amount of apparatus necessary to take photographs with this film. Kodak 5247 film is available by mail order. It was originally made for the motion picture industry but now is packaged in cassettes for 35 mm slide photography. Most camera magazines contain advertisements for this product.

Faster films, with ASAs up to 1,000, have not proved to be better or brighter on testing this environment.

TABLE 5-1. Photographic film for use in arthroscopy (35 mm)

Light source	Type	ASA
Flash generator	Kodachrome	64
	Ektachrome	64
Available light	Ektachrome	400
	Kodak 5247	400

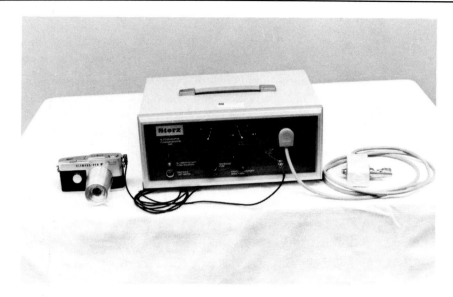

FIG. 5-10. Storz flash generator.

Some consideration must be given to the color balance of the light source, the arthroscope light transmission, and the film. Some film will produce a more yellow color; others will produce more bluish white light in a given system.

Flash generators

The flash generator is a little more difficult to use than available light because of the time lag necessary for regeneration of the flash and elaborate setup of the apparatus. The best photograph slides I have seen have been taken with the Storz flash generator, which produces abundant light for photograhy and has the advantage of flash units attached to the endoscope (Fig. 5-10).

Flash units in which the origin of light is within the light box lose considerable light in transmission. A percentage of effective light is lost for every foot it travels down a fiber-optic cable. Most cables are 6 feet long; therefore a flash unit located within the box loses 48% of its potential light. In addition, 30% of light is lost at each interphase. These highlight losses are reduced by the Storz flash generator, because the source is attached directly to the endoscope.

MOVIE PHOTOGRAPHY

Movie photography has a definite advantage over slide photography for high-quality documentation. It records motion as well as the sequence of the total examination (Fig. 5-11). Composition that is not possible with still photography is quite effective by movie photography. The flow of fluid and the motion of the intraarticular tissues can be observed. Synovium, loose bodies and meniscus motion are demonstrable. However, this method of documentation is somewhat impractical because of the high cost of the film and the great expense and weight of the movie camera.

Good movie photography has been achieved with 8 mm, 16 mm, or even Super 8 cameras with Ektachrome 7241 high-speed, single-perforated film. However, because the 7241 single-perforated film did not lock solidly during exposure, I switched to a 16 mm Beaulieu camera with 7241 double-perforated film

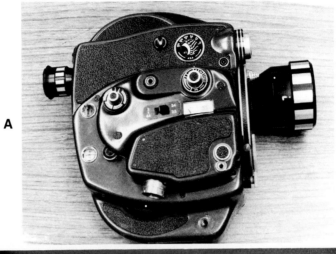

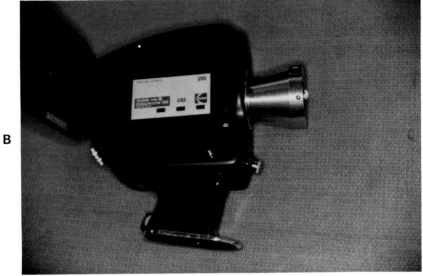

FIG. 5-11. Movie photography. **A,** Beaulieu 16 mm camera. **B,** Beaulieu 8 mm camera.

(see Fig. 5-14). This also allows flexibility for both right and left knees during the final editing process because the film can be reversed. That would not be possible with single-perforated film or video tape, unless it is transferred to film and the image reversed.

It is necessary to use the Dyonics 510 Fiberoptic 550K or a similar illuminator to achieve enough light for movie photography. With an additional light source, (i.e., a light wand) it is also possible to photograph with the 1.7 mm endoscope. Movie photography can be accomplished using the 2.2 mm diameter scope with light provided within a cannula. Movie photography with a Storz 3.5 and 5 mm endoscope produces a sharp, clear, well-illuminated image (Fig. 5-12).

A circumferential light source was devised. It increases the light 16 times, producing an excellent image for the Needlescope.

With the increasing quality of television cameras, use of movie photography

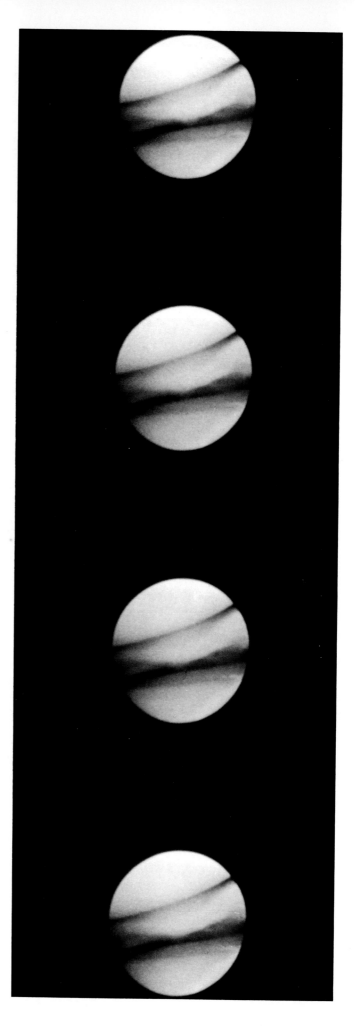

FIG. 5-12. Videotape transferred to movie film.

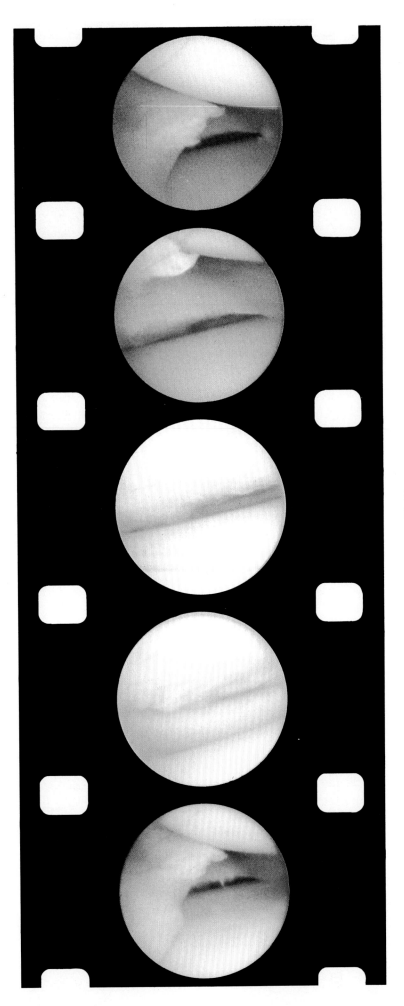

FIG. 5-13. Early television transfer to movie film.

313

has become infrequent. Videotape can be converted to movies. The reproduced picture is of excellent quality, but the process is expensive ($60 per minute) (Fig. 5-13).

TELEVISION

Modern videotape equipment makes it possible to document arthroscopic procedures while the image is simultaneously viewed for operative purposes.[1-3,5] Because there is no waiting time for videotape to be developed, the image observed through the arthroscope can be reviewed immediately. This can determine whether the document is adequate and whether the procedure has been fully recorded. If part of the document is not satisfactory, the recording can be repeated immediately. Some surgical findings have been observed by videotape review that were not seen during the arthroscopic procedure.

Since 1976 I have performed arthroscopic surgery with direct viewing from the television monitor. I have made a simultaneous recording of every arthroscopic procedure since that time, except when slide photographs were being taken for publication purposes.

Simultaneous monitoring and recording of arthroscopic procedures is a valuable technique. Operating while viewing the television monitor provides comfortable body position for the surgeon and frees both hands for manipulation of surgical instruments.

Operating room personnel can also view the procedure on the television monitor. This participation is good for morale. The electronically produced tape is immediately available for review.

A videotape record allows the surgeon at any stage of development to review operative procedures and techniques. Postsurgical viewing is similar to a football team's coaching staff reviewing films of a game, at their leisure, away from the heat of the competition. This way the coaches can pick up techniques and maneuvers that they otherwise may have overlooked. Self-study is good reason to use video recording.

Videotaped material can be edited for instructional programs or scientific presentations.

Video is useful in residency or fellowship teaching centers. Simultaneous viewing by the mentor provides instruction, guidance, and safety in the learning process.[4]

The saving of videotapes has provided excellent opportunities for comparison studies of disease processes and healing when subsequent second-look study is possible. Exact anatomical areas can be compared.

To my knowledge the medicolegal precedent of a videotape record has not been established. There could be some difficulty in proving that a given tape represented a procedure performed on a given patient. It is also doubtful that a jury or judge would understand what they were seeing. My contention is that this type of document serves the physician well where he or she has a good record of the lesion, the operative procedure, and the immediate postoperative status.

Another use for videotapes is the demonstration of problem cases to patients. Although I do not routinely view videotapes with patients, many arthroscopic surgeons do.

VALUE OF TELEVISION IN ARTHROSCOPY

Facilitation of technique
    Comfortable body position
    Freedom of both hands
Encouragement of surgical team
Production of a permanent record
    Self-study
    Educational purposes
    Scientific presentation
Potential medicolegal value
Patient review and education
Use in research

Some patients request a copy of their videotapes. Because the insurance companies in the state of Michigan do not pay for videotapes, they are made and stored at my expense for educational purposes. A nominal charge is made for videotape reproduction. Other medical records are sent without charge.

Arthroscopic television history

It has been my contention that video is an intricate part of arthroscopic surgery; it is neither a luxury nor an alternative. In 1981 approximately 25% of all surgeons who performed arthroscopic surgery used video. Those who did only diagnostic arthroscopy used it in 8% of their cases, and those who had over 400 case experiences used it 100% of the time. It appears that as the surgeons gained more expertise and had a greater volume of arthroscopic work, the videotape was used as an absolute routine. In 1983 80% of all arthroscopists used television. The video system becomes an integral part of the operating room environment. The system must fit the arthroscopic surgical environment of the institution.

In 1976 I used a large hand-held Hitachi 9017 camera. It was a single-tube Vidicon color camera attached directly to the arthroscope by a C-mount adaptor. A 15-foot interconnecting cable went around to the television set and/or recorder-player. It was housed in a specially made Formica-covered cabinet.

The camera weighed 4 pounds, and with a 38 mm C-mount adaptor I was able to record diagnostic work. There were approximately 250 television lines of horizontal resolution on this camera, which was a good match for both the player and the monitor.

Another camera that is practically the same size is the Hitachi GP 5. It is economical and a good-quality system; however, it is larger and heavier than the 9017. I then changed to a Hiatachi 9025 and a suspended system to regular operating room light handle. I now use a suspended JVC KY1900CH (Fig. 5-14), a 7-pound camera with three $^2/_3$-inch Saticon tubes. This offers high-quality color (500 lines at center G channel) and high sensitivity at minimum illumination, 150 lux. It produces a consistently bright, sharp color image.

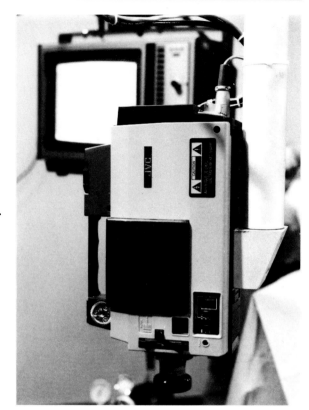

FIG. 5-14. JVC 1900 television camera.

Cameras

Hand-held cameras

All subminiature television tube cameras use a vacuum chamber tube that is ⅔ inch in diameter and 4 inches long. The tube houses a number of electronic parts that create an electronic image that is optically focused on the faceplate of the tube. The chemical layer of the photoconductive film on this faceplate determines the characteristic of that tube, and each is given a name such as vidicon, Newvicon, or Saticon. The internal characteristics of the tubes are similar, and each has the same life expectancy (about 2,000 to 3,000 hours), not including any standby modes. Tube life is determined by both mechanical shock and the tube's resistence to deterioration of the faceplate. The three types of tubes respond in different ways.

Vidicon tube. The vidicon (generic name) is the most popular type tube found in television cameras. It makes good-quality color pictures under ideal lighting conditions, and since it is the least expensive type tube it will be found in almost all the less expensive television cameras. Because of its tendency to be more sensitive toward the infrared spectrum, it will have a reddish cast, especially noticeable under lower light conditions. The vidicon camera tube cannot handle divergent light ranges simultaneously. As the scene changes, images appear to have a ghosting effect called lag. Bright highlights such as reflections or light bulbs will cause a comet-tail effect to the picture. This bright image can easily

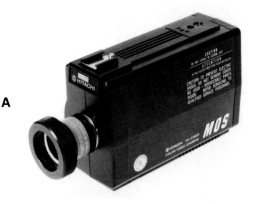

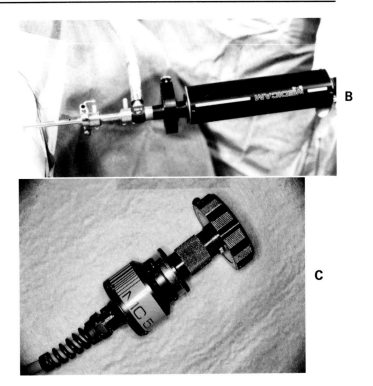

FIG. 5-15. Hand-held cameras.

A MOS camera.
B Tube-type camera.
C Chip (CCD-type) camera.

damage the faceplate phosphor, causing a permanent burn in the form of a blemish or a black and white spot. Bright reflections will often be enlarged, causing a washed-out effect referred to as blooming.

Newvicon tube. Although it has a faceplate similar to the vidicon, the Newvicon tube (trade name of Panasonic) is more light sensitive and less susceptible to image burn. Under low light situations, comet-tail effect will be present. Color quality is about the same as with the vidicon. This tube is most often used in low-light outdoor black-and-white television surveillance cameras.

The larger hand-held cameras use the Newvicon tube. One of the disadvantages of the Newvicon tube for general photography is that if the camera moves quickly across an object there is shadowing or tailing in the video field. This is not a problem when applied to close-ups in endoscopy. The camera weighs 4 to 5 pounds. Hand-holding it is difficult.

Saticon tube. The Saticon (trade name of Hitachi) is the most recently developed television tube. The spectral response of this tube is almost identical to that of the human eye. Its superb color retention (colorimity), its low light sensitivity and its resistance to burn, ghosting, and blooming have made this the most popular tube used in the new portable broadcast television cameras (Fig. 5-15).

The next generation of tube is the Saticon. It is used in lighter cameras, some as light as 6 ounces, and produces a very bright image. These cameras could be hand-held. They can now be soaked in Cidex or may be covered with a plastic sleeve. Although these cameras are very light, a 3-inch longmount on a 9-

inch arthroscope with a cord hanging on the end of the Saticon tube result in quite a lever arm and an instrument that was effectively heavier than its dead-weight.

The Saticon tube generally gives an excellent, bright picture. However, it does not compensate well for the bright femoral condyle and for shadowing into the posterior areas. Whiteouts with lag time for correction interfere with viewing. With burnout of the white flare areas on the femoral condyle, gaining control can be a problem. Careful composition editing is necessary to obtain an excellent video picture.

Solid-state camera (chip camera)

The solid-state camera replaces the vacuum tube with a tiny solid-state chip approximately 1 inch square. The ultimate benefits of this camera system will be smaller size and weight, better electronic tolerances, direct interface to computer systems, and mass production at lower cost. Black-and-white cameras have been available for the past few years, but color technology is now standard. Two types of devices are currently being marketed—the charge coupled device (CCD) (see Fig 5-15, C) and the metaloxide semiconductor (MOS) (see Fig. 5-15, A)

The Hitachi MOS camera weighs approximately 1 pound (see Fig. 5-15, A). This particular camera can be attached directly to the arthroscope by a C-mount. It produces an excellent picture, although it is not quite as bright as that produced by a Saticon or a Newvicon tube. It has good color, especially in the red ranges. One major advantage is that the cost for the entire camera system is under $2,000, compared to others up to about $12,000. This is a good choice for someone starting arthroscopic surgery or a surgeon with a lower volume of cases that could not justify the higher expense of the smaller cameras. This camera produces no less the quality of picture than a smaller chip camera. Because its electronics are not displaced away from the camera, it has virtually no service problems. However, it may no longer be available in the United States.

The same chips that are in the Hiatachi MOS camera have been incorporated into other chip cameras of a smaller size. These weigh as little as 2 ounces and are as small as 2 inches in diameter. The advantage is size and direct attachment to the arthroscope. The C-mount is often larger than the body of the camera. Many of these cameras were painted and not anodized; therefore paint chips in the operative area become a problem. If these cameras are not soakable they have the disadvantage of not being well sealed, and electronics that are exposed to salt water environment can cause service problems. A small soakable camera near an operative field where there is much saline is preferable to a nonsoakable camera.

There have been problems with the displacement of the electronics through a cord to the central control box.

When used with a variety of different light sources, the camera has not been easily color balanced. The ideal circumstance for a hand-held camera is one that is lightweight, easily balanced in the hand, and soakable. The electronics connections should be such that the cord which transmits from the small camera chip to the electronics main will not break down. The camera should be an integrated with the light source so that there is always a good color balance.

These major problems are being solved by the video companies, and the chip camera is increasing in popularity with orthopedic surgeons who do a considerable amount of arthroscopy in their practice.

Support electronics

The camera pick-up tube (Fig. 5-15, C) (or chip) is just the beginning phase of producing a television image. The ultimate picture quality is directly influenced by the electronic circuitry within the camera system, and care should be taken to select a camera that is designed around high quality circuitry.

Suspension system

I have continued with a suspended system in spite of the availability of small hand-held, direct-attached cameras. This is because I started with the suspended system and am comfortable with it. I own two articulating viewing devices that are in good condition although they are 8 years old.

I have had *no* service problems with my suspended cameras. I changed cameras only to upgrade picture. A suspended system does not limit the quality of the camera by size; even a three-tube camera, which has more lines of resolution than the best hand held camera. The suspended system is virtually weightless. The arthroscope attachment occupies less space in an operative field, especially if the chip camera cord and plastic cover are considered. It fits particularly well in an environment for arthroscopy of the shoulder and all other smaller joints. I work in a room dedicated to arthroscopy for all my cases, so transportation is not an issue.

Suspension systems can be mounted from the floor, arthroscopic table, or ceiling. They do increase the expense of the lens system, but with a trade-off decrease of expense in the camera. Camera size becomes unimportant in a suspended system. Larger, higher-resolution, three-tube camera systems (JVC KY1900CH) can be used by coupling them with an articulated viewing device.

The JVC KY1900CH is a lightweight (7.7 pounds), portable, three-tube ($\frac{2}{3}$ Saticon), professional quality (horizontal resolution 500 lines at center) video camera. It is inexpensive for television cameras of this quality ($4,000) and has built-in automatic white balance. There is also a built-in color bar generator.

If the operating room environment allows a ceiling suspension system, the camera is mounted to a pistoning system. It does necessitate a connecting articulated viewing device in which derotation of the picture proximally at the camera mount is required.

The arthroscopic Surgicenter (see Fig. 3-7, B) provides a means for a suspended camera system that can be moved from room to room. This has been popular with individuals using regular operating rooms for arthroscopy.

We encountered a considerable loss of light through the five-segment system, so we eventually changed to the three-segment system for suspension to have a brighter video image.

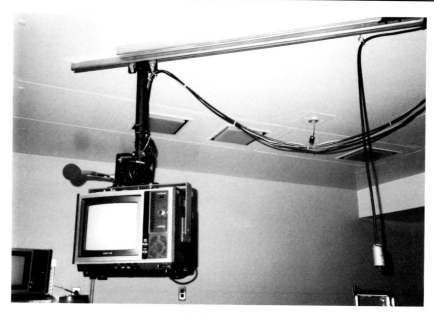

FIG. 5-16. Television monitor.

Monitors

The best television monitors are small. The 9-inch and 12-inch diagonal screens are best. Larger monitors expand the image and result in a loss of brightness and clarity. The small monitor is comfortable for viewing, because the surgeon is positioned only a few feet away.

The video picture is transmitted from the camera to the recorder to the monitor or from room to room. It can go to the monitor and from there to the recorder. When the image goes via the monitor to the recorder there is some quality lost in the recording; the best quality picture will be on the monitor. When the record is of utmost importance, the electronic impulse should be carried first to the recorder and then to the monitor (Fig. 5-16).

Recorders

Available videotape recorders accommodate ¾ or ½-inch tape formats. The ¾-inch machine made by Sony and is called U-Matics. The ¾-inch format can be edited for professional-quality presentations. The cassettes are larger for storage and more expensive.

For those who are interested in economy, the ½-inch format is available either in VHS (Hitachi, RCA, Panasonic) or Beta format (Sony). The VHS cassette is slightly larger for storage, and the image is not as sharp as the faster-running Beta I. The ½-inch format must be changed to ¾-inch for editing. VHS and Beta editors may be available soon.

At present I favor the ½-inch Beta I format for recording. It is economical and easily transferable to ¾-inch tape without loss of quality. Beta I tape moves at a faster rate than Beta II, Beta III, or VHS; therefore the image is sharper because there are more images per linear foot of film. It comes in a small package that is economical for both purchase and storage.

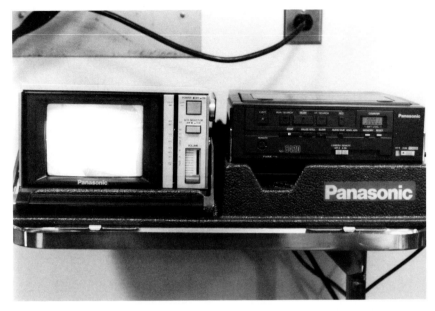

FIG. 5-17. Small monitor and recorder for nondedicated room environment.

A number of types of videotape player-recorders that use ½-inch tape are available. Smaller machines are being developed all the time so that the options range from a Beta I editing system down to a very small portable system. The self-contained systems are made to be battery powered and can be easily transported from room to room, or even hospital to hospital (Fig. 5-17).

The videotape cassette is less expensive in the ½-inch than the ¾-inch format.

Editing equipment

As the volume and number of arthroscopic cases performed and recorded have grown, the need for research and documentation has increased, especially with new operative techniques. The video editing system and a film library are added conveniences for rapid viewing and reviewing of the cases, as well as compilation of teaching material. The combining of ¾- and ½-inch formats, computer-synthesized grahics, and microscopic observations is possible with one system.

Storage

Storage of videotapes consumes considerable space, depending on the surgeon's case volume and the length of the procedure. The shelf life of color is limited but satisfactory through at least 9 years of my experience. The ½-inch format is smaller.

Scientific meetings

Projection systems are most commonly used during teaching seminars or scientific presentation. The Sony 5000 series player-recorders have fast-forward

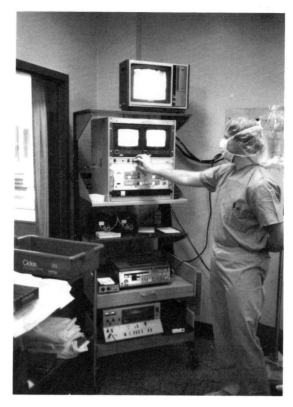

FIG. 5-18. Video tape mixer and monitors in arthroscopic suite permit simultaneous performance and inside-outside editing.

and reverse modes with scanning to facilitate searching or looking to certain segments. The Sony series ¾-inch player-recorder permits fast-forward and reverse scanning during projection.

OPERATING ROOM–TELEVISION STUDIO

The modern arthroscopic suite has become a television studio (Fig. 5-18). In my daily operations each case is recorded with simultaneous sound. A technician produces an edited version on ¾-inch tape. This version is a combination of inside and outside video. The use of dissolve and overlay techniques enhances the document's value for future education or scientific presentation.

As a result considerations were made for outside cameras. One is mounted high on the wall, and the other is portable on a tripod. These cameras, all JVC KY1900CH models, are electronically coupled at the monitor control deck.

The integration of the sound narration was best accomplished with the microphone attached to the surgeon's mask with direct connection to recorders and observation room speakers. Attempts at using a remote wireless system met with radio wave interference.

The regular operating room lighting system has been augmented with photographic balanced spotlights.

As in the recording studio, the operating room personnel must have discipline regarding talking and noise.

REFERENCES

1. Eriksson, E.: Problems in recording arthroscopy, Orthop. Clin. North Am. 10:735, 1979.
2. Jackson, D.W.: Video arthroscopy: a permanent medical record, Am. J. Sports Med. 6:213, 1978.
3. Jackson, D.W., and Ovadia, D.N.: Video arthroscopy: present and future developments, Arthroscopy, 2:108, 1985.
4. McGinty, J.A.: Closed circuit television in arthroscopy, Int. Rev. Rheumatology 33:45, 1976.
5. McGinty, J.A.: Photography in arthroscopy. American Academy of Orthopaedic Surgeons. Symposium on arthroscopy and arthrograhy of the knee, St. Louis, 1978, The C.V. Mosby Co.

CHAPTER 6

Arthroscopic surgical principles

Perspective
    Staged experience
    Patient's expectations
    Surgeon's expectations
    Personal preparation
    Organization and planning
        Environment
        Operating room team
        Instrumentation
    Plan of action
        Initial operative plan
        Alternative (contingency)
          plan
        Aborted procedure
        Fatigue and frustration
        Combined procedures
General surgical principles
    Asepsis
    Hemostasis
    Gentleness
    Working from known to unknown
Arthroscopic surgical principles
    Projection into joint
    Patient positioning
    Lens system
    Illumination
    Surgical exposure
    Surgical setup
    Distention with fluid
    Infusion system
    Inflow on arthroscope: smaller scope;
        small joints
    Separate superior portal inflow: knee,
        shoulder
    Inflow-outflow control: diagnostic
        phase
    No-flow viewing
    Operative outflow
    Postoperative inspection
    Suction pressure
    Fine tuning of flows
        Auxiliary inflow
        Joint position effects on flow
    Cleaning and vacuuming
    Distention with gas

Scope techniques
    Placement
    Fulcrum
    Replacement
    Direction
    Redirection
    Body control
        Lower body
        Upper body
    Hand control
        Palpation
        Pistoning
        Scanning
        Rotation
        Free hand activity
    Manipulation of joint
    Scope sweeping
    Composition
    Visual interpretation
        Illumination

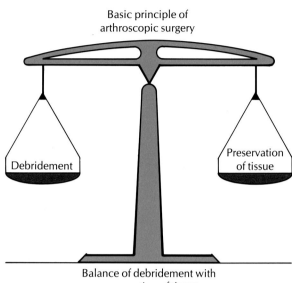

Basic principle of
arthroscopic surgery

Debridement

Preservation
of tissue

Balance of debridement with
preservation of tissue

PERSPECTIVE

Many principles must be established before the actual techniques of arthroscopic surgery are performed. The surgeon prepares himself or herself as team leader, not just surgeon-technician, because success in arthroscopy requires a team leader effort. Because arthroscopic techniques are still developing, all surgeons at all levels are learning and developing. Arthroscopy has always been and still is technically challenging. Careful consideration must be given to every detail that affects surgical judgment, technique, and result. These principles are not unique to arthroscopy. Arthroscopy demands attention to detail and surgical technique at a high level of control; thus, the emphasis on fundamental principles. "Good hands" will not compensate for the lack of surgical principles.

Joint surgery performed by open techniques can be the basis of knowledge, both anatomical and orthopedic, to form a foundation for arthroscopy. Arthroscopic technique should actually enhance or build on the previous experience of any orthopedic surgeon who cares for patients with synovial joint problems. It increases the surgeon's appreciation of anatomical structure, function, and relationships. The arthroscope allows access to areas of synovial joints not before seen by open methods.

No matter what or how vast the surgeon's experience or number of years in orthopedic surgery, he or she still will require specialized knowledge and training. Gradual, staged experience within the discipline of arthroscopic surgery is necessary to be successful.

The surgeon must prepare with the necessary knowledge and technical motor skills to accomplish the anticipated surgical procedure. Techniques the surgeon has yet to learn should not be applied to new procedures.

I believe in the old adage, pride precedes the fall. If one exalts himself, he will be humbled; if one chooses to humble himself, then he has a chance of being exalted. In arthroscopic surgery, the surgeon will be humbled in one way or another. The best choice would be to be humble going in.

The surgeon has certain confidence in his or her abilities, but this confidence can be challenged in arthroscopic surgery. There tends to be frustration and discouragement. The orthopedic surgeon who has performed well for many years in general orthopedics, or even specialized in the knee joint, finds his or her match in arthroscopic procedures. Exposure is difficult, the cutting proceeds slowly, and the OR floor is wet from fluid spillage. The surgeon is uncomfortable, and knows the procedure would have gone much faster by opening the joint.

The surgeon tends to expect too much. He or she must be realistic, because arthroscopy is a new discipline. Time and experience will be required to develop new skills. With patience and diligence, the surgeon will be well satisfied and well rewarded.

Staged experience

I enjoyed the luxury of learning diagnostic arthroscopy on thousands of cases (with relatively little pressure) before my first operative experience. My operative work developed slowly as the instrumentation became available, and I was intimately associated with introduction of new techniques.

The surgeon entering the field of arthroscopic surgery today is confronted with thousands of dollars worth of equipment (new toys), a new environment (a new field), and new personnel (new players); and somehow, this person expects to be an expert in arthroscopic surgery (a new ballgame). This expectation is unreasonable, unrealistic, and frankly, not possible.

The present dilemma results from consumer demand and intraprofessional competition. Even though this is a whole new ballgame, all the standards of surgery, patient care, and professional integrity cannot be abandoned.

The surgeon must accept staged development in arthroscopic surgery. Case experience over time will be necessary to achieve proficiency; a few successes are often followed by a frustration or two. This is to be expected in any growth pattern. Instrumentation will not do the job. I often point out that golf clubs do not play golf. The assistants (in the golf analogy, the caddy) cannot do it either. A continuing education course is only the lecture one attends before the laboratory experiment. What another surgeon can do may be different from you.

With that said, let us settle down to a basic approach that will provide ultimate success.

The beginner should select arthroscopic cases with a single, simple diagnosis, for example, meniscal flap tear or moderately degenerative joint.

The patient must be prepared with a comprehensive medical workup, including a physical examination of the joint (see Chapter 2). Just because the arthroscopic procedure will allow inspection of the joint, it does not mean that all the complaints arise within it. They could be in anatomical structures juxtaposed to the joint (e.g., shoulder pain of neck origin, knee pain of femoral, hip, or back origin).

Patient's expectations

The patient will arrive with high expectations concerning arthroscopic surgery. In his imagination, fostered by the lay press, he conceives that arthroscopic surgery is a cure-all. He may believe the surgery will be performed in the office, if not the waiting room, and that he will not only be healed but restored to normal. He may also believe that the recovery period will end when he leaves the operating table. He may be surprised that anesthesia is required or that a skin blemish results.

My experience has shown me that arthoscopic surgery requires more explanation to and "deprogramming" of patients than any type of orthopedic surgery. Ignoring this problem will only result in later, prolonged discussions with patient and/or family concerning their disappointments.

In addition, the patient should be prepared to understand there are alternate methods and other physicians from whom he might seek either treatment or a second opinion. Some cases require an open operation or a combined arthroscopic and open procedure. The arthroscopy may be the first of several operations in the patient's life.

The convalescence period and eventual return to work are important to the patient, but the desire to return to recreational and competitive sports is usually most important. He must consider the question, if the knee is opened, would the convalescence be prolonged?

What does all this discussion have to do with arthroscopic technique? Considerable! I will explain the worst possible case.

327

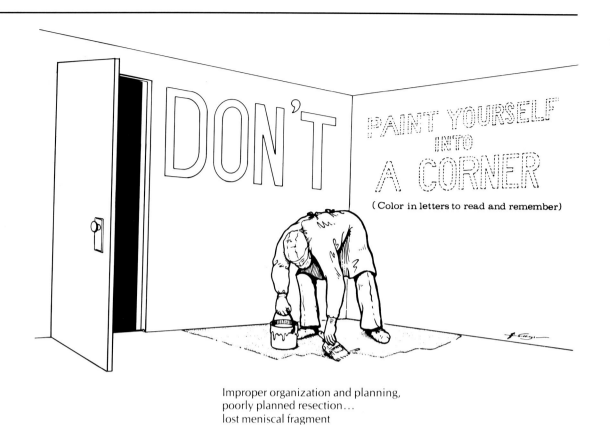

Improper organization and planning,
poorly planned resection...
lost meniscal fragment

FIG. 6-1. Don't paint yourself into a corner.

You are operating on a patient who expects the surgery will be performed without opening the knee. You identify a posterior tear of the meniscus. It appears complex in nature, possibly a double or triple bucket-handle tear. You have not performed this type of case before arthroscopically, though you could open the knee and remove front and back tears. The patient's expectations close this option, so you start the meniscus resection. You remove the first piece and find more tissue behind. The knee is tight. You find you have cut a portion of the second tear. The meniscus flap moves out of sight to the posterior and you cannot retrieve it. You try your first posterior puncture, and you finally get in. The extracapsular edema increases along with the operative and tourniquet times. You finally see the fragment but cannot get a second instrument in for resection.

The preoperative expectations of the patient have restricted the intraoperative alternatives. The pressure on the surgeon increases, and his or her technical performance is impeded in the face of frustration. The choices are to open the knee or abort the procedure. Either way, this patient will be unhappy.

Arthroscopic procedures, let alone mastery of technique, is difficult enough without the added pressures of patient's expectation pressures on the surgeon. Avoid painting yourself into a corner (Fig. 6-1).

Surgeon's expectations

The surgeon should know his or her limitations. Cases should be chosen by diagnosis, inherent joint laxity, and patient size to assure technical simplicity. A complex derangement in the tight knee of a fat patient would not be a good selection for the beginner. There is nothing wrong with selecting the tight knee in a thin person with simple meniscus tear, but not all difficult factors at once.

The surgeon should have complete candor about his or her level of arthroscopic development with the patient. What is the chance of opening the knee? What is your experience with anticipated diagnosis or operation? Have you performed similar operations.

A disappointing result can occur when the surgeon's or the patient's expectations are unrealistic. Both circumstances can be avoided.

Personal preparation

The organization necessary to be a team leader requires an attitude and presence not required for most open surgical procedures. The surgeon prepares with educational experiences, hands-on techniques, instrumentation, knowledge, and functioning television equipment.

Beyond the technical preparation is the emotional dimension. A disciplined, systematic, deliberate approach is tempered with exact execution and patience. The surgeon should share in the satisfaction of the team approach. Team members are encouraged by recognition of their meaningful contributions.

In general the arthroscopic surgeon renders to the patient an operation with lower morbidity and perhaps a better cosmetic result than an open procedure. With experience, I believe that the orthopedic surgeon has an opportunity to make a more careful diagnosis and perform a surgery on a very gentle microsurgical level, minimizing trauma to the joint and enhancing the repair or healing of tissues.

Organization and planning
Environment

The environment must be appropriate for the anticipated surgical procedure. The physician's staff should have at least minimal knowledge of arthroscopic techniques.

The environment must be appropriate for the anticipated procedure (see Chapter 3). Diagnostic arthroscopy by direct viewing is possible in a general operating room. Beyond that, the environment must be more elaborate and specific for arthroscopic surgery. The general operating room must be converted to accommodate the unique needs of arthroscopic techniques. The room lighting must be dimmed, and electrical outlets must be abundant. Electrical and radiowave frequency interference must be eliminated. The suspended fluids, suction outflow, collection bags for specimens, and fluid spillage on the floor must be managed. Television requires special stands, outlets, and connections.

This is why I recommend that a room be dedicated to arthroscopic procedures; there are already enough challenges for the arthroscopic surgeon. Organization and planning are necessary for an optimal environment.

Time should be well managed. In the ideal environment, one surgeon has a series of arthroscopic cases following each other to provide unrestricted block time. The surgeon should not bracket himself or herself with other cases or office hour commitments. The operating room staff should schedule ample time for each case and for room changeovers.

Operating room team

For simple direct-viewing diagnostic arthroscopy, an untrained assistant might be sufficient (see Chapter 3). For more advanced technical procedures, the staff should be knowledgeable and interested in arthroscopic surgery. There are those who, by choice or personality, have no interest in it, and should not be enlisted. They will not be of benefit to either the surgeon or the patient. Ideally, the staff will have a keen interest in arthroscopic surgery. The desire to learn and a spirit of cooperation create a pleasant environment.

Instrumentation

It is necessary to have the appropriate instrumentation (see Chapter 4). There should be a back-up for each instrument. They are fragile and they have the potential not only for breakage but for easy dulling. It is my opinion that a serious arthroscopist should have personal instruments. If they are shared, dull or broken instruments for a procedure will be the result, in which case the surgeon would simply have to make do.

If the hospital group has a common pool of instrumentation, it should include nonbreakable, nondulling tools, such as power sources, motors, probes, and television monitors.

Each surgeon should be assigned an arthroscope and alotted cutting heads for motorized instruments, knife blades, and basket forceps. Each becomes responsible and more interested in the care of the instruments and can monitor their gradual dulling. The administration can monitor the individual surgeon's use or abuse for accountability and cost effectiveness. This way no other surgeon's techniques or patient care is jeopardized or inconvenienced. The responsibility is properly placed on the individual surgeon.

The initial cost of duplicates would be compensated by better care, optimal function, and accountability, because they lessen total expense.

The instrumentation placed inside the joint should have magnetic properties. If there is breakage, retrieval is simplified. Magnetic devices are readily available in the marketplace (see Figs. 4-27 and 6-86). These devices should be available before any arthroscopic surgical procedure is initiated.

Proper care of instrumentation is absolutely necessary (see Chapter 2). These instruments cannot be dumped into a stainless steel tray, placed under hot water and soap, soaked, shaken, and sorted without being damaged. Careful maintenance is essential to proper arthroscopic surgical technique.

Plan of action

Initial operative plan

After the just-described conditions have been fulfilled, the scene shifts to the operating room. Based on the preoperative impression and the differential diagnosis, an operative plan is formulated. The various options are outlined in Table 6-1.

TABLE 6-1. Operative plan

Diagnostic arthroscopy	Operative arthroscopy	Combined procedure	Conventional open surgery
Now	Later	Later	Later
	Now	Later	Later
		Now	Later
			Now

The patient's expectations and the surgeon's ability condition the approach. The operating room staff must have proper set-up for anticipated open procedures to avoid delays and unnecessarily prolonged anesthesia time.

The routine of the diagnostic and operative system outlined in this text accommodates every technical eventuality of diagnosis and operation or intraoperative problem.

All anatomical compartments can be entered with instrumentation from primary and secondary portals. Any pathological condition is treatable, usually by arthroscopic or combined techniques.

Alternative (contingency) plan

No matter how sure the surgeon is of the diagnosis and his or her ability, a contingency plan is necessary. The surgeon, patient environment, instrumentation, and surgical team must be prepared for an alternate plan.

The procedure can be concluded following diagnostic arthroscopy. The operative arthroscopy may be completed, deferred, or referred. The same is so for combined or open procedures. Again, the procedure is conditioned by the patient's expectations and preparation.

It may be necessary to "change horses in midstream." For instance, it is common in anterior cruciate–deficient knees to find a torn meniscus that should and could be repaired. This could be done either arthroscopically or open. The ligament may be repaired or augmented. An extracapsular repair may be necessary after examination under anesthesia, and this may mean arthrotomy. Be prepared.

Aborted procedure

Any operative procedure can and should be aborted when it is in the patient's best interest. The usual reason to stop a procedure is when it exceeds a reasonable operative time. The limitations of tourniquet control (approximately 1½ hours) may be a factor. Procedures should not exceed 2 hours. It is reasonable to perform diagnostic and complicated operative arthroscopy, including combined open procedures, well within this time. If not, then staging or deferment of the operative dimension should be considered.

Prolonged operative times result in increased instrument passage, tissue damage, surgeon fatigue, and anesthesia risk.

As an operative procedure approaches 1 hour, the surgeon should formulate a plan to conclude. This may mean finishing the operative arthroscopy and leaving open surgery for another time. If meniscal repair cannot be accomplished arthroscopically, the knee should be opened early in the procedure.

If diagnostic arthroscopy exceeds 30 minutes, no operative work should be initiated. Diagnostic arthroscopy exceeding 1 hour is unnecessary when surgeons are available to perform with greater dispatch. Complicated operative work should not be initiated when a reasonable amount of time is not available for completion.

Arthroscopic meniscectomy should not exceed 1 hour. Surgeons with operative times that regularly exceed 1 hour for diagnostic and 1½ hours for operative work should limit their case selection to conform to reasonable operative times. Some should choose other interests within the field of orthopedic surgery.

The practice of operating without a tourniquet to allow longer than 2 hours safe operation time sacrifices the less bloody surgical field that could expedite the procedure. If the tourniquet is released and re-elevated in prolonged cases, the surgical field is compromised by bleeding and capsular edema.

I am an advocate of "how well" not "how fast." However, prolonged operative times often are a reflection of "how well" the procedure has progressed or been accomplished.

These opinions on time restrictions are intended as guidelines. Time is a measure of preparation, not just execution (see Fig. 2-46). When the surgeon has both, the operative times decline. Judgment precedes experience in the production of reasonable operative times.

Independent of time, if the surgeon is failing to make progress in any phase of arthroscopy, it is reasonable to conclude the operation. If the surgeon cannot see or make a diagnosis, the procedure should stop. If an arthroscopic diagnosis is made and the operative procedure is not within the skill level of the surgeon, then procedure should be aborted. The meniscus tear may be visible but not approachable in a tight knee. Simultaneous television monitoring resolves this question, clearly demonstrating the progress to all who are viewing.

Every attempt should be made to retrieve a broken instrument. Still, the operation should be aborted in the patient's best interest rather than use excessive time or create further tissue damage. A second look on another day is sound judgment.

In summary, if for any reason the surgeon is unable to complete the surgery safely for the patient, the operation should be aborted. This includes mishaps to the surgeon and any of the just-mentioned factors or anesthetic problems.

AN ABORTED PROCEDURE SHOULD REFLECT GOOD JUDGMENT, NOT FAILURE OF TECHNIQUE

There is always another day or another way. The case can be deferred or referred. Dogged determination to complete arthroscopic surgery without regard to time is not just unfortunate but unreasonable and unnecessary.

Fatigue and frustration

Fatigue and frustration are a dimension of arthroscopic surgery, no matter what the experience or skill level of the surgeon. If the operative progress is hampered, then concluding the procedure is sound judgment. These emotions can result in tissue trauma and inexact manipulation. Stopping for even 5 minutes early in the procedure will allow regrouping and subsequent progress.

The failure to make progress and the factor of fatigue may lead to loss of composure, self-control, or surgical imagination. Strife among the operating room team may have to be resolved. Good surgical judgment dictates concluding the surgery.

Combined procedures

Another plan of action is to combine arthroscopic techniques with conventional open surgery. The patient should recognize ahead of time that a combination procedure is being considered. This is the most common in the anterior cruciate–deficient knee with a torn meniscus.

The combined procedures are used in patellar alignment problems. An incision is used to reposition the tibial tubercle in patella alta and patella baja. In some cases of patellar dislocation the knee is opened for retinacular repair. Open repair is used in patients who are obese, who have severe chronic cases, and who have bone avulsed with retinaculum. In the latter case, the bone fragment is excised, and the retinaculum is resutured to the patella.

In unicompartmental degenerative arthritis the arthroscopic debridement is combined with high tibial osteotomy. In rotator cuff disease the patient is positioned on his side for arthroscopic work. This same position lends itself to open rotator cuff repair. Intraarticular work is done arthroscopically, thereby limiting the surgical exposure for cuff repair.

GENERAL SURGICAL PRINCIPLES
Asepsis

Infection is a rare complication of arthroscopy, although it does occur, especially when direct viewing immediately precedes open surgery. A complete skin preparation and sterile draping should precede open surgery if direct viewing is performed.

The system outlined in this textbook gives arthroscopic surgical sterile technique the same respect as in open procedures.

Hemostasis

Hemostasis is provided during the arthroscopy with tourniquet control. Operative techniques avoid or ligate vessels of significant size. Postoperative hemostasis is controlled with compression. Some surgeons use electrocautery in lateral capsular release to prevent postoperative hemarthrosis.

Air instillation can have a drying effect on tissues and cause hemostasis, which is especially useful in shoulder acromionectomy.

Gentleness

The restrictions of space, size of instruments, and delicacy of articular cartilage require maximum gentleness in arthroscopic surgery. Any lack of gentleness is magnified by the lens systems and projected on television for all to see. There is not much margin for error arthroscopically.

PROPER OVERVIEW

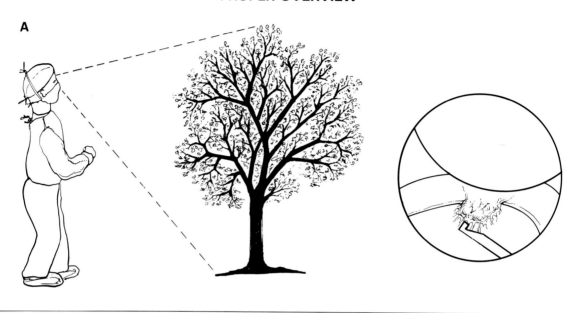

TOO CLOSE FOR COMFORT

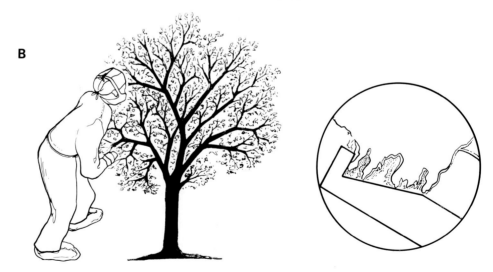

FIG. 6-2. Optimal position of arthroscope.

A Scope retracted to give overview.
B Surgeon and scope too close to lesion for comfort or instrumentation.

Working from known to unknown

The general surgical principle of working from known to unknown is absolutely necessary in arthroscopy. The arthroscopic view is small; if the view is up close to a structures, there is no adjacent landmark for orientation (Fig. 6-2). "Getting lost" is common. "Whiteout" and "redout" pictures confirm the lost position (Fig. 6-3).

During arthroscopy the view should be as wide as possible. This will show relative relationships. If a close-up is necessary, one may move in and out for perspective. In the knee joint, the femoral condyle serves a hozitonal reference point. Orientation is aided by locating tibial spine and moving into the selected compartment to see the inner edge of the meniscus. The horizon of the humeral head in the shouler or talus in the ankle may serve the same purpose. If lost, the surgeon should go back to the last known area.

The scope may scan back and forth from a known landmark to homogenous (i.e., articular cartilage), indistinct areas to maintain orientation. Retracing of steps may be necessary to regain position.

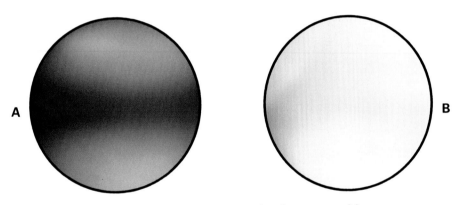

FIG. 6-3. Arthroscopic view of unknown position.

A "Redout."
B Whiteout.

ARTHROSCOPIC SURGICAL PRINCIPLES
Projection into joint

The surgeon must mentally project himself or herself into the joint (Fig. 6-4). He or she should ignore the body and hand position, seeking only to orient the image horizontally on the television monitor (Fig. 6-5). The surgeon must disregard position of the scope and instruments and focus only on the horizontal position on the television monitor. All other moves are made in relation to this orientation.

Repeated glances to outside positions distract and confuse orientation (see Fig. 6-44). Only when the surgeon is completely lost should he or she look at the hands or the instruments (see Fig. 6-26, *A*). The amount of angulation is best judged with direct viewing. The same is true for pistoning or rotation, once it is determined which direction the angled scope is facing. When the surgeon is reoriented, video monitoring can be resumed (see Fig. 6-44).

MENTAL PROJECTION

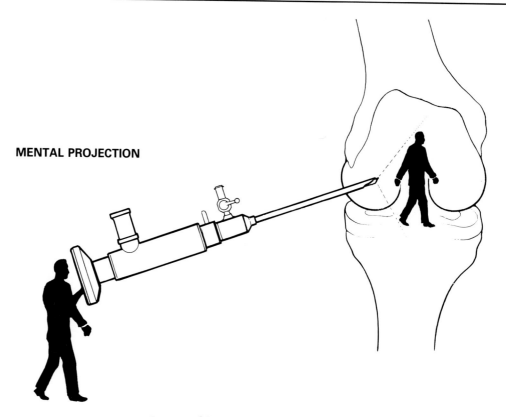

FIG. 6-4. Mental projection into joint.

ORIENTATION IN SPACE

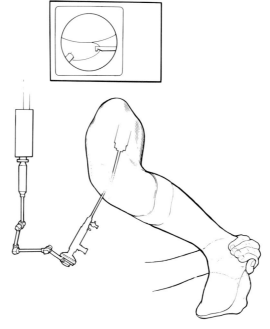

FIG. 6-5. Horizontal orientation of television image, without regard to body or scope position, is necessary to accomplish maneuver.

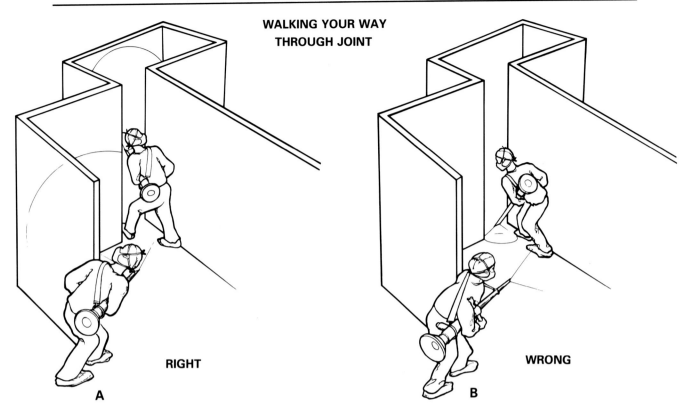

FIG. 6-6. Following light around corners.

A Right.
B Wrong.

As the surgeon progresses through the various recesses of the joint, he or she should shine a way through with the scope, as if with a flashlight (Fig. 6-6). The surgeon's head should be looking in the same direction as the light is shining. In case of arthroscopy, this is done by rotating the scope around corners.

Patient positioning

The patient is supine for all arthroscopic procedures except those in the shoulder, in which the patient is placed in opposite lateral decubitus position. A fracture table is used for hip arthroscopy to facilitate traction and x-ray control.

Lens system

A lens system is used in open surgery; it resides within the surgeon's eye. In addition, corrective lenses are used by some surgeons, in the form of conventional eyeglasses (Fig. 6-7, A and B).

The operating microscope used in eye, ear, and hand surgery is another example of surgical lens system (Fig. 6-7, C).

In arthroscopy, further lens systems exist within the arthroscope to visualize the operative site (Fig. 6-7, D to F).

The arthroscopic lens also magnifies. Further magnification occurs with an electronic image on a television monitor with minimal loss of optical clarity.

The arthroscopic lens system provides only a two-dimensional image, compared to the binocular vision at open surgery. The spatial relationships of expo-

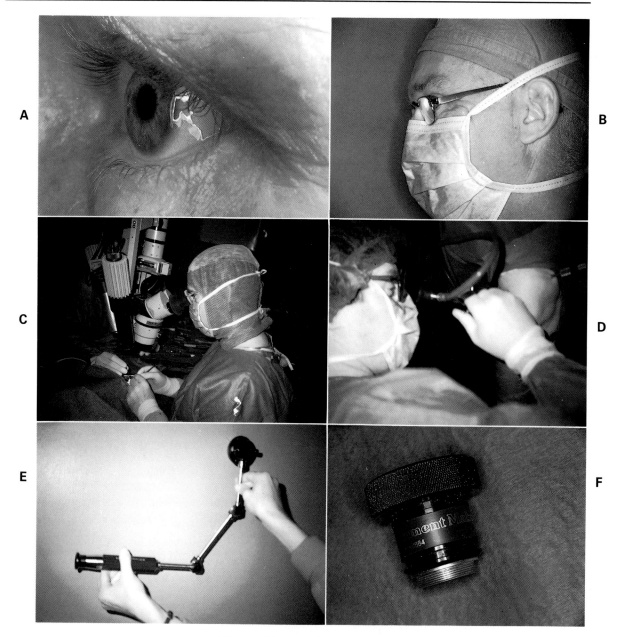

FIG. 6-7. Various lens systems.

A Surgeon's eye.
B Eyeglasses.
C Microscope.
D Arthroscope.
E Articulated viewing device.
F Camera lens adaptor.

sure are gained by shadowing, relative size, and position, and these are assisted by probing and palpation.

Illumination

All surgical procedures are performed with supplemental light. The requirements of open surgery are met with suspended lamps or head-mounted lights. Intraarticular spaces are dark requiring a powerful light supplement for surgical exposure (see Fig. 5-10).

Surgical exposure

The principle of a secured extremity is very important in arthroscopic surgery. Firm fixation of the proximal body part is needed to manipulate against to gain maximal mechanical access to small joint spaces (Fig. 6-8, *A*).

In the knee joint this is best accomplished with a mechanical device to secure the thigh. The Surgical Assistant thigh holder was the first such instrument. It was safe and effective. The Surgical Assistant is also used to secure the proximal arm in elbow athroscopy and the middle of the leg for ankle procedures. In shoulder operations the patient is secured to the table, but the scapula is stabilized by manual counterpressure at the time of operative work on the glenoid (stapling). In hip operations the patient is on a fracture table.

A

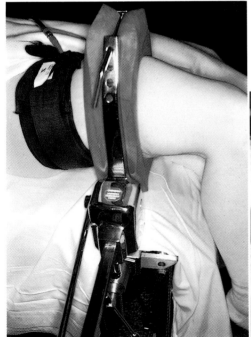

B

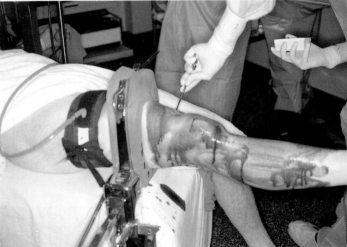

FIG. 6-8. Surgical setup and draping for knee joint.

A Thigh in Surgical Assistant.
B Skin preparation after application of tourniquet and mechanical device.

Continued.

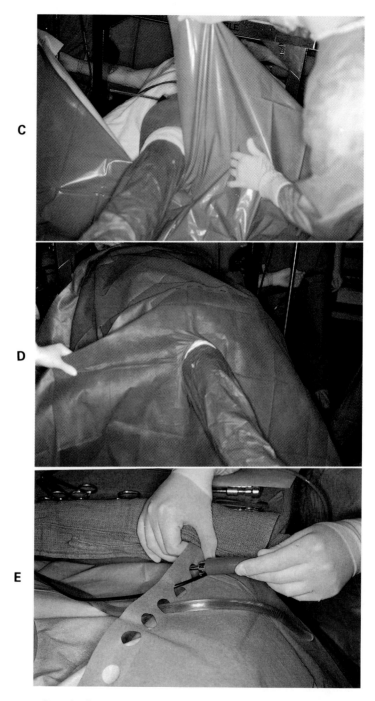

FIG. 6-8, cont'd. Surgical setup and draping for knee joint.

C Sterile draping over extremity and plastic barrier seals of patient and table.
D Wide paper drape over entire end of table has absorbent surface.
E Tubing through tabs in drape avoids falling to side of table.

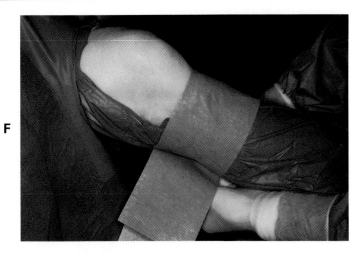

FIG. 6-8, cont'd. Surgical setup and draping for knee joint.

F Area exposed for surgical field. Wrap at lower end prevents fluid from running inside plastic bag to foot.

Surgical setup

The surgical setup includes a secured extremity, Betadine preparation, and sterile water impervious draping (Fig. 6-8, *A* to *D*). The Johnson & Johnson Arthroscopy Pack has special loops to hold various tubes and cords (Fig. 6-8, *E*). Adhesive wrap is applied to the extremity to secure unsterile areas for exposure (Fig. 6-8, *F*).

Distention with fluid

The synovial joint is normally in a decompressed state unless there is pathological effusion. Distention is necessary for access and visualization. This is usually accomplished with sterile normal saline or lactated Ringer's solution.[9] The theoretical value of Ringer's lactate has been demonstrated in the laboratory. I have observed no clinical problem with normal saline.

Originally I delivered saline into the joint via the arthroscope. A 60 ml syringe was attached to a K-52 plastic catheter, which was connected to the spigot of the arthroscope cannula. With this technique, the joint was penetrated and intraarticular placement confirmed before distention. This technique is still used for small joints.

The beginning arthroscopist may choose to distend the joint with a needle and syringe to facilitate entry. The maximal distention enlarges the target for the arthroscopic cannula. Fluid backflow through the cannula confirms entry. In small joints, preliminary distention is routine. In knee arthroscopy, I initially distend with a superomedial inflow cannula.

Infusion system

Traditionally the infusion system for diagnostic arthroscopy was brought through the arthroscope via one of the side spigots of the cannula system. This was adopted from a urological technique. In addition, the traditionalists used what was called a Verres needle in the suprapatellar pouch. They insisted that

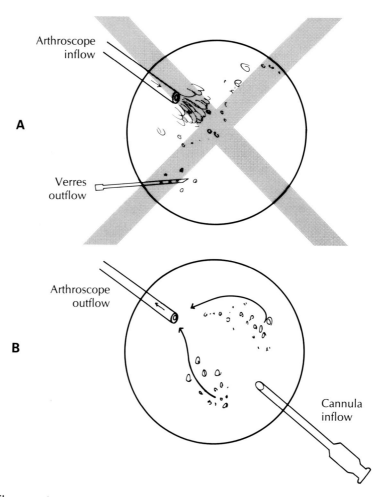

FIG. 6-9. Flow systems.

A Impractical inflow on arthroscope and outflow via Verres needle.
B Large cannula inflow and intermittent outflow on arthroscope during diagnostic phase.

small particles were blown from in front of the scope and moved 2 or 3 inches up into the suprapatellar pouch, where they flowed out of the knee joint from one of the many tiny holes in the Verres needle (Fig. 6-9). I doubt this was the case.

In the past, some surgeons simultaneously opened both inflow spigots on the arthroscopic cannula. They insisted the fluid would flow in along the arthroscope, into the joint, back out the joint, and into the opposite spigot. Of course, fluid flows to the area of least pressure; in this case, that was directly across the cannula. No fluid flowed into the knee joint. It was a nonexistent irrigation system.

Inflow on arthroscope: smaller scope, small joints

The delivery of fluid through the arthroscope during either diagnostic or operative arthroscopy is limited by small spigot openings. The spigot opening is approximately 1 to 2 mm in diameter. This is a cross-sectional area far less than that of a 4.2 mm cannula used in the suprapatellar pouch. Unless pressure was applied by pump or to the fluid reservoir by mechanical means, the amount of fluid delivered would not be comparable.

Inflow on the arthroscope produces turbulence in the field of views, and concentration is disrupted by constant motion of synovium. If loose fragments exist, swirling of the pieces adds further distraction, and they are transported out of sight to recesses of the joint rather than removed.

Under local anesthetic technique, intermittent distention of the joint was originally alternated with vacuuming. Subsequently an inflow via a separate cannula in the suprapatellar pouch was combined with an outflow and intermittent suction on the arthroscope.

Separate superior portal inflow: knee, shoulder

During the development of the Intra-articular Shaver System, a heart-lung machine was used to measure flows and pressures as well as record volumes. The patient's fluid intake and output during the preoperative and postoperative course were also measured. We settled on the following irrigation method as being simple, safe, rational, and effective.

Each knee operative case in the knee begins with the insertion of a 4.2 mm inside diameter cannula into the suprapatellar pouch (Fig. 6-10). This cannula comes with the Dyonics Intra-articular Shaver System. In shoulder surgery the inflow comes through the superior supraspinatus portal.

Malposition of the cannula may compromise fluid flow (Fig. 6-11). It may be placed out of the joint or above the suprapatellar bursa. A poor direction is proximal. It is not proper to have the cannula pushed against the far joint wall. The latter problem prompted the two small openings in the end of the inflow cannula.

Two 3-liter bags are attached via a sterile Y-tube to an adaptor on the cannula. The bags are placed at least 1 meter above the patient (Fig. 6-12).

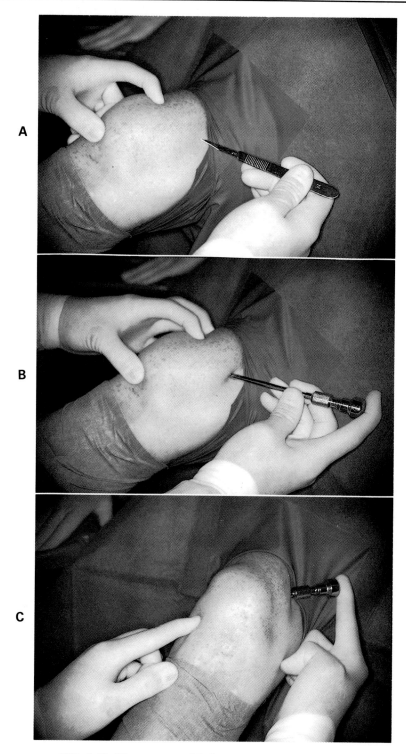

FIG. 6-10. Placement of inflow for knee joint.

A Site of skin incision.
B Cannula placed parallel to undersurface patella.
C Cannula tip palpated laterally.

D

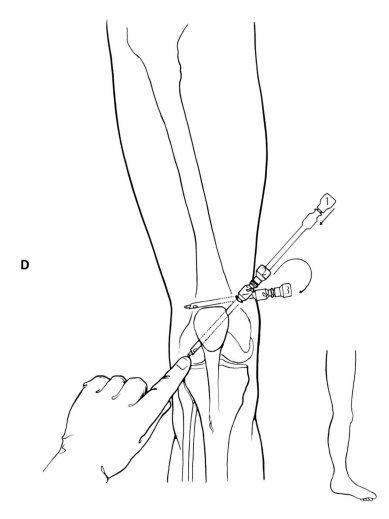

FIG. 6-10, cont'd. Placement of inflow.

D Drawing of inflow cannula insertion.
E Fluid removed from joint.
F Inflow tubing attached via adaptor.

E

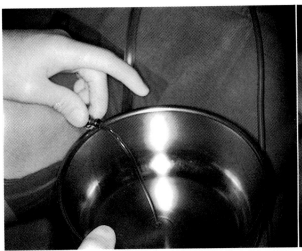

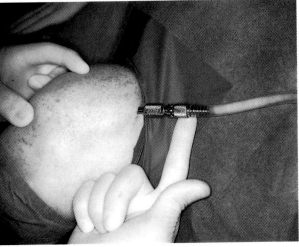

F

A

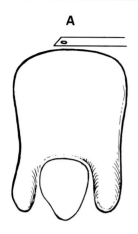

B

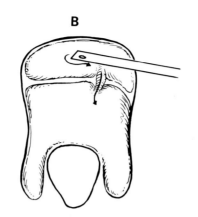

C

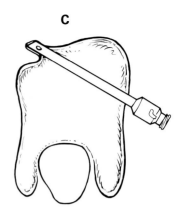

FIG. 6-11. Malpositions of inflow placement.

A Superior to pouch.
B Above plica in suprapatellar bursa.
C Proximal angulation against opposite wall.

Inflow-outflow control: diagnostic phase

The arthroscope is placed in the joint, and the suction apparatus is attached to one of the spigots of the arthroscope. Inflow on arthroscope moves tissues or fragments out of sight and is counterproductive (Fig. 6-12, *A*). During diagnostic arthroscopy, the distention is controlled by balancing inflow and outflow (Fig. 6-13). This can be done by continuous flow (Fig. 6-13, *B*). If suction exceeds inflow, the joint is decompressed (Fig. 6-13, *C*). The outflow spigot may be closed (Fig. 6-13, *D*). This method has some advantages. Particles are drawn into view and out of the joint rather than being blown away (Fig. 6-14). Fragments or loose pieces are drawn toward the arthroscope for identification and removal. If the pieces are very small and supple, they can be removed by the suction alone. If large, they may cover the end of the arthroscope and block visualization. Simply removing the arthroscope from the cannula and letting the fluid rush out removes the piece (Fig. 6-14, *C*). With only a momentary delay, inspection can proceed by replacing the arthroscope.

A piece too large for the cannula is delivered by suction to a site for easy removal. For instance, a loose body from the posterior aspect of the joint can be moved to the anterior aspect of the intercondylar notch. This space is anterior, has bony confines, and is easily exposed and entered with forceps.

Using suction on the arthroscope allows recessed areas to be vacuumed, such as under the meniscus, the popliteal sheath, or a Baker's cyst. In addition, turbulence created by external ballotement from the posterior aspect of the joint moves particles to the arthroscope.

One disadvantage of this system occurs when suction draws synovium over the end of the arthroscope, obscuring the view. Simply turning off the suction and moving the arthroscope will release the synovium and allow visualization to commence.

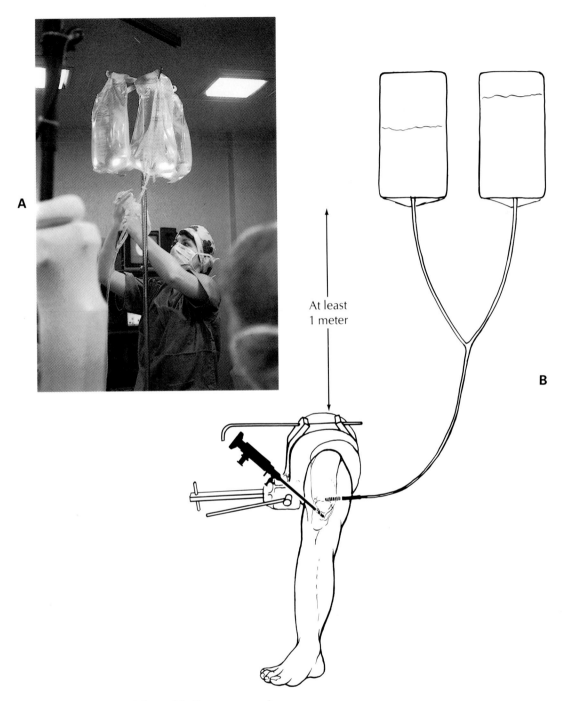

A

At least
1 meter

B

FIG. 6-12. Position of inflow reservoir.

A Bags allow manual compression to increase pressure and flow when needed.
B Reservoir suspended at least 1 meter above joint.

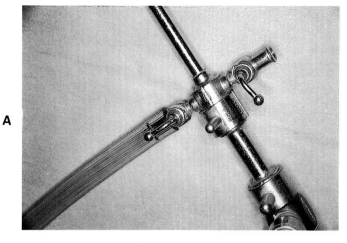

FIG. 6-13. Various inflow-outflow combinations.

A Suction attached to arthroscope spigot.
B Inflow should exceed outflow with outflow open.
C Outflow greater than inflow results in joint collapse
D No outflow, no flow is the situation during some of the diagnostic phase

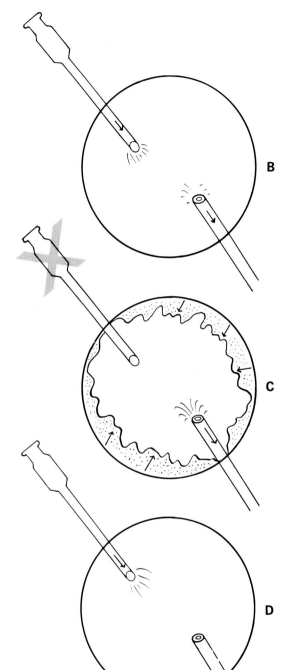

E There is considerable mobility to lateral meniscus, seen here in maximal distension.
F With inflow clamped off and suction applied to arthroscope spigot, lateral meniscus collapses inward from posterior and anterior, hinging immediately anterior to popliteus tendon.

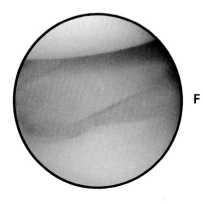

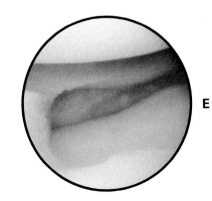

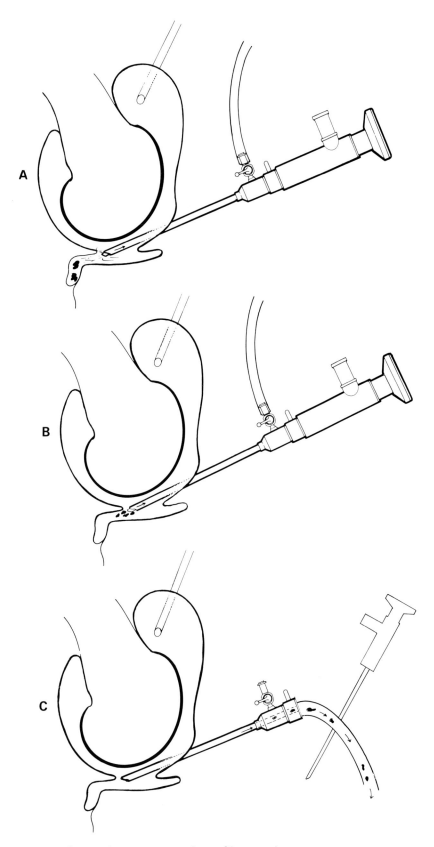

FIG. 6-14. Intermittent vacuuming of loose pieces.

A Suction on arthroscope.
B Small fragments move out between cannula and scope.
C Large fragments removed out of cannula when scope is removed.

No-flow viewing

After the compartments have been examined and cleansed, the outflow spigot is closed (see Fig. 6-13, *D*). The inflow remains open via cannula for maximal distention.

There is not flow during most hand instrumentation. After hand instrumentation (basket forceps), small fragments are removed by insertion of cannula and gravity flow. Outflow is used during use of motorized instrumentation.

Operative outflow

The effectiveness of motorized instruments is based on flow, both to move material into the cutting device and remove it from the joint by suction.

Postoperative inspection

Postoperative inspection is accompanied by reapplication of vacuum suction to the arthroscope to remove any remaining surgical debris.

Suction pressure

Gravity outflow is not adequate to mobilize intraarticular fragments or maximize motorized instruments. Suction is required.

In 1975 to 1976, during the development of the Intra-articular Shaver System, we tested all the various pressure suction apparatus. The wall vacuum system in our operating room was measured at 14 and 16 inches of mercury (40 cm Hg) (see Fig. 4-20).

It is important that this be measured in-line and not end-on. End-on measurements will tend to falsely elevate the value of the suction over the in-line test (Fig. 6-15). Most operating rooms suction systems measure between 14 and 16 inches of mercury.

The Dyonics Intra-articular Shaver System (window size, and diameter) was calibrated for this in-line suction pressure. I am not familiar with calibration of replicas.

Suction can be used intermittently throughout the procedure to vacuum any small particles from any and all recesses of the joint (see Fig. 6-14). Free-hand ballottement or even the probe to elevate areas to remove debris could be done within any recess of the joint.

Suction can also be valuable in gaining access to a suprapatellar plica area so that when the joint is distended the plica appears as a very sharp structure that is displaced from the joint. If the joint is decompressed, which is the normal joint situation, the medial plica will be seen to move in between the patella and femur and show its juxtaposition to rough areas. Even suprapatellar plicae can be large enough to cause patellofemoral arthralgia and can mimic chondromalacia by coming down all the way in a decompressed joint between the patella and the femoral articulation.

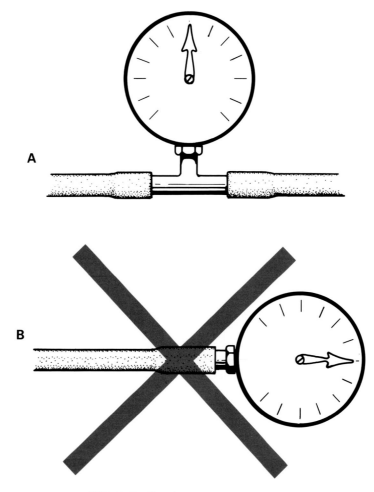

FIG. 6-15. Suction measurements.

A In-line.
B End-on.

Fine-tuning of flows

Careful attention is given by the circulating nurse to avoid an empty fluid reservoir (see Fig. 6-12, *A*). One bag usually empties before the other. If not, one bag is clamped off as they empty. Pressure is applied to the other bag until it is empty. The first bag is unclamped to maintain flow during change of the second bag. An alternating emptying system is most functional.

In some cases, extra pressure is required to overcome synovial encroachment. Increased flow may be necessary when motorized instruments are used in the lateral compartments of the knee with capsular compression from the figure-4 position. In either case, intermittent pressure created by clamping one bag and squeezing the other solves the problem.

The outflow may not be in perfect balance with the inflow. The joint may be overvacuumed (see Fig. 6-13, C). This happens in small joint arthroscopy and with small intraarticular fluid reservoirs. The arthroscopic view is obliterated by the rush of air bubbles and by joint lining encroachment. The second assistant can partially restrict outflow by bending the outflow tubing (Fig. 6-16). The experienced assistant can perfectly coordinate (fine-tune) the flow by watching the surgical field on the television monitor. In some cases, both pressure on bags and restriction of outflow are necessary.

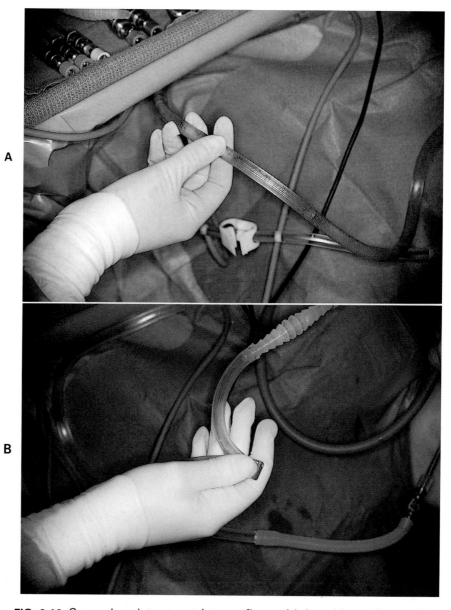

FIG. 6-16. Second assistant restricts outflow with bend in outflow tubing.

A Partial measured restriction.
B Clamped off to redistend joint.

Auxiliary inflow

Additional cannulas or attachments to the arthroscope are sometimes used as auxiliary sources of inflow to tight or small reservoir spaces.

The inflow system can be attached to the arthroscope with use of an adaptor for gravity flow (Fig. 6-17, *A*). A K-52 catheter may be attached to the arthroscope spigot and fluid delivered under pressure with 60 ml syringe (Fig. 6-17, *B*).

An additional cannula may be placed in the same compartment or an adjacent area to provide unobstructed flow to motorized instrumentation.

Joint position effects on flow

In the knee joint, acute flexion or figure-4 position will obstruct flow from suprapatellar area to the lower compartment operative site. In that case, increased pressure is applied to the bags and knee is taken into flexion to expose the operative lesion. The flow is cut off and the compartment is vacuumed dry, which results in ineffective cutting. This problem is overcome by starting with

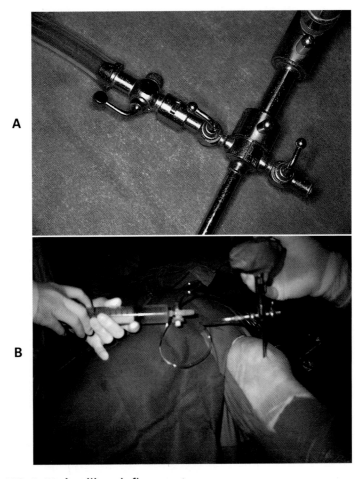

FIG. 6-17. Auxiliary inflow system.

A Gravity flow to arthroscope via adaptor.

B 60 ml syringe drivers fluid under pressure via K-52 catheter.

the knee in slight extension to provide flow. The knee is flexed slowly to the point of decompression. Just before the compartment is dry, the leg is extended briefly to re-establish flow. The motorized instrument is run continuously, and the inflow of fluid to the compartment is regulated by gently moving the knee back and forth.

If this method fails, an alternate method of resection with hand instruments without flow may be necessary.

Cleaning and vacuuming

The liquid medium lends itself well to dilution of joint effusion and mobilization and removal of loose fragments. Surgical exposure and visualization are enhanced by cleansing and vacuuming joint fluid and fragments. The joint is then filled with clear liquid. Even massive hemarthrosis can be cleansed with proper technique and volume exchange with saline.

Joint cleansing is enhanced by large-volume inflow on a separate cannula. Suction vacuuming on the arthroscope draws fragments to the scope for removal. Small, soft pieces fold up and are removed along the scope. Medium-sized pieces come out of the cannula with momentary scope removal. Suction can be applied directly to the end of the scope cannula. Large pieces may require forceps or motorized instrument removal.

Ballottement of a joint, especially on the posterior aspect of the knee, creates turbulence and mobilizes fragments from joint recesses to the force of suction on the arthroscope (Fig. 6-18).

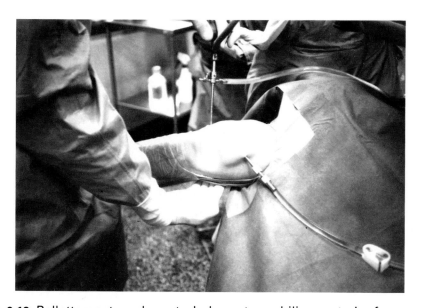

FIG. 6-18. Ballottement produces turbulence to mobilize posterior fragments.

Distention with gas

The joint can be distended by room air or CO_2 delivery systems.[3,10] For diagnostic purposes, the field of view is optically wider in air than in a liquid medium (Fig. 6-19). CO_2 must be used for laser surgery. It has some advantage over sterile water for lateral release by electrocautery, but no other advantages. I have used room air for joint distention to enhance a slide photograph with a wider angle of view. The practical value of intermittent distention with room air is to control bleeding. The drying effects of air cause a clot to form. This is most often used in shoulder and subacromial bursa surgery. Room air is delivered via a 60 ml syringe via a K-52 catheter attached to the arthroscope spigot. The air quickly dissipates, and a repeat volume is delivered.

I have seen no complications of infection, air embolism, or troublesome subcutaneous emphysema. The concern over injecting nonsterile room air is no more hazardous than the same air coming into contact with the wound at open surgery. Gas infusion under mechanical pressure could result in subcutaneous or tissue emphysema.

One disadvantage of air distention is the absence of liquid circulation for mobilization of loose fragments. Also, operative motorized instruments are designed for fluid medium and fragment removal by suction.

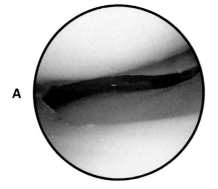 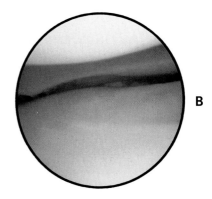

FIG. 6-19. Wider angle of view in air than in fluid medium of lateral compartment.

A Air medium.
B Fluid medium.

SCOPE TECHNIQUES
Placement

Proper placement of the arthroscope is essential to successful arthroscopy (Fig. 6-20). It constitutes the surgical approach. If an incision is misplaced in open surgery, a correction is possible. In arthroscopic surgery, a separate puncture or redirection is required to correct. A scope placed too superior does not enter into the slot of the intercondylar space. Access for viewing the posterior meniscal horn is obstructed. A scope placed too far inferior could go through or under the meniscus, impeding movement and subsequent viewing, not to mention rendering tissue damage.

The skin only is lacerated with a No. 11 blade (Fig. 6-20, C). Care is taken not to penetrate into the joint or articular cartilage. The puncture should be only wide enough to accept the cannula. Otherwise, fluid leaks out and causes joint decompression, wet feet, and a wet floor.

A cannula with a sharp trocar pierces the skin and capsule. The trocar is replaced with a blunt obturator for synovial penetration and joint entry. The commercially available cannula systems have trocars that are too sharp and obturators that are too blunt. I have smoothed a sharp trocar, and it serves both functions to allow a single joint entry.

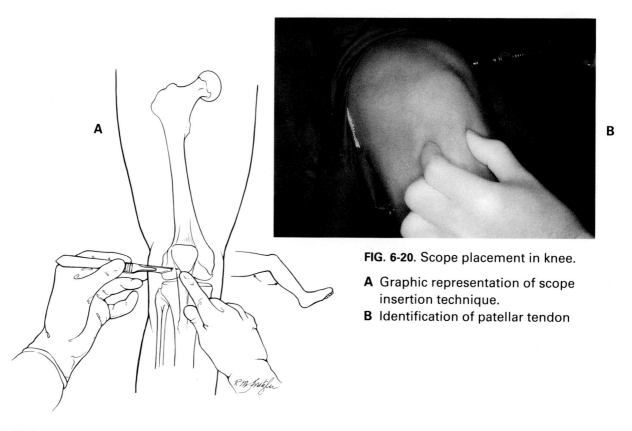

A

B

FIG. 6-20. Scope placement in knee.

A Graphic representation of scope insertion technique.

B Identification of patellar tendon

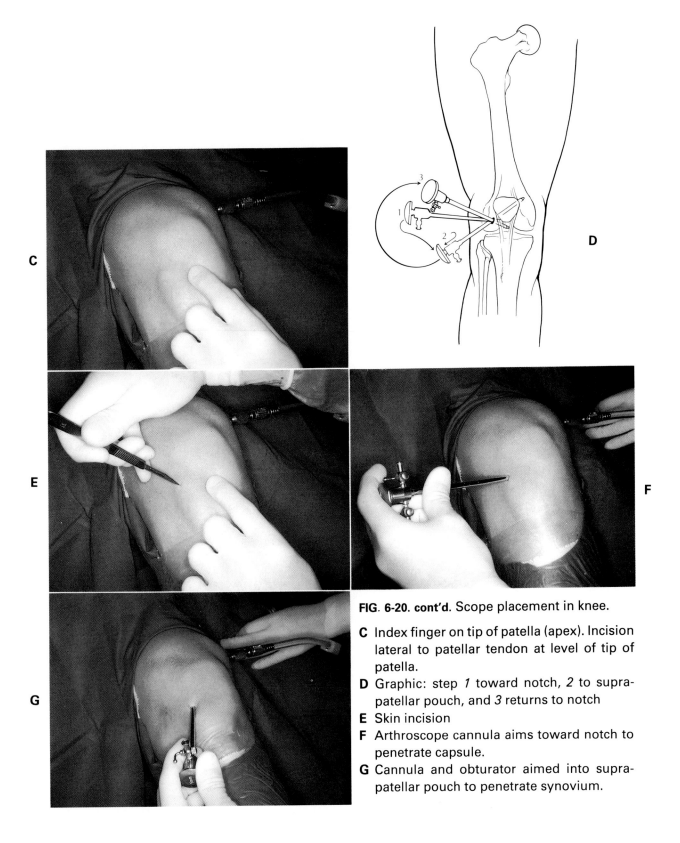

FIG. 6-20. cont'd. Scope placement in knee.

C Index finger on tip of patella (apex). Incision lateral to patellar tendon at level of tip of patella.

D Graphic: step *1* toward notch, *2* to suprapatellar pouch, and *3* returns to notch

E Skin incision

F Arthroscope cannula aims toward notch to penetrate capsule.

G Cannula and obturator aimed into suprapatellar pouch to penetrate synovium.

The hand control for penetation is forward pressure with rotation (Fig. 6-21). The rotation motion works cannula and obturator into the joint. This controlled technique avoids "plunging," mishap, and joint surface injury (see Fig. 6-21).

Complete penetration gains maximum entry of the instrument into the joint. Slow retraction without rotation hangs up the synovium and capsule on the instrument shaft. This avoids accidental exit and covering of the end of the scope with tissue, obscuring the view (Fig. 6-22).

The inexperienced arthrocopist is so intensely focused on difficulties of viewing that he or she fails to recognize incorrect placement. Perhaps another site should be selected. It is considered good technique to either replace or redirect an arthroscope. This avoids struggling with poor exposure.

ARTHROSCOPIC INSERTION

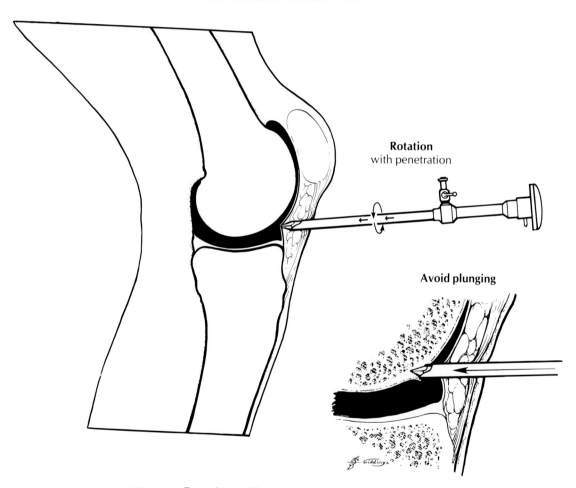

Rotation
with penetration

Avoid plunging

FIG. 6-21. Rotation with penetration avoids plunging.

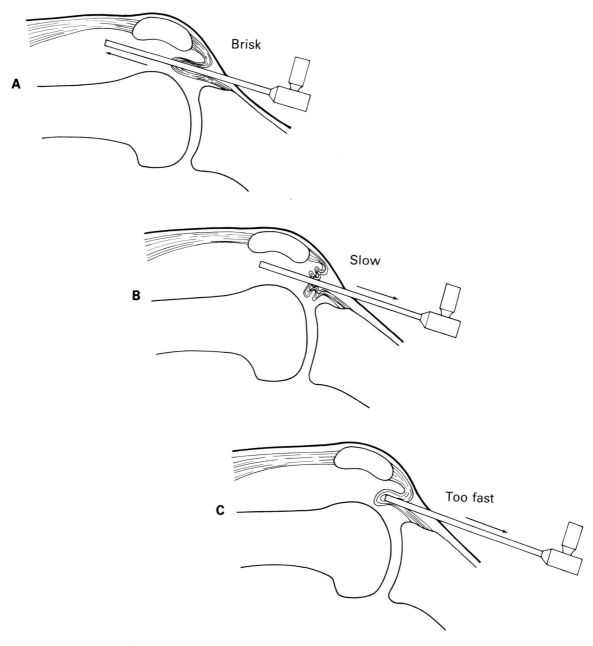

FIG. 6-22

A Brisk motion will penetrate fat pad and suprapatellar pouch, hanging fat pad synovium on shank of cannula.

B Very slow retraction of cannula and endoscope will prevent fat pad from slipping over end of scope.

C Fast retraction will pull endoscope into fat pad and obscure viewing.

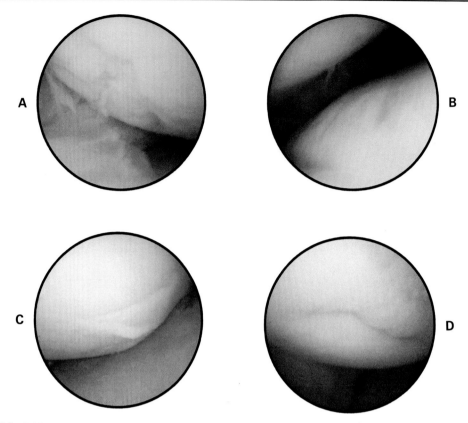

FIG. 6-23

A Iatrogenic traumatic arthritis after failed attempt at medial meniscectomy.
B Gouges in femoral trochlea 6 months after diagnostic arthroscopy.
C Scrape on femoral condyle with scope entry in wrong direction.
D Defect on femur after failed arthroscopy of surgeon in self-training.

Poor placement sites are commonly seen in patients seeking second opinions after failed arthroscopic surgery. I have seen some placed as much as 2 inches below the joint line. No amount of manipulation could produce proper surgical exposure from this position. Reoperation usually shows unrecognized lesions and iatrogenic articular cartilate damage (traumatic arthritis) (Fig. 6-23).

Fulcrum

All instrumentation placed arthroscopically operates off a fulcrum principle. The skin and capsular tissues hold the instrument in one place for side-to-side motion. Therefore motion on the outside to the right moves the instrumentation on the inside to the left and vice versa.

Small puncture wounds provide firm fulcrum fixation and exacting motions. A large portal incision not only allows the instrument to slide side to side, but in and out, thus losing manipulative exactness. Troublesome leakage may also occur around a large opening. If the hole is large, hand pressure may be necessary at the skin level to stop the leak and keep the instrument from plunging.

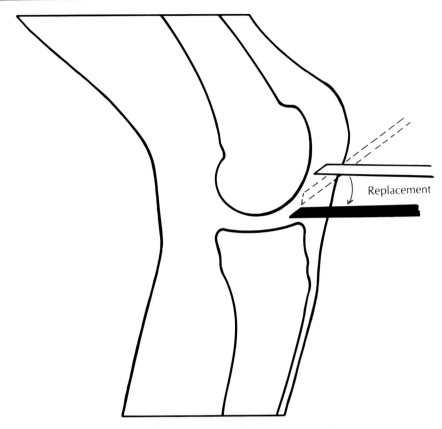

FIG. 6-24. Replacement for proper viewing.

Replacement

If surgical exposure is not optimal, the scope should be removed and another site selected (Fig. 6-24). Attention to proper sites is mentioned under specific techniques.

If the site appears close to optimal, then the same skin incision could be used. The skin is moved sideways up or down, and another capsular penetration is accomplished.

Replacement is chosen if either scar tissue or depth of tissue decreases instrument mobility. If compartment visualization is compromised, an alternate portal is chosen.

Direction

The scope or instrument is directed toward a known anatomical target. It is helpful to view the surface anatomy with bony landmarks. However, the internal structures are still not seen as in open surgery, with layer by layer exposure.

Palpation is the sense that is of greatest value in proper direction. To enhance palpation, it is helpful to look away; this removes the useless temptation to visualize. This technique is used in shoulder portal placement of the scope. After entry is sensed by palpation the scope is placed for confirmation. This same technique is valuable for placement of instrumentation. Specific portals are discussed in the chapters on specific joints.

Redirection

If the position is acceptable and failure of proper placement seems to be directional, the redirection should be tried before portal position is changed. The instrument is withdrawn through the capsule, not the skin, and reinserted by palpation in another direction.

Patients who are obese give a wide fulcrum in the tissue for the arthroscope (Fig. 6-25). Scars of previous surgery or injury make it difficult to move the arthroscope. Redirection should be considered in these cases. Forcing the arthroscope through a wide fulcrum or through tough tissue can only result in injury to the arthroscope and/or the patient's articular tissue. In some patients with a very tight or scarred joint, it may be necessary to redirect as many as three times to view a single compartment. This should be considered good technique, not failure of the initial placement. This also can be the case in moving from the suprapatellar pouch down into the medial or lateral compartment. In addition, it may not even be possible to see the suprapatellar pouch from below if there are large osteophytes on the patella. This may necessitate redirection or use of a different portal to visualize the area.

Redirection to an area is simple. It produces less tissue injury than does forceful angulation. Redirection facilitates complete inspection of all the chambers of the joint.

If redirection fails, then a minor change of portal position will be necessary. In some cases, an alternate portal at another area of the joint will be necessary.

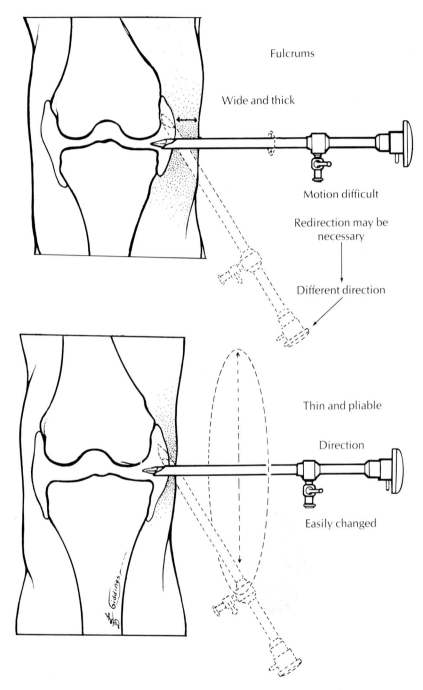

Fulcrums

Wide and thick

Motion difficult

Redirection may be necessary

Different direction

Thin and pliable

Direction

Easily changed

FIG. 6-25. Redirection necessary in scarred or thick fat capsule.

Body control

Lower body

The arthroscopist may appear as a one-man-band with all body parts being involved (Fig. 6-26, *A*). The feet must be firmly planted on the floor or the surgeon firmly seated on a stable stool. This is the platform from which various maneuvers take place. One foot secures balance as the other operates the foot pedal.

During knee joint arthroscopy, the surgeon secures the patient's leg against his or her thigh, thereby freeing both hands for surgical manipulation (Fig. 6-26, *B*). Joint flexion and extension are controlled with the flexion-extension of the surgeon's knee. This often requires that the table be lowered so the surgeon does not have to stand on tiptoe, thereby losing balance and fine control. Varus and valgus are applied by lower body pressure. A gentle, continuous force will open the medial or lateral compartment the millimeter that is necessary for adequate visualization.

Upper body

Although the grip on the arthroscope is firm, it is important that the rest of the body remain relaxed. The intensity of the procedure may cause unconscious tenseness and fatigue. The surgeon's wrist, elbow, and shoulder make up universal joint for scope manipulation.

The firmness of the grip allows precise movements and prevents any slippage or inadvertant joint injury. Dexterity is provided by the wrist, elbow, and shoulder. Lack of precision in handling the endoscope and cannula and/or trocar could result in quick motion and potential abrasions to the intraarticular structures, especially the articular cartilage. Damage to the arthroscope is also possible.

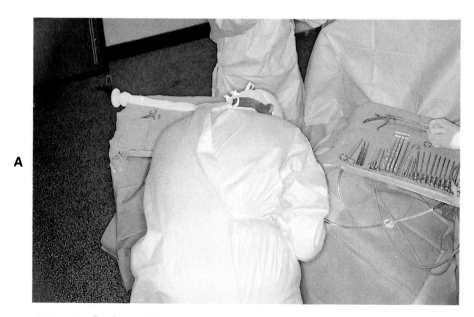

A

FIG. 6-26. Body position.

A Bending over for direct viewing is uncomfortable and unnecessary.

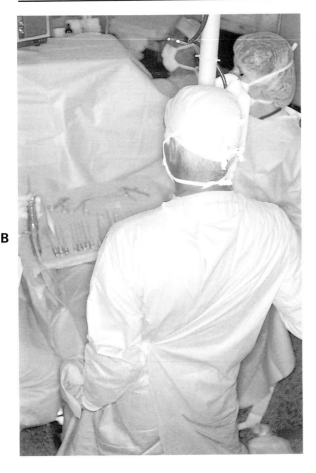

B

Fig. 6-26, cont'd

B Video viewing in good body position.

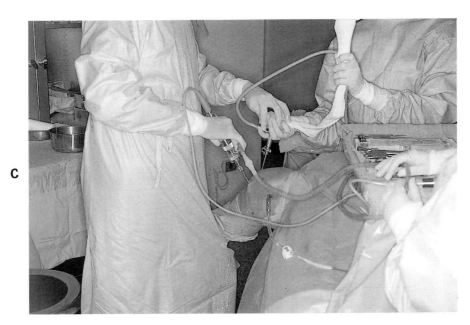

C

Fig. 6-26, cont'd

C Patient's leg held with surgeon's thigh and valgus force.

Continued.

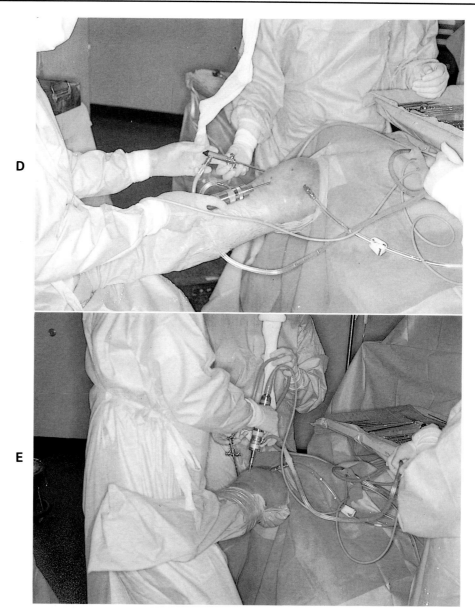

FIG. 6-26, cont'd. Body position.

D Patient's leg in surgeon's lap for suprapatellar viewing.

E Patient's leg held with surgeon's thigh in varus for lateral compartment approach.

Hand control

With direct viewing the scope is handled firmly, like a pencil, between the thumb and fingers (Fig. 6-27). When using video projection, the hand is cupped around the scope occular and articulated viewing attachment (Fig. 6-28). This leaves the fingers free for manipulation. The scope is controlled with very slow, deliberate motions to allow time for assimilation of the image. Quick motions lead

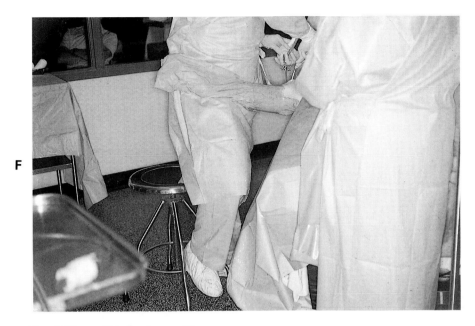

Fig. 6-26, cont'd. Body position.

F Hyperextension necessary to reach posterolateral in particular patient.

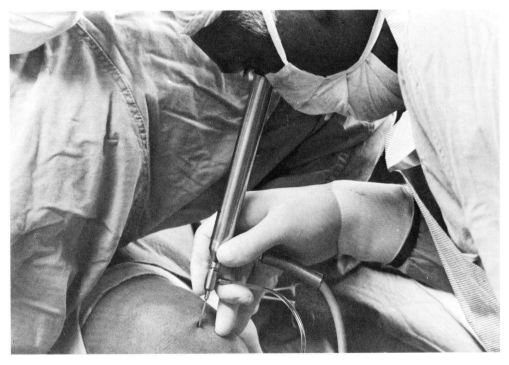

FIG. 6-27. Fingertip control during Needlescope arthroscopy.

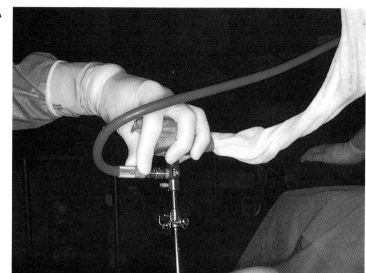

FIG. 6-28. Single-hand control of arthroscope couple to AVD.

A Index finger and thumb initiate rotation.

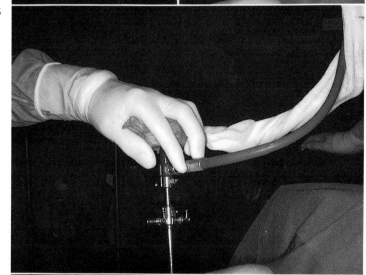

B Index finger moves side arm of scope to ring and little fingers.

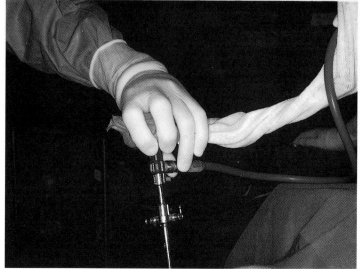

C Thumb and ring finger control scope after 180 degrees of rotation.

to disorientation or even joint damage. The motion can be likened to that used to smooth frosting in cake decoration. The pressure is firm but gentle and rythmical (Fig. 6-29).

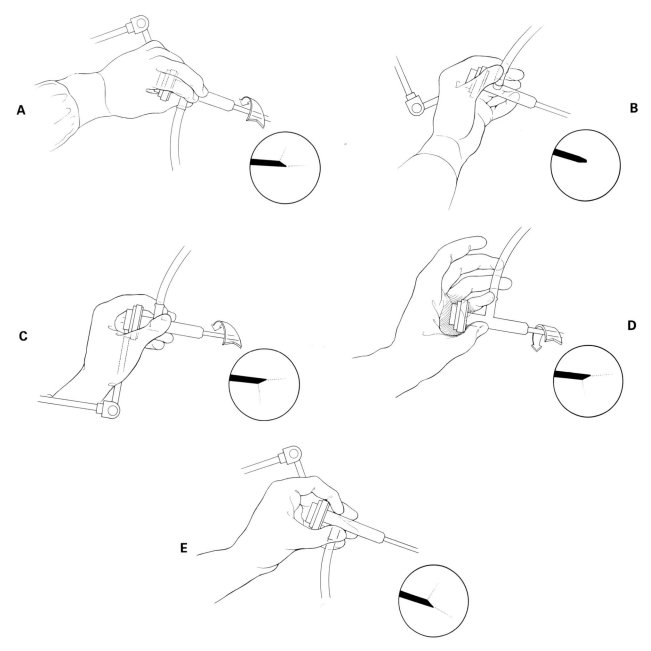

FIG. 6-29. Diagram of hand control on arthroscope. Rotational movement.

A Rotation to left.
B Scope faces away to left.
C Continuation of rotation so scope looks inferior to opposite light cable in this particular model.
D Little finger catches cable attachment to continue scope rotation
E Regripping of scope with cupped hand after 360 degrees of rotation.

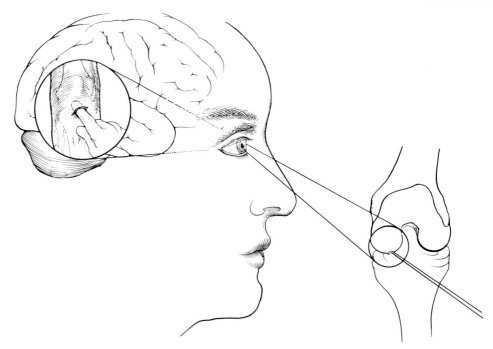

FIG. 6-30. Palpation in joint.

Palpation

Although endoscopists emphasize hand-eye coordination, palpation skill is also important (Fig. 6-30). As one's technical skills improve, so does the ability to sense by palpation the proper location within the knee joint. Visualization follows that placement or sense of placement. For instance, one learns to sense by drag and palpation the different layers of fat, capsule, and synovium during joint penetration. Palpation is used to determine the position of the arthroscope in relation to the various intraarticular parts, whether the patella, suprapatellar pouch, biceps tendon, or glenoid. After some experience, it is even possible to palpate soft tissue structures such as an anterior cruciate ligament in the knee or biceps tendon in the shoulder. The skill of palpation is essential as one advances to arthroscopic inspection of the smaller joints, that is, the elbow, the hip, or the ankle.

A well-placed endoscope, with the surgeon keeping an awareness of the sense of palpation and not just emphasizing or attempting the visualization, will facilitate the arthroscopic examination.

Pistoning

The most primitive motion of the arthroscope is penetration into the joint. The scope is moved forward, then retracted backward (Fig. 6-31). This back-and-forth motion is described as pistoning. It can help establish location and dimension, and it is most valuable in trying to determine the size of an object. A magnification factor is seen arthroscopically. While pistoning in and out, one can view the size of the object in question in its relation to the other articular surfaces.

The beginning arthroscopist generally makes very gross movements. Brisk withdrawal of cannula or scope will slide the instrument out of joint cavity, ob-

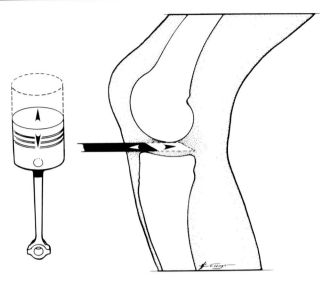

FIG. 6-31. Pistoning in joint.

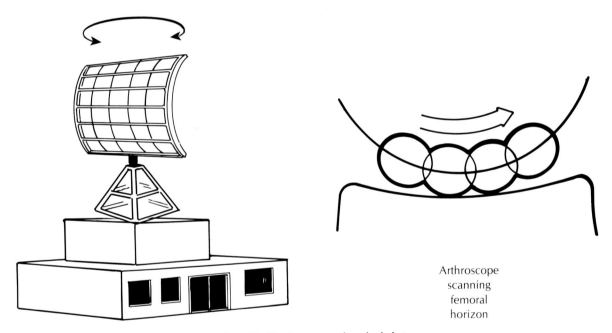

Arthroscope
scanning
femoral
horizon

FIG. 6-32. Radar scanning in joint.

scuring the view or causing loss of knowledge of placement of the cutting edge (see Fig. 6-22).

Scanning

A second basic manipulative procedure involves moving the scope from side to side (Fig. 6-32). Its most valuable use is in identifying the horizon of an articular surface, the tangential portion of the joint, and then the joint space and adjacent structures. The edge of the condylar horizon is kept in the edge of the image for orientation.

As in any type of surgery, it is important to work from known to unknown. When there is an identifiable structure, the most obvious are the horizon of a condyle in the knee joint, the glenohumeral articulation in the shoulder joint, or the tibiotalar joint in the ankle. Finding these important landmarks arthroscopically, even if they are not the focus of the inspection, restores confidence to the surgeon concerning landmarks and anatomy. He or she can then move to the various structures from that point. If the surgeon became lost or disoriented, he or she could move back to where there was a known horizon and move back to the area in question, thereby re-establishing position in the joint.

Rotation

Scope rotation is probably the most valuable of the individual techniques. I prefer, as many arthroscopists do, an endoscope that has a 30-degree fore-oblique field of view. In a direct-viewing arthroscope, rotation will not change the view (Fig. 6-33). Without moving the 30-degree inclined arthroscope from side to side or in and out, rotation gives a much wider view of the entire area to be inspected. It does not necessitate any motions of the joint and/or the arthroscope to view areas to one side to the other, above, or below. This can be a distinct advantage in a circumstance in which one does not want to or cannot change position. Scope rotation can accomplish what otherwise would not be achievable by either pistoning or scanning (Fig. 6-34).

Although this was clearly illustrated in the first edition of this textbook, it continues to be a technique overlooked even by experienced arthroscopists.

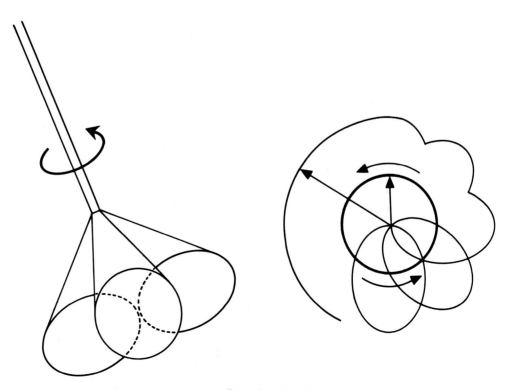

FIG. 6-33. Rotation in joint.

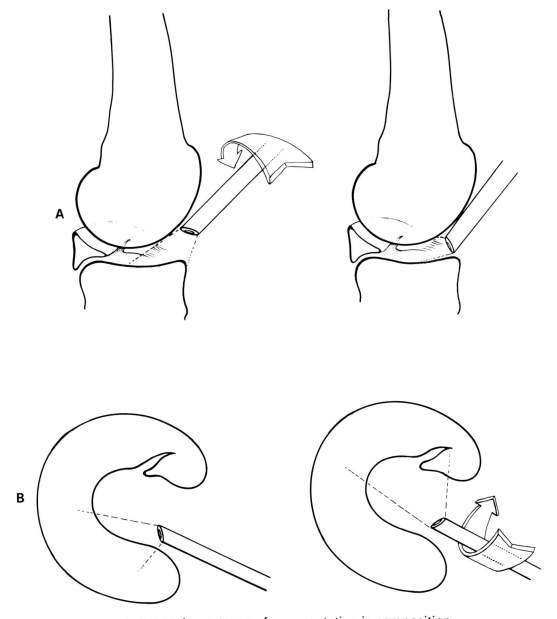

FIG. 6-34. Importance of scope rotation in composition.

A Rotation necessary to see between condyles.
B Rotation necessary to see meniscus tear.

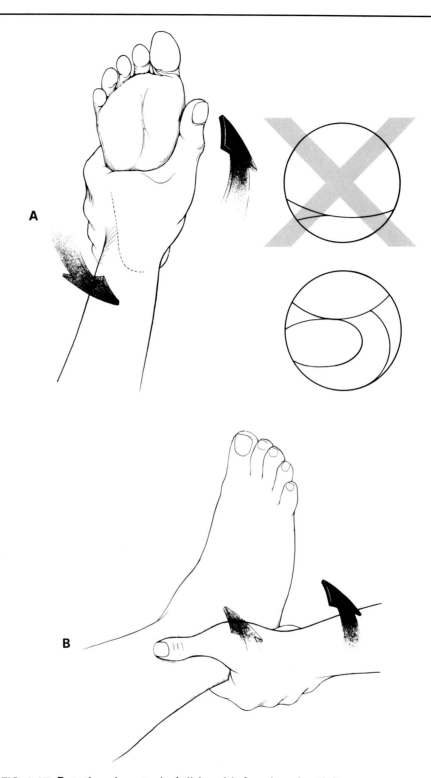

FIG. 6-35. Rotational control of tibia with free hand activity.

A External rotation force on foot. Less exposure without rotation control.
B Internal rotation of foot and ankle.

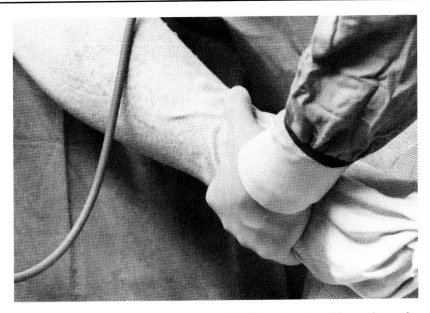

FIG. 6-36. With free hand, arthroscopist can hold patient's ankle and monitor tightening of Achilles tendon. Any tightening of knee or apprehension of patient is quickly discerned through Achilles tendon tenseness, allowing arthroscopist to be sensitive to patient's comfort under local anesthesia. In addition, with internal and external rotation, flexion and extension, abduction and adduction, arthroscopist can compose clear-cut endoscopic picture.

Free hand activity

The other hand, the surgeon's body, an assistant, or even mechanical traction techniques can be used to manipulate the distal portion of the joint.

In the knee joint, the surgeon can hold the patient's ankle with one hand and thus apply varus or valgus, or the surgeon can use his or her own thigh or hip to do the same thing. He or she also may use the free hand to internally or externally rotate the tibia (Fig. 6-35).

With the patient under local anesthesia, it is possible to monitor the patient's tightness or anxiety by noting spontaneous tightening the Achilles tendon (Fig. 6-36). This can alert the surgeon to any quick motion by the patient and thus avoid damage to the joint or the endoscope.

Varus or valgus strain or rotational stress can be applied in the joint and coordinated with pistoning of the endoscope to construct the arthroscopic composition.

The arthroscope can be fixed within the joint and the joint moved to create

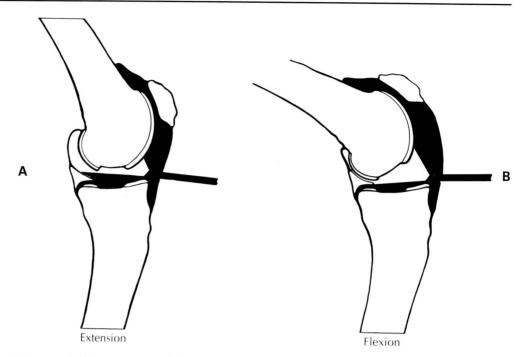

A — Extension

B — Flexion

FIG. 6-37. With scope position steady, flexion and extension of knee change arthroscopic view. **A** Extension. **B** Flexion.

the view in front of the arthroscope (Fig. 6-37). In procedures on the knee, the arthroscope can be placed in the joint and the knee taken into flexion and extension without moving or penetrating the scope. The tissues carry the arthroscope proximal and distal, which allows viewing from anterior to posterior.

Too much emphasis has been placed on scope manipulation and too little on manipulation of the extremity to gain arthroscopic composition (Fig. 6-38).

In addition, the extremity can be manipulated with the side of the surgeon's hip or thigh. This frees the second hand for manipulation, vacuuming, suctioning, a pushing behind the joint for ballottement (Fig. 6-39). Ballottement or palpation with the free hand can be done either posteromedially or posterolaterally when viewing from the anterior position. It can push loose bodies or fluid up into the anterior compartment for visualization. Constant manual pressure in the posterior aspect will bring the posterior horn of the meniscus forward to allow a better inspection (Fig. 6-40).

The free hand holds the leg in internal or external rotation by manipulation of the foot and ankle (see Fig. 6-39, *E*).

The most common use of the free hand for rotation is in the knee with a pivot shift. When valgus is applied, the knee shifts. To be kept in control, the knee has to be flexed and externally rotated at the foot to keep it in its valgus position with opening of the medial joint line. Otherwise a shift occurs and closes up the space (see Fig. 6-35).

The opposite is true for the lateral side in a cruciate-deficient knee. When varus is applied up into flexion in a knee it tends to externally rotate, thus closing the space. Internal rotation is required to open the knee for adequate visualization into the lateral compartment when varus force has been applied.

376

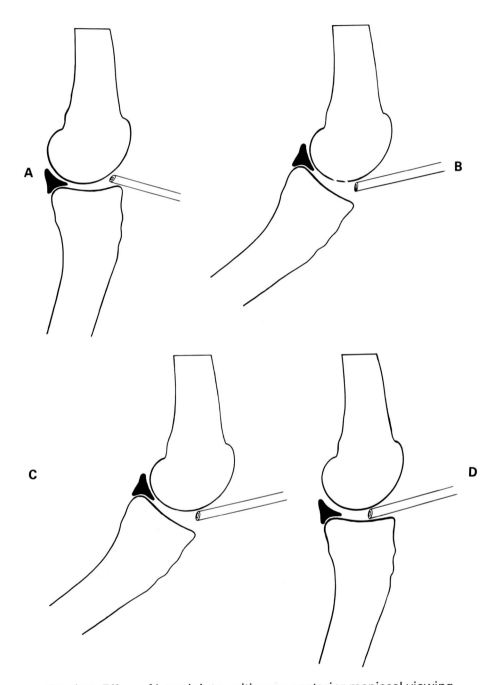

FIG. 6-38. Effect of knee joint position on posterior meniscal viewing.

A Cannot see in extension.
B Can see in flexion.
C Cannot see in flexion.
D Can see in extension.

FREE HAND MANIPULATION

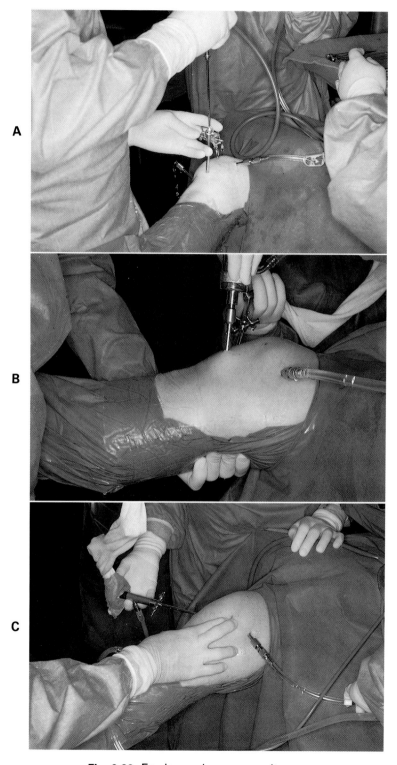

Fig. 6-39. For legend see opposite page.

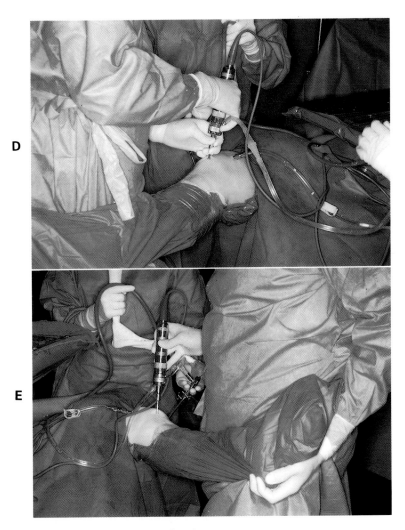

FIG. 6-39. Free hand contributions.

A Inserting instruments.
B External posterior pressure or ballottement.
C External palpation to locate site of lesion or instrument portal.
D Two hand control of surgical instrument.
E Rotational and varus-valgus flexion-extension control of leg.

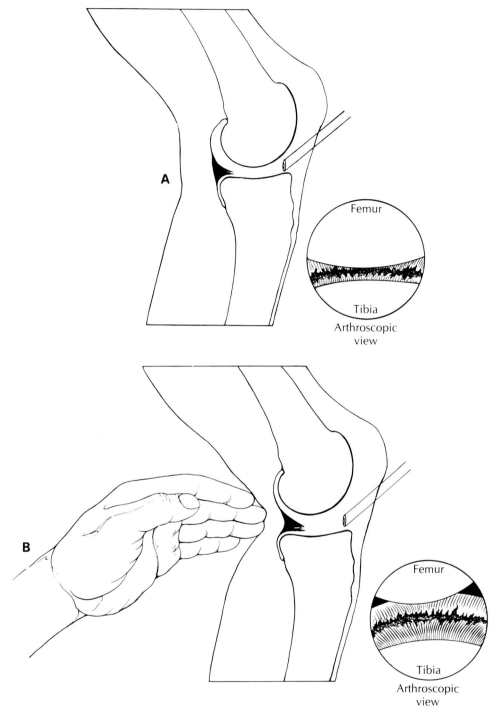

FIG. 6-40. External pressure posterior brings meniscus forward in joint.

A No pressure.
B Pressure.

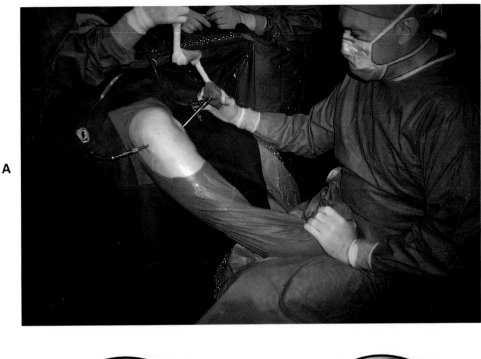

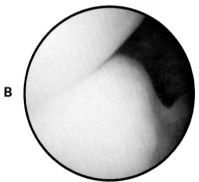

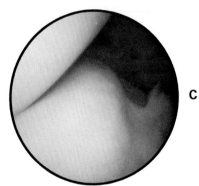

FIG. 6-41

A Surgeon internally rotates tibia on femur.
B Arthroscopic view of meniscus before rotation.
C Meniscus drops off tibia with internal rotation.

Just placing the knee in a figure-4 position, in the absence of a leg holder, is not adequate. In the presence of a pivot shift, this position would not open the space as adequately as it could be done with the leg secured in a Surgical Assistant thigh holder with varus, flexion, and internal rotation.

Posterior compartment viewing is aided by internal (medial) or external (lateral) rotation that drops the meniscus away from the femoral condyle (Fig. 6-41).

Manipulation of joint

The surgical exposure is facilitated by application of various forces to open or distract the joint. The shoulder is exposed by suspension, rotation and flexion,

TABLE 6-2. Combined motions of scope and extremity

Scope motion	Joint manipulation	Knee example
Yes	No	Suprapatellar pouch
Yes	Yes	Posterior horn meniscus
No	Yes	Viewing entire medial femoral condyle

and abduction. The knee joint is opened by varus-valgus and varying positions of flexion and internal and external rotation. Flexion and extension are used in smaller joints.

The composition is affected by external manipulation (see Figs. 6-37 and 6-38). In one situation, the joint is held still and the scope is moved. The joint may be manipulated with extremity motion to valgus force and the scope also moved within the joint. The third action is to hold the scope still and move the joint in front of the scope (see Figs. 6-37 and 6-38). This is a common means of observing the femoral condyle from front to back (Table 6-2).

The positioning becomes quite complex when various combinations of forces are applied to scope and the extremity. Although exact awareness of individual factors is not possible during surgery, it may be helpful to review the graphic illustration of various combinations.

Scope sweeping

Scope sweeping, jumping from side to side with very rapid motions, injures the joint and allows visualization of nothing (Fig. 6-42).

The instrument is like a pencil pushed through a cardboard sheet. A move to the right on one side (on one end of the pencil) creates a move to the left on the opposite side, as it does inside the joint.

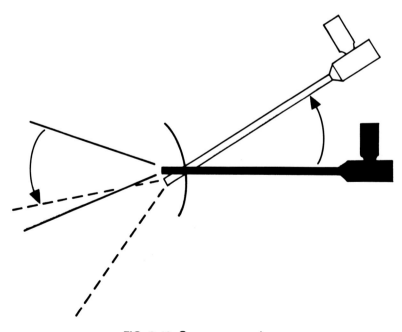

FIG. 6-42. Scope sweeping.

If a move is made very rapidly, it is impossible either by direct or video screen veiwing to even observe what passes in front of the arthroscope, let alone comprehend it. Gross movements of the scope during repositioning should be avoided. The observations made during quick movements are useless, as well as potentially damaging to the joint or scope (see Fig. 6-23).

When the scope is moved very slowly, the actual sequence of images is observed or comprehended by the surgeon. Although there is no depth perception, because the scope is a single lens, slow movements combined with manipulative procedures make it possible to fully comprehend and create sequentially organized images for storage in the surgeon's brain (Fig. 6-43).

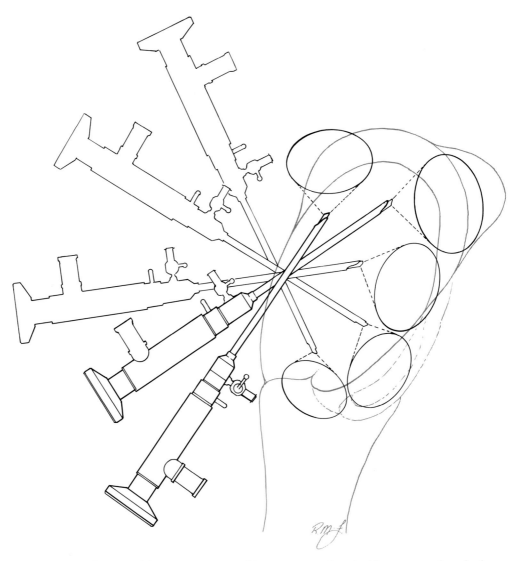

FIG. 6-43. Composition: sequence of images constructed in surgeon's mind.

Composition

The single arthroscopic view cannot visualize a joint in its entirety. A single view encompasses part of a compartment or anatomical structure. Appreciation for the entire joint is accomplished intellectually after proper techniques are mechanically executed. This is similar to the construction of photographs taken from outer space, in which individual electronically produced dots are printed in an orderly manner, line after line. The printout of these various bits of information illustrates the entire image.

There are many mechanical factors. They include the arthroscope, light, nature of patient, adherence to principles, and performance of techniques. In addition, the proper combination of factors influences the arthroscopic picture. For example, a bright light up close to the condyle blanches out any detail. This could be corrected by retracting the scope away from the object or by dimming the light. Another surgical approach would provide a tangential view of the same area. Flexion and extension show various contact areas. Palpation with a probe determines the texture of tissue. These experiences are all just for one area of the joint seen at one time during arthroscopy.

The summation of all visual, position, and palpation experiences is recorded on television. The television records, but it cannot conceptualize. The imagery is simulated and constructed in the surgeon's mind.

The quality of the composition is affected by the surgeon's ability, capacity, discipline, and willingness to follow strict protocol yet allow for surgical imagination.

Arthroscopic technical ability is not solely dependent on intellect. It is a motor skill. Certain skills can be improved by education and motor skills training. There is no direct correlation between athletic skills and the intellect; you either run fast or you don't. Techniques and training will maximize natural abilities. There are some limitations, however. Lack of innate abilities for arthroscopy should not reflect poorly on a surgeon. A certain natural endowment makes arthroscopy easier for one surgeon than another.

Given the ability, the surgeon must have an emotional capacity for arthroscopic surgery. The qualities of patience, gentleness, and self-control are needed, and the surgeon must have a willingness to discipline himself or herself and the staff. The delicate tools, small spaces, and remote control of manipulations are demanding. Repeated practice will cause discipline to become natural and satisfying.

The surgical imagination of the physician is the intangible ingredient that aids in overcoming the unexpected and even the unknown. This is the design, the dance, the excitement, and the sound that is recognized in other art forms.

There are not shortcuts or tricks to arthroscopic surgical success. The arthroscopic procedure requires careful preoperative organization and planning. There is not time or space to ignore protocol.

The arthroscopic composition is a matter of penetration, rotation, scope sweeping side to side, or any variety of these techniques. The beginning arthroscopist generally uses a lot of scope sweeping, jumping from side to side with very rapid motions. The observation made during that quick movement is virtually useless, as well as potentially damaging to the joint or scope.

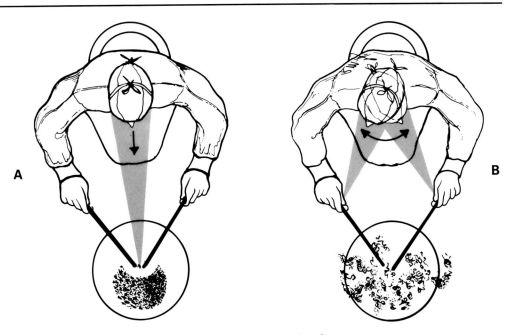

FIG. 6-44. Surgeon focus on inside of knee.

A Inside focus gives best control.
B Outside look causes loss of control and position.

When the scope is moved very slowly and the actual sequence of images is observed or comprehended by the surgeon, slow movements combined with the manipulative procedures described make it possible to fully comprehend or make composition arthroscopically (Fig. 6-44).

Visual interpretation
Illumination

Varying illumination is necessary with television viewing. If the camera does not have automatic gain control, some areas will be too bright and others are too dark. Manual control of light source intensity may be necessary. Articular cartilage requires less light than the cavernous, synovium-lined suprapatellar space. A decrease in light is necessary to properly evaluate subtle changes in articular surfaces.

The color balance of a television camera may require attention to maintain realistic colors of tissue. Most system manuals outline the procedure for correction. The JVC KY1900CH has built-in color bars and an external button for ease of light balance correction.

Contrast dye

In some cases a contrast dye may assist in highlighting intraarticular structures (Fig. 6-45). The determination of the amount of roughening or fragmentation or of fissure depth may be enhanced.[5] I have used methylene blue, 1 mm injected along the scope to the exact site. It clears easily from the joint for further arthroscopy. It selectively stains fibroid exudate or loose bodies (see Chapter 13). I have seen no complications with its use in hundreds of cases.

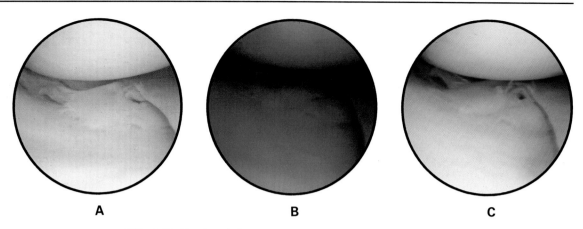

A   B   C

FIG. 6-45. Contrast dye.

A Arthroscopic view.
B Bolus of 1 ml methylene blue placed into joint along arthroscope.
C Cleared, contrast dye shows subtlety of tear.

Two-dimensional image

Arthroscopic viewing is two dimensional in a three-dimensional field. Using shadowing, relative size, scope movements, and palpation allows the surgeon to perceive in three dimensions (Fig. 6-46).

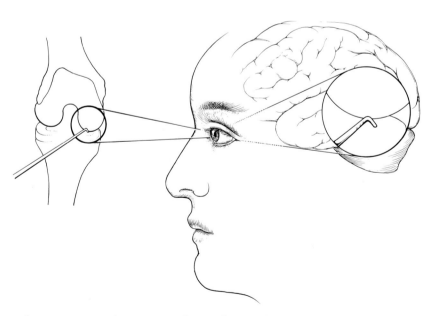

FIG. 6-46. Instrument and scope motions of scanning, pistoning, plus rotation create a continuous video recording. However, the concept must be in the surgeon's mind.

Orientation

Orientation begins with body and eyes in line with the scope (Fig. 6-47, A). The television monitor is perpendicular to the axis of the scope. The angle of the arthroscope's inclined view is oriented with the side arm of the light guide attachment. Some scopes angle toward, others away. This is a necessary reference for scope manipulation when the angled end of the scope is in the joint and out of sight.

With some approaches it is not possible for the surgeon to position his or her body along the axis of the arthroscope. The monitor should be rotated perpendicular to the scope. The surgeon enhances orientation by viewing the monitor with his or her head rotated, even facing another direction toward the monitor, though the body cannot gain complete reorientation (Fig. 6-47, B and C).

Orientation is challenged when arthroscope is viewing from the surgeon's side, but the instrumentation entering via a portal opposite (180 degrees) the arthroscope and arthroscopist. Instrumentation movements are opposite those used when an instrument enters from the same side (simple triangulation). The coordination is enhanced by starting slowly, testing motions and results, and then commencing with surgery. Rotational direction has to be figured out. This is the standard position for shoulder and elbow arthroscopic surgical procedures.

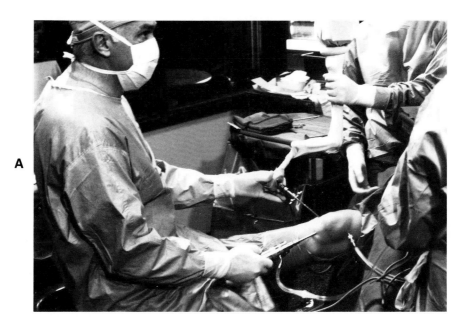

FIG. 6-47. Orientation.

A Ideally, the body and hands are behind the arthroscope and surgeon is looking forward toward television monitor.

Continued.

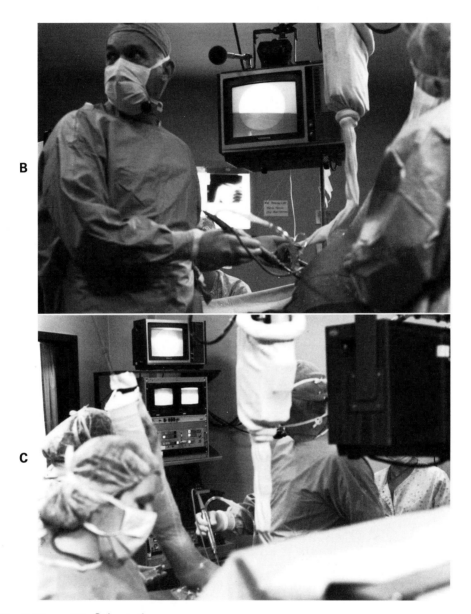

Fig. 6-47, cont'd. Orientation.

B In shoulder arthroscopy, scope is switched to far side and surgeon remains on side opposite monitor. He or she must look away to place body in line with arthroscope, looking at second monitor (seen in **C**).

C Look-away viewing is off recording monitors in room.

The most difficult maneuver during which to maintain orientation is when the scope enters from the side opposite the surgeon yet the television monitor remains behind rather than in front of the scope (see Fig. 6-47, *B* and *C*). When instrumentation is placed on the surgeon's side, the matter is further complicated. This positioning is unnecessary and should be avoided. The surgeon should take time to reposition his or her body and the equipment. If not, then a slow approach, and testing of the movements of instruments, is necessary. Rotation of the television to 90 degrees removes some disorientation if the surgeon's head also faces the monitor.

If this explanation is not clear, imagine the difficulty in orientation during actual arthroscopy.

Disorientation and vertigo

On rare occasions, I have experienced momentary disorientation and even vertigo. It has happened during complex cases with multiple portal changes. I was operating from all possible perspectives. Fatigue usually preceded the vertigo experience.

I stopped, waited, relaxed, rested, reoriented choosing simpler approaches, and completed the procedure without incident. There were no further problems on that day or subsequent days. Vertigo problems can be avoided by systemtic approaches and proper position of the surgeon, arthroscope, and television monitor.

Surgical imagination

Surgical imagination is the key ingredient of surgery. The small confines, the use of television, the different hand position, and looking up not down requires considerable imagination.

Visitors often ask me how many times I have performed a certain technique. In one case, I tried seven different ways to get the fat pad down on a repaired anterior cruciate ligament. When I finally figured out the technique, it went very easily. The second time I did the operation in front of visitors, they asked me how many times I had done it. I told them I had done it seven times, but all on one patient. The eighth time I performed the technique was on the second patient. Some inherent surgical imagination and self-learning has to go on in virtually every kind of operation.

Surgical conductor

Not only is the surgeon "playing" many instruments and thinking, but he is also responsible for teaching and directing the surgical team. It is easy to see why arthroscopic surgery is so challenging.

SURGICAL PORTALS
Multiple portals

Diagnostic arthroscopy requires use of multiple portals to see or triangulate.[11] Arthroscopic surgical procedures use multiple portals for inflow, scope, and instrumentation. Specifics for joints other than the knee are outlined in each specific chapter.

Anterolateral (inferior) portal

The anterolateral portal is located by taking the knee into 45 degrees of flexion. A site is located lateral to the patellar tendon at the level of the tip of the patella. In a thin patient with prior joint distention, this area may bulge because the capsule is thin.

This is the common portal for arthroscope placement. It provides access to most areas of the joint for viewing with a 30-degree inclined scope. It also serves as an instrument portal for lateral meniscectomy, patellar debridement, and lateral retinacular release.

I have seen laceration of the patellar tendon lateral margin at the time of combined open surgery. This could be the cause of persistent incisional tenderness in some patients. This is also why I avoid the central patellar tendon approach.

Some portals are routine (primary) and others are used only in special approaches (secondary) (Fig. 6-48). The portals are named in relation to the patella or joint compartment. In some cases, they are named for a specific anatomical structure (e.g., transpatellar tendon).

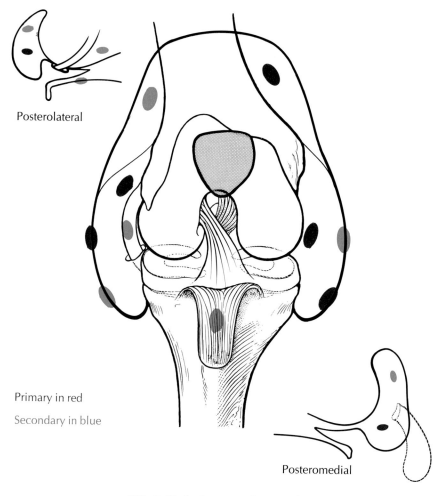

Posterolateral

Primary in red

Secondary in blue

Posteromedial

FIG. 6-48. Arthroscopic portals.

Superomedial portal (anterior)

The superomedial portal is approximately 1 inch above the patella and posterior and medial at the level of the undersurface of the patella. The approach takes a distal and lateral course.

It is used for the initial inflow cannula and for suprapatellar viewing in patellar surgery and tracking.

It is preferred over the superolateral portal because the tissue is thicker, reducing fluid leakage. The medial position allows viewing of the lateral retinacular release procedure. If the lateral portal is used the cut of release approaches the scope, causing poor view and leakage.

This portal through the vastus medialis has not caused a problem with pain, fibrosis, or lack of extension. On one occasion I placed the inflow too far posterior, resulting in postoperative bleeding and ecchymosis. Posterior placement is near larger vessels at the medial intramuscular septum and should be avoided.

Superolateral portal (anterior)

The superolateral portal is above and lateral to the patella. Because the patella rests superior and lateral in extension, placement will be eccentric from the joint. The portal courses distal and medial through the tough tendon of the vastus lateralis.

This portal is used for medial joint observation, especially for medial gutter synovectomy and osteophyte resection.

The disadvantages are a tough, thin tissue, which results in easy leakage. With valgus force on the Surgical Assistant, the cannula bumps the leg holder as held in rigid tendon tissue. It is not a good site for lateral release observation, because the incision approaches a portal, which compromises the view.

Anteromedial (inferior) portal

This portal is determined after the diagnostic portion of the procedure has been initiated. If the major pathological lesion has been determined to be in the medial compartment, the knee is taken into slight valgus and flexion. The site is determined with a No. 18 spinal needle. The position for medial meniscal work is usually slightly inferior to the arthroscope placement (Fig. 6-49). It is more medial than the medial puncture wound previously used for Needlescope arthroscopy.

If the diagnostic portion of the procedure demonstrates a major lesion within the lateral compartment, the knee is taken over into varus flexion position (see Fig. 6-73). The needle is placed more superior and lateral than for the medial compartment and is directed toward the lateral compartment. As with any other portal, redirection from a given portal is possible but it may be necessary to have two medial portals, especially in the degenerative joint, to facilitate entry into both the medial and lateral compartments. This may be because of tibial osteophytes in the intercondylar notch, joint instability, or collapse caused by articular cartilage loss.

Redirection from the anteromedial portal to the patellar area may not be possible because of osteophytes. An auxiliary portal more proximal and posterior

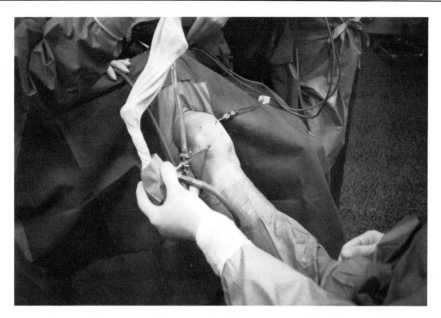

FIG. 6-49. Suprapatellar pouch. Scope rotated looking to left.

may be necessary to enter the patellar area (see Fig. 6-74, *B*). There are no disadvantages to medial portals if the surgeon remains flexible and varies placement.

Posteromedial portal

This site is posterior to the femoral condyle and superior to the medial meniscus and goes through the posterior oblique ligament.[1,6] In a thin patient, the area may be seen to bulge and may be palpable. Otherwise a No. 18 needle is used to determine a soft spot.

It is used for both diagnostic and surgical exposure in the posterior compartment and for Baker's cyst exploration.

The area may be difficult to locate in an obese person. The saphenous vein and nerve course over the area and must be protected. A small, shallow skin laceration helps avoid vessel and nerve if they are not visualized.

Posterolateral portal

The site for the posterolateral portal is posterior to the lateral femoral condyle and superior to the lateral meniscus. The opening is small. It is approached from a point at the intersection of the posterior fibula and lateral intermuscular septum (see Fig. 6-58). A needle directed anterior and inferior determines entry direction.

This portal is used for diagnostic and operative intervention. The main problem is difficulty of entry, often requiring maximal joint distention and high technical ability of the surgeon.

Transpatellar tendon approach

With the knee at approximately 45 degrees of flexion, a point is selected approximately 1 cm distal to the tip of the patella. A transverse skin incision and a vertical patellar tendon incision are made.[2,4] The obturator then enters the joint. This particular approach, popularized by Nils Oretorp and Jan Gillquist of Sweden, has given it the name, the "Swedish technique."[8]

The advantage of this particular technique is that it allows the use of both a medial and lateral portal for instrumentation with central viewing. It also facilitates passage into the posteromedial and posterolateral compartments from a single puncture. Visualization of the suprapatellar pouch is also facilitated, in that the properly placed puncture is superior to the area of the fat pad. Of course, difficulty would be encountered in seeing this area in patients with large distal pole patellar osteophytes.

The disadvantage of this procedure is that the tissue in the patellar tendon is thicker than the tissue adjacent to it, and manipulation through this area is somewhat impeded by the thicker tissue. Although a clean passage can be made, a short passage can be placed through the patellar tendon. Manipulation over any prolonged operative time would cause compression or tearing due to the angulation and pistoning back and forth of the arthroscope through the patellar tendon.

Patients may complain of postoperative irritation in the area of the patellar tendon.

I do not favor this as a routine approach. I have abandoned the transpatellar tendon approach for use of the arthroscope and only occasionally use it for instrumentation in an extremely tight knee. Placing the arthroscope anterolaterally allows visualization similar to that with the transpatellar tendon approach, yet without injury to the important patellar tendon.

Midpatellar lateral approach

The midpatellar lateral portal is opposite the midpoint of the patella. The scope is directed distally to see compartments.

Patel advocates this portal for optimal viewing of anterior compartments and three instrument manipulation, a scope, a grasper, and a cutting instrument.[7,8] I rarely use this portal, because it has no advantages over a portal slightly distal opposite the tip of the patella. This midlateral portal does not allow transcondylar access to the posteromedial compartment.

Accessory portals

Accessory portals can be made at virtually any anatomically safe position in the knee joint, with a No. 18 spinal needle to determine the passage. The most commonly used accessory portal is one to approach the patella for debridement. In an obese patient or one with an osteophyte, passage is difficult from the routine anteromedial portal.

It should be noted that this accessory portal will be more proximal, and surprisingly posterior so as to pass the instrumentation parallel to the patellar surface. Again, this can be established by trial and error with a No. 18 spinal needle while visualizing from either the superomedial or the inferoanterior and inferolateral portals. The No. 18 spinal needle is seen to pass parallel to the patellar area; the cannula system can then be placed along the same course.

An operative portal to the popliteus sheath can be established by viewing from anteromedial or preferably anterolateral. The passage of the No. 18 spinal needle is from proximolateral to inferior along the course of the popliteus sheath and can actually enter into the sheath for removal of loose bodies or synovial resection.

A posterolateral accessory approach can be placed into the posterolateral compartment for synovectomy while viewing from anteromedial. With the knee in varus–external rotation and flexion, the No. 18 spinal needle can be placed posterior to the popliteus tendon, but not as far posterior as in a normal posterolateral approach. This facilitates operative work in the posterolateral compartment both above and below the meniscus and is most often used for synovectomy and/ or loose body removal.

Accessory passage can come under the meniscus at the junction of the middle and posterior thirds of the meniscus.

In tight knees, this accessory portal provides access for resection of the inner border of posterior meniscus without having to traverse the condyles.

DIAGNOSTIC TECHNIQUES
Routine diagnostic arthroscopy of the knee (general anesthesia)

The diagnostic techniques for the right knee are outlined here. I emphasize the coordinated team effort. Consult Chapter 7 for various views. The basic principles of knee joint arthroscopic techniques carry over into the other joints. Techniques concerning other joints are described in each specific chapter.

Coordinated team effort

In preparation, the patient is placed on a regular operating room table in the supine position. A physical examination is performed with the patient under anesthesia. A tourniquet is placed high on the thigh. A determination is made of patellar and joint stability, and the passive range of motion is recorded. An elastic wrap is placed on the lower extremity. The tourniquet is pressurized to 450 mm Hg. The elastic wrap is removed, and an over-the-top arthroscopy table is positioned.

The thigh is secured in a mechanical device (the Surgical Assistant) placed at least 6 inches above the superior aspect of the patella with the leg in extension (see Fig. 6-8, A). The technique of application of the Surgical Assistant is outlined in Chapter 4. The Surgical Assistant creates a maximum pressure of 350 mm Hg. The thigh, when secured, assumes a quadrilateral shape.

The foot of the table is dropped, creating space for a circumferential instrument approach.

The foot is held by the circulating nurse. An antiseptic agent is applied to the skin (see Fig. 6-8, B). The Johnson & Johnson arthroscopic knee disposable drape creates a sterile, water-impervious barrier (see Fig. 6-8).

The leg is brought through the hole in the broad main sheet that covers the operating room table. The excess drape hanging down on the floor is swept under the table in a coordinated effort by both the assistant and the surgeon. This clears the floor for the surgeon and for foot pedals or power source controls.

A simultaneous coordinated effort of the team brings the instrumentation into place. The electrical cords are positioned through the loops in the arthroscopy drapes (see Fig. 3-13). To decrease clutter, the cords and inflow-outflow tubes come under the Mayo stand.

The tables with the instrumentation are brought into place. The surgeon places the inflow cannula into the suprapatellar pouch as the assistants set up the inflow system (see Fig. 6-10). The sterile Y-tube is handed to the circulating nurse. The circulating nurse suspends and attaches the 6 L of fluid via the sterile Y-tube (see Fig. 6-12, A). The surgeon attaches the inflow tube to the suprapatellar cannula and the joint is distended.

The suprapatellar portal is used routinely for the inflow cannula system (see Fig. 6-11). It is located at a point approximately 1 inch proximal to the patella and 1 inch deep to the anterior portion of the knee joint or the skin over the patella. This allows the cannula system to enter the space between the patella and the femur with the knee in extension.

The initial placement is through the capsule with a sharp trocar at a distal angle of approximately 45 degrees. A change to a blunt obturator allows the cannula to pass between the patella and the femur without injury; it also allows the cannula to be palpated with the fingertips of the opposite hand, anterolaterally and inferiorly.

The cannula system is then allowed to rest on the suprapatellar pouch. However, a result of this oblique passage, the distal opening of the cannula points inferior toward the compartments with all positions of the knee.

If the cannula system is taken from the superomedial portal perpendicular to the axis of the knee joint, it is possible to pass it outside to the suprapatellar pouch or above the imperforate suprapatellar plica. When the knee is taken into other positions, the attitude of the cannula could be superior or be blocked off in the suprapatellar pouch, aiming away from the desired area of flow or pressure.

While that is taking place, the first assistant prepares the television system. I use an articulated viewing device to connect to a camera suspended from the ceiling (see Fig. 3-3, A).

Arthroscope placement

The distended knee joint is flexed to 45 degrees. The surgeon's index finger identifies the tip of the patella (see Fig. 6-20, B). A No. 11 blade is used to lacerate the skin and capsule (see Fig. 6-20, C). Care is taken not to enter the joint. The arthroscope cannula with semisharp obturator is inserted and directed toward the intercondylar notch (see Fig. 6-20, D). An incision is made at a point lateral to the patellar tendon at the level of the distal pole of patella. This provides the thinnest fulcrum for manipulation of the scope. In thin patients a bulge is seen at the point of entry. This is created by intraarticular pressure and thin capsular tissue lateral to the fat pad and the patellar tendon. The entry portal is lateral to the fat pad. This position keeps the arthroscope from encroaching on the instrument portals. The 30-degree inclined arthroscope facilitates a good view from this eccentric position. With a direct-viewing scope, a more central position is required, in the absence of obliquity.

After the cannula has entered the suprapatellar area, it is moved to the intercondylar notch. If this direction is used for synovial penetration, subsequent redirection becomes necessary for multicompartmental viewing.

This method avoids the common problem of getting lost in the fat pad or tissue. First, the joint is maximally distended before entry. The inflow is via a separate cannula. Inflow on the arthroscope is avoided, because it may cause extravasation of fluid when the end of the scope unintendedly exits the joint. The entry incision is purposely smaller than the diameter of the cannula, restricting interstitial leaks or extravasation. The arthroscopic portal is lateral to most of the fat pad.

The course is through the capsule and downward toward the notch. Before synovial penetration, the knee is extended. Synovial penetration is into the suprapatellar pouch (see Fig. 6-20, E). The cannula is returned to the intercondylar notch to demonstrate freedom of motion.

With the scope resting in the intercondylar notch, the obturator is removed and replaced with the arthroscope. For the learning arthroscopist, a look into the scope confirms entry; there is more intimacy or confidence to direct viewing. Only the simplest operative work should proceed under direct viewing. Viewing from the television monitor facilitates body position and use of both hands. Television viewing is then instituted. The intercondylar notch is seen, confirming entry. The scope is returned to the suprapatellar pouch. Television recording commences.

Suprapatellar space

To view the suprapatellar pouch, the scope is rotated up and to the left (in a right knee) (see Figs. 6-49 and 7-2). The arthroscope is horizontal. A view is captured through the patellofemoral joint. Further penetration enters the suprapatellar pouch. The suprapatellar plica guards suprapatellar bursae at both the medial and lateral walls. (see Chapter 13) It can be seen with scope rotation to the right and with retraction (Fig. 6-50). The continuance of the suprapatellar

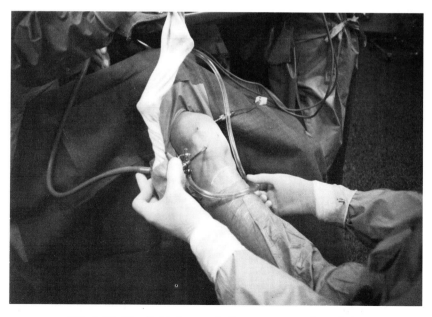

FIG. 6-50. Medial joint wall. Scope rotated to right.

plica with a medial shelf is demonstrated. The viewing follows the medial plica to the fat pad. With the knee in extension, the fat pad covers the femoral condyle. The knee is flexed to 60 degrees. The arthroscope faces downward and the membranous ligament and the entire intercondylar notch can be seen. From that position, the leg can then be brought back up into extension. The arthroscope is slowly rotated toward the patella as the knee is carried into extension.

In extension, the patella has a position superior and lateral to the femur, and normally overhangs the femur above the lateral gutter. Diminution of the light enhances viewing of the bright patellar surface. The inflow cannula may be used to palpate the patellar surface and femoral trochlea. A search is made for fissures or soft articular spots. Patellar tracking can be viewed from below to 45 degrees of flexion.

Patellar tracking

The arthroscope is retracted slightly and positioned to view the patellofemoral articulation. The patella is superior and lateral to the condyles and appears to overhang laterally (Fig. 6-51, *A*). The knee is flexed to 20 degrees. The patella moves distally and medially. Contact is initiated on the lateral facet of patella and the femoral condyle (Fig. 6-51, *B*). The vertical wall of the medial patella covers the medial femur. The medial facet does not touch (Fig. 6-51, *C*).

At 45 degrees of flexion, the patella centers in the femoral groove (Fig. 6-51, *C*). Compression of anterior tissues and of the fat pad often obscures this observation at greater degrees of flexion. Patellar tracking is best observed from the suprapatellar portal.

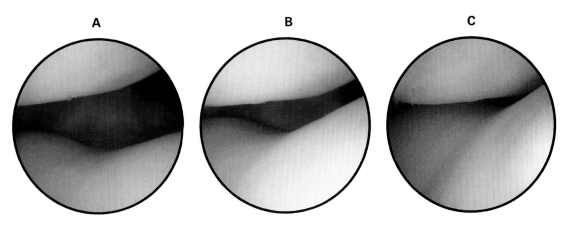

A   **B**   **C**

FIG. 6-51. Patellar tracking: viewed from below.

A With knee in extension, distention causes wide patellofemoral space and patella is lateral and superior to femur.
B At 20 degrees of flexion, lateral patella contacts lateral femoral condyle.
C At 45 degrees patella centers, but is often obscured by tissue compression.

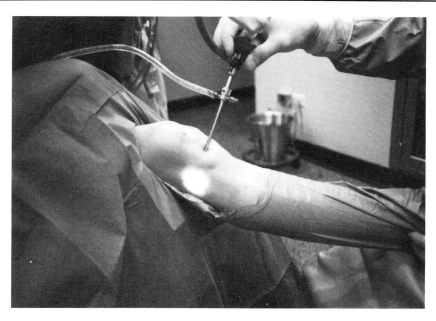

FIG. 6-52. Lateral gutter viewing. Arthroscope in popliteus sheath with transillumination.

Lateral and medial gutters

The knee is returned to extension. The scope is angled toward the lateral gutter, then rotated from the patella superiorly, 180 degrees to the left into the lateral femoral recess (see Fig. 7-6). With scope retraction, the recess is viewed from proximal to distal. Valgus force allows the lateral capsule to move away from the condyle. Penetration posteriorly identifies the popliteus tendon and sheath. The popliteus sheath is entered with suction activated, because this is a possible site of loose bodies (Fig. 6-52). The meniscal ligaments are observed above and below the sheath.

The steps are retraced to the patellofemoral area. The scope is rotated to view the medial plica again (see Fig. 6-50). From there the scope is advanced over the condyle. With rotation of the 30-degree inclined scope downward, the medial gutter comes into view (see Fig. 7-5).

With angulation, the scope moves from proximal to distal over the medial femoral condyle.

Medial compartment

The surgeon assumes the standing position. The knee is flexed to 20 degrees. A valgus force is applied by pressure from the surgeon's hip and thigh (Fig. 6-53, *A*). The scope is retracted following the horizon of the medial femoral condyle into the medial compartment. The anterior horn of the meniscus, the adjacent femur, and the underlying tibial condyle comes into view (see Fig. 7-7).

The scope is rotated to look posterior to and under the medial femoral condyle. The scope follows the landmark of the inner meniscal border. As the posterior horn is approached, a greater amount of valgus pressure is necessary. The scope is carefully advanced between the condyles. Rotation of the inclined view

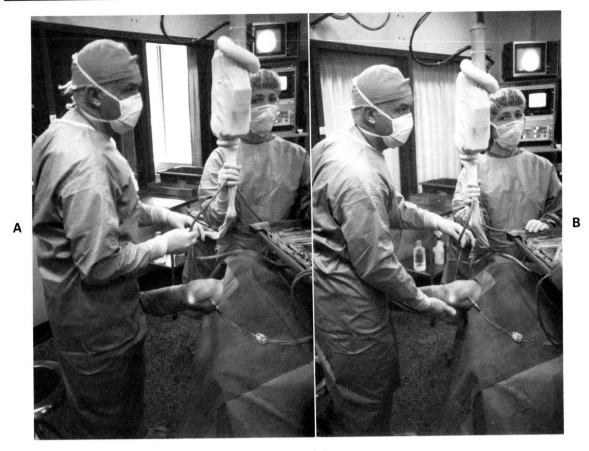

FIG. 6-53. Medial compartment.

A Direct viewing: notice light.
B Free hand pushes meniscus foward.

continues to the position of looking up under the femoral condyle to the meniscus. Varying degrees of flexion, even to hyperextension, may assist in obtaining this access. In some cases external rotation and flexion move the meniscus forward with the tibia. In other cases external pushing from the posterior will move the meniscus forward into the view of the arthroscope (Fig. 6-40 and 6-53, *B*).

Position of arthroscope

If the resultant image shows mostly femur, some meniscus, and no tibia, the scope is rotated too superior (see Fig. 6-34). On the other hand, if little femur shows and the entire meniscus and a large area of the tibial plateau are seen, the scope is looking down. Proper rotation places the meniscus in the midfield, with equal amounts of femur and tibia showing.

The tibia is inspected with scope manipulation. The femoral condyle is viewed by scope motion or by steadying the scope and moving the condyle in front of the scope with flexion and extension.

Varying the intensity of illumination enhances the appreciation of subtle articular changes.

If the patient has lost the anterior cruciate ligament, a straight valgus force in extension will cause a pivot shift, compromising the medial compartment view. Flexion of the knee and forceful external rotation of the tibia with the free hand maintains joint reduction and medial exposure (see Fig. 6-35).

Posteromedial (transcondylar) viewing

The surgeon is in a standing position. The scope is moved to view the slot between the tibial spine and the lateral border of the medial femoral condyle (Fig. 6-54; see Figs. 7-10 and 7-11).

The scope is rotated to view the medial border of the posterior cruciate ligament. The scope is advanced. The sulcus around the ligament comes into view before the posteromedial compartment does. Knee flexion to 35 to 40 degrees facilitates entry. The arthroscopic view is momentarily obscured by tight passage. A sense of palpation is helpful in this situation.

The transcondylar approach may be accomplished by replacement of the scope with a blunt obturator. Gentle rotation and penetration secure posteromedial entry. Forceful penetration with or without the scope should be avoided.

In some cases, transcondylar entry may not be possible. This occurs in small people or those with osteophytes in the area of the intercondylar notch. A transcutaneous method is an alternative.

On transcondylar entry, the scope is rotated 180 degrees to the right. The scope is positioned to view the meniscofemoral junction. This is facilitated by flexion of the knee to 45 degrees.

Combining flexion-extension, scope penetration, and rotation allows a view of the entire compartment. If a Baker's cyst is present, the opening will be on the posterior wall. The outflow suction is applied to the arthroscope spigot to mobilize any loose bodies. The scope is removed with gentle rotation and retraction.

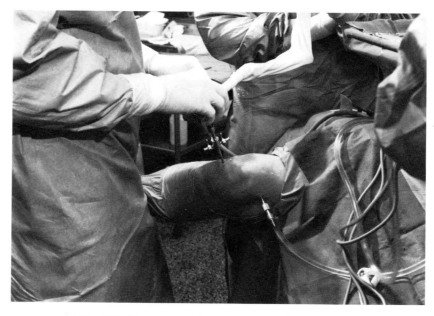

FIG. 6-54. Transcondylar posteromedial viewing.

Intercondylar notch

The surgeon assumes the sitting position (Figs. 6-55 and 7-13). The outflow suction is shut off to avoid attracting the ligamentum mucosa over the scope and thus obscuring the view. The knee is taken to 45 degrees of flexion.

The ligamentum mucosa is anterior and superior in the intercondylar notch. It varies in size and contour (see Fig. 7-13). Scope positioning over or under this ligamentum mucosa is necessary to see the compartment. In some cases, surgical release of the synovial ligament from the femur is necessary to gain exposure of the remainder of the structures in this compartment.

The anterior cruciate ligament is easily identified by its position and size and the vessel on its surface. The ligament is observed with external pull on the tibia (drawer sign). This is performed at various positions of knee flexion.

The posterior cruciate ligament attaches to the medial femoral condyle. It is less distinct, because it is covered with subsynovial fat.

Anterolateral compartment

The surgeon assumes the standing position. He or she moves to the lateral side of the leg so that the varus force can be applied (see Fig. 6-56, *B*, 7-19, and 7-20).

The scope focuses on the slot between the lateral tibial spine and the femoral condyle. The surgeon keeps an eye on the television monitor while applying

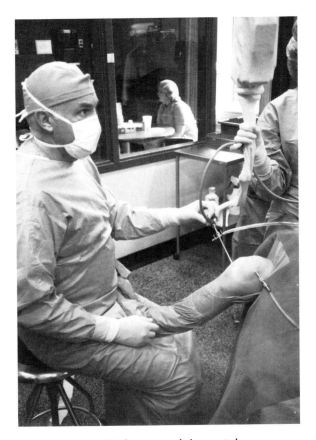

Fig. 6-55. Intercondylar notch.

increased varus on the patient's leg with the free hand under the lateral malleolus. The scope follows the horizon of the lateral femoral condyle over to the inner rim of the lateral meniscus.

Lateral compartment viewing is facilitated by taking the knee into slight flexion, placing the free hand under the lateral mallelous, and lifting the entire leg toward the ceiling. This opens the joint in a way similar to the figure-4 position. In an anterior cruciate–deficient knee, it may also be necessary to apply internal rotation to control the shift of the knee. Tibial rotation reduces exposure of the lateral compartment.

The scope is rotated to direct the 30-degree inclined view to the anterior horn of the lateral meniscus. From that position the inner margin of the meniscus is followed around to the popliteus tendon. This is accomplished by scope rotation and penetration. At this point, increased flexion and forceful varus are allied with the free hand lifting under the lateral malleolus toward the ceiling. The remainder of the meniscus is visualized by combining scope rotation toward the posterior horn with a gradual reduction of varus-flexion force.

Suction is applied to the arthroscope throughout the entire time of the lateral compartment viewing. Ballottement is used behind the knee to bring any loose tissues from the posterior for removal.

The posterolateral bundles of the anterior cruciate ligament course above the extreme posterior horn of the lateral meniscus (see Fig. 7-18, *E*).

The scope is positioned to view over the meniscus to the posterolateral compartment. The suction outflow is re-established on the scope spigot to draw any loose fragments into view.

The direction is then reversed. The meniscus is followed to return to obtain an overview of the lateral compartment. The inflow is clamped off, and suction decompression shows normal mobility of the lateral meniscus. The femoral condyle is viewed in flexion-extension of the knee. A reduction of light intensity enhances appreciation of the articular surface. Scope manipulation is used to scan the tibial surface.

Transcutaneous posteromedial approach

The surgeon assumes the sitting position, facing the medial aspect of the knee. The patient's knee is flexed to 90 degrees, and his foot rests in the surgeon's lap (see Figs. 6-58 and 7-11). The arthroscope and cannula are removed from the anterolateral portal. The arthroscope is replaced in the cannula with a sharp trocar.

The inflow remains in the superomedial portal. Manual pressure distends the joint. A palpable bulge may be palpated in thin patients. The posteromedial portal may be identified with a No. 18 spinal needle (Fig. 6-56). Palpating with the needle identifies the femoral condyle, and "marching" posteriorly enters through the posterior oblique ligament into the compartment. Removal of the stylet demonstrates the flow of saline, which confirms entry. This needle is removed, and cannula follows the same plane into the maximally distended joint. The scope replaces the trocar. The surgeon must be sensitive to the depth of the tissue before entering the posterior compartment (see Fig. 6-59). It is usually between ½- and 1-inch deep, depending on the patient's body fat. Placing the trocar at a depth of 2 inches without entry indicates that the trocar is posterior to

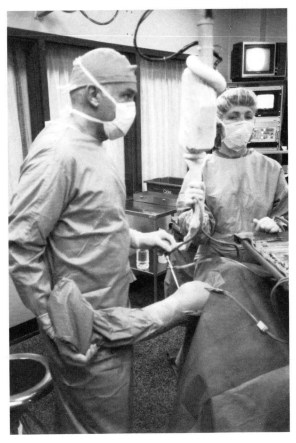

FIG. 6-56. Lateral compartment. Free hand under lateral malleolus opens joint.

the space and in the area of the neurovascular bundles. At the landmark constituted by the junction of the femoral condyle and the meniscus, the remainder of the compartment is visualized by scope manipulation. Maximal internal rotation of the tibia drops the meniscus off the femur to visualize the superior meniscal surface, which is not as easily seen from the anterior portal.

A false passage may enter a Baker's cyst, especially in an obese person in whom palpation is difficult. This does not produce any morbidity, but neither does it provide visualization.

The Baker's cyst can be entered intentionally, either viewing through the posteromedial compartment into the opening of the cyst (see Fig. 7-11) or, in the case of large loose bodies, through a separate entry by the transcutaneous inferomedial portal (see Fig. 9-29).

The Baker's cyst is on the posterior wall above a horizontal ridge of capsule (see Fig. 7-11).

There are two other ways to locate the posteromedial portal, and both require a previous transcondylar approach. In one, the arthroscope is left in the compartment. The illumination of the scope directs transcutaneous placement and direction. In the other method, while viewing the posteromedial compartment from notch, a needle is passed from the outside. This is confirmed by ar-

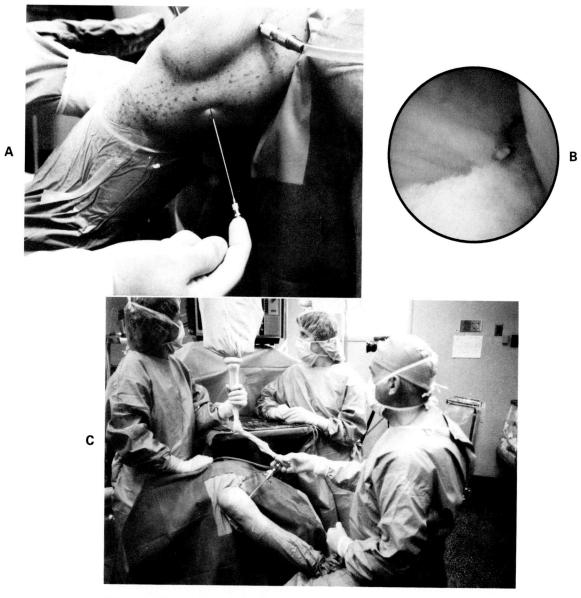

FIG. 6-57. Posteromedial portal.

A Needle identification of site.
B Arthroscopic view of needle from transcondylar approach.
C Arthroscope and surgeon's positon.

throscopic viewing (Fig. 6-57). An operative cannula is placed in the same position. The later change to an arthroscope cannula is facilitated by switching sticks.

At the conclusion of the posteromedial transcutaneous inspection, the portal is preserved with the cannula and obturator if surgery is anticipated. Otherwise, the instruments are removed. Also, keeping the hole plugged avoids leakage and preserves the portal for possible instrumentation.

Transcutaneous posterolateral approach

The posterolateral approach is facilitated by the surgeon moving around the lateral aspect of the knee (Fig. 6-58, *D*). The table has to be slightly elevated and the knee brought into about 100 degrees of flexion. Compression of the inflow bags creates maximal distention for entry into the small potential space.

At the point where a line drawn along the lateral intermuscular septum intersects a line drawn up from the posterior aspect of the fibula, a No. 18 spinal needle with a stylet is inserted (Fig. 6-58, *A*). The needle is aimed anterior and slightly inferior into the posterior compartment. Palpation of the femoral condyle helps locate the space. The stylet is removed to demonstrate backflow (Fig. 6-58, *C*). In some cases backflow may not be abundant because of synovitis in the posterolateral compartment.

A small laceration in the skin with a No. 11 blade is followed by placement of an arthroscope cannula and a sharp obturator. Using palpation to march off

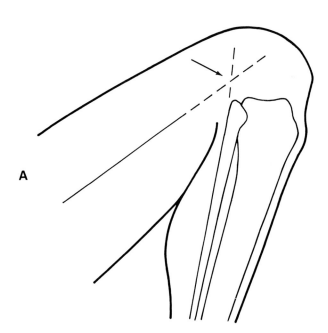

FIG. 6-58. Posterolateral view.

A Point of posterolateral entry where line drawn up from lateral intermuscular septum intersects with line drawn up from posterior aspect of fibula. Trocar and sharp cannula are placed, then directed slightly inferior and anterior to enter posterolateral compartment.

Continued.

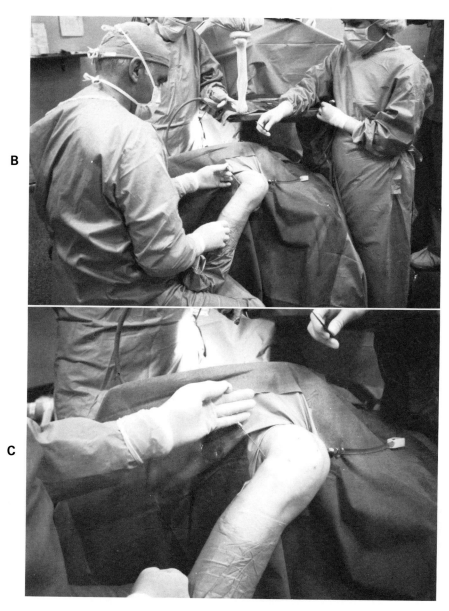

FIG. 6-58, cont'd. Posterolateral view.

B Needle identification of site.
C Fluid backflow through needle confirms entry.

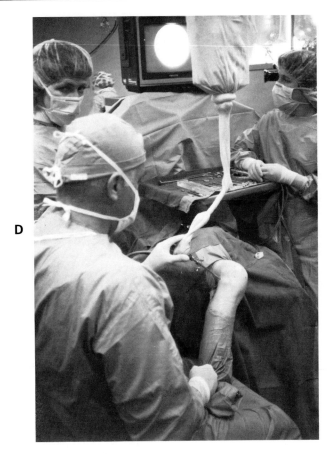

D

FIG. 6-58, cont'd. Posterolateral view.

D Surgeon's position and arthroscopic placement.

the posterolateral aspect of the femur, the space can be entered with the assistance of maximal distention. Without distention, entry is difficult and unconfirmed by outflow.

The arthroscope is placed to confirm entry (Fig. 6-58, *D*). If distention is lacking, a K-52 catheter with a syringe can be attached to the arthroscope to instill saline and thereby distend the posterior compartment.

After entry through this portal has been confirmed, the junction between the meniscus and femoral condyle is an identifiable landmark (see Fig. 7-22). The meniscus does not bulge as it does posteromedially; it has more of a vertical nature. External rotation sometimes, but not always, will drop the meniscus off the condyle for better visualization. Intermittent pressure and vacuuming can cleanse the posterior compartment for better visualization. It may be possible to follow along the course of the meniscofemoral junction to the popliteus tendon. Entry into the popliteus sheath is difficult from posterior and lateral.

If there is going to be no operative procedure from the posterolateral portal, the arthroscope can be removed. Otherwise the position should be secured with a cannula system and obturator.

Suprapatellar viewing

It may be necessary to lower the table and move the inflow system to accommodate a repositioning. The joint is redistended.

The surgeon moves to the medial side of the knee and takes it into extension. The television monitor is positioned in front of the surgeon (Fig. 6-59).

It may be necessary to redirect the 30-degree inclined scope to see the entire patellofemoral articulation. A 70-degree scope is a possible alternative for a better view.

I prefer the superomedial approach because it enters through a wide base of tissue, including the vastus medialis in some cases, and therefore does not leak. In addition, if patellar alignment is being done, the arthroscope position is opposite the area of the lateral release rather than in the site. It allows for visualization of the lateral release, and, if there is a superolateral puncture nearby, the area of tissue is so thin that it will leak anyhow. With the addition of a lateral release, one ends up with massive leakage in an inadequately distended joint. Distention is necessary for operative procedures of this nature.

Although I have seen some cases of ecchymotic anteromedial puncture (see Fig. 11-49). I have not observed complaints of vastus medialis pain or discomfort nor findings of lack of extension or fibrotic adhesions as a result of the superomedial approach. In summary, because this portal facilitates any anticipated operative procedures, avoids excessive leakage, and provides for continued distention, I use it.

When patellar tracking is viewed from the superomedial with the knee in extension, the patellar rides superior and lateral to the femur (see Fig. 10-33). When the knee is in 20 degrees of flexion, the lateral aspect of the patella touches the lateral femoral condyle and, although there may be an opening to the medial side, the edge of the medial patella would be in line with the medial aspect of the femur.

A   B

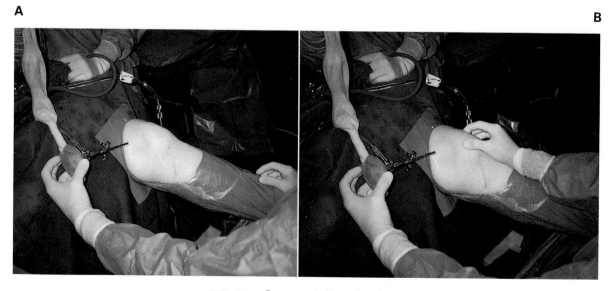

FIG. 6-59. Suprapatellar viewing.

A Positioning.
B Free hand control on patella.

At 45 degrees of flexion the "keel" of the patella is well centered and the patella is in contact both medially and laterally with the condyles. At 60 degrees of flexion it is further and more firmly centered in the notch, and only a small ellipse of patella is seen superiorly. At 90 degrees of flexion the patella is virtually out of sight except for a very tiny proximal lip seen in the intercondylar notch.

After going through incremental flexion and extension positions and checking each one, the surgeon takes the knee dynamically or actively through flexion-extension maneuvers to see if there are any abnormalities in patellofemoral articulation, its contact or movement.

Anatomical structures to be seen from the superior include the lateral retinaculum. With rotation of the arthroscope the lateral recess and fold will be seen. Angulation of the left or medial will make it possible to see a portion of the medial gutter and the medial plica. The pathological plica will come all the way across the fat pad. The tongue of the fat pad is easily and more adequately visualized from the superior.

It also should be stated that many lesions not seen from inferior on the patella or the trochlea are more easily visualized from the superior. Manual tipping of the patella with the opposite hand during visualization and palpating with the inflow cannula, which is now located anterolaterally, greatly enhance inspection of the patella.

With the completion of the superomedial inspection and evaluation of tracking, the knee has been completely visualized and, it is hoped, conceptualized.

OPERATIVE PORTALS
Needle placement

The needle is placed with the knee in slight flexion and valgus, with the surgeon viewing from lateral and placing a No. 18 spinal needle by trial and error into the anteromedial compartment (Fig. 6-60). This site is usually on a line about 1 cm distal to the placement of the arthroscope or 1 cm distal to the tip of the patella. It is more medial and away from the edge of the patellar tendon. By trial and error, the No. 18 needle spinal needle is placed. A position is desired from which the posterior horn of the meniscus and any other areas that will be operated on can be easily palpated with a No. 18 spinal needle. If the area of anticipated surgery or inspection cannot be palpated or touched with a No. 18 spinal needle, it will not be reachable with a larger instrument. In some cases, it is possible to elevate or depress the menisci or even to probe with the No. 18 spinal needle to assist in visualization of various parts. The lateral compartment approach has a different placement site (see Fig. 6-73.)

During this positioning it is important to avoid the neurovascular bundles, which are near the veins and the cutaneous nerves. The placement should not be through one of these veins, but adjacent to it (Fig. 6-61). Transillumination shows cutaneous vessels and accompanying cutaneous nerves.

Probing

The probe, although it is not considered a surgical "instrument," is an integral tool of the arthroscopic procedure (Fig. 6-62). Visualization of the parts

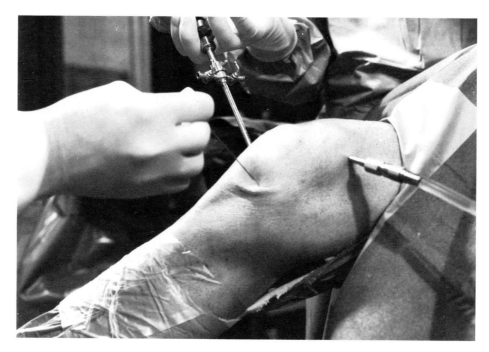

FIG. 6-60. Needle placement determines exact operative site at anteromedial portal.

FIG. 6-61. Transillumination.

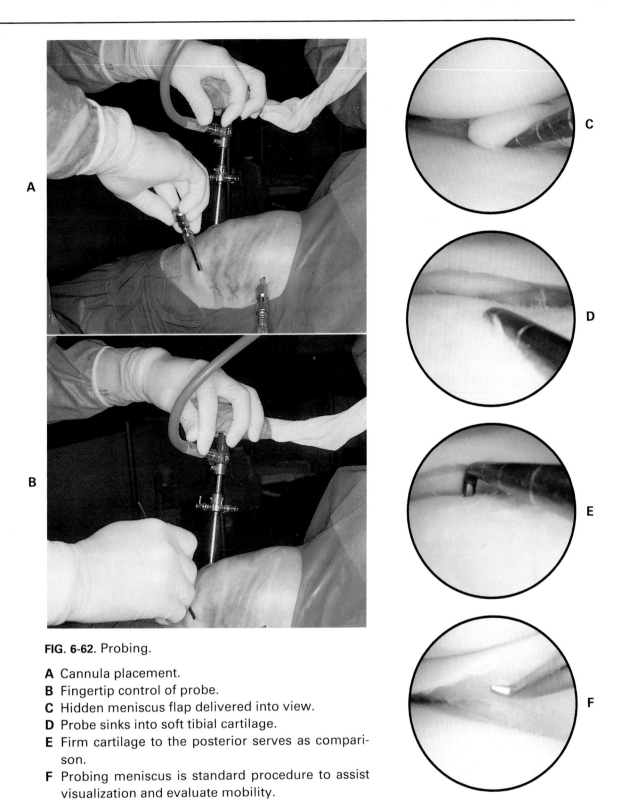

FIG. 6-62. Probing.

A Cannula placement.
B Fingertip control of probe.
C Hidden meniscus flap delivered into view.
D Probe sinks into soft tibial cartilage.
E Firm cartilage to the posterior serves as comparison.
F Probing meniscus is standard procedure to assist visualization and evaluate mobility.

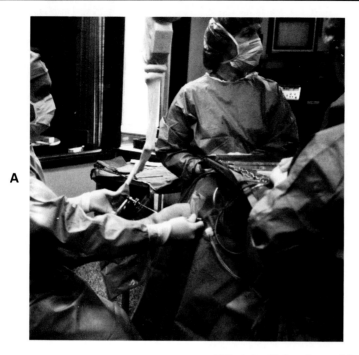

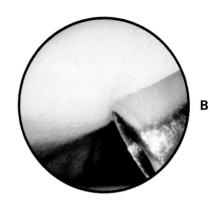

FIG. 6-63. Palpation with inflow cannula.

A Outside view of position.
B Inside view of patella and cannula.

will give only a portion of the information that one hopes to gain, and palpation is essential. Some palpation can be attained, as mentioned previously, with the use of the inflow cannula (Fig. 6-63). However, it may also be necessary to use a probe (see Fig. 6-66).

In the routine case, after I have run through all the visualization or determined a point at which probing should be introduced before complete visualization of all compartments, I usually place the arthroscope from anterolateral and bring the probe into the anteromedial compartment.

A small nick is made in the skin with a No. 11 blade, and the cannula system is placed along the area. First the sharp trocar and then the blunt obturator is placed to enter the joint. The obturator is removed. With the cannula in the joint, the probe is placed in the cannula. After the tip of the probe is seen in the joint, the cannula is removed and placed back on the Mayo stand. There is no leakage around the probe or cannula, and free palpation is allowed within the joint.

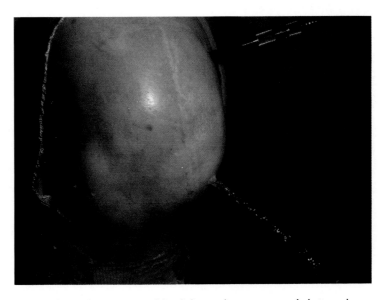

FIG. 6-64. Leakage from large portal incisions decompress joint and aggravate surgeon.

Control of joint leakage

If an incision made for portal placement exceeds the diameter of the cannula, leakage occurs (Fig. 6-64). Leakage out of the joint may cause decompression. Even worse is extravasation into the capsule and skin, obstructing the views on manipulation. Cannula systems decrease fluid leakage by creating a single hole of entry. The obturator placed in the cannula preserves the portal for subsequent use and control of leakage. When instrumentation is passed through the cannula, the cannula is removed over the instrument and returned to the Mayo stand. When instrumentation is complete, the cannula is placed back over the probe or knife for interchange to another instrument. Passage without cannulas is necessary with the use of forceps, but the small incisions still reduce leakage.

Care must be taken to avoid injury to the joint surface with the edge of the cannula when reaching to the extreme posterior regions from the front. The cannula may need to be removed for this maneuver.

Diagnostic probing

The probe can be used to elevate the meniscus and bring the arthroscope in underneath (see Fig. 6-62, *F*). Suction on the scope removes loose pieces. Turbulence can be created by palpating up and down the menisci with a probe to wash loose bodies out from under the menisci.

The meniscus can also be depressed. Pushing down on the posterior aspect makes it possible to see over the meniscus in loose-jointed people. The area of the tibial collateral ligament can thus be palpated.

It should be noted that the posterior horn of the medial meniscus is not very mobile. The anterior horn will move into and away from the joint approximately the width of the meniscus, and this can be done with a probe.

The tip as well as the knuckle of the probe can be used to palpate any interstitial tears or disruptions in the meniscus substance. These are not easily visualized because the skin of the meniscus is intact and there would be no entry point (Fig. 6-65).

Probing of the intercondylar notch can facilitate visualization of the cruciate ligaments by holding the ligamentum mucosa to one side or the other. It is possible to create a drawer sign and then palpate the anterior cruciate to see if it has

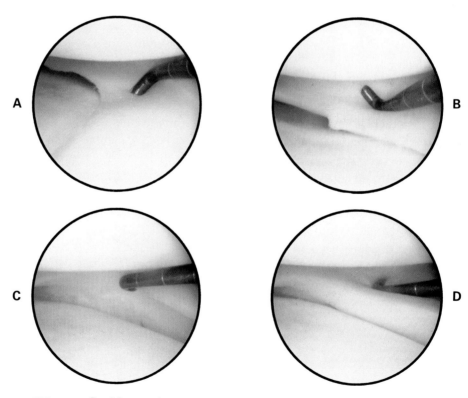

FIG. 6-65. Probing technique.

A Tip.
B Knuckle.
C Probe lifts meniscus.
D Probe depresses meniscus, surgeon sensing tissue consistency.

integrity during the drawer sign. With the knuckle of the probe it is possible to delineate between the anteromedial and posterolateral bundles of the cruciate ligament.

The knee is then taken into the varus position, as just mentioned, by viewing the slot between the tibial spine and the lateral femoral condyle. Without losing sight of this landmark, the probe is placed into the lateral compartment. Then the surgeon takes the knee into varus with his or her body, and moves over to the lateral side of the leg, still viewing from the inferior anterolateral portal. Probing of the lateral compartment can be carried out completely in most knees from the anteromedial portal. In some knees there is a very prominent tibial spine or osteophytes in the notch that mechanically block this maneuver; therefore it would be necessary to switch the arthroscope to medial and the probe to lateral. Probing in the lateral compartment can elevate the meniscus to view the meniscotibial ligament. Depression of the meniscus shows the meniscosynovial ligaments and the popliteus sheath (see Fig. 7-19). Probing of the mobility of the anterior and posterior horns can give the surgeon a sense of normalcy. It must be remembered that suction decompression may cause complete collapse of the lateral meniscus (see Fig. 6-13, *E* and *F*). This kind of mobility of the posterior and anterior horns is normal, not hypermobile. Checking this on all normals will help the surgeon in detection of an abnormal by giving him or her a sense of what normal is; there is no exact measure.

The knee can then be taken out into extension and probed. Perhaps even by redirection, it can be carried into the suprapatellar area.

Probing of the posterior compartments is facilitated by viewing from one portal and probing from the opposite (Fig. 6-66). The scope and probe approaches can be reversed.

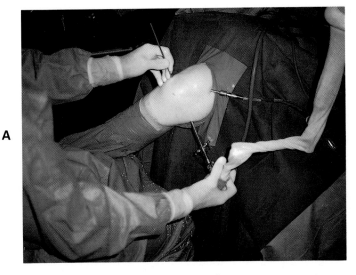

A

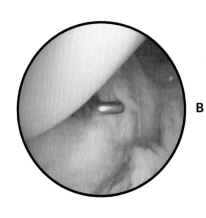

B

FIG. 6-66. Probing in posterior compartment.

A Probe placed from lateral through intercondylar notch with arthroscope from posteromedial portal.

B Arthroscopic view **(A)** with probe through notch on posterior cruciate ligament.

Continued.

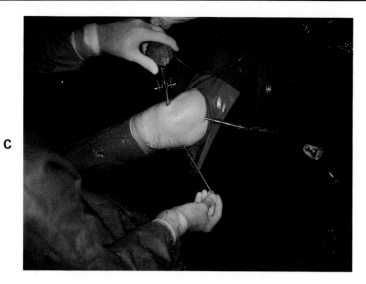
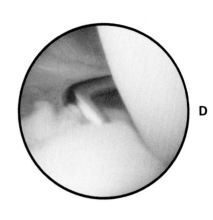

FIG. 6-66, cont'd. Probing to the posterior.

C Probe placed from posteromedial transcutaneous and scope from lateral via intercondylar notch.

D Arthroscopic view **(C)** with scope through intercondylar notch and probe on posterior horn of medial meniscus.

DIAGNOSTIC ARTHROSCOPY
Local anesthesia

The technique of local anesthesia is presently performed in the same surgical setup as for general anesthesia, including tourniquet, thigh holder, and television monitoring. The environment that is necessary for operative arthroscopy facilitate the diagnostic procedure. The techniques learned with local anesthesia have been combined into the present diagnostic routine just described in this chapter on general anesthesia. This section will detail features unique to the procedure under local anesthesia.

For local anesthesia to be possible, the surgeon must have the ability, capacity, and confidence to perform the procedure with dispatch. An operative time of up to 15 minutes is tolerable.

The surgeon should have established a good physician-patient relationship. Local anesthesia is best chosen for a patient from the local community or for a previous patient. Local anesthesia techniques necessitate selecting a patient who requests local anesthesia or accepts the technique because of medical reasons. The factors of general medical risk or necessity of travel on the same day may be important. Local anesthesia is not well suited for the apprehensive, emotional, or unstable patient. Any patient with a known low threshold of back pain should be excluded.

The patient's instructions concerning the procedure are reinforced by written information (see box on p. 417). At the first reading of instructions, apprehension may increase. This same material proves valuable during the procedure. Apprehension is reduced when procedure events proceed as outlined. The patient becomes relaxed and cooperative.

ARTHROSCOPY: LOCAL ANESTHETIC INSTRUCTIONS

Arthroscopy (looking into the joint) is a surgical procedure performed with a small-diameter telescope. The procedure may be performed with local anesthetic, similar to dental techniques that cause numbness in the area of the teeth. In the case of arthroscopy, the areas to be probed in the joint are deadened in a similar manner.

A local anesthetic method is chosen over putting the patient to sleep (general anesthesia) when the anticipated procedure is short or the necessary general medical conditions dictate this type of anesthetic.

The procedure is performed in a general hospital (Ingham Medical Center) to provide the optimal environment for the arthroscopy. In some cases, we schedule an anesthesiologist to "stand by" if further anesthetic is necessary.

The procedure usually requires the use of a tourniquet and a holding device on the patient's thigh. The tourniquet tightness is probably the most uncomfortable part of the procedure, but the procedure is usually of short duration (10 to 15 minutes) and is tolerable. If the patient relaxes the thigh and leg, the pressure of the tourniquet is less uncomfortable.

The leg is painted with antiseptic solution, which feels cool and wet. Sterile sheets are applied to reduce the chance of infection. The extremity will be well supported.

There is some discomfort from the "freezing" feeling of the joint, similar to dental techniques. The sites of entry will be numb, but not the entire extremity. The joint will be swollen with salt water as air distends a "balloon," to allow seeing inside the joint. This will give a sensation of fullness.

There are complications to any procedure, and so it is with arthroscopy. There is less than 1% chance of complication. The known problems have been breakage of the fiberoptic scope, infection, allergic reaction to the medicines used, and knee effusion (swelling). These are rare, and we take measures to prevent them.

Now for your part:
1. You will be called by the hospital regarding your time of arrival.
2. Please shave your leg (groin to ankle) and shower prior to the test.
3. Bring a list of any known allergies to medicines and/or general medical problems for our information.
4. Anticipate 1 to 2 hours total time to get in and out of the hospital.

Thank you.

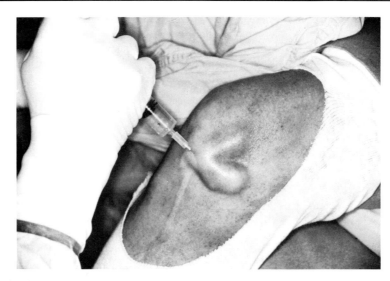

FIG. 6-67. Plain lidocaine, 1%, blocks infrapatellar branch of saphenous nerve. This decreases patient's proprioception and anxiety and increases comfort during procedure.

Preoperative medication is rarely necessary in well-selected cases with a short operative duration. I originally used medication for cases in the early 1970s. The side effects of medication were worse than the medication effects were advantageous, even delaying discharge because of nausea and vomiting.

When local anesthesia is desirable but reservations exist concerning the length of the procedure, an anesthesiologist may stand by if further measures are necessary. Standby anesthesia may be chosen in patients with a medical risk. This anesthetic assistance may determine the success of arthroscopy.

The anesthetic agent is 1% plain lidocaine. It is injected with a syringe and needle in the skin down to synovium, but not into the joint. The anesthetic is locally infiltrated along the anticipated course of the scope or instruments. In the knee joint, blocking of the intrapatellar branch of the saphenous nerve decreases the patient's proprioception to surgical manipulation (Fig. 6-67). Intraarticular anesthetic is not necessary for the patient's comfort with gentle surgical technique. It also provides a means of testing tender areas in the joint to correlate with clinical symptoms. This is especially indicated in plica syndromes.

Marcaine, 0.25% plain, is used in operative arthroscopic procedures such as lateral release. It would facilitate prolonged diagnostic procedures, but it should not be placed in the joint because of its demonstrated adverse effects on articular cartilage. It also is destructive to muscle.[7]

I have used normal saline for local anesthetic effects. I was confronted with an out-of-town patient referred for diagnosis only in the 1970s who was allergic to all "-caines." During my residency, Dr. Fred C. Reynolds had mentioned the possibility of saline during a historical discussion of local anesthetic agents. I used normal saline in massive amounts. Distention of skin and soft tissues provided the sole anesthetic effect.

Most patients will tolerate an environment with a tourniquet and the Surgical Assistant mechanical thigh holder. The tourniquet pressure is uncomfort-

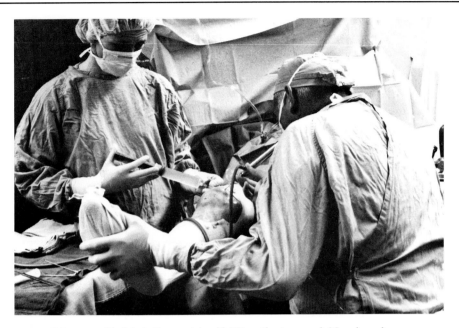

FIG. 6-68. Fluid delivered by K-52 catheter and 60 ml syringe.

able. If the patient understands that the avascular field provided by the tourniquet speeds the procedure and enhances the accuracy of diagnosis, the pressure is tolerable for 10 to 15 minutes for most patients. I have gone as long as 45 minutes with a tourniquet in an unanesthesized patient. After 20 minutes an anesthetic effect occurs from ischemia. The patient's discomfort is worst when a prolonged tourniquet time is concluded and circulation is restored.

The thigh holder has a compression pressure less that of the pneumatic tourniquet (350 mm Hg). In some cases in which I started with both the tourniquet and thigh holder, I have deflated the tourniquet for comfort. The patient tolerates the lower pressure of the Surgical Assistant as the procedure is completed, with the avascular surgical field maintained.

The inflow for the local anesthetic is attached to the arthroscope to simplify the system in diagnostic arthroscopy. A 60 ml syringe with a K-52 catheter delivers the fluid (Fig. 6-68). Most knee joints hold 90 ml of fluid. If the joint shows effusion, repeated distention and vacuumings cleanse for viewing. If joint clarity is not possible or if operative work is performed, a separate infusion inflow cannula is placed with the patient under local anesthesia.

The original local anesthetic procedures were performed with a small arthroscope and direct viewing. In the early 1970s operative arthroscopy was not yet developed, and open surgery was the usual alternative. The small scope was well tolerated by the patient. It provided access to all compartments for comprehensive arthroscopic inspection. The small scope still has the same advantages for diagnostic arthroscopy.

As experience in arthroscopic techniques was gained, the maneuvers previously thought possible only with a small scope became routine with scope of 4 mm diameter.

The success of diagnostic arthroscopy was based on continual monitoring of the patient's comfort. The circulating nurse sits and converses with the patient

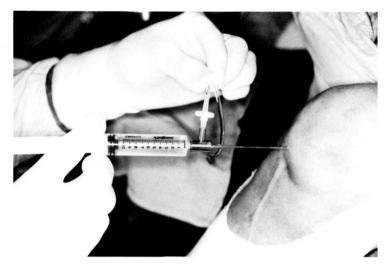

FIG. 6-69. Anesthetic agent delivered to tip of cannula via cannula.

to distract him, with the patient keeping the surgeon apprised of any discomfort. The local anesthetic is injected in sufficient amounts and the necessary time is allowed for effect. Some patients require more anesthetic or time. Repeat injections may be necessary.

If the scope cannula is being inserted but is not yet in the joint, and the patient complains, the following technique delivers anesthesia to the exact point of pain (Fig. 6-69). The cannula remains in place and the obturator removed. The thumb is placed over the end of the cannula. The anesthetic agent is delivered via an inflow spigot at the end of the cannula. Instillation of lidocaine permits resumption of penetration and the procedure.

The surgeon can monitor patient discomfort with the free hand on the ankle (see Fig. 6-36). The patient will tighten the Achilles tendon as the first response to apprehension or pain.

Postoperative care

At the conclusion of the diagnostic procedure, a sterile dressing is applied with Webril cotton wrap, which the surgeon or patient can remove without scissors. It is removed the next day, and Band-Aids are applied.

Instructions are given for wound care, potential complications, and time of repeat office visit.

ARTHROSCOPIC SURGICAL TECHNIQUES

The principles of diagnostic technique are carried over into the surgical dimension.

Surgical approaches to compartments

All portals of entry can be used in various combinations for surgical approaches. The most common combination is the superomedial approach for the inflow cannula, the anterolateral inferior approach for the arthroscope, and the anteromedial approach for instrumentation. The posteromedial approach is next most common. The less commonly used portals are the posterolateral, the superomedial anterior, the transpatellar, and the accessory approaches.

By using the inherent integrity of the tissues with the techniques outlined here under the various operative procedures, a three-portal technique is routine. It is possible to use the tissue's own tension for appropriate cutting. Vacuum suction puts tissue under tension for the use of motorized instruments.

This eliminates the necessity of placing a third instrument in the joint to create tissue tension for cutting. These techniques remove the crowding of three instruments, which makes manipulation difficult and visualization impossible sometimes. Further, the techniques avoid the bumping or injury to the articular surfaces. I have not had any cases that necessitated the use of the superior midpatellar approach when these methods were adhered to.

Medial compartment approaches

Visualization is from anterior lateral and instrumentation from anteromedial to approach the medial compartment (Fig. 6-70). For extreme anterior horn tears, it may be necessary to switch the arthroscope to medial and view downward. The surgeon should operate from the lateral to have an instrument that parallels the course of the anterior meniscus. This is more commonly necessary in the anterolateral compartment.

The posteromedial area of the meniscus is most often approached from anterolateral with the knee in slight flexion or in extension and valgus, depending on the contour on both the femoral and tibial condyles. The medial needle placement to the posterior horn has to be carefully selected, not only its proximodistal position but its position around the arc of the knee joint between the patellar tendon and the tibial collateral ligament. This is done to palpate all the extremes of the posterior horn of the meniscus.

An exceptionally loose knee, which is often seen in patients with genu valvum may allow access to the posterior from anterior approaches. A transcondylar or posteromedial approach will be necessary to visualize beyond the lead edge of the meniscus.

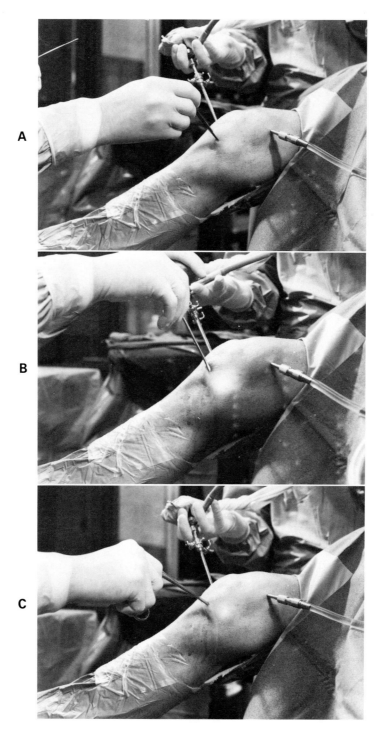

FIG. 6-70. Medial compartment approaches.

A Small skin incision.
B Knife blade.
C Forceps.

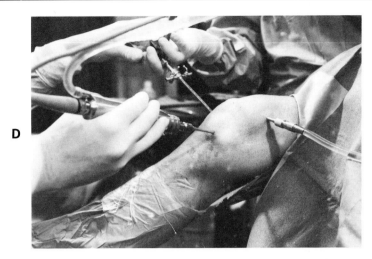

FIG. 6-70, cont'd. Medial compartment approaches.

D Motorized instrumentation.

Intercondylar notch approach

The intercondylar notch can be approached with the arthroscope from any anterior portal and the instrumentation placed from the opposite direction (Fig. 6-71).

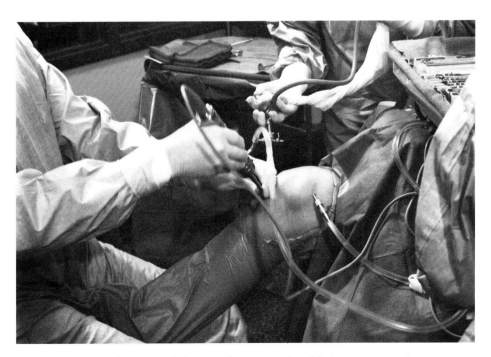

FIG. 6-71. Intercondylar notch approach with instrumentation.

Lateral compartment approach

The anterolateral compartment is most easily operated on while viewing from lateral with instrumentation placed from an anteromedial portal. An exception is the extreme posterior horn of the meniscus (Fig. 6-72). In some cases with either a large tibial spine or an osteophyte in that area, the arthroscope has to be placed to the medial side and the instrumentation to the lateral side. It should be noted that the anterior horn is most easily operated on while viewing from lateral and the instrumentation portal to the medial side.

Also, as mentioned previously, the selected portal for the instrumentation is more superior and nearer the patellar tendon than that which could be chosen specifically for the medial portal (see Fig. 6-72). On a loose knee with no scar or obesity, it may be possible to carry out the operative procedure using one surgical portal for the lateral meniscus.

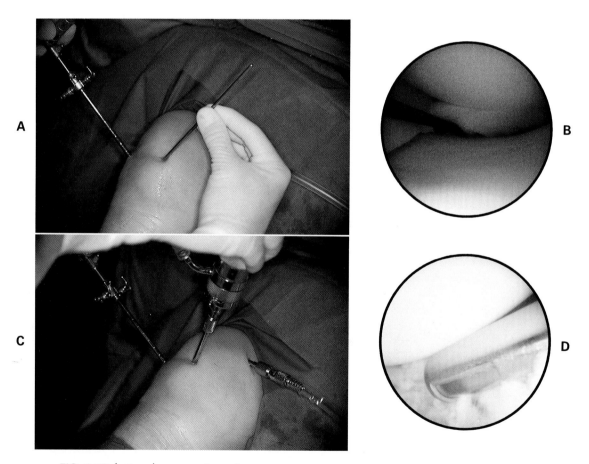

FIG. 6-72. Lateral compartment surgery.

A Medial instrument portal is more proximal and lateral than for procedure in medial compartment.
B Arthroscopic view of probe.
C Motorized instrument clean-up of synovium.
D Arthroscopic view of motorized instruments.

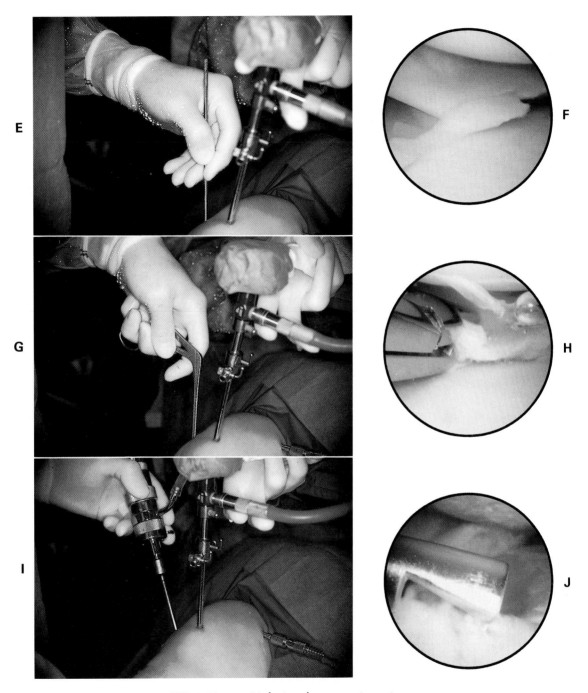

FIG. 6-72, cont'd. Lateral compartment surgery.

E Scope to medial and knife lateral.
F Arthroscopic view of knife cut.
G Basket forceps removal of fragment.
H Arthroscopic view of basket forceps.
I Final clean-up with motorized instrument.
J Arthroscopic view.

Patellofemoral approach

The best arthroscopic approach to view patellar work is from the supero-medial position (see Fig. 6-72, *B* and *C*). It gives a better view of the patella in its entirety, especially with the opposite hand manipulating the patella. It is possible to view tracking as well as the entire patellar surface from this position, and operative work on the patella can also be done.

Medial plica resection would not be possible with a 30-degree inclined scope, but interchange with a 70-degree arthroscope would allow not only ease of visualization for lateral release and/or medial imbrication. The new 30-degree inclined, 120-degree of field of view Storz scope yields an entire view.

The Surgical Assistant occupies space. Space limitations exist with this portal in a very short and fat person, but in most cases it would be possible to carry this out with an arthroscope attached to video. Direct visualization would not be possible with the thigh holder on, because the limited space for the surgeon's head would result in contamination of the operative field.

With the arthroscope proximal, the medial approach to the patella from below can be blocked by the contour or tightness of the joint or by osteophytes. In that case the instrument approach is more proximal and posterior than tha used for the medial compartment. A trial approach with a No. 18 spinal needle will locate the exact spot. It is a surprise to find a portal so posterior, with the instrument angled anteriorly, and yet observe the cutting head parallel to the patellar surface (Fig. 6-73, *B*).

A routine lateral original arthroscope portal gives the best access to the lateral facet and the entire patella. Aside from the ease of this approach via the original arthroscope portal, access is provided to femoral trochlea and lateral gutter (Fig. 6-73, *C*).

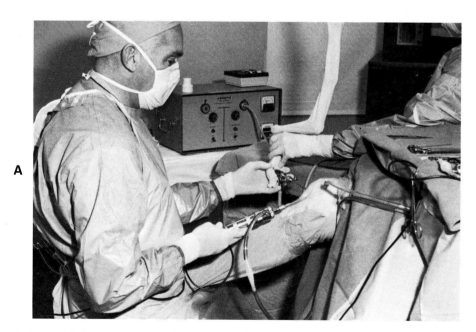

FIG. 6-73. Patellofemoral surgical approach.

A Comprehensive arthroscopic surgical position facilitates patellar shaving from below. Interchangeability of cannula and surgical instruments is also possible.

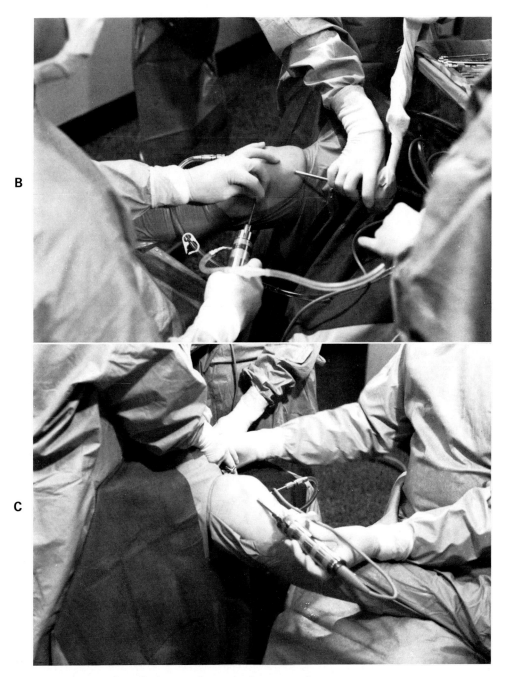

FIG. 6-73, cont'd. Patellofemoral surgical approach.

B Scope moved superomedially, and instruments shifted more proximally and posteriorly.

C Scope placed superiorly and motorized instrument laterally.

Approaches to posteromedial compartment: combined transcondylar and transcutaneous

The arthroscope can be placed transcondylarly across into the posteromedial compartment and instrumentation transcutaneously by the posteromedial portal (Fig. 6-74).

It is possible to interchange an arthroscope with instrumentation by using switching sticks through cannulas. This method reduces tissue trauma, operative time necessary for switching portals, and leakage of fluid. It also secures position for each new instrument, placing the scope transcutaneous and the instrument transcondylar (Fig. 6-75).

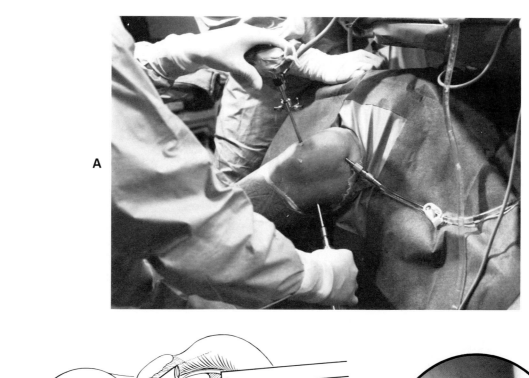

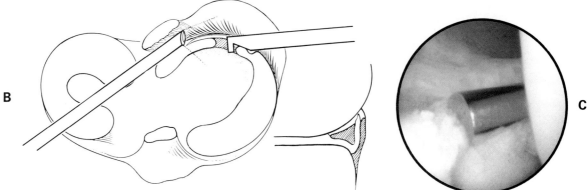

FIG. 6-74. Posteromedial compartment approaches.

A Scope placed through intercondylar notch.
B Graphic illustration of approach.
C Arthroscopic view of cutter entering through notch below posterior cruciate ligament and posterior to femoral condyle.

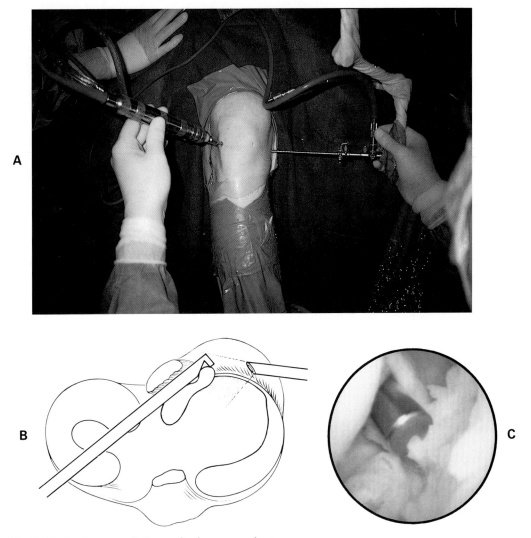

FIG. 6-75. Posteromedial surgical approaches.

A Instruments placed from anterolateral portal through notch to posteromedial area.

B Graphic representation of motorized instrument in posteromedial compartment.

C Arthroscopic view from transcutaneous position of cutter coming through notch.

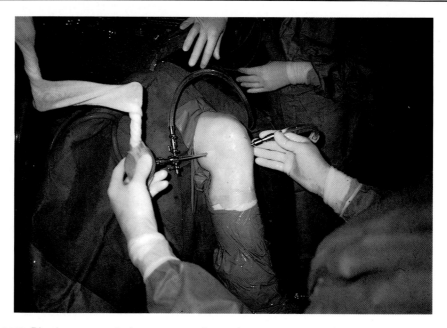

FIG. 6-76. Placing cannula into posterolateral compartment from anteromedial (inferior) portal.

Posterolateral compartment: combined transcondylar and transcutaneous

Combined transcutaneous and transcondylar approaches are used in the posterolateral compartment, just as in the posteromedial.

Access is not as easy because of the restricted space. The best procedure is to start with the scope in the posterolateral compartment and place the cannula into the compartment from the anteromedial (inferior portal) (Fig. 6-76). This second portal provides access for a probe or for inflow. Often the transcondylar approach is too narrow for the cannula, and only the probe can traverse the space.

An auxiliary approach paralleling the lateral meniscus, placed from the lateral side above and the posterior to the popliteus tendon, may give another cannula site.

Double transcutaneous posterior approaches

Posteromedial. The posteromedial compartment can be approached by placing two instruments posteromedially (Fig. 6-77). The arthroscope is placed from the extreme superior approach, and the instrumenation allows one to view down on that compartment, which facilitates entering the Baker's cyst. The instrumentation is placed slightly anterior and inferior to the arthroscope placement. The positions can be reversed with switching sticks (Fig. 6-77, C). Care should be taken in approaching the posteromedial portal to avoid puncturing the saphenous vein.

Double transcutaneous approaches are often limited by small space. Fortunately, access is often possible from the anterior portals.

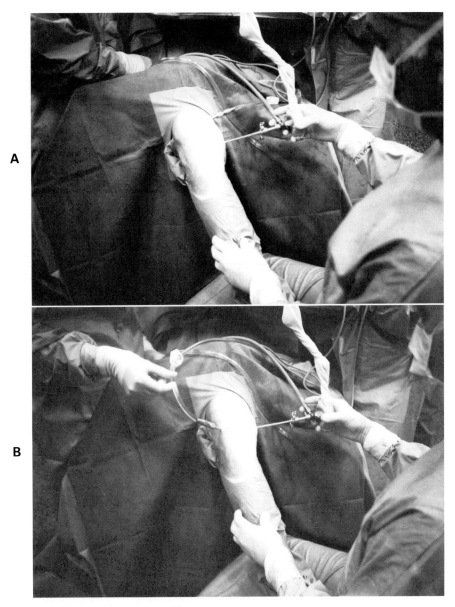

FIG. 6-77. Posteromedial surgical approach.

A To start, inflow is placed above and scope posteromedially.

B Inflow placed through intercondylar notch to posteromedial compartment.

Continued.

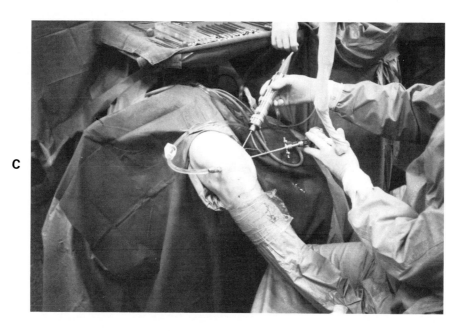

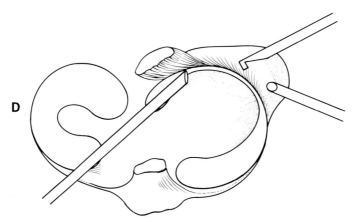

FIG. 6-77, cont'd. Posteromedial surgical approach.

C All three cannulas in posteromedial compartment with scope and cutter transcutaneous.

D Graphic illustration of approach.

Approach to popliteus sheath

The popliteus sheath is approached arthroscopically from the routine antero-lateral portal (Fig. 6-78). Using a No. 18 spinal needle from the proximal, a site is selected for an instrumentation portal to provide access down the sheath (Fig. 6-78, *B* and *C*).

This provides access for synovectomy and/or loose body removal.

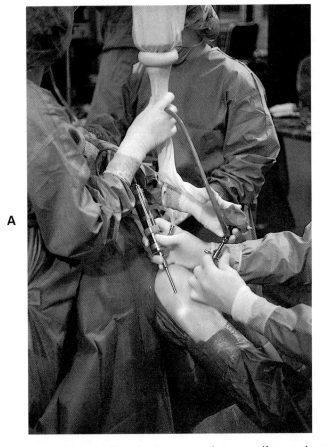

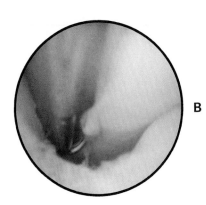

FIG. 6-78. Surgical approach to popliteus sheath.

A Scope placed from routine portal and instrument from proximal portal.
B Arthroscopic view of cutter cannula to left of popliteus tendon.

ARTHROSCOPIC OPERATIVE PRINCIPLES
Cannula system

The cannula system used in arthroscopic surgical work is the same as that used in diagnostic arthroscopy. In fact, the cannula system can be used and interchanged between the three routine portals: the superomedial, the anteroinferior medial, and the anteroinferior lateral. The cannula systems can be used posteromedially and posterolaterally or obliquely placed across the joint from the anterior to posterior. For the area of the popliteus sheath or into the posterolateral compartment, the cannula approach is used. A superolateral portal could also be used with a cannula system.

The system is used for the initial insertion, and then the position is preserved so that if there is some leakage of saline, reidentification of the passage is not difficult (Fig. 6-79). Interchangeability of the cannula system is facilitated by using switching sticks.

Surgical exposure

Exposure is developed in the same way that is mentioned in the section on diagnostic arthroscopy. With the secured thigh, distended joint, and proper placement, the synovial resecter is used to achieve surgical exposure if synovium blocks the view. In cases of anterior cruciate ligament tears, bucket-handle tears, or work in the intercondylar notch, the ligamentum mucosa can be resected from its femoral attachment. Existing distention will push the fat pad away from the intercondylar notch, improving visualization. In addition, it may be necessary to vacuum loose bodies from the joint or cleanse it. There may be a single or multiple loose bodies in front of the meniscus, and the posterior horn may not allow visualization. These loose bodies are vacuumed from the joint.

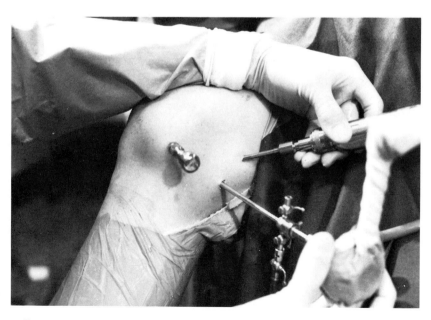

FIG. 6-79. Preservation of previous portal with cannula and obturator while doing posterior surgery.

Another general principle of exposure is to debride near the point of entry and work into the joint to obtain a view. The anterior portion of a compartment is cleaned first, then the surgeon works his or her way to the posterior. In some cases of degenerative meniscus, exposure can be facilitated by first carrying out careful condylar debridement; this gives a wider exposure, especially in a collapsed degenerative joint. With this method the surgeon will be able to see the posterior portions of the meniscus.

Debridement and tissue preservation

Debridement is a common denominator of all arthroscopic surgery. It is balanced by tissue preservation (see Fig. 6-81). The surgeon's powers of discernment have to be used concerning the limitations of the resection, whether it be extent of meniscus removal or depth of articular cartilage debridement.

One of the difficult decisions is determining an acceptable extent of debridement. The general principle is to debride less rather than more. For example in the case of a degenerative medial compartment with a degenerative torn meniscus, preservation of meniscal tissue, even with a small posterior horizontal cleft tear of 1 mm, could be more acceptable than resection of all the tissue.

Resection principles

Instrument portals

Traditionally meniscectomy work was done by grasping the anterior horn of the meniscus with a large meniscus clamp through an arthrotomy and then cutting the tissue. This could be done in arthroscopic work, but it would require three instruments—an arthroscope, a grasping forceps, and a cutting instrument—all in the same compartment. Patel has modified his placement of the arthroscope to a more superior position so as to displace the arthroscope from the compartment and thus allow space for two operating instruments, a grasping and a cutting instruments, in the same compartment. The Swedish technique places the arthroscope through the tendon and the instruments on both sides of the patellar tendon, one for grasping and one for cutting.[8]

Order of resection

The first principle of resection in arthroscopic surgery is to remove the soft parts. This can be done with a synovial resector and an Intra-articular Shaver with a trimmer or a cutter head on the meniscus. After the soft parts are resected, leaving the firmer tissue behind, the firm tissue is then more amenable to cutting with hand instruments (a knife blade or a basket-type forceps). The firm or larger pieces of tissue must be cut under tension.

The three-instrument technique is not necessary except for a medial bucket-handle tear.

Tissue tension

With the technique of motorized debridement of the soft parts to create excellent exposure, the meniscus tissue itself is under tension. If the meniscus tissue is cut in the appropriate manner, using and maintaining tissue tension

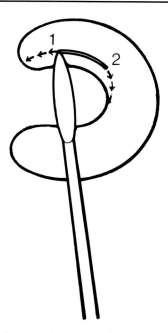

FIG. 6-80. Medial meniscus cutting toward notch first.

within the meniscus itself, a grasping forceps is not necessary until after the tissue has been released.

The other method of cutting tissue under tension is to use motorized instruments or any other type of instrument with suction. The suction itself creates tissue tension. The tissue is simultaneously resected and removed.

Plan of attack

The surgical protocol should have a design; it is important to plan every cut. A typical error occurs with posterior longitudinal tear of the meniscus. If the tear is freed to the medial side, then it is difficult to cut the posterior horn. There is no tissue tension unless a grasper were to be placed in the joint. I have learned that the normal tissue tension can be used by first cutting the side toward the notch (Fig. 6-80). It is easy then to cut the proximal side; pressing down on the meniscus tissue with gentle pressure and dragging the knife blade back and forth creates the cut.

Experience, planning, and surgical imagination can prevent "painting yourself into a corner" (see Fig. 6-1).

Incisions, inscriptions, excisions, and removal

Incisions using the knife blade, basket forceps, or any other type of instrument should be designed for complete resection or removal. Traditionally the surgeon using a knife blade would cut the entire fragment to be removed all the way through. In arthroscopic surgery, there is an advantage to an incomplete incision, a so-called inscription, with a knife blade. The inscription in the meniscus will clearly outline the pattern to be resected. Either basket forceps or motorized instruments can go up to the line of inscription, which is perhaps two thirds to three fourths of the way through the meniscus. When resecting the meniscus with the knife blade, it is good to leave a very tiny fragment on either end intact. The piece will not float away in the joint if the inflow on the arthroscope is eliminated.

After it has been incised, only a small tag is still intact. The fragment can be grasped and removed with an avulsion of the tag. The clean-up can be done with a motorized system. Complete cuts are carried out on the anterior and posterior horns. A bucket-handle tear of the medial or lateral meniscus is then grasped with the forceps. A complete cut is used in quadricepsplasty or lateral release and medial imbrication.

INSCRIBE—RELEASE—GRASP—CLEAN-UP

Attention should be given to the contour of the cut. The contour of the menisus is looked at from superior to inferior and from inside to outside. In this way, both dimensions of the contour are considered, and there will be no offending irregular shapes for the articular surface.

Techniques

Technique by location

When an extreme posterior horn tear has been identified diagnostically, the lesion may be so far posterior that it is not reachable from the anterior. In that case a posteromedial puncture and a transcondylar arthroscopic approach could allow the posterior horn of the medial meniscus to be resected via a posterior compartment (see Figs. 6-75 and 6-76) with the knee in flexion. Interchange of portals facilitates a tangential position of the shaft of the motorized instrument to the condyles.

Technique by depth

In synovial lesions the depth of the resection can be controlled to remove only villi, the entire synovial layer, or portions of underlying capsule. Invading synovial pannus can be removed from the underlying bone. The superficial synovectomy is common in degenerative villous synovitis. In cases of pigmented villonodular synovitis the entire synovium is resected. A wide synovectomy with capsulectomy is indicated in a loose type of destructive rheumatoid arthritis or in previously failed synovectomy (see Chapter 13).

The depth of resection in hyaline cartilage disease is minimal. Partial-thickness lesions should not be converted to full thickness except when lack of viable tissue is demonstrated by the most gentle nonagressive instrumentation (whisker).

When bone is already exposed in a degenerative joint, the depth of debridement need only be 1 to 2 mm to expose intracortical blood supply. Deeper cutting or drill holes are unnecessary and contraindicated (see Chapter 8).

Technique by tissue type

The articular cartilage is more safely cut with a trimmer head; in articular cartilage the cutter head is too aggressive and can cause tissue injury. The meniscus is resected with a cutter head.

In tight spots it is also beneficial to use a well-housed cutting shape when working near the articular cartilage.

The synovial whisker is best for synovial villi and careful debridement of furry articular cartilage.

The full-radius synovial resector will cut even bone, but bone is best resected with an abrader.

Technique by shape of lesion

If the lesion is well circumscribed with firm articular cartilage adjacent to the edges, the surgeon might use a knife blade or a curette. For a lesion that is spread out and has a gradation of softness at the center to a gradual healing or fissuring at the margins, the Intra-articular Shaver trimmer or whisker head is more appropriate than a knife blade. Only the degenerative articular tissue can enter into these resectors, and the resection is limited to reshaping into the contour of a saucer.

Instrument selection

A specific instrument can be used if the surgeon has knowledge of that tool and of the pathological lesion being managed.

Hand instruments

Cannula. The cannula with an obturator can be used to probe articular surfaces or menisci and give a sense of palpation of softness or firmness of any given tissue.

Probe. The probe is used for probing under or above menisci or to catch an articular piece. It can also be used as a retractor; the menisci can be lifted up so as to pass an arthroscope underneath and palpate the anterior cruciate ligament for tightness while a drawer tests is being performed. The probe can be used as an internal retractor to move the ligamentum mucosa from side to side in the intercondylar notch.

The probe can also be used to determine the mobility of a meniscus or the accessibility of a plica for resection.

Knife blade. The knife blade is used most to cut the firm tissues. It can also be used to perform an inscription or complete release of tissue.

Knife blades are passed through cannula systems to minimize trauma to soft tissues of capsule and to protect articular cartilage (Fig. 6-81, *A*). The blade is observed as it enters the joint from the cannula (Fig. 6-81, *B*). The cannula is removed and placed on Mayo stand (Fig. 6-81, *C*). The knife is held with a fingertip grip for precision (Fig. 6-81, *D*).

Basket forceps. The basket forceps is most useful in resecting meniscal tissue, especially in a tight knee with too little fluid flow for motorized instruments (see Figs. 4-32 and 4-33). If the tissue is facing directly end-on and is not removable by slight angulation with an Intra-articular Shaver cutter or with a knife blade, a basket forceps is used. In some extreme posterior horn lesions, it

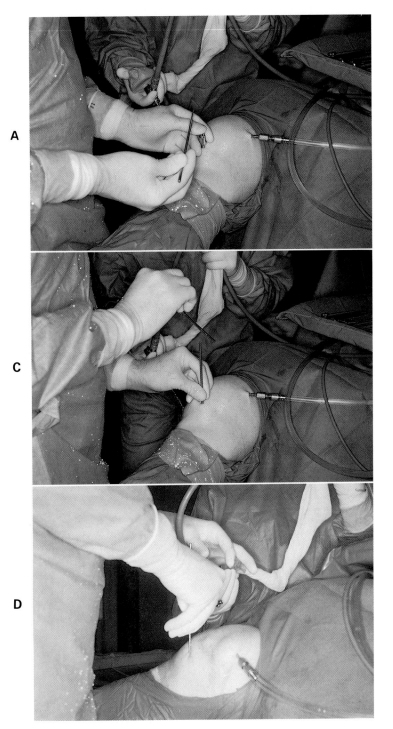
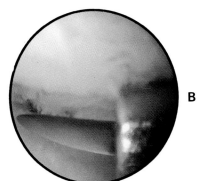

FIG. 6-81. Knife blade technique.

A Cannula system covered with surgeon's thumb to prevent leakage as knife is ready to enter cannula.

B Arthroscopic view of tip of knife entering safely via cannula.

C Cannula is removed and placed on Mayo stand.

D Knife is held with fingertips for precision and control.

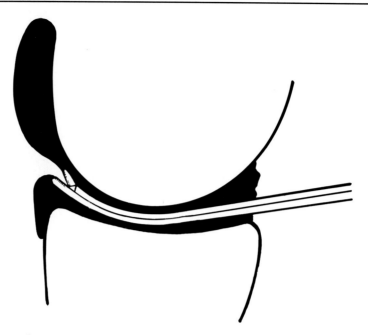

FIG. 6-82. Posterior extremes reached by using curved basket forceps from anterior portal.

is possible to pass a curved basket forceps from front to back through the joint. The posterior horn rim to be trimmed is located beyond the flair of the condyle (Fig. 6-82), and this allows the basket forceps to be opened.

Basket forceps are placed transcutaneously. They are not placed through a cannula system. For operations on the posterior horn in a tight knee, the basket forceps is rotated to the vertical position after it is over the meniscus and used to bite down on the meniscus. The basket forceps is then retracted and rotated. This procedure is then repeated, advancing gradually from one side to the other, with the forceps resecting adjacent to the last cut (Fig. 6-83).

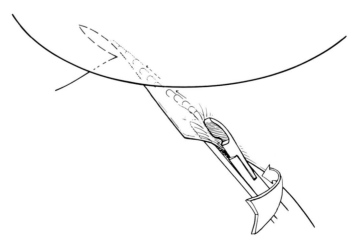

FIG. 6-83. Basket forceps gradually advance from side, resecting adjacent to the previous cut.

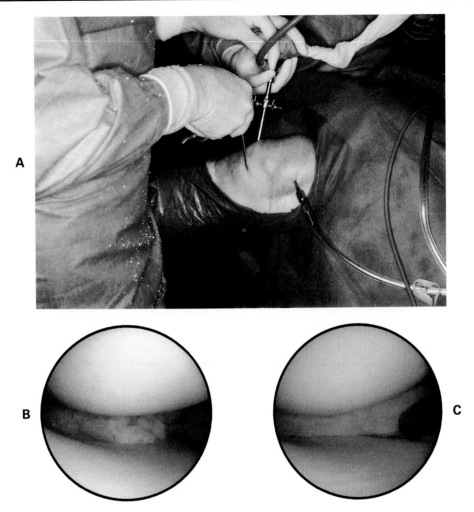

FIG. 6-84. Basket forceps technique.

A Instrument passed transcutaneously.
B Cutting off flow at time of resection allows fragments to stay put for removal.
C Clean-up with motorized instruments.

The basket forceps can be used as a scissors. It removes pieces along the line of the incision to allow for better visualization along the cut. The two pieces do not overlap as with scissor cutting (see Fig. 6-83).

The disadvantage of using a basket forceps is that it requires multiple passes and leaves multiple pieces. If space restrictions are such that the forceps cannot be opened, resection is impossible.

The basket forceps is best used with the flow system turned off. The pieces will stay in place for removal with cannula suction or motorized instrumentation (Fig. 6-84).

Scissors. The hand scissors is beneficial for resecting bucket-handle tears and for resecting plicae. It can also be used like a basket forceps, especially when there is firm, mobile tissue that has to be cut sharply. For soft tissue that is too mobile to be cut with a knife blade, the scissors of the variable axis system is effective (see Fig. 4-33).

Graspers. The graspers are used either with or without a ratchet. I favor using the graspers without a ratchet for quick release. Although the ratchet holds well, it does not release easily. The graspers can be used with rotation to avulse small pieces (see Figs. 4-24 to 4-26).

Switching sticks. Switching sticks are useful for interchanging cannulas of various lengths and diameters (see Fig. 4-21). These simple straight rods, which are blunt on the end, provide for change of portals without loss of position (Fig. 6-85). The technique is simple and effective.

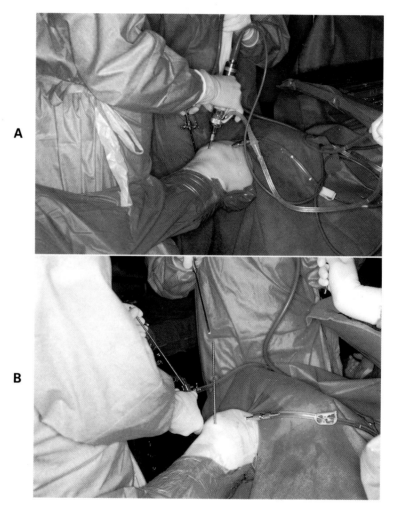

FIG. 6-85. Switching sticks.

A Scope placed laterally, instruments medially.
B Scope removed, switching stick placed. Instrument removed, other switching stick placed.

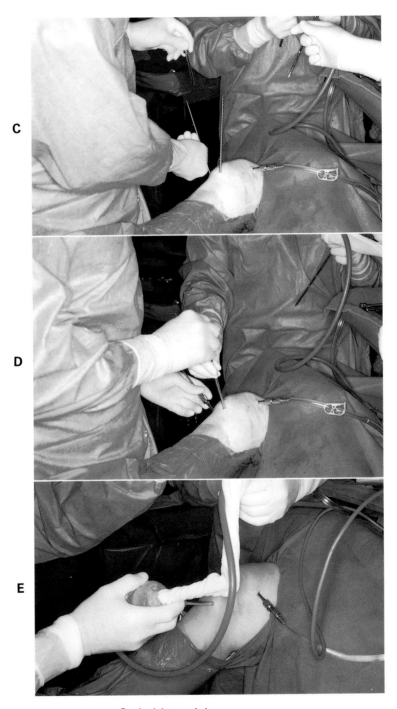

FIG. 6-85, cont'd. Switching sticks.

C Interchange of cannulas off the lateral side.
D Scope cannula on medial side. Switching stick removed.
E Scope in medial portal. Instrument cannula in lateral portal.

Golden Retriever. The Golden Retriever is used to retrieve loose, metallic fragments with magnetic properties (see Fig. 4-27). When an incident of breakage occurs, the surgeon should pause and collect his or her thoughts. The gold-colored retriever is easily identifiable in a surgical pan of silver-colored instruments.

The device is inserted via the cannula system (Fig. 6-86, *B*). The fragment is manipulated end-on to the magnet for removal through the cannula (Fig. 6-86, *D*). With the cannula in the joint, the Golden Retriever and fragment are removed (Fig. 6-86, *E*). *Do not* remove the fragment transcutaneously, because it may be lost in tissues.

The suction will aid in retrieval, but suction that is too strong will bring soft tissue in between the magnet and fragment. This is why a tight suction connection is not possible while using the Golden Retriever.

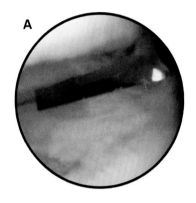

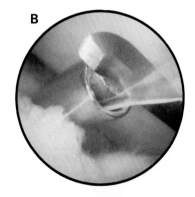

FIG. 6-86. Golden Retriever.

A Fragment broken off in joint.
B Golden Retriever passed via cannula. Magnet attracts fragment on side. Notice effect of suction on tissues.
C Cannula pushed over Golden Retriever into view.
D Fragment end on magnet to facilitate cannula removal.
E Fragment seen in cannula opening.

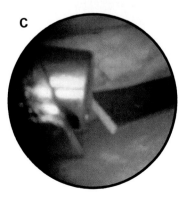
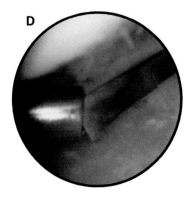
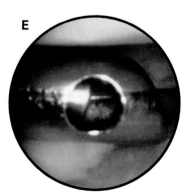

Motorized instrumentation

Motorized instrumentation facilitates simultaneous resection and removal, and it reduces the number of entries necessary into the joint (see Figs. 4-41 to 4-43). There is less risk of articular cartilage injury or scuffing. It decreases the amount of hand activity necessary by the surgeon, and minimizes his or her fatigue (Fig. 6-87). It is especially effective in articular cartilage debridment and synovectomy, which could not be as easily accomplished in any other way.

A motorized instrument is handled very much like a pencil. To use one that has a "gun" or pistol grip, the surgeon has to supply rotation with forearm rather than motion with the hand. Some systems rotate by manipulation of the barrel with the second hand. The axial alignment of the Dyonics system allows for greater ease of handling and encourages precision gripping. A second hand may be necessary for control (Fig. 6-87, *A*).

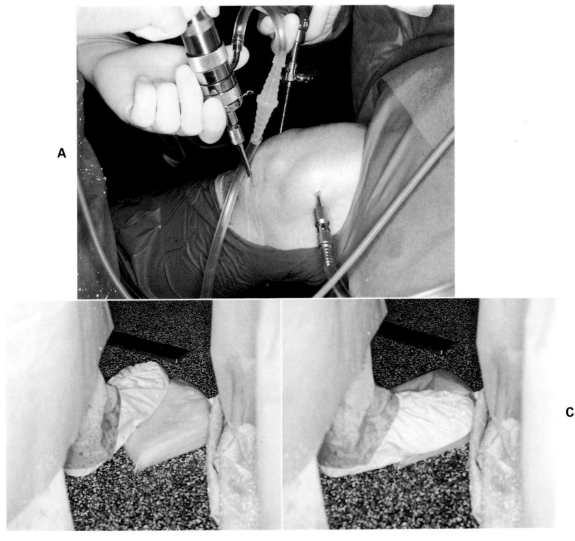

FIG. 6-87. Motorized instrumentation. **A** Two-handed control of motorized instrumentation. **B** Foot pedal forward control. **C** Foot pedal reverse control.

On the original Dyonics system there was a side spigot that could mechanically block the angle of access to joint (Fig. 6-89, *A*). Rotation of the spigot with a second hand permits axial alignment with the patella for continued cutting (Fig. 6-88, *B*).

Technique by manipulation

Shaving. Shaving is the technique that started the development of motorized instrumentation. The shaver or cutter head is moved back and forth across a surface very much as electric razor is guided across a beard. The tissue comes into the instrumentation by suction. The rotating-cutting device removes the soft articular parts. The shaving technique is basic, and instrument head changes are made based on tissue type (Fig. 6-89).

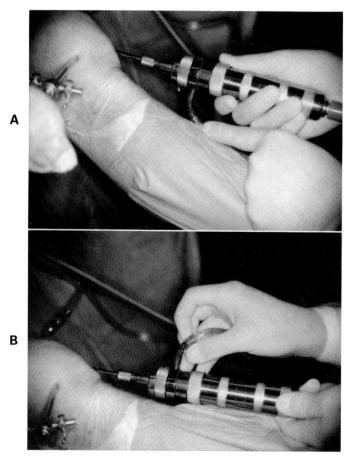

FIG. 6-88. Mechanical block from side spigot with IAS or AS.

A Angle of access to patella blocked by spigot.
B Angle improved after rotation of spigot.

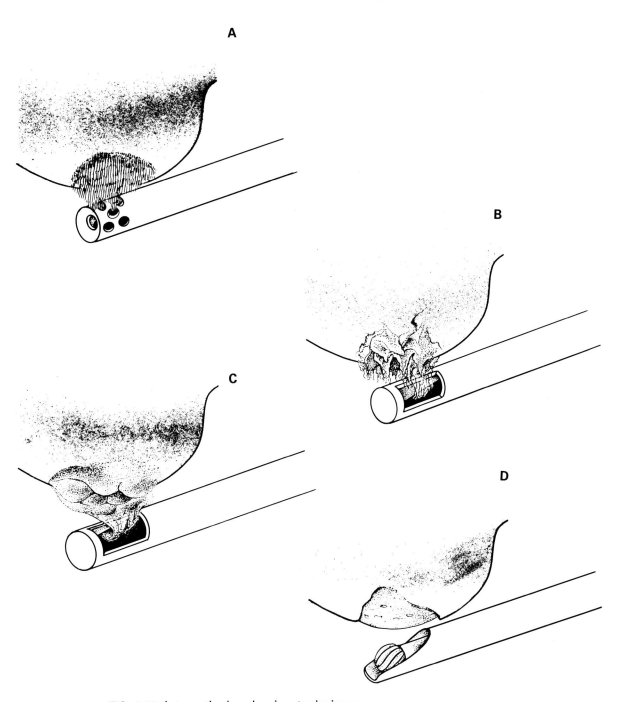

FIG. 6-89. Intraarticular shaving technique.

A Whisker head used for furry material.
B Trimmer head used for shaggy material
C Trimmer head used for bulky surface.
D Shaving motion of abrader head on exposed bone.

Dabbing. Dabbing is an oscillating action that can be likened to blotting spilled fluid with a towel (Fig. 6-90). The towel is placed on the fluid repeatedly until the water is drawn up into it. As the towel approaches, the fluid will seem to jump up into it. This is actually the case with arthroscopic dabbing; the instrument is held away from either synovium or the soft part. The suction is open on the instrument. As the instrument moves towards the object, the material is moved under tension into the instrumentation. This suction tension permits sharp cutting action.

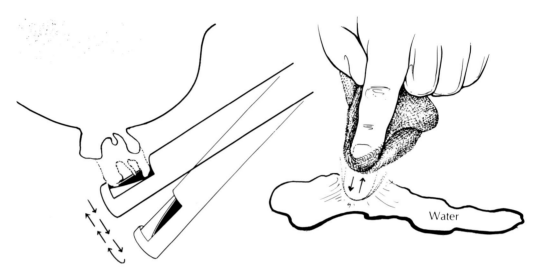

FIG. 6-90. Dabbing motion.

Pawing. Another technique is the use of pawing (Fig. 6-91). Pawing is used in the Intra-articular Shaver System, with a trimmer head for use on articular cartilage or the cutter head on meniscus. The motion is as if one were pawing or scratching in the dirt. It is a very slow motion, and the surgeon can pull down toward his or her body, go back, and pull toward the body again several times. Repetition of pawing and pulling goes over the same part. It is used on meniscus and articular cartilage flaps.

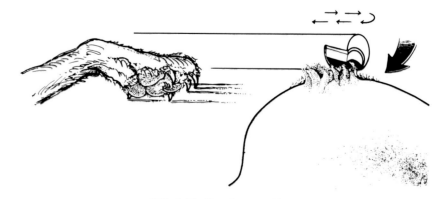

FIG. 6-91. Pawing motion.

Whittling. Whittling is a technique of using the foot pedal on motorized instrumentation, forward, then reverse, back and forth (see Fig. 6-87). This technique is likened to whittling wood (Fig. 6-92). Whittling on one side of a green stick bends it over without further resection; reversing the twig provides an angle for cutting. A more effective method of resection is to alternate whittling from one side of the stick and then from the other side. The foot pedal is used in the same way, alternating forward and reverse on any given fragment, to produce the whittling effect.

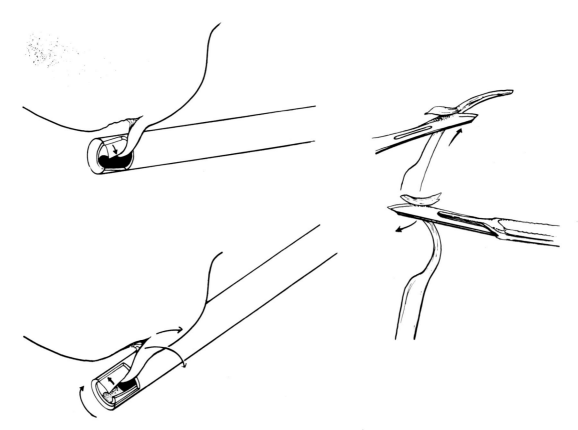

FIG. 6-92. Whittling motion.

Scooping. The scooping action is like that used in scooping ice cream (Fig. 6-93). The open portion of the cutter head rests along the edge of tissue to be resected. The motor is activated, and cutting is initiated. The instrument is rotated to lift material with a scooping motion as it is resected. This motion is used on irregularly shaped tissue of hard consistency.

Joint manipulation. The surgical instrument can remain stationary with the knee joint taken into flexion and extension to cause a change in the position of the cutting head on the femur (Fig. 6-94). The same method is used in the shoulder with passive humeral rotation.

Technique by cutting head

Shaver. The shaver is used with a side-to-side motion; this is analogous to mowing the lawn. The bullet-nose prevents an effective pawing motion, but dabbing is possible (Fig. 6-95).

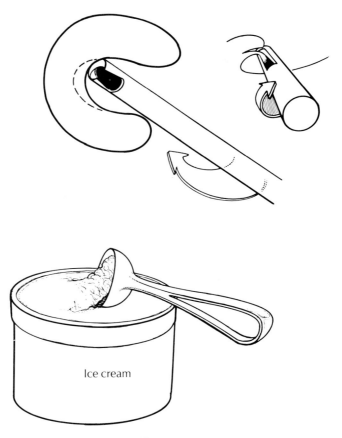

FIG. 6-93. Scooping motion.

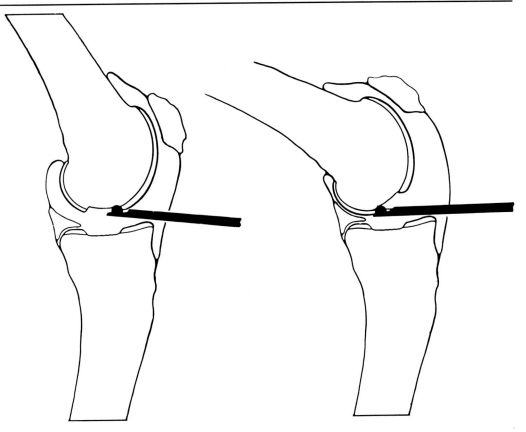

FIG. 6-94. Knee action.

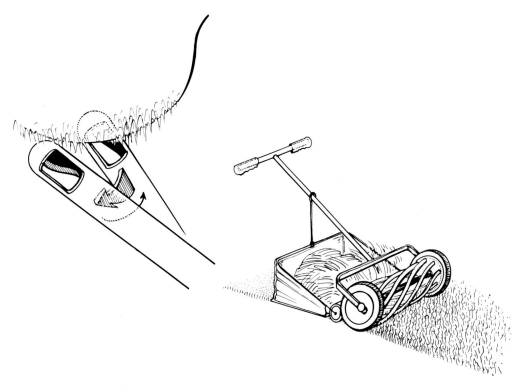

FIG. 6-95. Shaver head.

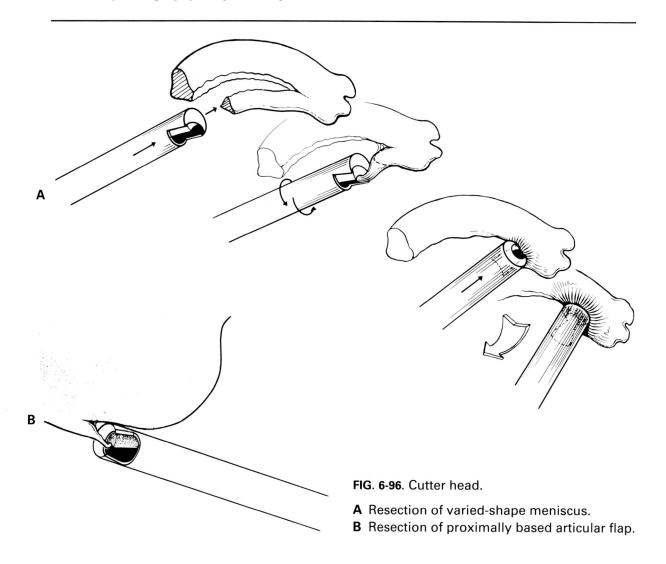

FIG. 6-96. Cutter head.

A Resection of varied-shape meniscus.
B Resection of proximally based articular flap.

Cutter. With the cutter head, both pawing on hard parts and dabbing on soft free edges are used on the meniscus (Fig. 6-96). If the cutter is used on undermined edges of articular cartilage, scooping is the proper technique. Whittling is a function of all of these motions. Scooping is used when working under the edge of the meniscus, at the junction of a tear and normal meniscus tissue.

Trimmer. The shaving motion is the most common for the trimmer head (Fig. 6-97). A combination of pawing and scooping facilitate resection of tissues.

Whisker. The whittling, side-to-side motion clears small holes of tissue. The instrument is held off of the synovium and draws in villae with a dabbing motion.

Abrader. With the abrader the action is shaving, with an even pressure to progressively resect bone. The reverse mode is less aggressive than the forward angle of the cutting edges. A combination shaving and scooping or pawing action gives even control to resection. The whittling action cleans the burr of bony debris. A curetting motion is used on deep holes. The scooping motion elevates and resects the edges of osteophytes.

Synovial resector. The nature of the cut in synovial resection is affected by shaving and dabbing. The distance from the synovium determines the depth of

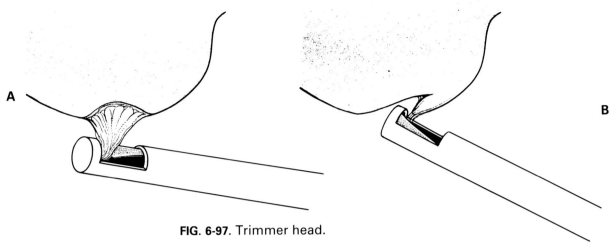

FIG. 6-97. Trimmer head.

A Removal of long, loose fragment.

B Resection of proximal-based articular flap.

the section. When held off the villae and slowly moved by dabbing, only the villae are resected. A closer position removes synovial membrane. A pawing action with pressure will resect the capsule or even muscle.

Final operative steps

The final step of any arthroscopic technique is to repeat the diagnostic review of the joint. The areas of meniscus resection or articular debridement are reprobed to see that all the remaining tissue is firm and of the proper shape. A motorized instrument is used to vaccum or debride and clean-up the area to leave behind the cleanest possible wound. This reduces the amount of work that the joint itself has to do in cleaning-up.

Host tissue response

One factor that surgeons tend to ignore is that the body responds not only to disease or injury but also to surgery (see Chapter 8). Any debridement and/or repair has to be thought of in terms of the opportunity for the tissue to respond. For instance, a semitendinosus graft from the tibia to the femur placed to augment the anterior cruciate ligament demonstrates excellent intraoperative fixation. There is no motion, and the Lachman test is normal. What happens to the tissue? It is covered with clot. Synovial and vascular covering surrounds the tendon tissue mass. An amalgamation of harvested anterior cruciate ligament and tendon graft forms. The tendon graft remains unchanged, as demonstrated by biopsy (see Fig. 8-81).

In the case of a torn meniscus, the possibility of repair is first priority, followed by resection, and perhaps a combination of both techniques. With resection, the edges will smooth, and a fibrous tissue will form on the surface. Both cellular and angioblastic responses occur with repair.

Careful debridement of a partial-thickness lesion removes potential fragments from the joint. Often, fibrous repair is seen on the surface without drilling to the bone (see Fig. 8-23).

453

If sclerotic exposed bone is debrided, hemorrhage occurs and is followed by spindle cell formation. If the area is properly protected, reparative fibrocartilage will develop (see Fig. 8-39 and 8-40).

During any operative procedure, the diagnosis is maximized as the surgeon considers the adequacy of the surgical repair or resection. But he or she must always consider the great potential the body has for repair. The resection of tissue should be adequate but not excessive or unnecessary.

INTRAOPERATIVE COMPLICATIONS

The only way to avoid surgical complications is to avoid surgery. The issue then becomes recognition of the potential for complication and minimization of its occurrence. Knowing this potential, proper preparation for complications with backup instruments, retrieval tools, and alternate or additional procedures is mandatory. Recognition of complications is based on knowledge of their potential. The exercise of sound judgment in management is based on the surgeon's previous experience or that of others.

Instruments

All optical, electrical, or mechanical devices are subject to breakage or failure of function. Therefore backup devices or methods must be available to substitute or compensate for the problem.

A fractured arthroscope can occur when the scope is dropped before or during the procedure. The arthroscope can also be fractured during intraarticular manipulations. The arthroscope is not a crowbar; it is a fine surgical-optical instrument and should be handled as such. The surgeon should recognize that the scope is bending if an elliptical picture is seen either on direct visualization or on the video screen (see Fig. 4-9). With all the distractions of the operation, the elliptical fracture of the arthroscope will go unnoticed by the surgeon. Assistants are trained for observation, and they will bring it to the surgeon's attention.

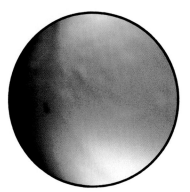

FIG. 6-98. Elliptical arthroscopic image indicates bending of scope and impending breakage.

The arthroscope coverplate is subject to fracture or scratching. Also, a piece of glass could drop into the joint. From a visual standpoint, the scope maintains its integrity, but clear visualization is lost. A change of arthroscope is necessary in this instance.

You must have a backup arthroscope.

Fractured instruments

It is imperative that all instruments placed within the joint have magnetic properties. This allows retrieval by a magnetic-suction device (see Fig. 6-86). Such a device must be in the arthroscoic surgical setup. The major problems occur when too great a rotational or angulatory stress is placed on the instrument. With small arthroscopic instruments, breakage can occur with a powerful grip on the handles. The surgeon must have a sense of the magnitude of pressure these instruments can tolerate.

Virtually all instruments made for arthroscopic surgery are breakable. They need not be broken if the surgeon is familiar with the instrument's proper use and tolerance.

Technical problems
Scuffing

The most common interoperative complication is injury to the articular surface, so-called scuffing (see Fig. 6-24). This can happen accidentally, unknowingly, or inadvertently. Scuffs are permanent articular cartilage injuries. Although they seal with fibrous tissue and smooth away, they are permanent. The hyaline cartilage is not replaced. Every effort should be made to avoid scuffing. This can be done by minimizing the number of passes of instrumentation, and also by exercising gentleness, "treading light," and conceptually placing yourself on the end of the instrument (see Fig. 6-5).

Ligament injury

It is possible to tear the tibial collateral ligament with valgus stress on the knee. A leg holder provides a fulcrum. I have had two such experiences. Both patients were over 70 years old. There was a slight audible pop with stretching. These injuries were treated with splint immobilization for 1 week and early motion and healed without problems.

A ligament may be lacerated during operative resection. The tibial collateral ligament is adjacent to the medial meniscus. The posterior cruciate ligament is close to the posterior horn of the medial meniscus. The posterolateral bundles of the anterior cruciate ligament cross above the posterior horn of the lateral meniscus. The cruciate ligaments fill the intercondylar notch in small people or those with osteoarthritis. Care should be taken to control the knife blade or basket forceps. No undue pressure should be applied to pass the arthroscope through a tight intercondylar notch. Pressure from the scope through that area can cause an attentuation of the cruciate fibers by compression. These incidences can be avoided by knowledge of the placement of these ligaments and careful control of instruments.

Popliteus tendon

The popliteus tendon courses through the posterior attachments of the lateral meniscus. Care must be taken not to injure this tendon during lateral meniscectomy.

The patellar tendon approach is avoided to protect the integrity of this important structure.

Vascular injury

Transcutaneous surgical approaches cannot identify vessels. The common arthroscopic portals are near the inferior genicular vessels, but bleeding or false aneurysms are uncommon complications. The cannula system establishes a portal to the side of these veins by pushing them aside during entry.

Care is taken during placement to avoid cutting the cutaneous veins. The saphenous vein courses over the posteromedial portal. Transillumination or preoperative identification and marking with a skin scratch locates the vein during surgical approach.

The popliteal vessels are posterior and central to the knee joint. Laceration would occur only with extraarticular instrument penetration. Having cutting tips in view of all times avoids this mishap. Knife blade cutting should be careful, slow, and measured. Fingertip control avoids "plunging." Resting the hand on the patient further stabilizes it.

If major vessel injury occurs, its recognition is followed by repair, even with vascular surgical consultation.

Transillumination assists direct visualizations of venous landmarks. In obese patients such location is not possible. The approach technique of skin laceration and cannula insertion pushes neurovascular structures out of the way. If laceration of the saphenous or cephalic vein occurs, suture ligation is sufficient.

Lost tissue in joint

A frustrating intraoperative complication is sudden loss of a tissue fragment (Fig. 6-99). The surgical technique of inflow on the scope draws pieces toward the view, not away from it. The use of motorized instruments with suction assists in controlled removal; knife blade inscription, not resection, techniques keep the piece in place. Infrequent use of the basket forceps reduces the potential for multiple fragments.

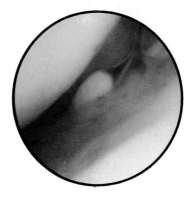

FIG. 6-99. Arthroscopic view of lost piece of meniscus seen at time of repeat arthroscopy.

When a piece is lost, it may be in the joint, part of the way out into the tissues, or even out of the joint. I look at the easiest place first. Inspection of the drapes, gowns, floor, graspers, and Mayo stand eliminates that position. Inspection of instrument exit portals from the inside may show the "tail" of the fragment. If so, the piece should be placed back into the joint before removal. Attempts at removing it from its position in the capsule may lose piece altogether. If a fragment is completely lost in the capsule or subcutaneous tissue, a motorized instrument is pistoned in and out, widening the hole and freeing the fragment from its attachments. The force of fluid flow may push it out of the joint. In another case, the fragment may be caught in the window of the cutter head and thence moved into or out of the joint. Finally, after the portal is widened, an open forceps pushes through the portal to dislodge fragments back into the joint. I have not yet had a fragment lost in the capsule or subcutaneous tissue that was not retrievable by this method.

However, before extensive enlargement of the portal, a search should be made throughout the joint. The enlarged portal causes leakage that decompresses the joint.

If the fragment is believed to be in the joint, the inflow cannula is opened and suction is applied to the arthroscope. All recesses of the joint are vacuumed. Ballottement is helpful to mobilize the pieces.

Intermittent clamping of the inflow tubing will decompress the joint, creating movement of fluids and hopefully of the fragment to the arthroscope. Finally, a trimmer head on the motorized instrumentation is placed into the joint and used as a vacuum cleaner, probing every recess. When the fragment is identified, it is brought into the intercondylar notch for retrieval with knee at 45 degrees flexion.

Fluid leakage

Leakage from various puncture wounds has two disadvantages: it decompresses the joint, compromising visualization; and it is a nuisance to have fluid flowing over the surgeon and on the floor. Fluid leakage interferes with concentration.

Leakage is prevented by making small puncture wounds and using a cannula system. The large puncture wounds made for transcutaneous placement of instruments result in leakage. When multiple punctures are used, the cannulas can be left in place with their obturators, reducing the leakage from any given portal.

Leakage that does not come out of the joint can be an even worse problem if it enters the synovium and causes compression of the fat pad or of other areas. It can compress the joint so that intraarticular visualization is not possible. This is one of the main disadvantages of having the inflow on the arthroscope. If the arthroscope is retracted out of the joint the extravasation causes tissue edema, and visualization is compromised.

If leakage occurs around an instrument and the operation is to continue, a suture ligature may be placed adjacent to the scope or instrument to control the leak. A small leak that is spouting fluid can be controlled by gauze around the instrument to dampen or redirect the flow.

Extrasynovial compartment extravasation of fluid may cause temporary (a few minutes) of blanching of the area or the distal parts. This problem resolves. The potential for compartment syndrome exists, but an occasional case of even massive extravasation has resolved in 30 minutes. I have seen this in the quadriceps with hip arthroscopy and in the calf with knee procedures.

Intraarticular bleeding

Intraoperative bleeding is controlled distal to the knee or elbow by use of a tourniquet.

Epinephrine solution (1 mg per ml) is used in the shoulders and the hips during the diagnostic phase *only*. A continuous infusion of adrenalin solution could cause extravasion and delay absorption, resulting in cardiovascular problems. This may occur especially in elderly patients or those with existing medical problems. No epinephrine (Adrenalin) is used, especially in the elbow or ankle or other distal parts.

Injection or distention with room air controls bleeding through its drying effect. Electrocautery may also be used.

Laceration of the cutaneous vein may require ligation. I have not had a case with major vascular injury.

Postoperative care

The success of surgical technique does not end at the operating room or recovery room door. Preoperatively, the patient is instructed on what to anticipate. Postoperatively, he is given both verbal and written instructions (see under specific operations). I do not use suture material in routine puncture wounds. The larger wounds of loose body retrieval are sutured. I use a soft dressing with a wrap of webril so that it is easily removed by the patient or by me without scissors. Band-Aids are applied the next day. I give patients color-coded instruction sheets (Fig. 6-100).

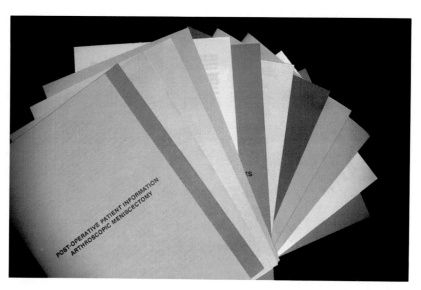

FIG. 6-100. Patient information forms. Forms are color coded for easy identification and reference.

REFERENCES

1. Dahefsky, J.H.: Arthroscopic visualization of the "blend area" in the posteromedial compartment of the knee, Orthop. Rev. **5**(9):51, 1976.
2. Eriksson, E.: A comparison between the transpatellar tendon and the lateral approach to the knee joint during arthroscopy, Am. J. Sports Med., **8**:103, 1980.
3. Eriksson, E., and Sebik, A.: Arthroscopy and arthoscopic surgery in a gas versus a fluid medium, Orthop. Clin. North Am. **13**:293, 1982.
4. Gillquist, J., Hagberg, G., and Oretorp, N.: Arthroscopic visualization of the posteromedial compartment of the knee joint, Orthop. Clin. North Am. **10**:545, 1979.
5. Guten, G.S.: Methylene blue staining of articular cartilage during arthroscopy, Orthop. Rev. **6**:59, 1977.
6. Lewicky, R.J., and Abeshaus, M.M.: Simplified technique for posterior knee arthroscopy, Am. J. Sports Med. **10**:22, 1982.
7. Nole, R., Munson, N.M.L., and Fulkerson, J.P.: Bupivacaine and saline effects on articular cartilage, Arthroscopy **1**:123, 1985.
8. Oretorp, N., and Gillquist, J.: Transcutaneous meniscectomy under arthroscopic control, Int. Orthop. **3**:19, 1979.
9. Patel, D.: Proximal approaches to arthroscopic surgery of the knee, Am. J. Sports Med. **9**:296, 1981.
10. Patel, D.: Superior lateral-medial approach to arthroscopic meniscectomy, Orthop. Clin. North Am. **13**:299, 1982
11. Peek, R., and Haynes, D.W.: Compartment syndrome as a complication of arthroscopy, Am. J. Sports Med. **12**:464, 1984.
12. Reagan, B.F., et al.: Irrigating solutions for arthroscopy, J. Bone Joint Surg. **65A**:629, 1983.
13. Sherpak, R.C., Schuster, H., and Funch, R.S.: Airway emergency in a patient during CO_2 arthroscopy (letter), Anesthesiology **60**:171, 1984.
14. Whipple, T.L., and Bassett, F.H.: Arthoscopic examination of the knee: polypuncture technique with percutaneous intraarticular manipulation, J. Bone Joint Surg. **60A**:444, 1978.

Arthroscopic anatomy

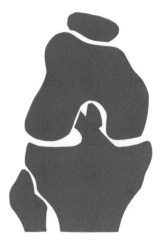

Recognition of the normal arthroscopic anatomy and its variations is essential to any interpretation of pathological conditions.[4-6] The illustrations and descriptions offered here should help to establish a basis from which change or pathological alteration can be recognized. The opportunity for arthroscopy on patients as young as 18 months and as old as 89 years has provided an understanding of the normal anatomy by age. An appreciation of the expected degenerative changes provides a standard by which pathological lesions can be judged.

The techniques outlined in the previous chapter provide for adequate visualization of and access to the various anatomical compartments. The individual anatomical structures can then be inspected or treated.

Describing the arthroscopic anatomy by compartments correlates well with the various surgical approaches. This format helps the surgeon conceptualize individual anatomical structures. The borders and contents of each compartment are presented in this chapter. There is some overlap when certain anatomical structures form the border of adjacent compartments. For example, the medial meniscus forms a portion of the anterior border of the posteromedial compartment but also forms the posterior portion of the anteromedial compartment.

First the various compartments, then individual structures, and finally common anatomical variations are presented here. See Chapter 6 for technical details to demonstrate anatomy.

NORMAL ARTHROSCOPIC ANATOMY BY COMPARTMENTS
Suprapatellar pouch

The suprapatellar pouch is initially viewed from the anterolateral portal with the knee in extension. The superomedial arthroscope portal is an important adjunct used in delineating patellofemoral problems.

To view through the anterolateral inferior portal, the arthroscope is moved medially to show the normal relationships of the patellofemoral joint in extension (Fig. 7-1). Flexion causes compression from the anterior tissues, and the fat pad usually obscures patellofemoral visualization. Patellofemoral tracking is best viewed from a superomedial portal.

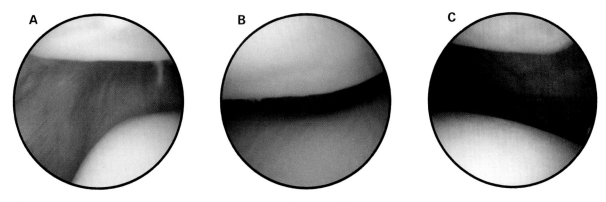

FIG. 7-1. Arthroscopic views of patellofemoral joint in extension.

A Lateral.
B Central.
C Medial. Note that medial patella covers femoral condyle.

When the arthroscope penetrates beyond and beneath the patella, the suprapatellar pouch is entered. It is possible to see the suprapatellar plica, which usually forms an arc or a circle by its synovial fold (Fig. 7-2, *C* and *D*). Penetration past the opening within the suprapatellar plica enters into the area of the suprapatellar bursa, which is lined with synovium (Fig. 7-2, *E*).

Retraction of the 30-degree inclined arthroscope coupled with upward rotation shows the undersurface of the patella. The patellar surface is normally smooth in contour and without any synovial encroachment. It is firm but not hard to palpation with an inflow cannula or probe.

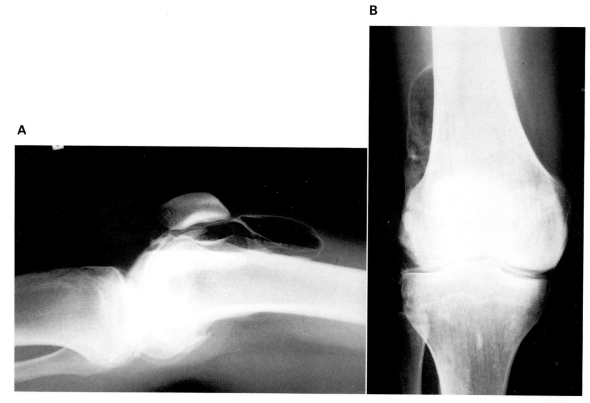

FIG. 7-2. Suprapatellar space.

A Lateral air contrast arthrogram shows extent of suprapatellar pouch and plica.
B Anteroposterior air arthrogram shows extent of suprapatellar bursa.

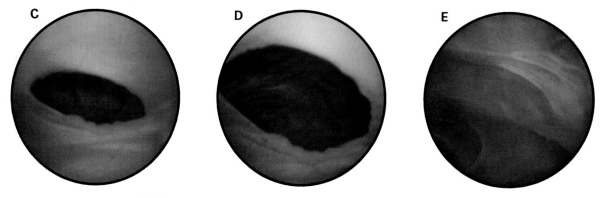

C Suprapatellar plica with opening to superior bursa.
D Scope approaches opening to suprapatellar bursa.
E Arthroscope enters suprapatellar bursa.

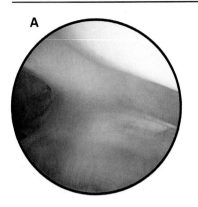

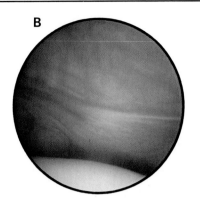

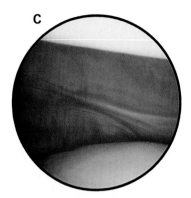

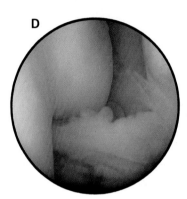

FIG. 7-3. Medial wall of knee.

A Junction of medial plica with medial suprapatellar plica.
B Central area of small medial plica.
C Distal plica as it forms reflection on fat pad.
D Continuation of fold to ligamentum mucosa.

Further scope rotation to the medial side demonstrates the medial plica (Fig. 7-3, *A* to *C*). The plica usually can be followed from its superior origin near the suprapatellar plica to the fat pad, and then continues around to the ligamentum mucosa at the superior attachment of the intercondylar notch (Fig. 7-3, *D*). This view is facilitated by slight flexion of the knee and scope rotation.

Superior and proximal scope rotation shows the femoral trochlea and the patella above. Extension of the knee accompanies this scope maneuver.

The superomedial portal clearly shows the medial and lateral femoral condyles, the trochlear area, and the patella (Fig. 7-4). This portal provides an overall view of the patellar surface position and the dynamics of tracking. Tracking is evaluated by flexion and extension maneuvers (see Chapter 10). The patellar and femoral articular surfaces are smooth.

Beyond the patella, it is possible to see the small fronz, or "tongue," of the fat pad. If ideally positioned, a medial plica can be visualized. A 70-degree inclined view scope provides a better overview of this area, because the shaft of the arthroscope can be placed more nearly perpendicular to the thigh.

Viewing into the medial and lateral gutters is also possible from the superior portal.

463

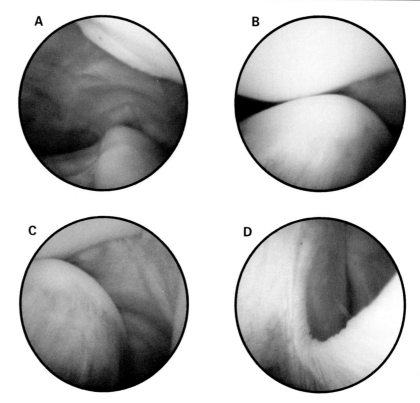

FIG. 7-4. Patellofemoral joint viewed from above (superomedial portal).

A Medial femoral condyle below and patella above.
B Patellofemoral joint at 20 degrees of flexion shows lateral contact.
C Lateral gutter: femoral condyle to left and patella above.
D Penetration into lateral gutter shows normal fold.

Patellar position and tracking

The normal patellar position with the knee in extension is superior and lateral to the lateral femoral condyle (see Fig. 10-21). There is no contact in the fluid-distended knee (see Chapter 10).

Medial gutter (Fig. 7-5, *A*)

The medial gutter may be viewed from the anterolateral, anteromedial, and superior positions. Frequently multiple portals are necessary to completely view the medial gutter. A fascial fold is often on the medial wall (plica).

The normal anatomy shows a smooth junction of synovial reflection at the femoral condyle with a minimal condylar prominence and no osteophytes. It is not possible to see any other ligamentous structures along the wall without adding stress. With application of valgus force, the tibial collateral ligament may become prominent (Fig. 7-5, *B*). The space is free of synovial folds below the medial plica.

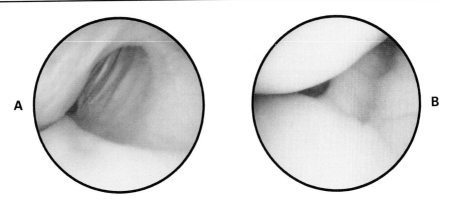

FIG. 7-5. Medial gutter.

A Medial femoral condyle meets medial meniscus with gutter seen to right or medial.

B Tibial collateral ligament seen elevated above meniscus when valgus force is applied to knee.

Lateral gutter (Fig. 7-6)

The lateral gutter is viewed from the superomedial and lateral portals. The normal gutter has one large, prominent, wide, thick fold. Unlike the thin medial plica, it is perpendicular to the gutter.

It is not uncommon, even in a normal case, to see synovial villi in the depths of the gutter near the popliteus tendon sheath (Fig. 7-6, *B* and *C*). These probably represent response to normal wear particles collecting in a posterolateral, gravity-dependent area.

The popliteus tendon is followed from its femoral attachment down the sheath. Entry from the anterolateral approach shows the meniscosynovial and meniscotibial ligaments (Fig. 7-6, *C* to *E*). The popliteus tendon, posterolateral meniscus, and lateral femoral condyle make up the other borders of this recess.

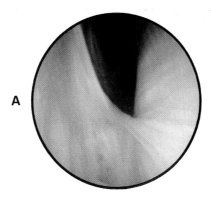

FIG. 7-6. Lateral gutter.

A Superior view in lateral sulcus shows normal fold of synovium, which could be considered a plica. It is a normal variant and never seems to be symptomatic.

Continued.

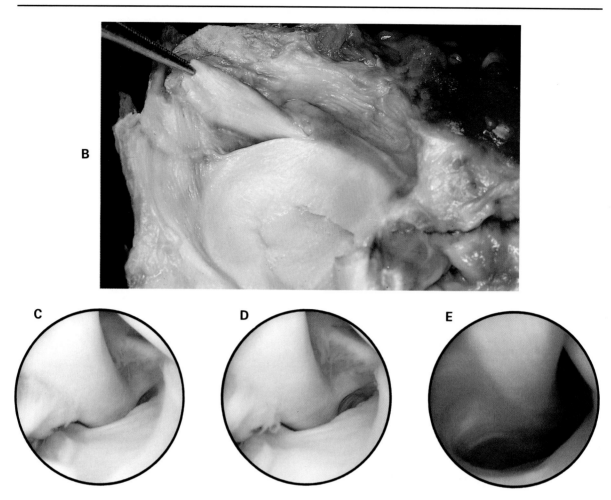

FIG. 7-6, cont'd. Lateral gutter.

B Gross anatomical dissection of lateral gutter and popliteus tendon sheath.
C Scope enters popliteus tendon sheath. Tendon is to left. Broad inferior tissue is lateral meniscotibial ligament.
D Further penetration shows arch of superior meniscosynovial attachment.
E Penetration to depth of recess shows popliteus tendon exiting joint.

Anteromedial compartment (Fig. 7-7)

The anteromedial compartment is usually viewed from the lateral portal with a 30-degree inclined view arthroscope.

Inspection shows a smooth surface on both the femoral condyle and the tibia. The surfaces are white, glistening, and firm, yet they yield to the probe.

The meniscus can be visualized from anterior to posterior. Usually only the anterior portion of the posterior horn is visualized from this compartment.

Anteriorly the meniscosynovial reflection shows some evidence of vascularity. As the examiner proceeds posteriorly, the reflection at the meniscus becomes more distinct, and fewer vessels are observed. The anterior horn is movable (up to 1 cm) by distention or probing (Fig. 7-8). The posterior horn is immovable.

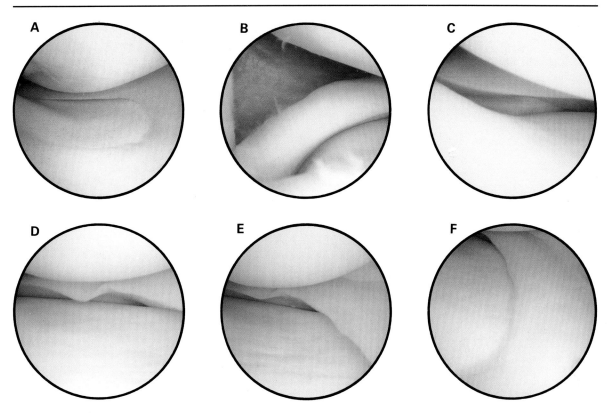

FIG. 7-7. Anteromedial compartment.

A Arthroscopic overview of compartment showing femoral condyle, entire medial meniscus arch, and tibial surface.

B Close-up of posterior horn of medial meniscus near posterior cruciate ligament.

C Overview of tibial spine, femoral condyle, and meniscus in background.

D Medial meniscus has serpentine border as result of valgus stress.

E Midportion of medial meniscus.

F Anterior horn of medial meniscus.

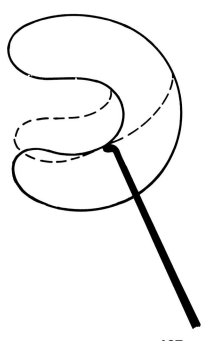

FIG. 7-8. Normal passive movement of medial meniscus when probed.

In a lax knee, it is possible to see both under and over the meniscus when the thigh is mechanically secured and appropriate flexion and valgus stress are applied.

Arthroscopic viewing under the medial meniscus is achieved by application of valgus force with the knee in 15 degrees of flexion and by gentle penetration of the area with the arthroscope (Fig. 7-9). The area of the meniscotibial ligament then comes into view.

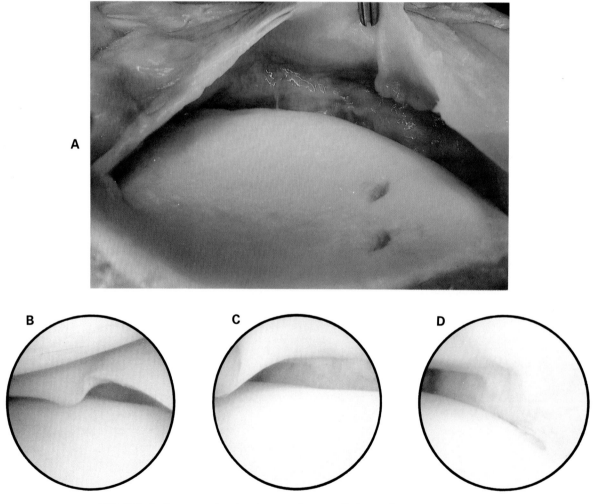

FIG. 7-9. Arthroscopic viewing under medial meniscus

A Gross anatomical dissection of region under meniscus.
B Arthroscopic view of meniscus showing effects of valgus force.
C Scope penetration under elevated meniscus.
D Meniscotibial ligament.

Posteromedial compartment (Fig. 7-10)

In most patients the transcondylar or transcutaneous posteromedial approach provides access to the posteromedial compartment. On the transcondylar view, the femoral condyle is seen to one side and the posterior cruciate ligament to the opposite side (Fig. 7-10, *C*) The posterior cruciate ligament has a fatty synovial covering that thins as the ligament courses posteriorly. A sulcus surrounds the posterior exit toward its tibial attachment (Fig. 7-10, *D*).

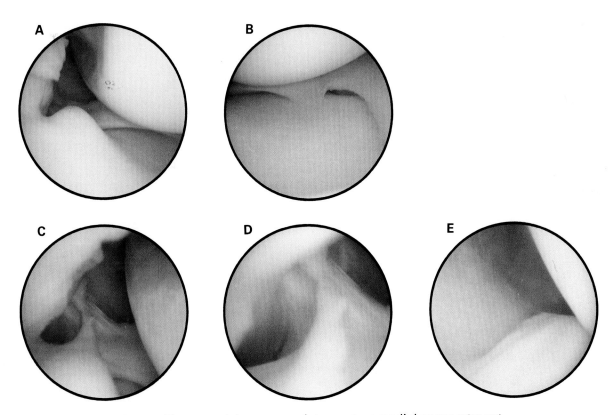

FIG. 7-10. Transcondylar approach to posteromedial compartment.

A Landmark for approach to posteromedial compartment is over medial aspect of tibial spine.

B Overview of medial compartment for anatomical relationship.

C Penetration with scope shows medial femoral condyle to right, posterior cruciate sulcus to left, and posterior horn medial meniscus deep in field.

D Scope incline to left shows sulcus around posterior cruciate ligament as it courses over tibia.

E Meniscofemoral junction with posterior compartment to left.

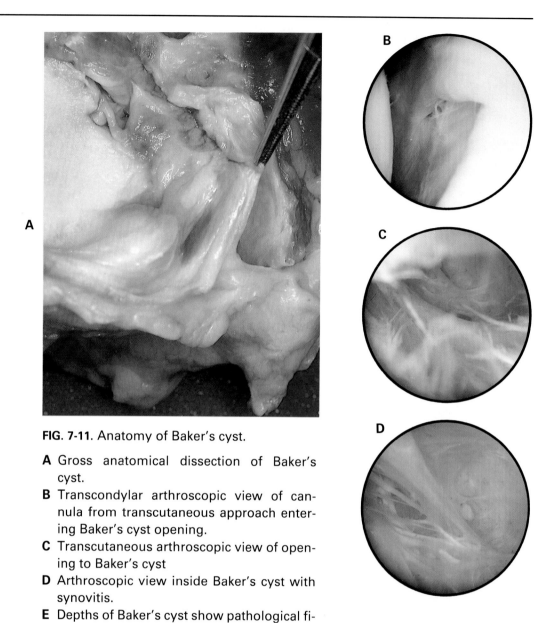

FIG. 7-11. Anatomy of Baker's cyst.

A Gross anatomical dissection of Baker's cyst.

B Transcondylar arthroscopic view of cannula from transcutaneous approach entering Baker's cyst opening.

C Transcutaneous arthroscopic view of opening to Baker's cyst

D Arthroscopic view inside Baker's cyst with synovitis.

E Depths of Baker's cyst show pathological fibrous adhesions.

Penetration in the posterior compartment requires scope rotation to the medial side and flexion of the knee to see the femoral-meniscal junction (Fig. 7-11, *E*).

Further use of scope rotation allows positioning to see the area of Baker's cyst opening (Fig. 7-12).

The transcutaneous portal to view the posteromedial compartment demonstrates a well-defined junction between the meniscus and the condyle (Fig. 7-12, *B*) that is enhanced by internal rotation of the tibia (see Fig. 6-41). The posterior cruciate ligament is easily visualized from this portal (Fig. 7-12, *B*). It is at the depth of the compartment, has an oblique course from proximal to distal, and is often covered with prominent vessels.

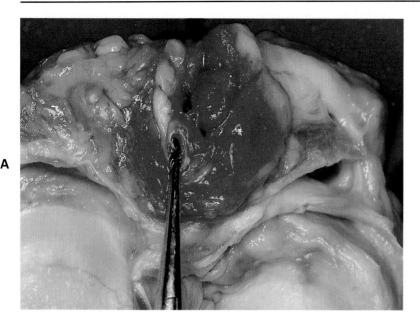

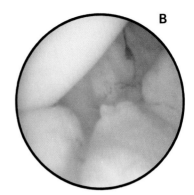

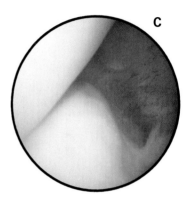

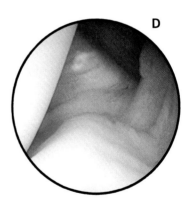

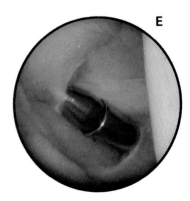

FIG. 7-12. Transcutaneous approach to posteromedial compartment.

A Gross anatomical dissection shows probe on popliteal artery. It is remote from posterior compartments at level of joint line.

B Posterior cruciate ligament deep in field, covered with synovium and vessel.

C On retraction scope shows overview of compartment and meniscus to left below femoral condyle.

D Further scope retraction shows close-up of meniscus-condyle junction. This is important landmark for orientation.

E Transcutaneous cannula seen from transcondylar view.

Superior scope rotation shows the synovial reflection with gastrocnemius tendon beneath. It may be possible to see and enter the opening into a Baker's cyst (Fig. 7-12, *D*).

The normal opening to a Baker's cyst shows a smooth lining with only occasional folds or fenestrations. A Baker's cyst usually accompanies some other pathological abnormality, such as a torn meniscus, degenerative arthritis, or synovial disease.

Intercondylar notch (Figs. 7-13 to 7-16)

The intercondylar notch is bordered by the medial and lateral femoral condyles. They join superiorly at the arch of the intercondylar notch. The tibia and the tibial spine are inferior, covered by the cruciate ligaments. The ligamentum mucosa is a band that spans the intercondylar notch (Fig. 7-13). Occasionally it forms a solid partition (Fig. 7-23, *B*). It courses from the superior aspect of the intercondylar notch anteriorly to the fat pad. In some instances, it may be more developed and actually be a continuation of a sickle-shaped structure from the medial plica all the way to the ligamentum mucosa attachment (see Fig. 7-3, *D*).

The two most important structures seen in the intercondylar notch are the anterior and posterior cruciate ligaments.

Anterior cruciate ligament

The most prominent anatomical structure is the anterior cruciate ligament (ACL), which is identified by its borders and its oblique course from the anterior aspect of the tibia to its posterolateral position on the femur. Often, it is identifiable by a blood vessel along its surface (Fig. 7-13, *C* and *D*).

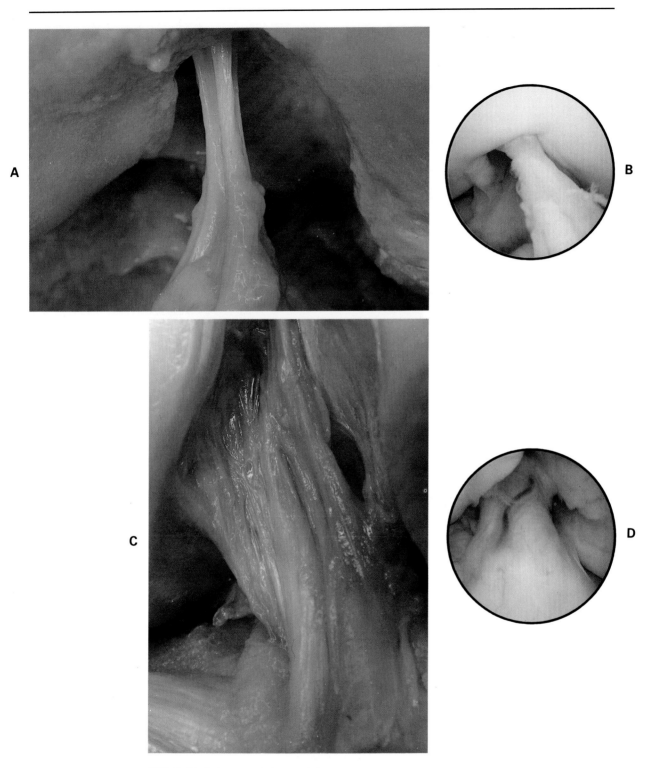

FIG. 7-13. Intercondylar notch.

A Gross anatomical dissection of ligamentum mucosa
B Arthroscopic view of ligamentum mucosa.
C Gross anatomical dissection of ACL.
D Arthroscopic view of ACL. Note blood vessel on surface.

The ACL attaches to the tibia opposite the medial meniscal attachment and anteriorly to the lateral meniscal reflection of the tibia (Fig. 7-14 *A*, *B*, and *D*). The ligament may be divided into three bundles: anteromedial, intermediate (often indistinct from anteromedial) and posterolateral[8] (Fig. 7-14, *C*).

The femoral attachment of the ACL is high on the lateral aspect of the femoral intercondylar notch (Fig. 7-15). There is also a band of ACL that courses behind the posterior cruciate ligament to the medial femoral condyle (Fig. 7-16). It varies in size but is a consistent finding. This attachment to the femur gives stability to the joint when the ACL is separated from the lateral femoral attachment.

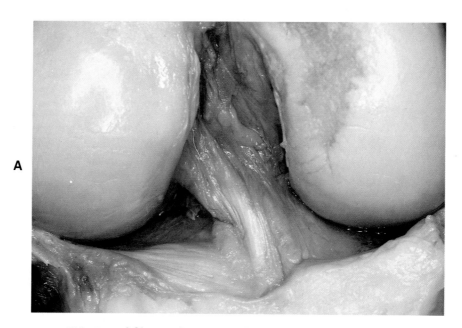

A

FIG. 7-14. ACL attachment to tibia.

A Gross anatomical dissection of ACL showing bundles.

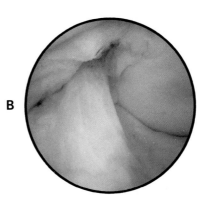

B

B Arthroscopic view of tibial attachment of ACL.

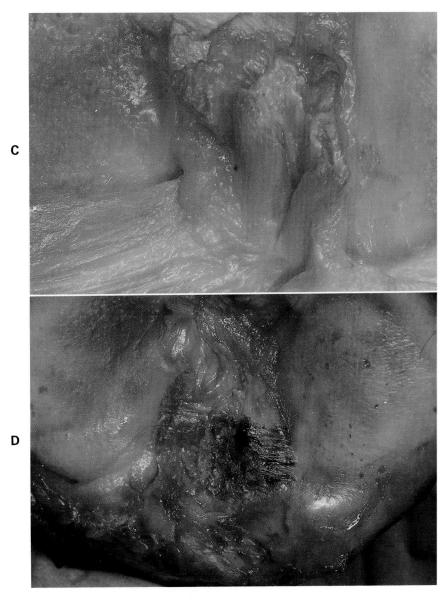

FIG. 7-14, cont'd. ACL attachment to tibia.

C Gross dissection of ACL bundles at tibial attachment.
D Green mark on tibial attachment of ACL after gross anatomical resection.

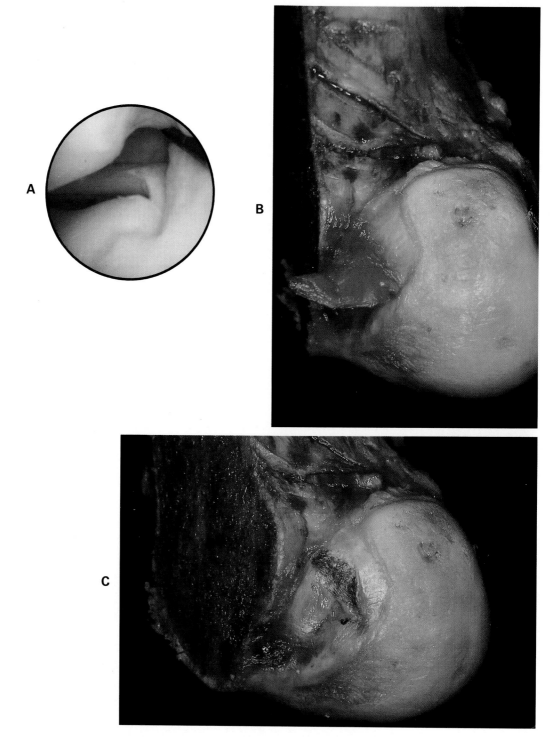

FIG. 7-15. Femoral attachment of ACL.

A Arthroscopic view with probe retracting ACL to show attachment.

B Gross dissection shows stump of ACL at attachment from posterior view.

C Femoral attachment site of ACL marked in green after gross anatomical resection.

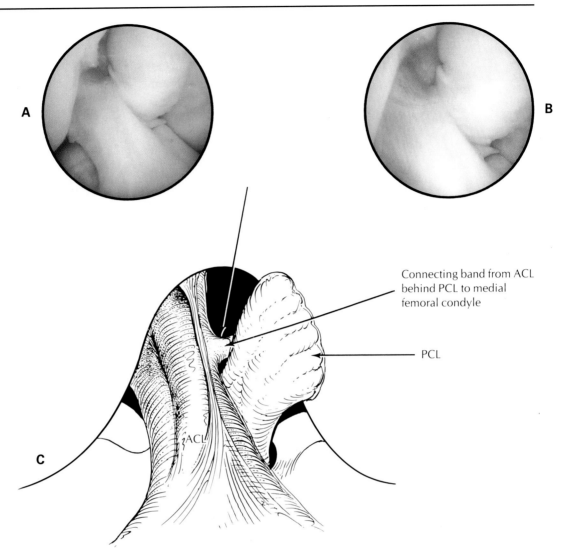

FIG. 7-16. Medial femoral attachment of PCL.

A Arthroscopic view of intercondylar notch shows crossing pattern of cruciate ligaments, their common synovial covering, and ACL accessory bundle coursing behind PCL.
B Close-up of ACL bundle coursing behind PCL to medial femoral condyle.
C Graphic illustration of medial femoral extension of ACL.

Posterior cruciate ligament

Penetration along the medial wall of the intercondylar notch shows the posterior cruciate ligament (PCL), its sulcus, and its recess adjacent to its tibial attachment (see Fig. 7-10, C and D). The PCL courses behind and medial to the ACL. It has a thick, fatty synovial covering (Fig. 7-16). The synovium is continuous over the ACL and PCL. An extension of the ACL courses adjacent to and behind the PCL and attaches to the medial femoral condyle. The definition and development of this extension vary. The PCL attaches to the tibia outside of the joint (Fig. 7-17, C and D).

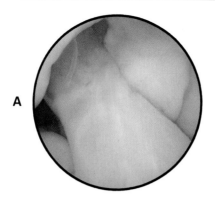 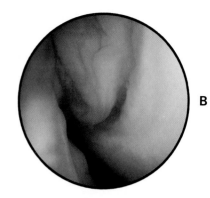

FIG. 7-17. Posterior cruciate ligament (PCL).

A Arthroscopic view shows outline of PCL as less distinct than that of ACL.

B Fatty synovial covering on PCL attachment to medial femur.

C Gross anatomical dissection shows PCL tibial attachment from posterior perspective. Note thin posterior meniscofemoral ligament.

D Gross anatomical specimen shows extra-synovial area of PCL attachment to tibia marked with green.

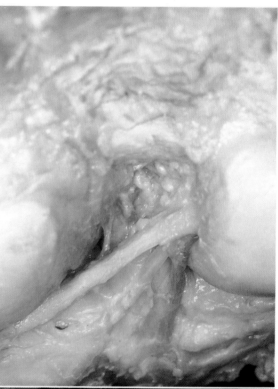

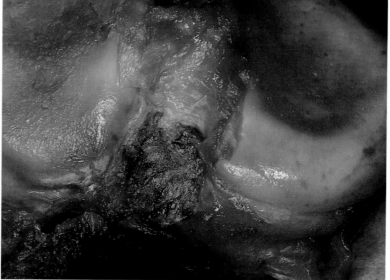

Lateral compartment (Fig. 7-18)

The lateral compartment is visualized either from an anteriomedial inferior or an anterolateral inferior portal (Fig. 7-18).

The femoral condyle and its articulation with the tibia are easily visualized. Anterior to these structures is the meniscus, which originates near the intercondylar notch (Fig. 7-18, *D* and *E*). The meniscus courses around laterally and then out of sight under the lateral femoral condyle (see Fig. 7-13, *A*). During further varus stress, the junction of the middle and posterior horns of the lateral meniscus is seen (Fig. 7-18, *B*). The popliteus tendon is posterior and lateral to the meniscus (Figs. 7-19 and 7-20). Rotation of the scope toward the posterior meniscal horn with slight retraction and then extension of the knee crosses the midportion of the lateral meniscus and extends to the posterior horn (Fig. 7-18, *C*). The ACL courses up to the posterolateral aspect of the femur.

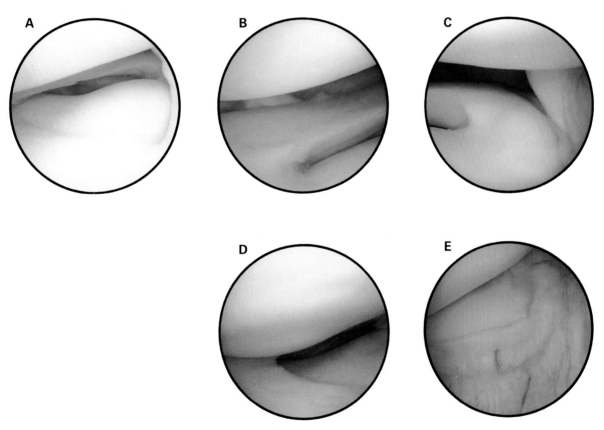

FIG. 7-18. Lateral compartment.

A Overview.

B Close-up of posterior meniscus in front of popliteus tendon. Femoral condyle is seen above.

C Extreme posterior horn attachment of lateral meniscus. Note ACL to right and above.

D Anterior horn of lateral meniscus.

E Vascularity on surface of lateral meniscus near ACL attachment to tibia.

With extension to the knee and varus positioning, the meniscus tends to elevate off the tibia, and it is possible to see under the meniscus to the meniscotibial ligament (Fig. 7-20). There is an oval window in the meniscotibial ligament, and the popliteus tendon courses deep to this opening. The meniscosynovial ligaments are situated above the meniscus and course to the posterior wall (Fig. 7-19).

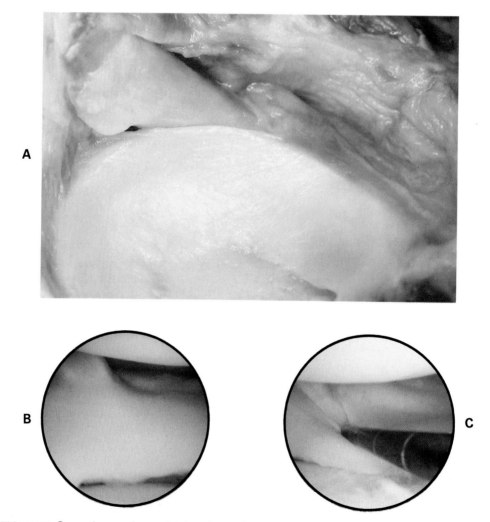

FIG. 7-19. Superior surface of lateral meniscus.

A Gross views of superior surface of lateral meniscus, popliteus tendon, and meniscosynovial ligament.
B Arthroscopic view of same area.
C Probe in popliteus sheath on top of meniscus.

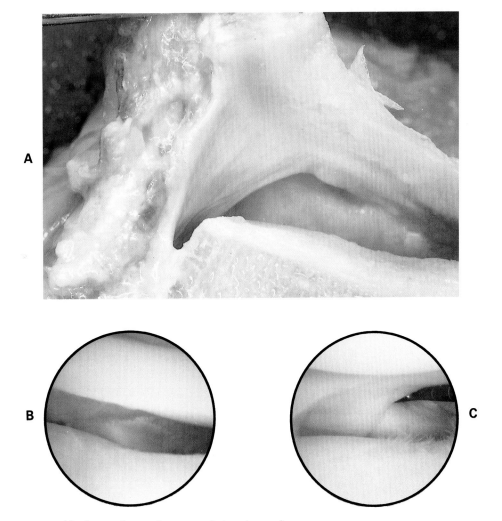

FIG. 7-20. Undersurface of posterolateral meniscus.

A Gross anatomical dissection with cutaway showing meniscotibial ligament lateral to window in popliteus tendon sheath.

B Arthroscopic view of same area.

C Probe on meniscotibial ligament.

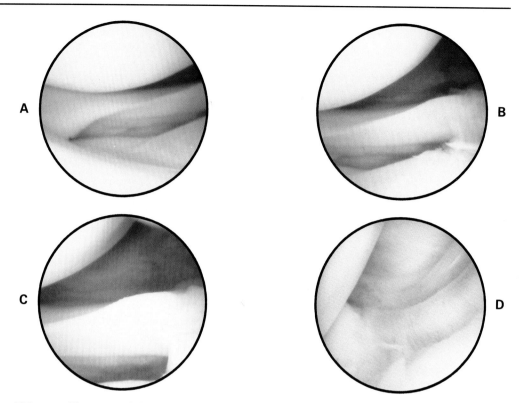

FIG. 7-21. Transcondylar approach to posterolateral compartment.

A Arthroscopic overview of entire lateral compartment for orientation.
B Lateral meniscus of posterior horn.
C Penetration over posterior horn.
D Scope rotated to left, viewing posterolateral compartment and meniscofemoral junction.

Posterolateral compartment (Fig. 7-21)

A transcondylar approach to the posterolateral compartment starts with an anterior orientation overview (Fig. 7-21, *A*). The arthroscope penetrates to and over the posterior horn of the lateral meniscus (Fig. 7-21, *B* and *C*). After entry, the inclined scope is rotated left to see the landmarks for orientation of the meniscofemoral junction (Fig. 7-21, *D*).

A separate transcutaneous posterolateral approach is carried out as illustrated in Chapter 6. The first landmark seen is the meniscotibial junction (Fig. 7-22). The meniscus normally sits flatter and has less bulge than on the medial side. Rotation superiorly shows the same type of synovial arching on the medial side.

Rotation of the arthroscope with slight retraction and angulation anteriorly provides another view of the popliteus tendon and sheath.

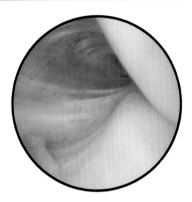

FIG. 7-22. Transcutaneous view of posterolateral compartment shows mensico-femoral landmark and synovial reflection posteriorly.

NORMAL ARTHROSCOPIC ANATOMY BY STRUCTURE
Synovium

A young person's synovium is flat, thin, and transparent and has minimal vascularity. Normal synovium will readily absorb saline solution. It is visible as small shiny balls within the villi. It should not be mistaken for crystalline synovitis.

The first sign of synovitis or villi is seen in the lateral gutter adjacent to the popliteal sheath. This area collects articular debris, even wear particles, hence the synovial change. This villous proliferation is seen in most patients of any age who come for arthroscopic examination.

Villous proliferation seems to be proportional to degenerative changes. The medial plica and anterior chamber synovium, become thick, even edematous, when adjacent articular cartilage degenerates. Diffuse nonvascular changes are common in elderly patients.

Synovial folds (plicae)

The *suprapatellar plica,* when present, is a crescent-shaped, thin sharp-margined structure in the suprapatellar compartment (see Fig. 7-2). It serves as a demarcation between the main knee joint and the suprapatellar bursa. It varies in size from a thin projection to a complete barrier with a separate suprapatellar bursa above.

Histologically it is a thin fibrous tissue fold with a synovial covering (Fig. 7-23, *A* and *B*), and it is attached to the joint capsule. During arthroscopic inspection with joint distention, it appears as a taut, firm tissue. This misleading impression is overcome during joint decompression (the normal state). The plica is soft, pliable, movable, and folded on itself. It is firm to arthroscopic palpation only when distended or stretched.

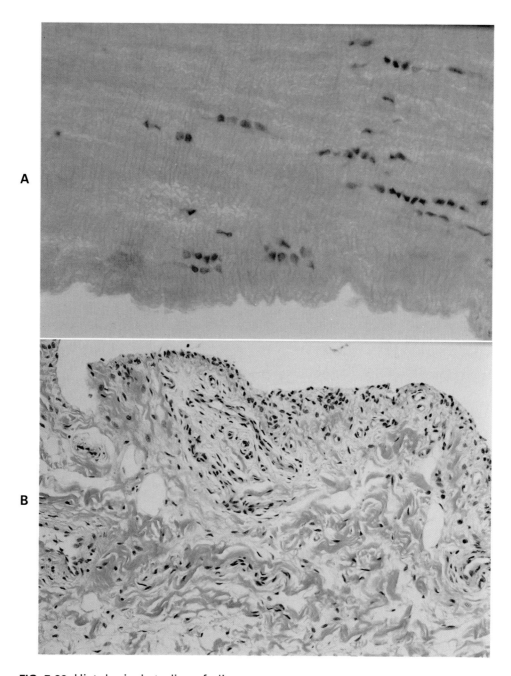

FIG. 7-23. Histological studies of plica.

A Photomicrograph shows fibrous tissue, chains of cells, and minimal synovial covering. (Hematoxylin and eosin stain; ×400.)

B Photomicrograph of plica with minimal; yet normal, synovial reaction. (Hematoxylin and eosin stain; × 100.)

The *medial plica*, or medial shelf, is an extension of a thin, broad fascial tissue on the medial wall of the knee joint (see Fig. 7-3). The structure is seen as a continuation of the suprapatellar plica to the fat pad and ligamentum mucosa attachment at the intercondylar notch of the femur. Dissection shows it to be a broad band sweeping down to the medial patellar retinaculum. It is covered with synovium.

In extension it courses horizontally and parallel to the patellofemoral joint. With flexion, it becomes more perpendicular and moves across the medial femoral condyle.

It varies in size from nothing to a 2 to 3 cm wide, protruding fold (Fig. 7-24). It is usually only a few millimeters thick and is soft, white, and pliable to probing. With joint decompression, it folds to look less ominous and assumes a position between the patella and medial femoral condyle. This arthroscopic maneuver is essential to evaluation of the plica's possible clinical significance.

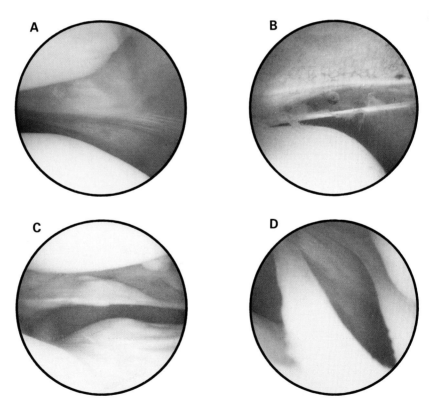

FIG. 7-24. Variations in medial plica.

A Small medial plica.
B Large medial plica.
C Fenestrated plica (small band).
D Fenestrated plica (large band).

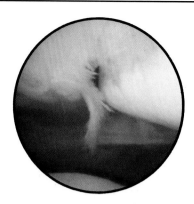

FIG. 7-25. Arthroscopic view of parapatellar fold appears like the fringe on a surrey.

The *parapatellar fold* attracts arthroscopic attention when the edges have reactive synovial villi (Fig. 7-25). Otherwise the fold is flattened with joint distention and is of no clinical significance.

It is only 2 to 4 mm deep and 1 mm wide. It completely encircles the patella about 0.5 mm from its margins.

The *lateral synovial fold* is perpendicular to the patellofemoral joint. It is broad, has a short circumference, and contains more fibrous tissue base than the medial wall plica. It is changed little by distention-decompression maneuvers. I have never observed any pathological significance to this plica.

I have seen three cases of a lateral gutter plica similar to the medial plica, but smaller, thinner, and very mobile. These plicae were not adhesions. They coursed from the lateral wall over the lateral femoral condyle to the ligamentum mucosa.

Patella

The patella is located in the suprapatellar compartment. It is approximately 5 by 7 cm in size. It is crescent shaped with a central keel that corresponds to the concave femoral trochlear surface (see Fig. 7-1). The surface is white and smooth, firm but compressible. There should be no fissures or alterations on the articular surface.

The quadriceps tendon attaches to the superior patellar anatomical base, and the patellar tendon attaches to the distal apex. The quadriceps tendon, especially the varus lateralis, is identifiable arthroscopically (see Fig. 10-115, *C*). Distally, the fat pad covers the patellar tendon.

A parapatellar synovial fold encircles the patella. The patella is movable by external pressure in extension. A surgeon can manipulate the patella to tip it side to side or push it proximally, distally, or side to side.

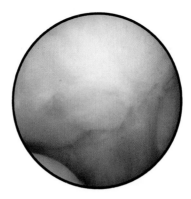

FIG. 7-26. Bipartite patella viewed from superior portal. Notice separate facet in center of field on superolateral aspect of patella.

As the position of flexion increases, the patella's passive mobility is decreased; it becomes mechanically secure in the femoral trochlea at 45 degrees of flexion beyond it. Normal patellar tracking is best observed from a superior portal (see Chapter 10). A common variation is congenital separation of fragments, that is, bipartite patella (Fig. 7-26).

Articular cartilage

In preadolescents the articular cartilage is absolutely smooth, white, and firm. In teenagers the patellar surface may show a "bacon-strip" shagginess at the superior aspect (Fig. 7-27). In other individuals there may be a parapatellar synovial fringe (see Fig. 7-25). These are usually asymptomatic.

The articular surfaces lose their brilliance with age. The first sign of degenerative change is lack of luster or reflection of the articular surfaces. The smooth surface becomes irregular, grows fuzzy, or has fissures. Small articular pieces may be free in the joint. Thin strips of articular cartilage lift up, producing a furry, even granular surface. Complete loss of articular cartilage indicates a pathological process.

The color changes from white to opaque to yellow with aging. The normal degenerative process can include development of small osteophytes at the joint margins.

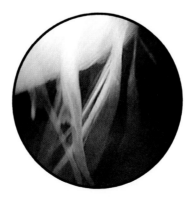

FIG. 7-27. Bacon-strip fragments hanging down from superior pole of patella.

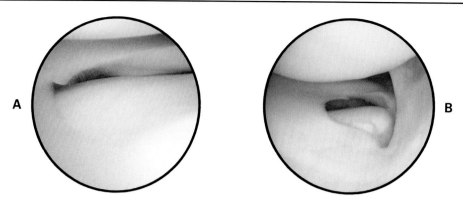

FIG. 7-28. Variations of lateral compartment.

A Arthroscopic view of longitudinal fissure of lateral tibial plateau.
B Variant of diskoid lateral meniscus; almost diskoid in nature.

A fissure is common on the lateral tibial condyle in women with genu valgum and/or patellar malposition (Fig. 7-28, A). The fissure is shallow and is located in the portion coursing from front to back. Its pathological significance is not clear to me; it does not produce symptoms by itself.

Femoral and tibial condyles

The normal condylar surfaces are glistening white (see Fig. 7-7, A). They are gently curved on tangential viewing. The surface is smooth and firm, compressible, yet with elastic properties to regain shape after temporary application of local pressure. The medial and lateral reflections show rolled edges. The synovial refractions are gradually flat and minimally vascular.

Meniscus

The meniscus is a fibrocartilaginous, semilunar-shaped spacer between the tibia and femur. It is intimately attached to the capsular and ligamentous tissues. The meniscus is triangular in cross-section, having a thin inner margin.

A thin, synovial covering blankets the meniscus at the transition area with the joint wall. The inner margins are dense connective tissue. Often the inner margin is thin enough to be transilluminated.

The vascularity normally involves the outer one third of the meniscal substance[1,2,9] (see Fig. 8-63, A). The anterior horns are more vascular than the posterior horns. The lateral meniscal bridge in front of the popliteus tendon is notably avascular. This fact should influence repairs and resections of meniscal tissue. The meniscus functions in load shock absorption, joint lubrication, and stability.

The *medial meniscus* is shaped like the letter C (Fig. 7-7, A). It is securely attached at the posterior by meniscotibial and meniscosynovial ligaments. Its fibers blend with those of the deep portion of the tibial collateral ligament, making this area very secure to probing. Anterior to the tibial collateral ligament, the meniscus is attached to both the capsule and tibia, but it has more mobility.

The *lateral meniscus* is smaller and more oval than the medial meniscus (see Fig. 7-18, *A*). The anterior horn attaches via the meniscotibial ligament and to bone. The posterior horn courses under the oblique course of the ACL. The posterior horn attaches into bone. The superior meniscosynovial ligament is medial and the meniscal tibial ligament anterior to the popliteal fossa. The lateral meniscus is more mobile than the medial meniscus. When suction decompression of the joint is applied to the arthroscope, the normal lateral meniscus collapses inward, with the fulcrum lateral (see Fig. 6-13, *E* and *F*). The inner rims of the anterior and posterior horns touch each other. Probing shows the same mobility. These rims should be observed routinely to develop an appreciation for normal appearances and probed to recognize normal mobility.

Further inspection of the meniscotibial and meniscosynovial ligaments can be made from the lateral gutter approach to the popliteus sheath (see Fig. 7-6).

The lateral meniscus may have rather large openings in the meniscotibial and meniscosynovial areas, mimicking a tear. Probing the meniscus for its basic stability assists in determining whether there is an abnormal response to mobility or attachment in that area.

The meniscus may vary in size approaching form frust or diskoid shape (Fig. 7-28, *B*).

Effects of age

In the knee joint of a person under 15 years of age, the meniscus is thin in its anterior, posterior, and vertical dimensions. It has a sharp inner margin without any degenerative changes or irregularities. The meniscus appears white and lies flat and very close to the tibial condyle. Even with valgus strain, the meniscus elevates only slightly off the tibia. The exception to this would be a young woman with hyperextensible genu valgum. There is more joint and meniscus mobility in this particular situation.

Viewing the meniscus from the posteromedial and posterolateral compartments shows a clean junction with the articular cartilage (see Fig. 7-11, *E*). There is no pile-up of synovium at the posterior slope of the meniscus, and the contour is smooth with no irregularities. The meniscus fits snugly against the condylar surface, and there is no synovitis. Rarely is there an opening to a Baker's cyst.

During adolescence the meniscus shows signs of wear. The first sign is a translucency along its inner border with no other significant variations from normal. It should be noted that vigorously athletic individuals appear to have premature degenerative meniscal changes, probably resulting from multiple microtrauma. Even fringe degeneration of the meniscus will be observed.

In the third decade of life, degeneration of the meniscus usually includes fragmentations or breaking down into tags. This process can be symptomatic and result in progressive small tears, which cause catching and popping. Usually these are self-limiting conditions related to contraction of tissue.

The normally brilliant white meniscal cartilage seen in young patient's knees starts to take on a yellow tone. Also, the synovium becomes more villous and vascular in nature.

Over subsequent decades, it is common for degenerative changes of the meniscus to increase. Of autopsy specimens, 69% show degeneration of the posterior meniscus.[7] The meniscus may develop yellow streaks or even have deposits of degenerative crystalline material, yet the patient may be asymptomatic. Initial thickening of the meniscal substance may progress to meniscus that is firm or hard to palpation, although the surfaces may appear smooth. The edges are frequently rounded on the inner border as a result of wear. There appears to be an increased width and breadth to the meniscus accompanying the decreased elasticity to probing or palpation. Posterior punctures may show angular or bulbous deformation of the meniscus.

Anterior cruciate ligament

The ACL is in the intercondylar notch area behind the ligamentum mucosa (see Fig. 7-13). The presence, size, and extent of the ligamentum mucosa affect the ease of ACL visualization. In some cases, a probe is used to move the ligamentum mucosa to the side. In others, resection of the femur is necessary to expose the ACL.

The ACL courses from an anterior position on the tibia obliquely to a posterior position on the inner aspect of the lateral femoral condyle.[7] It is composed of three bundles named after their tibial points of origin: anteromedial, intermediate, and posterolateral[8] (see Fig. 7-14). Clear distinction of these bundles may not be possible except by palpation and assigning a geographical location.

The ACL usually has a prominent vessel on the anterior surface running down its length (see Fig. 7-13, *D*). The two-dimensional arthroscopic view may give the appearance of a wide tibial attachment and narrowing of the ligament toward its femoral attachment.

Examination of the ACL at different positions of flexion and extension shows the posterolateral bundle to be lax at every position, except under varus stress.[3,8] The intermediate and anteromedial bundles tighten only in the extended and hyperextended positions. This is determined by positioning the knee and probing the ligament.

Anterior translation of the tibia on the femur tightens the entire ligament at any position. It is lax to anterior displacement up to 1 cm. Examination of the ACL with the patient under local anesthesia shows increased tension at 45 degrees or more of extension when tightening the quadriceps against resistance. Even straight leg raising or isometric contraction places tension on the ACL greater than the tension at rest.

Posterior cruciate ligament

The PCL is seen both at its anterior attachment in the intercondylar notch and through the posteromedial compartment (see Figs. 7-11, *B*, and 7-17, *C*). Anteriorly, it attaches to the femur and has a fatty synovial covering. It courses posterior to the ACL and exits via a synovial sulcus to its extrasynovial tibial attachment.

When viewed from the posteromedial transcutaneous portal, the PCL has better definition and is covered with thin synovium and a few small vessels. It is rigid to posterior displacement and firm to probing. It appears to vary only in relation to how distinctly it is visualized relative to its synovial and fatty covering.

ATHROSCOPIC VARIATIONS IN COMPOSITION, SIZE, AND SHAPE
Anatomical differences

There are specific anatomical variations in size and shape that must be differentiated from pathological or symptom-producing conditions.

Synovium

A common variation in the synovium is the ligamentum mucosa, which can be seen in all different sizes, shapes, thicknesses, and widths. It can also be completely imperforate, which in fact makes visualization in the intercondylar notch impossible in some cases (Fig. 7-29, *B*). The ligamentum mucosa attaches to the intercondylar notch above the cruciate ligaments. Another common variation is a small separate synovial band paralleling the lateral aspect of the ACL.

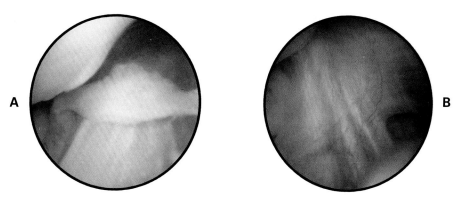

FIG. 7-29. Variations in ligamentum mucosa.

A Small synovial band over lateral aspect of ACL.
B Almost imperforate ligamentum mucosa makes thin covering over ACL.

Synovial folds

The synovial folds, or plicae, present the greatest variations in size and shape (see Figs. 7-24 and 7-30). The suprapatellar and medial plicae are the most common. There may be no plica, one or the other, or both; all these findings may be normal. Their size varies greatly. The suprapatellar plica may be so large that when the joint is decompressed, the plica fold into the patellofemoral joint. If it does and symptoms are correlated, resection should be considered. All medial plicae come over the medial condyle with joint decompression.

The thickness of the plica varies from transparent to opaque in appearance. Only cartilaginous or fibrous change should be considered pathological. Some plicae are so thick that they are palpable on physical examination, yet the patient remains asymptomatic. The plica can be solid or split. Openings or fenestrations are normal in suprapatellar plicae; they create separate bands, usually on the lateral side (Fig. 7-30). These fenestrations are less common on medial plicae and are perhaps normal, but they are routinely resected when observed because of the high correlation with symptoms.

Tibial condyle

A common variation of the medial tibial plateau is depression of the posterior one third. It is not pathological. It often is not seen on plain x-ray films. It can make the surgical approach to the meniscus difficult (7-31, *D* to *F*).

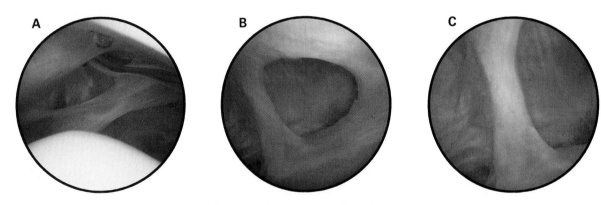

FIG. 7-30. Variation in suprapatellar plica.

A Arthroscopic view of transverse fenestration.
B Arthroscopic view of vertical lateral fenestration.
C Close-up of view in **B**.

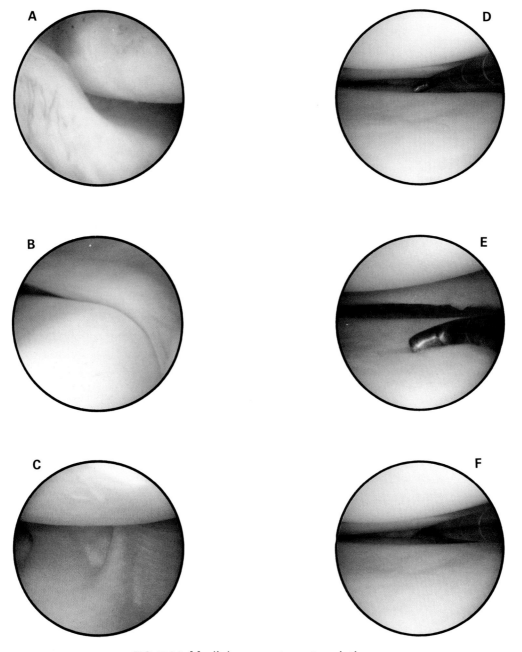

FIG. 7-31. Medial compartment variations.

A Arthroscopic view of anterior horn of medial meniscus continuing onto ACL.

B Arthroscopic view of short anterior horn that does not cover anterior tibia.

C Fibrous band parallels medial meniscus front to back and covers inner side of tibial collateral ligament.

D Probe on middle medial tibia.

E Probe over ledge of posterior offset.

F Probe over posterior tibial condyle.

Patella

Common patellar variations include superior pole "bacon strips" of articular cartilage, parapatellar synovial folds, synovial villi, and bipartite patella (see Figs. 7-25 to 7-27). Bipartite patellae have bony separation with or without articular cartilage inscription.

The same patellar size and shape variations demonstrated on x-ray films are seen arthroscopically. Consideration of the vertical medial patella is important when surgically repositioning the bone.

Condyles

There are considerable variations in bony size and contours. These differences are recognized when difficulty is encountered in exposing a posteromedial meniscal tear. The matching convexity of tibia and femur may require a medial shift of portal to gain entry by a straighter approach to the meniscus.

Meniscus

The lateral meniscus varies in width (see Fig. 7-28, *B*). It may cover all but the central portion of the tibial condyle. The meniscosynovial attachments vary only in size of opening for the popliteal tendon. The meniscotibial ligaments may fluctuate from a continuous sheet to openings of varying size. Often two openings may be seen in the ligament to the popliteal sheath. The anterior attachment may appear continuous with the ACL. Mobility of these structures will be discussed in relation to distention-decompression.

The anterior horn of the medial meniscus is the site of most variation; it varies in mobility and in attachment. In most mobile menisci, joint distention will displace the rim over the tibial condyle. The attachment of the anterior horn can appear continuous with the ACL (see Fig. 7-31, *A*). In another variation, the anterior horn does not cover the anterior tibia (see Fig. 7-31, *B*).

Cruciate ligaments

The most common variation is a connection to the PCL and a fibrous strand across the lateral aspect of the ACL (see Fig. 7-16). A minor variation of the ligamentum mucosa is an extra band coming from a superoanterior to posterolateral direction across the ACL (see Fig. 7-29, *A*).

Differences in response to various influences
Tourniquet

The use of a tourniquet to cut off the blood supply results in a better opportunity to visualize the joint structures. The tissues are blanched, there is greater reflection within the joint, and there is no cloudiness in the synovial fluid from microscopic bleeding.

Without a tourniquet, the synovium shows normal vascularity. Better visualization of the vascular pattern clearly outlines the synovial articular cartilage reflections (see Fig. 7-7). Pannus that goes across the articular surface is more easily visualized.

Visualization of blood vessels on the ACL or vascularity on meniscosynovial reflections can be identified with release of the tourniquet.

Medium of distention

Arthroscopic anatomy is virtually the same whether the knee is distended with a fluid or with air. The air medium provides a wider optical field of view.

In a fluid medium, a syrupy material may be seen. This represents aggregates of synovial fluid floating within the saline medium. The advantage of a liquid medium is that it allows any particles to float or to be mobilized and visualized better than in an air medium. Removal by suction is easier in a fluid medium than in a gas medium (Fig. 7-32). With a gas medium, there is more glistening and convolution seen in the synovial tissue than with a fluid medium.

Joint distention and decompression

In the distended knee the tissues are pushed away from the bony structures to their maximal extent. Correction for that distortion has to be made in visualizing patellofemoral tracking or meniscal position. Distention makes the plicae appear more ominous in appearance than when the joint is decompressed. Decompression is important to determine the actual position of the patella, anterior horn meniscus, and plica. Alteration of distention-decompression demonstrates the collapsibility and mobility of the lateral meniscus. Decompression can show areas of bleeding or irritation. Normal arthroscopic distention can blanch vessels and create hemostasis through pressure.

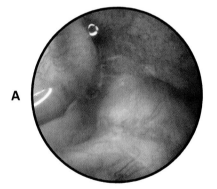 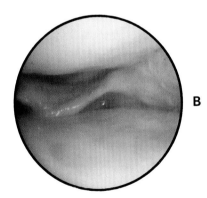

FIG. 7-32. Influence of physical conditions on arthroscopic view. Notice vascularity and glistening appearance of tissues.

A Intercondylar notch view with tourniquet released and with room air distention.
B Medial compartment in same environment. Postoperative open meniscectomy with regrown small vascular rim.

Light intensity

Varied light is important for visualization of the surfaces. If the light intensity is too great, viewing on a white surface results in a whiteout that does not show any of the natural convolutions. Bright light could give a false negative impression of articular surfaces. In visualizing the large cavity of the suprapatellar pouch, maximal light intensity is necessary to see the detail of the synovial areas.

Dyes

Various dyes can be used and are especially helpful in evaluating degenerative changes within the joint. The dye flows into various crevices, and the extent of the crevices or the depth of any variations can be interpreted. Use of dye also allows the perception of the magnitude of various defects of articular and meniscal tissue for the purpose of documentation. Methylene blue dye is particularly useful and safe.

Application of force

The application of force is necessary for proper arthroscopic inspection. The leg and foot are positioned and manipulated during knee joint arthroscopy. The shoulder is suspended, and distraction, rotation, flexion, and abduction are applied. The results of these various forces must be appreciated to avoid misinterpretations.

Valgus stress on the knee causes a minimal fold in the medial meniscus. In the absence of valgus stress, the same fold suggests a torn meniscus. A varus force causes the lateral meniscus to elevate off the tibial condyle. Folding does not occur on the lateral side.

The normal cruciate ligament response to position and force must be appreciated to recognize injury. The PCL remains tight throughout flexion and extension. It shows no laxity to passive posterior pushing on the tibia with the knee in flexion. The exactness of these observations is hindered by a thick, fatty synovial covering.

The ACL is lax in 90-degree flexion and tight in extension.[3,8,10] The posterolateral bundle is tight only with varus force or hyperextension. The amount of laxity or tibial displacement measured with the drawer test varies with the position of flexion. At 90 degrees of flexion, a maximal pull on the tibia will cause minimal motion change. The ACL is entirely lax to probing. The tension is assumed in the capsular ligaments, preventing complete stretch of the ACL.

As the knee position exceeds 45 degrees of extension, the tension is gradually taken up in the ACL. At 30 degrees, the ACL becomes tight with tibial pull. At 20 degrees and beyond, the ACL is so tight that further stretch is not possible by tibial pull. These observations influence passive ligament testing, interpretation, and postoperative positioning. Similar tests have been performed with the patient under local anesthesia and with the added dimension of active muscle contraction. The passive observations were the same as in the anesthetized patient.

Maximal quadriceps contraction with or without resistance with the knee at 45 degrees or more of flexion does not stretch or tighten the ACL. Beyond the 45-degree position, quadriceps contraction against resistance tightens the ACL, and the straight leg position shows a passive increase in ACL tension. Quadriceps contraction in extension maximizes tightening of the ACL, and this occurs against resistance to hold the 0-degree position without resistance and moving into hyperextension.

This information should greatly condition postoperative rehabilitation exercise formats for the ACL. Tests in vitro give similar results.

REFERENCES

1. Arnoczky, S.P., and Warren, R.F.: Microvasculature of the human meniscus, Am. J. Sports Med. **10**:90, 1982.
2. Day, B. et al.: The vascular and nerve supply of the human meniscus, Arthoscopy **1**:58, 1985.
3. Fischer, R.A., et al.: Knee anterior cruciate ligament strain, Presented at the 29th meeting of the Orthopaedic Research Society, Anaheim, Calif., 1982.
4. Harty, M.: Arthroscopic anatomy. In American Academy of Orthopaedic Surgeons Symposium on arthroscopy and arthrography of the knee, St. Louis, 1978, The C.V. Mosby Co.
5. Johnson, L.L.: Arthroscopic anatomy and how to see it. In American Academy of Orthopaedic Surgeons Instructional course lectures, vol. 27, St. Louis, 1978, The C.V. Mosby Co.
6. Joyce, J.J.: Arthoscopic anatomy, Orthopedics **6**:1115, 1983.
7. Meachim, G.: The state of knee meniscal fibrocartilage in Liverpool necropsies, J. Pathol. 119:167, 1976.
8. Norwood, L.A., Jr., and Cross, M.J.: The intercondylar shelf and the anterior cruciate ligament, Am. J. Sports Med. 5:171, 1977.
9. Odensten, M., and Gillquist, J.: Functional anatomy of the anterior cruciate ligament and a rationale for reconstruction, J. Bone Joint Surg. **67A**:257, 1985.
10. Rosenberg, T.D., and Rasmussen, G.L.: The function of the anterior cruciate ligament during anterior drawer and Lachman's testing: an in vivo analysis in normal knees, Am. J. Sports Med., **12**:318, 1984.
11. Scapinelli, R.: Studies on the vascularity of the human knee joint, Acta Anat. **70**:305, 1968.

Pathology of the knee

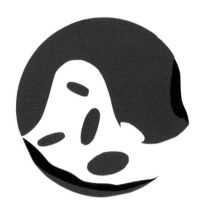

In this chapter the pathological bases or rationales for various arthroscopic surgical procedures will be discussed. Illustrative histopathology, as it relates to diagnostic arthroscopy, will be covered in the individual chapters as will the pathology of joints other than the knee.

My medical practice philosophy involves cooperation with the natural healing process. Observation of the body's response to injury or disease is the basis of successful medical treatment. Any medical or surgical procedure should stop a destructive process, remove dead tissue, and create an environment for natural repair.

Stopping the destructive process may mean stopping bleeding by ligation of large blood vessel. At the same time, bleeding subsequent to tissue resection is necessary for clot formation, the precursor to fibrous repair. An anticoagulant medication may be desirable in the same patient to reduce the risk of thromboembolism. A varied and balanced attack is necessary.

The source of cellular repair and the means of tissue nutrition are important in surgical procedures. This is especially notable in discussions on articular cartilage healing and anterior cruciate ligament grafting.

Pertinent experimental evidence that has bearing on clinical practice is mentioned here. This evidence is placed in perspective by arthroscopic observations.

In the absence of his or her own experiments or clinical observations, the surgeon is restricted by the experiences or beliefs of others. This is why arthroscopy has satisfied my curiosity and raised challenges to "established" ways and means.

The technique of arthroscopy provides an unparalleled opportunity for a study of synovial joints and their changes subsequent to age, disease processes, and trauma. The opportunity for documentation by either slide or movie photography or routine videotaping provides exact comparisons of the areas in which lesions are located. Observation before, during, and immediately after treatment may be compared to treatment response. Routine storage of videotaped material allows exact identification of the areas treated for subsequent documentation or biopsy.

Arthroscopic biopsy and surgical specimens provide opportunities for pathological studies.

GLOSSARY

A review of common terms and their definitions as they apply to tissue healing will help to clarify the discussion of pathology that follows.

Many words concerning healing have been used interchangeably or incorrectly. It is common to hear, "The pathology was in the meniscus"; this says that the *study* of the disease process was in the meniscus. The speaker means, "The lesion (abnormality) was in the meniscus."

More confusion occurs when healing is discussed, especially healing of articular cartilage. What do I mean when I say *healed*? Does it mean returned to the normal state? If so, is everything else not healed? Not really.

The following glossary will aid in semantics and communication in the discussion of healing.

CARTILAGE

Articular cartilage: Cartilage found in an articulation of joint; usually refers to the hyaline cartilage covering of bone. It does not designate biochemical character (hyaline or fibrous). Technically, the meniscus could be considered articular because of location. I prefer to use the term with further definition: *hyaline, reparative, meniscal,* or *fibrous.*

Hyaline cartilage: Normal hyaline cartilage derives its name from its "glassy" appearance (Fig. 8-1). Hyaline cartilage is normally avascular and composed of cells and a gel-like matrix.[86] The morphological appearance of the cells includes characteristic lacunae around the nuclei. They are arranged in orderly patterns in clumps or chains and are relatively large in size when mature (see Fig. 8-39, *A, C,* and *E*). The matrix consists of a network of collagen fibrils embedded in a gel-like substance of polyanionic proteoglycans and water. The collagen protein is found to be 90% alpha-1, type II, based on the amino acid arrangements. This is in contrast to the alpha 1, type I, collagen found in skin, bone, and fibrocartilage and the alpha 1, type III, collagen found in retinacular connective tissue. Embryonic hyaline cartilage has both types I and II collagen.[21,86,77] The proteoglycans (a combination of protein and carbohydrates) are elastic molecules that strongly resist compression. The matrix is a complex gel of proteoglycans entangled with collagen fibrils that is 75% to 80% water. Water content contributes to the tissue's resiliency.[36]

Fibrocartilage: Fibrocartilage exists at normal tendon-bone attachments. It is positive on histochemical staining for proteoglycans but contains no type II collagen; rather, there are types I and III collagen.

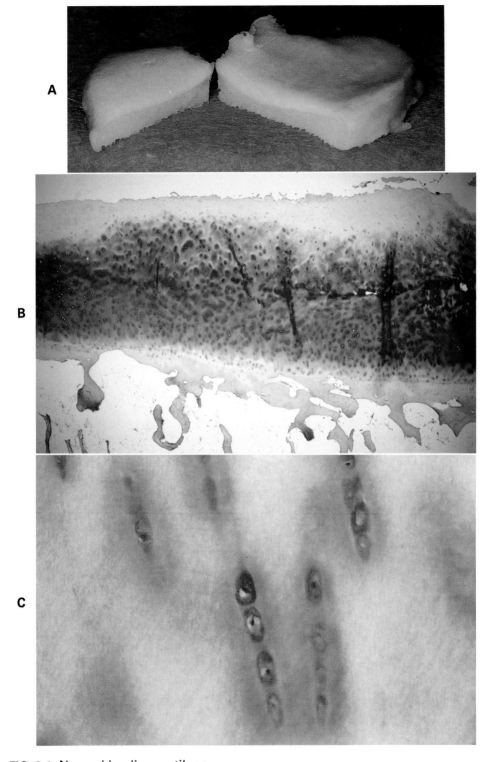

FIG. 8-1. Normal hyaline cartilage.

A Gross cross-section.

B Photomicrograph of same specimen showing pale blue staining on surface, red staining of mucopolysaccharides showing cellular pattern, and blue staining of bony trabeculum below. (Safranin O stain; ×40.)

C Photomicrograph of normal hyaline cellular pattern with surrounding dense-staining mucopolysaccharide. (Safranin O stain; ×400.)

Reparative fibrocartilage: Reparative fibrocartilage forms following full-thickness injury to hyaline cartilage (see Fig 8-39, *C,D,* and *F*). It occurs as a natural repair process in joints with degenerative arthritis. The process of repair is enhanced by surgical treatment and joint protection. Cartilage cell types are indentified by the histological characteristics of a plump oval nucleus and pericellular lacunae. Proteoglycan production is identified by histological staining properties with safranin O. Little type II collagen has been found in reparative fibrocartilage (see Fig. 8-41).

The use of the word *reparative* indicates a putting-together, or replacement of destroyed cells or tissues by new formation. Reparative fibrocartilage restores the integrity, not the nature, of the injured tissue. It does not restore the tissue to its previous state or to normalcy. By contrast, restoration of the natural state does occur in bone.

Debridement: A French word meaning the removal of foreign matter and contaminated or devitalized tissue from or around a lesion until surrounding healthy tissue is exposed.

Disease: A morbid process, often with a particular progression of symptoms.

Epidemology: The science dealing with the cause of disease.

Granulation: Formation of small, rounded masses of tissue during repair; consists of fibroblasts, inflammatory cells, and vessels.

Heal: To make sound or whole; to restore to health; to cause an undesirable condition to be overcome; to patch up; to breech a division; to restore to original purity or integrity. Synonym: *Cure.*

Healing: The process of cure; the return of integrity to diseased or injured tissue.

Healing by first intention: A union that restores continuity without intervention of granulation.

Healing by second intention: A union with granulation.

Lesion: Natural pathological or injurious interruption of tissue or loss of function of a part.

Mend: To cure; to put in good health. Synonyms: *Repair, patch, rebuild.*

Metaplasia: The transformation of fully differentiated cells of one kind into fully differentiated cells of another kind (e.g., columnar to squamous cells).

Norm: A model, an average, or a fixed, authoritative, or ideal standard. Synonyms: *Regular, standard.*

Normalcy:	The state of being normal.
Pathology:	The Greek root *patho-* means disease. Pathology is a branch of medicine that studies the essential nature of disease.
Primary lesion:	The original lesion that manifests a disease or injury.
Regeneration:	Healing by proliferation of parenchymal elements. The result is complete restoration of kind (i.e., epithelial cells, bone, lymph).
Repair	(Verb): To restore by replacing a part or putting together what is torn or broken. Synonyms: *Fix, renew, remedy.*
Repair:	(Noun): The replacement of destroyed cells or tissues by new formation of nonspecialized elements of connective tissue with fibrosis; *also,* the physical or mechanical restoration of damaged or diseased cells by growth of new cells or surgical apposition.
Response:	Any action or change of condition evoked by a stimulus.
Restore:	To renew; to rebuild; to alter; to get back; to return; to put or bring back into existence; to put back to original state.
Restoration:	Healing by proliferation of the parenchymal elements with the result of complete regeneration (e.g., epithelial cells or bone, liver, pancreas, adrenal gland).
Syndrome:	A set of symptoms recognized to be the hallmark of a specific disease process.

After reviewing these definitions, it is obvious that the word *healing* does not mean restoration to the preexisting state. Healing implies a process of cure. Restoration of integrity to the injured tissue is not synonymous with restoration to the previous state. The word *restore* means to return or to bring back into existence. In its strictest sense this definition means "to put back to the original state." This is not what occurs in most tissue healing. Healing is usually a repair or return of tissue integrity or continuity. Perhaps the best word for tissue healing is the noun *repair*, which means "replacement by new formation." Tissue repair, not restoration, takes place in most instances.

PATHOLOGICAL CHANGES IN ARTICULAR CARTILAGE
Laceration

Laceration of articular cartilage is produced by trauma or surgery (Fig. 8-2, *A*). Experimental studies show no adjacent tissue response up to 1 year later.[42,44,45] In humans the lesion response is similar (Fig. 8-2, *B* to *D*). The lacerated edge shows no repair, flattening of cells, or empty lacunae. The biopsy incision shows clumping common to degenerative change.

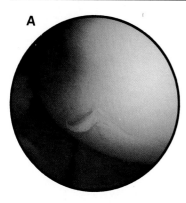

FIG. **8-2.** Intraoperative laceration of articular cartilage.

A Arthroscopic view of "scuffing."

B Photomicrograph of biopsy of edge of laceration. (Hematoxylin and eosin stain; ×100.)

C High-power photomicrograph of laceration edge. (Hematoxylin and eosin stain; ×100.)

D Opposite side of biopsy shows margin of biopsy incisional site on specimen. (Hematoxylin and eosin stain; ×100.)

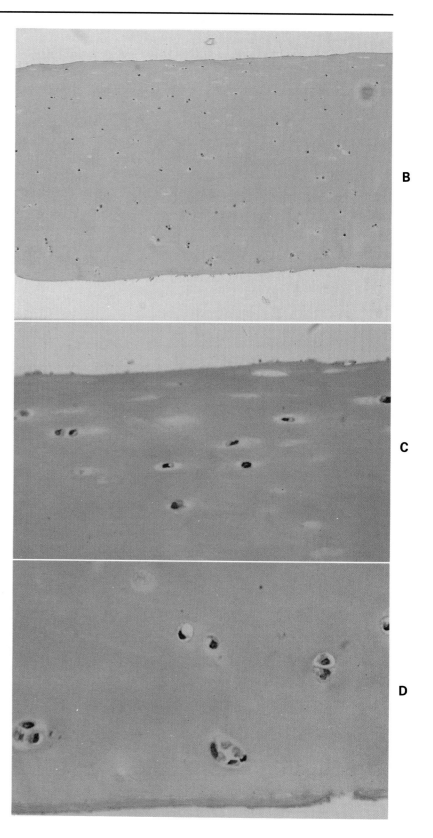

B

C

D

Contusion

Direct blows are the most common cause of contusion. The skin may show injury, but not necessarily (Fig. 8-3, *A*). The surface of the articular cartilage is disrupted. There are signs of degeneration, acellularity, and fragmentation (Fig. 8-3, *B*).

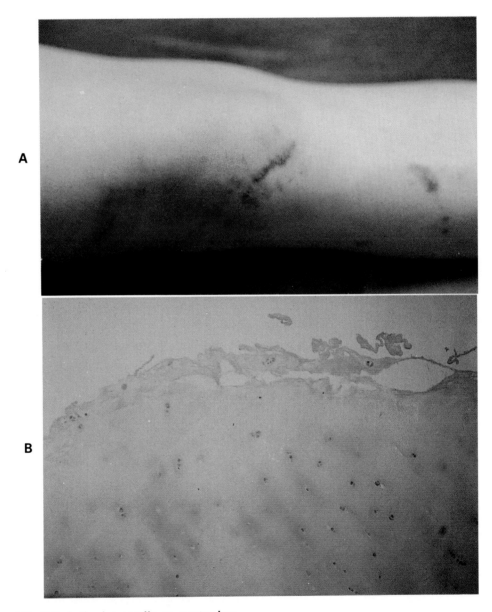

FIG. 8-3. Articular cartilage contusion.

A Skin may show effects of direct blow, but this is not necessary for deep joint injury.

B Photomicrograph of lesion showing surface disruption and decreased cellularity.

Blunt trauma

In experiments, blunt trauma causes little reaction in adjacent cartilage.[19,24,38,64] If an underlying bone is fractured, healing occurs by a method similar to that which occurs in full-thickness lesions.[44,45]

Bubble

The swelling of articular cartilage appears as a "bubble" arthroscopically (Fig. 8-4, *A*). The lesion is soft and compressible. Careful inspection may show fissuring on the surface or a deeper area of cartilage separation (Fig. 8-4, *B*), not visible on the surface.

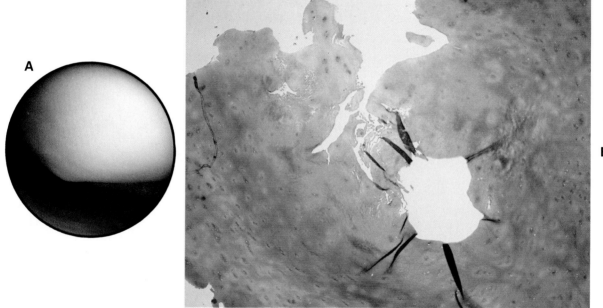

FIG. 8-4. "Bubble" on articular surface.

A Arthroscopic view of bubble, which is soft and compressible to probing. Resection is performed only in movable lesions.

B Photomicrograph of bubble lesion with fissure to surface and central tissue disruption. Lesion was resected because of size of fissure and mobility of edges. (Hematoxylin and eosin stain; ×40.)

Fissure

The fissure is a common lesion in the lateral tibial plateau (Fig. 8-5, *A*). It occurs in women and persons with genu valgum. Fissures are a common finding in the patella of an otherwise normal knee. The base of a fissure often shows translucent tissue. On biopsy it shows its avascular fibrocartilaginous nature (Fig. 8-5, *B* to *D*).

506

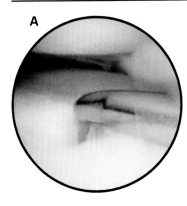

FIG. 8-5.
Articular cartilage fissures.

A Arthroscopic view of probe in lateral tibial plateau fissure.

B Photomicrograph of tooth-shaped tissue dislodged from microbiopsy of fissure. (Hematoxylin and eosin stain; ×100.)

C Photomicrograph healing fibrocartilage in fissure. (Hematoxylin and eosin stain; ×200.)

D High-power view shows plump fibrocartilage cells. (Hematoxylin and eosin stain; ×400.)

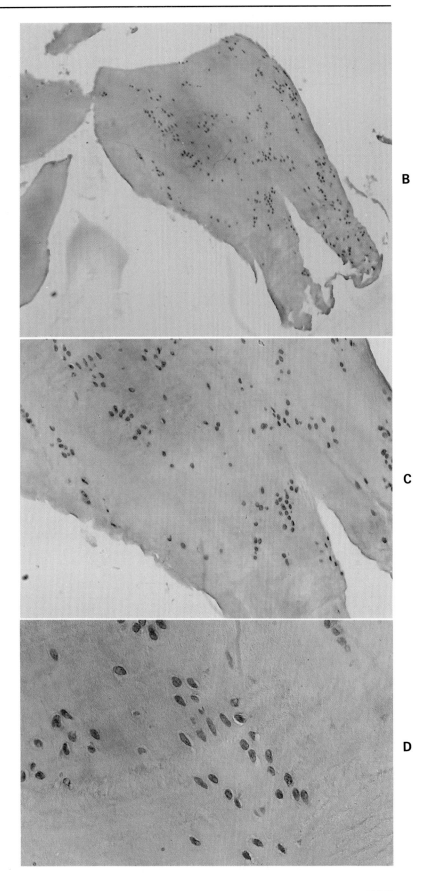

507

Furry degenerative changes

An arthroscopic view of fragmentation shows a "furry" appearance of the articular surface (Fig. 8-6, *A*). The lesion shows multiple cleft disruptions of the articular surface (Fig. 8-6, *B* and *C*). The cellular pattern is disorganized in clumps and aggregations. The cellular characteristics are still cartilaginous, and no evidence of repair is seen. Fragments that are removed by wear become loose bodies (see Fig. 8-7, *C* and *D*).

The surface is pale and stains blue with safranin O, indicating the absence of glycosaminoglycans. The deeper tissue adjacent to the bone shows an increased uptake of the red stain adjacent to normal cartilage cells (Fig. 8-6, *D* and *E*). The cellular clumping at the surface does not have the same cellular characteristics or pericellular staining properties. There is no evidence of cellular repair.

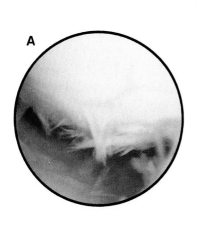
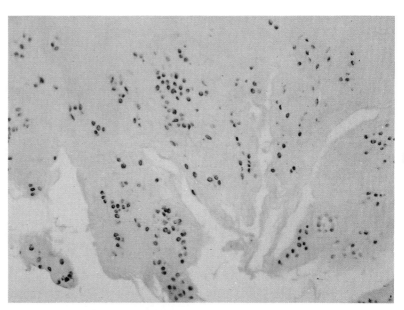

FIG. 8-6. Arthroscopic "furry" degenerative changes.

A Arthroscopic view of "furry" femoral condyle degeneration.

B Photomicrograph of similar lesion showing clefts and fragmentation. (Hematoxylin and eosin stain; ×100.)

C Photomicrograph shows cartilage cellular clumping and aggregates. No signs of repair. (Hematoxylin and eosin stain; ×400.)

D Loss of staining of surface in areas of fragmentation. (Safranin O stain; ×100.)

E Erosion of articular mass and surface cellular clumping, fragmentation, and lack of surface staining for glycosaminoglycans. (Safranin O stain; ×40.)

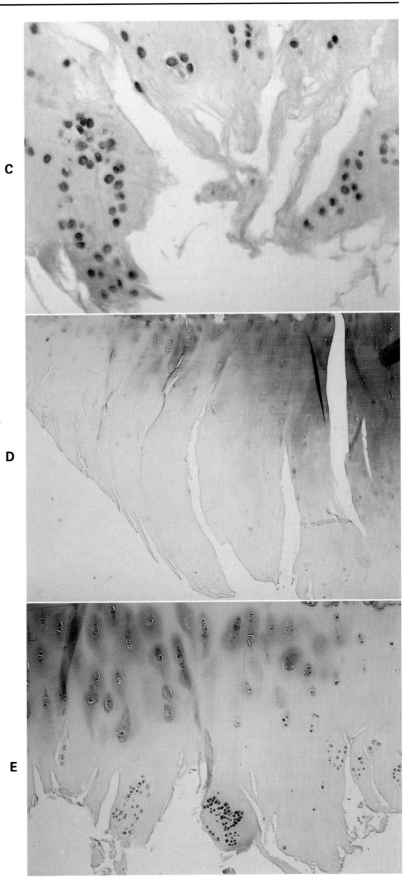

FIG. 8-6, cont'd. For legend see opposite page.

Articular debris

Articular surface fragmentation results in loose bodies.[17,30,56] The loose bodies are first observed as small flakes of tissue in synovial solution during arthroscopy (Fig. 8-7, *A*). As they become larger and more numerous, they cannot be overlooked (Fig. 8-7, *B*). Aspiration by arthroscopy or needle arthrocentesis shows multiple fragments (Fig. 8-7, *C*). It is even therapeutic. A cell block of aspirate shows synovial debris (Fig. 8-7, *D*).

Larger loose bodies are engulfed in synovium (Fig. 8-8, *A* to *C*). There is a reactive vascular synovitis (see Fig. 8-8, *C*). The capsular tissue becomes thickened (see Fig. 8-7, *A*). The larger pieces may be clinically palpable (see Fig. 8-8, *C*). The engulfment may cause loose pieces to be located out of the joint and out of the view of the arthroscope.

As the cartilage is surrounded with reactive synovium it loses its cells (Fig. 8-8, *D* and *E*). Eventually tissue is removed by the inflammatory process (Fig. 8-8, *F*). Loose body removal relieves the joint of this effort.

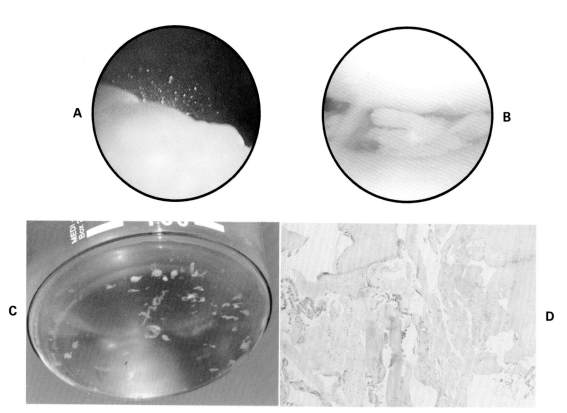

FIG. 8-7.

A Stardusting. Loose synovial and articular fragments seen in suprapatellar pouch with transillumination.

B Multiple loose bodies between tibia and femur in medial compartment. Methylene blue enhances visualization.

C Loose bodies vacuumed from joint through cannula.

D Photomicrograph of synovial fluid cell block, including articular cartilage synovial debris.

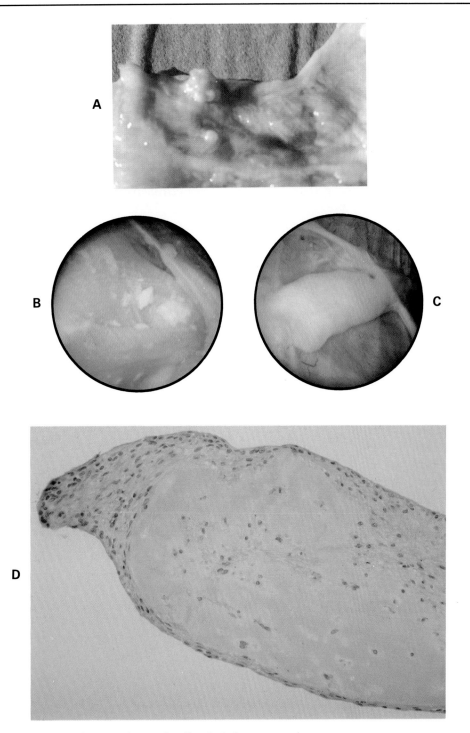

FIG. 8-8. Fate of larger loose bodies is left to synovium.

A Gross photograph of articular cartilage engulfed by synovium if not removed from joint. May thicken synovial capsule.

B Arthroscopic view of engulfed articular cartilage in synovium. Notice fibrous bands as well.

C Arthroscopic view of large piece of articular cartilage attached to synovium.

D Photomicrograph of fragments engulfed in synovium. (Hematoxylin and eosin stain; ×40.)

Continued.

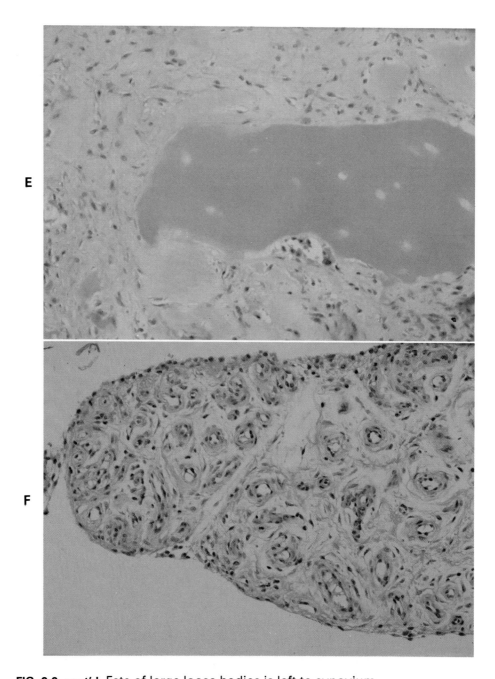

FIG. 8-8, cont'd. Fate of large loose bodies is left to synovium.

E Photomicrograph shows acellular necrotic articular debris. (Hematoxylin and eosin stain; ×200.)

F Photomicrograph of typical synovial hyperemia. (Hematoxylin and eosin stain; ×200).

The fragmentation is reduced on the surface after surgical debridement or wear (Fig. 8-9, *A* and *B*). The base is still degenerative, but the fragments are shortened and the clefts are shallower. Motion of the surface tissue is mechanically decreased. This explains the reduction in crepitus after arthroscopic surgical surface debridement.

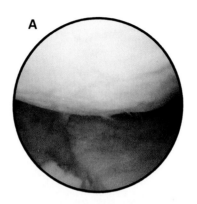

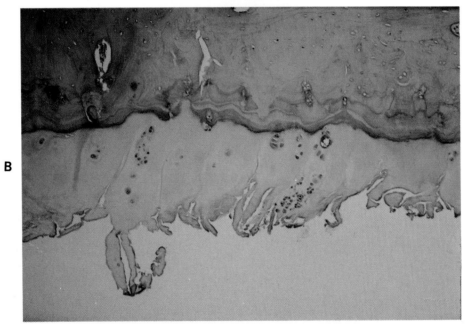

FIG. 8-9. Loss of surface with wear or surgical debridement.

A Arthroscopic view of debrided area immediately after procedure.

B Biopsy shows decreased fragment length and shallow clefts. (Hematoxylin and eosin stain; × 100.)

Degenerative process

Further progression of the degenerative process results in thinning of articular cartilage. The arthroscopic appearance is granular or in a cobblestone pattern (Fig. 8-10, *A*). On histological examination a loss of hyaline cartilage shows a reduction depth of tissue, in the number of cells, and in staining properties (Fig. 8-10, *B*). Mitosis occurs in early phases of degenerative arthritis.[31,79,65]

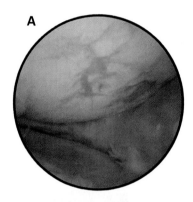

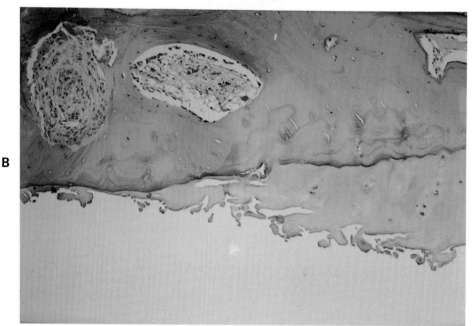

FIG. 8-10. Granular or cobblestone arthroscopic appearance with loss of hyaline cartilage.

A Arthroscopic view of cobblestone appearance on medial femoral condyle.
B Photomicrograph with loss of tissue, cells, and normal staining properties. (Safranin O stain; ×20.)

The cortical bone becomes exposed with progressive loss of hyaline cartilage. Areas of pink bone tissue are seen arthroscopically between white or yellow degenerative cartilage (Fig. 8-11, *A*). The lesion shows absence of cartilage and increased density to subchondral bone. There is also increased vascularity as well as subchondral aggregation of fibrous tissue (Fig. 8-11, *B*). These may become cysts that are even visible by x-ray examination.

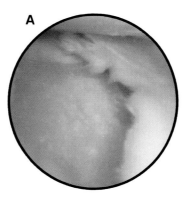

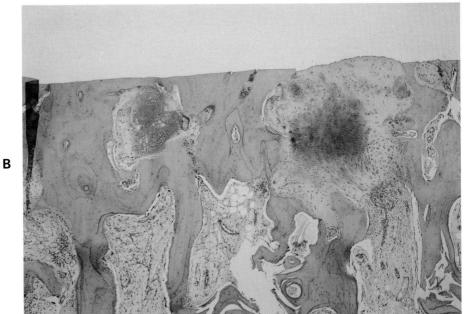

FIG. 8-11. Evidence of exposed bone on joint surface.

A Sclerotic area of exposed bone in degenerative arthritis. Arthroscopic view of sclerotic area on tibia. Meniscus is fragmented.

B Low-power histological view shows sclerotic surface with aggregates of repair fibrocartilage. (Safranin O stain; ×40.)

THE SCLEROTIC LESION IN DEGENERATIVE ARTHRITIS

Little attention is given to the sclerotic lesion in the literature.[5,26,34,52]

Arthroscopic examination shows areas of exposed yellow bone with adjacent degenerative cartilage and fragmentation. The surface is covered with dead osteons with islands of fibrocartilage in varying amounts (Fig. 8-12). The cortical bone is increased in density with thickened trabeculae. The vascularity in the sclerotic area is increased. The vessels penetrate through the cortex to the surface (Fig. 8-12, *D*). Arthroscopically they are seen as small, dark specks. The

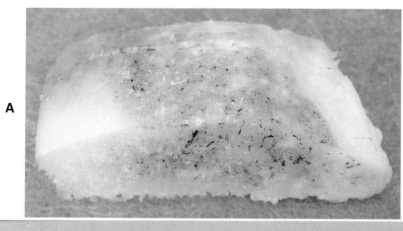

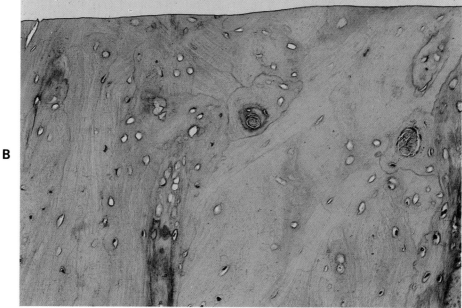

FIG. 8-12. Sclerotic lesion showing dead osteons on surface.

A Gross specimen from total knee surgery. Darkened surface of lesion is caused by blood clot in abundant subchondral and cortical vascularity. Notice vessels on cut surface.

B Photomicrograph shows dense bone, empty lacunae, and vessels. (Hematoxylin and eosin stain; ×100.)

presence of the white fibrocartilage patches and dark vessels gives a salt-and-pepper appearance to the sclerotic surface. In some cases focal areas of hemorrhage are seen on the surface (Fig. 8-13).

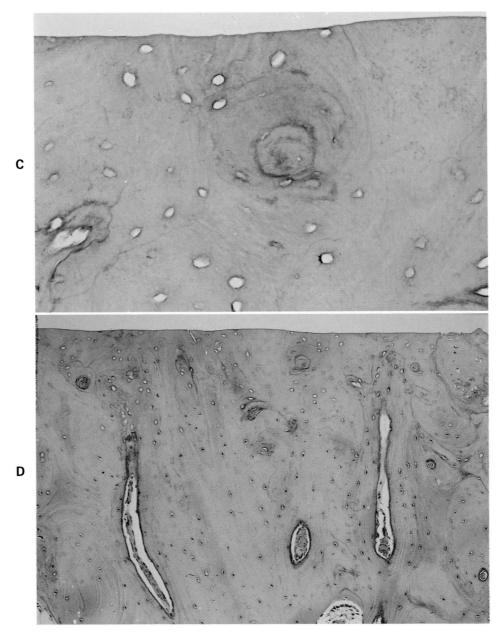

FIG. 8-12, cont'd. Sclerotic lesion showing dead osteons on surface.

C Higher power of sclerotic surface with dead osteons. (Hematoxylin and eosin stain; ×200.)

D Photomicrograph shows vessels on surface. (Hematoxylin and eosin stain; ×100.)

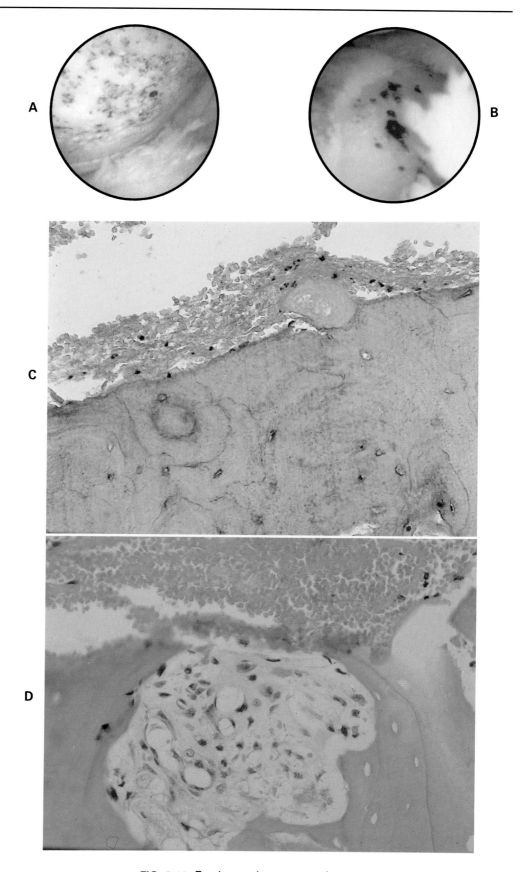

FIG. 8-13. For legend see opposite page.

FIG. 8-13. Vascularity of sclerotic lesion; natural process.

A Arthroscopic view of femur with multiple puncture surface vessels, each with blood clot.

B Arthroscopic view of tibial sclerotic lesion in 70-year-old woman. Notice not only vessels at surface, but also hemorrhage.

C Photomicrograph biopsy of lesion shown in Fig. 8-12, **B**. Notice hemorrhage on surface of sclerotic bone. (Hematoxylin and eosin stain; ×100.)

D High-power photomicrograph of same specimen with hemorrhage and vascular bed at surface within sclerotic cortex. (Hematoxylin and eosin stain; ×400.)

Analysis of the natural history of the complete loss of articular cartilage shows abortive attempts at repair (see Fig. 8-16). The bone thickens with absence of the articular cartilage cushion. The exposed osteons become necrotic, as does exposed bone in other areas.[54] The hypervascularity penetrates the surface, resulting in hemorrhage. The focal area of the blood clot undergoes an inflammatory response, and organization results in fibrous tissue. With time the fibrocartilage island develops. It is not possible for live tissue to grow over dead tissue unless the area of necrosis is removed by inflammatory cells or by surgical debridement. This also holds true for other tissues.

Reports of fibrocartilage growth following osteotomy are probably the result of an improved environment for natural tissue response.[14,15,22] These reports had no preoperative control, but postoperative x-ray films showed wider joint spaces after realignment procedures. The second-look arthroscopic inspections had no preoperative exact-site comparison for biopsy.

Inspection of normal hyaline cartilage surfaces gives a basis for comparison of the sclerotic lesion of degenerative arthritis (see Fig. 8-11). The gross specimen of hyaline cartilage shows the full bone surface covered with white, glossy hyaline cartilage (see Fig. 8-11, *A*). The hyaline cartilage tissue is thick, and the surface is smooth. The cells are arranged in orderly vertical rows. There is an abundance of pericellular material that stain positive for glycosaminoglycans (see Fig. 8-11, *B*). The tidemark is evident. The subchondral bone is cancellous with thin trabeculae. Osseous vascularity is minimal.

The sclerotic lesion of exposed bone in degenerative arthritis has the same histological characteristics of dense bone trabeculae of the cortex in the subchondral areas.

The vascularity of the lesion is abundant both in the cancellous area and on the surface.

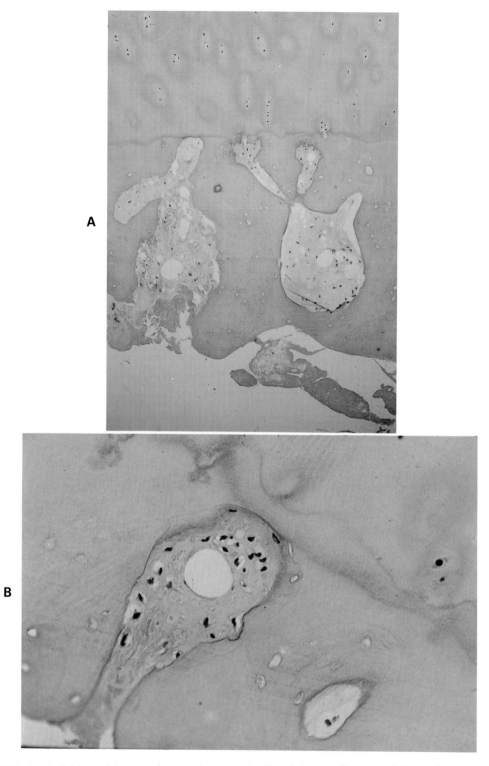

FIG. 8-14. Early evidence of vascular penetration into cartilage to tidemark.

A Photomicrograph shows tidemark as well-defined barrier at base of hyaline cartilage. (Hematoxylin and eosin stain; ×100.)

B In degenerative process, vessels have penetrated through calcific layer to tidemark. (Hematoxylin and eosin stain; ×400.)

The cancellous vascularity remains in normal bone. As the degenerative process progresses in hyaline cartilage, the vessels penetrate through basal cartilage layers to the tidemark (Fig. 8-14). As the degeneration proceeds, vascularity penetrates the tidemark invading the deep layers of articular cartilage, often with fibrous tissue (Fig. 8-15).

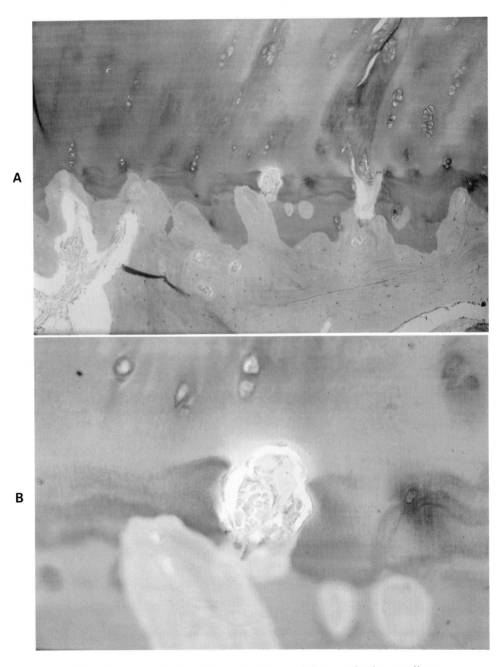

FIG. 8-15. Vascular penetration through tidemark into articular cartilage.

A Low-power photomicrograph shows vessels through tidemark area. (Safranin O stain; ×100.)

B Higher power shows vascular penetration. (Safranin O stain; ×400.)

Continued.

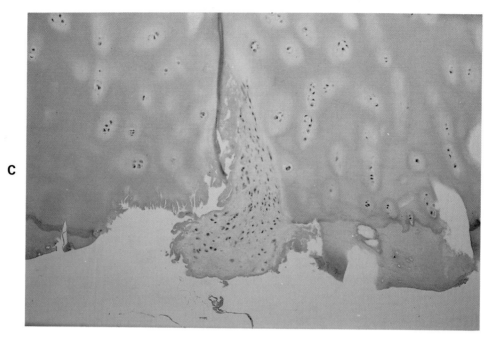

FIG. 8-15, cont'd. Vascular penetration through tidemark into articular cartilage.

C Fibrovascular penetration into hyaline cartilage tissue. (Hematoxylin and eosin stain; ×200.)

The other characteristics of the sclerotic lesion are islands or patches of cartilage dispersed on and in the surface. They stain positively for glycosaminoglycans (see Fig. 8-11). The shiny sclerotic surface shows punctured white patches (Fig. 8-16, *A*). This tissue is usually fibrocartilage (Fig. 8-16, *F* to *I*). It is the natural healing process following hemorrhage. There also are islands of normal degenerative hyaline cartilage (see Fig. 8-16, *C* to *E*).

The naturally appearing fibrocartilage is localized to the cortical level and does not appear as a drill hole (Fig. 8-17). The patches are well secured both biologically and mechanically to the cortex. The relationship of vessels in juxtaposition to the base of fibrocartilage patches suggests the formation of the patches is a result of hemorrhage (Fig. 8-17, *D*). The regrown tissue remains an island because of the adjacent surface of the dead osteons.

Text continued on p. 529.

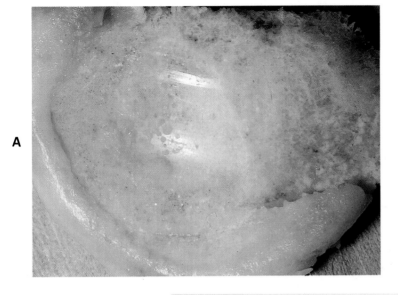

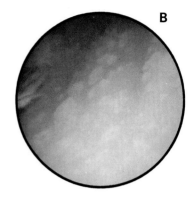

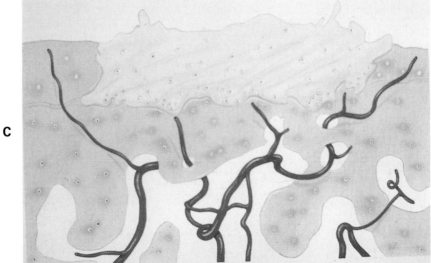

FIG. 8-16. Islands of cartilage, both hyaline and fibrous, are seen in sclerotic surface. Natural history

A Gross specimen of sclerotic femoral surface from total knee surgery.
B Arthroscopic view of islands of cartilage on sclerotic tibial surface.
C Artist's conception of histopathology of lesion with fibrocartilage patch. (Courtesy Dyonics Corp. and Lewis Saddler, Ph.D., Dallas, Tex.)

Continued.

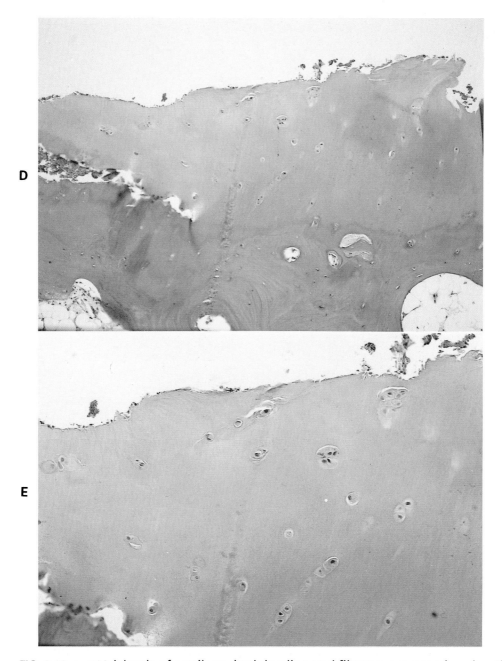

FIG. 8-16, cont'd. Islands of cartilage, both hyaline and fibrous, are seen in sclerotic surface. Natural history.

D Low-power photomicrograph of island of degenerative hyaline cartilage. (Hematoxylin and eosin stain; ×100.)

E Photomicrograph of degenerative hyaline cartilage patch. (Hematoxylin and eosin stain; ×200.)

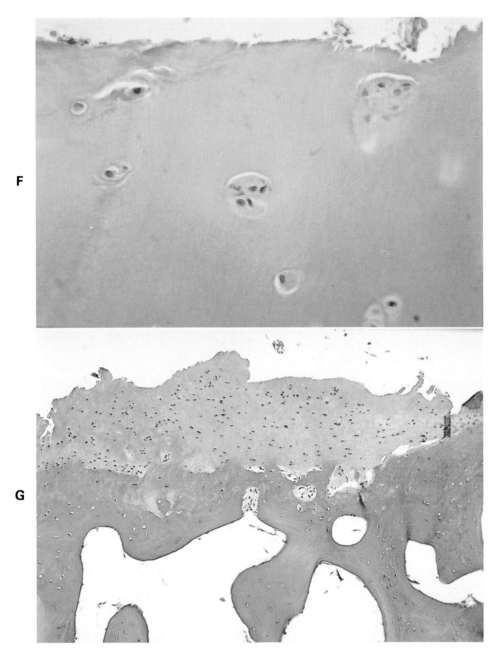

FIG. 8-16, cont'd

F Cellular pattern is that of degenerative hyaline cartilage. (Hematoxylin and eosin stain; ×400.)

G Low-power photomicrograph of reparative fibrocartilage. (Hematoxylin and eosin stain; ×100)

Continued.

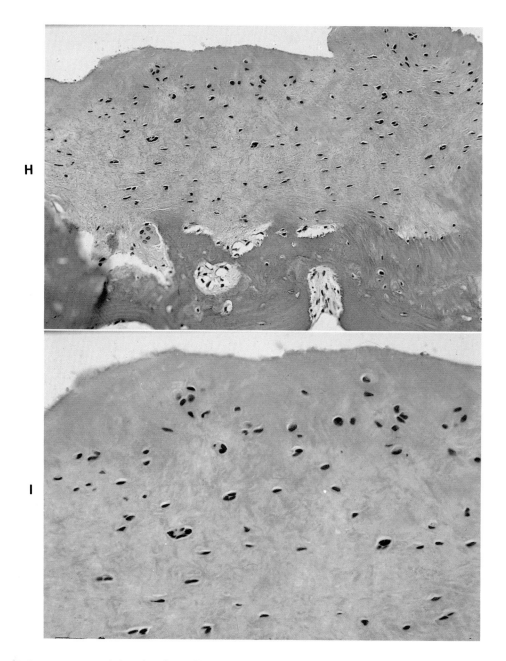

FIG. 8-16, cont'd. Islands of cartilage, both hyaline and fibrous, are seen in sclerotic surface. Natural history.

H Fibrocartilage well adhered to bone with vascularity at base; no previous surgery.

I High-power photomicrograph of naturally occurring fibrocartilage.

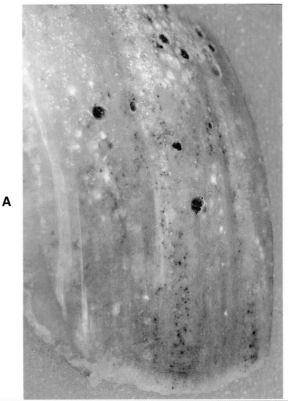

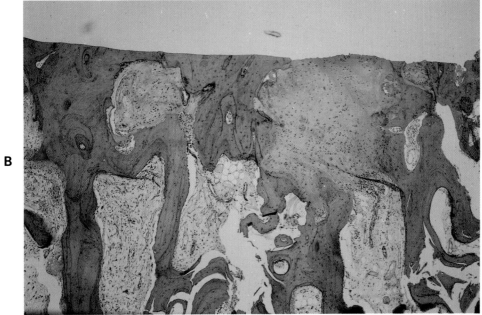

FIG. 8-17. Natural pathological history of islands of reparative fibrocartilage.

A Gross femoral specimen from total knee replacement shows shiny surface of sclerotic lesion.

B Photomicrograph shows islands of fibrocartilage at surface of sclerotic lesion. (Hematoxylin and eosin stain; × 100.) *Continued.*

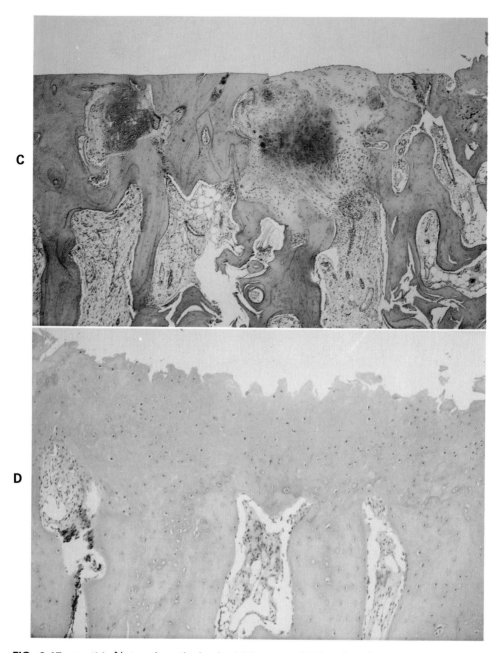

FIG. 8-17, cont'd. Natural pathological history of islands of reparative fibrocartilage.

C Special staining shows glycosaminoglycans in fibrocartilage. (Safranin O stain; ×100.)

D Photomicrograph of biopsy specimen from another patient shows relationship of cortical vascularity to naturally occurring surface fibrocartilage repair.

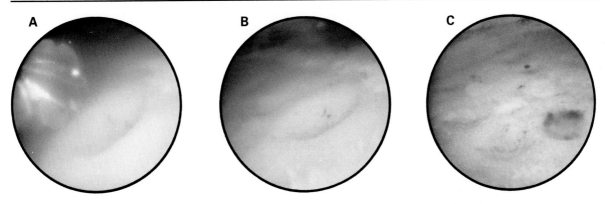

FIG. 8-18. Arthroscopic demonstration of vascularity at surface in cortex.

A Arthroscopic view of motorized burr creating 2 mm deep cut in cortex, but not into cancellous bone.
B Arthroscopic view of vascularity in cortex. Notice small red specks in crater.
C Arthroscopic view 5 weeks after localized cortical abrasion, vascular fibrous patches are seen. Some avascular patches are on posterior aspect of tibia.

Surgical disruption of the cortex with a rotating burr shows blood vessels within (Fig. 8-18, *A*). Decompression of the joint causes blood to ooze from the surface (Fig. 8-18, *B*). These superficial defects in the cortex heal within 5 weeks with hemorrhage and fibrovascular response, becoming avascular by 8 weeks if the joint is protected (Fig. 8-18, *C*). Preexisting normal hyaline patches probably produce findings of type II collagen after various drilling procedures or osteotomy. This is not regrown hyaline cartilage but rather preexistent.

Arthroscopic surgical perspective

In 1979 I recognized that areas of exposed bone did not heal following generalized arthroscopic debridement including 1 month of postoperative non-weight-bearing crutch walking. The patients' symptoms returned, and there was no relief from pain. The x-ray films were unchanged. Second-look arthroscopy and comparison videotapes showed an unchanged sclerotic lesion.

Consideration was given to arthroscopic drilling procedures to stimulate fibrocartilaginous growth as advocated in the literature.[32,33,52]

I was curious as to how deep a drill hole must be made to create bleeding. I was not aware at the time of the pathological nature of sclerotic lesions. With 3 mm curettage of the sclerotic surface, the intracortical vessels were observed within 1 to 2 mm of the surface (Fig. 8-18).

I created small dimple defects in those areas I was unable to reach with a drill. Second-look arthroscopy performed for academic purposes showed surface fibrous tissue repair (Fig. 8-18, *C*). I next placed multiple dimples on a single surface lesion and observed no clinical problem and similar islands of healing. There was minimal clinical improvement and no coalescence at second look.

To obtain complete surface healing I abraded the entire sclerotic lesion on the tibial side only. I was concerned with intracondylar fibrous adhesion and ankylosis. I therefore avoided doing the opposite area on the femur. Remember, all this occurred before literature reports on motion studies with cartilage healing were performed. I did know that immobilization resulted in adhesions. The patients' condition improved after a 2-month non-weight-bearing intermittent active range of motion regimen.

The next step was to create surface debridement on sclerotic lesions of opposing surfaces. To avoid intraarticular adhesion, intermittent active motion was recommended. Second-look arthroscopy showed hypervascular fibrous tissue coalescence of the cartilage surface. This is in contrast to Ghadially's avascular repair in animal drill holes at cartilage level.[23]

I theorized that non-weight bearing would protect this healing surface. Second-look arthroscopy with biopsy showed avascular spindle cells at 2 months when a patient protected the joint yet used intermittent active motion exercises. I have no comparative clinical experience with continuous passive motion. The routine of 2 months with non-weight-bearing crutches was instituted. The patients were more comfortable, and the area of repair was avascular.

At this time some patients had both surface loss and alignment problems. I believed both the surface and alignment should be corrected. I was unable to technically perform both arthroscopic debridement and osteotomy in a reasonable operative time; the arthroscopic portion took me 1½ hours in early 1980. I was using primitive transcutaneous burrs without suction. Many patients were elderly or had medical problems that further restricted the extent of the surgical procedure.

I decided to do the arthroscopic procedure initially and keep the patient on non-weight-bearing crutches. The patient would then return for corrective osteotomy in 6 to 8 weeks. My patient volume for this procedure increased, because patients wanted an alternative to total knee replacement. The public recognized that the results of total knee replacement did not approach those of total hip surgery.

Many patients experienced immediate relief of pain after the abrasion arthroplasty. I theorize that this is a result of the removal of dead surface osteons. If so, it is similar to removal of bony sequestra elsewhere. The other possible cause of pain relief is debridement and coating of intraarticular ulcer with blood. This may be analogous to ulcers elsewhere in the body. A gastroduodenal ulcer is painful; hemorrhage coats the ulcer and reduces pain. A painful varicose ulcer on the leg is improved by debridement and skin graft application.

During the non-weight-bearing period the pain was so diminished that most patients declined the osteotomy. They opted for testing the result of arthroscopic procedure. I seized this opportunity to observe the results of the arthroscopic abrasion arthroplasty procedure (see Chapter 9). Biopsies at 4 to 6 months showed reparative fibrocartilage (see Fig. 8-35). In patients who did not or could not (i.e., bilateral cases) protect the joint, the tissue remained fibrovascular (see Figs. 8-44 and 8-45). This experience limited subsequent patient selection for this procedure to those who could and would protect the joint.

SOURCES OF CELLULAR HEALING IN SYNOVIAL JOINTS

The potential sources of repair of diseased or injured tissue within synovial joints are vascular and avascular.

Avascular source

Parent tissue

The parent tissue contributes to healing in the synovium and bone. The tendon contributes to healing by cellular proliferation in the synovial environment and in tissue culture.[3]

The hyaline cartilage adjacent to a laceration or partial-thickness lesion demonstrates no healing contribution to the lesion.[42]

There is adjacent cellular mitosis in the early stages of degenerative arthritis.[31,79] There is no cellular contribution demonstrated by some authors.[65]

Barrie suggests that local cartilage cells proliferate, causing fibrous tissue sealing of surface defects as seen in loose bodies.[2] Biopsies of the femur show a similar histological appearance (see Fig. 8-29).

Carlson reported "atypical chondrones"[8] adjacent to lesions.

Free synovial cells

Free synovial cells contribute to cellularization and fibrous tissue formation of acellular 14½-year-old freeze-dried tendon grafts placed free within the animal knee joint.[40] Potenza showed a contribution to both surface covering and filling of open spaces within the freeze-dried graft.[59]

This avascular source of cellular layers and fibrosis may contribute to sealing of the edge of the meniscus, healing loose bodies, articular cartilage partial-thickness lesions, and other disrupted intraarticular tissue (Fig. 8-19).

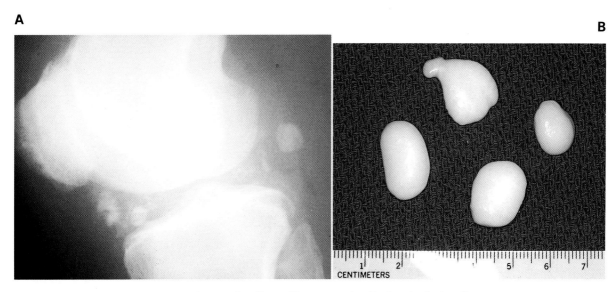

A   **B**

FIG. 8-19. Loose bodies offer opportunity to study healing.

A Lateral x-ray film of knee with loose bodies.
B Gross specimen.   *Continued.*

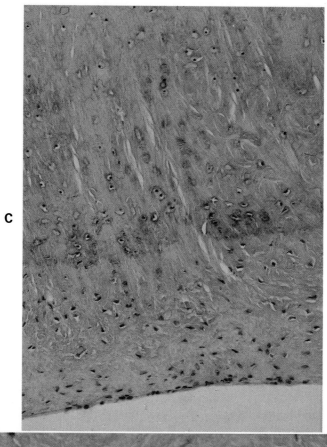

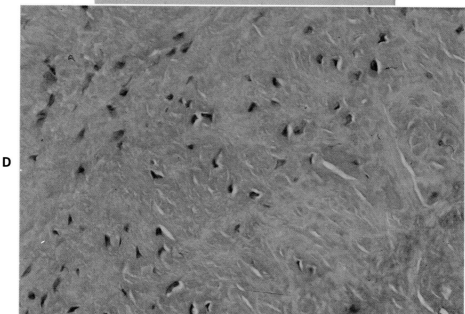

FIG. 8-19, cont'd. Loose bodies.

C Photomicrograph of surface of loose body. (Hematoxylin and eosin stain; ×100.)

D Photomicrograph of proliferating fibrocartilage on surface. (Hematoxylin and eosin stain; ×400)

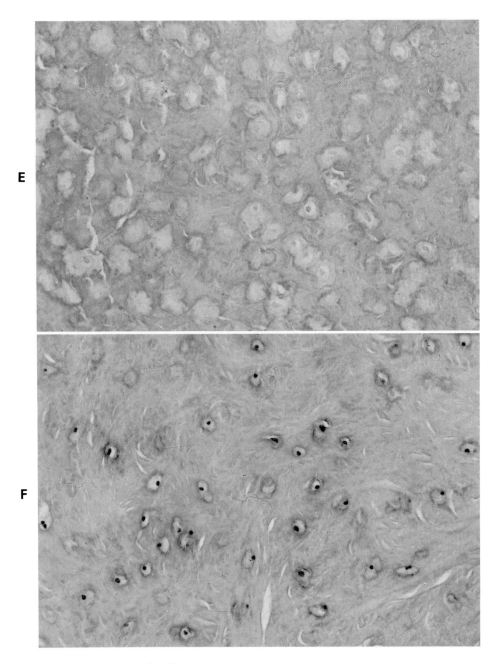

FIG. 8-19, cont'd. Loose bodies.

E Necrotic cartilage cells at center of loose body. (Hematoxylin and eosin stain; ×400.)

F Living cartilage cells near surface of loose body. (Hematoxylin and eosin stain; ×400.)

Vascular source

Hemorrhage and angioblasts

Disruption of vessels results in hemorrhage, inflammation, and cellular repair of tissue.[44,45] Vascular budding further contributes to repair of the injured area.[55]

Adjacent tissue

Adjacent tissue may contribute to the healing of the intraarticular lesion. Synovium grows over meniscal lesions, peripheral articular cartilage defects, and the covering of cruciate ligament tears (Fig. 8-20).

Excessive responses to injury or surgical intervention include the production of adhesions. This occurs most commonly after procedures that have the potential for excessive bleeding, such as lateral release or intraarticular exposure of bone. Postoperative joint immobilization promotes adhesions between articular surfaces or between the articular surface and capsule.[78]

Differentiation of the tissue occurs with maturation, as it does in a drill hole through articular cartilage to the cancellous vascularity.

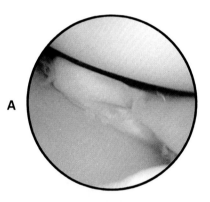

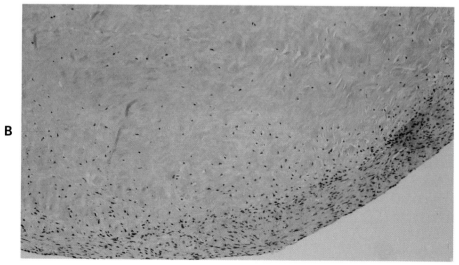

FIG. 8-20. Adjacent tissue source, nonangioblastic, covering meniscus.

A Arthroscopic view of meniscus stump.
B Photomicrograph of meniscus stump shows synovial cell covering. (Hematoxylin and eosin stain; ×100.)

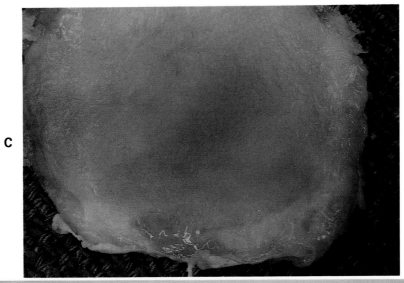

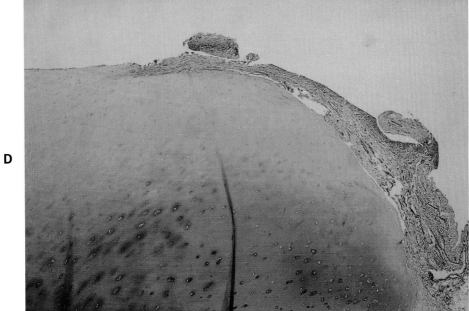

FIG. 8-20, cont'd

C Gross photograph of patella removed at time of total knee replacement with pannus covering marginal defect.

D Photomicrograph of pannus with vessels covering patella in **C** at margin.

Continued.

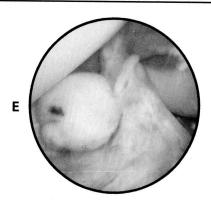

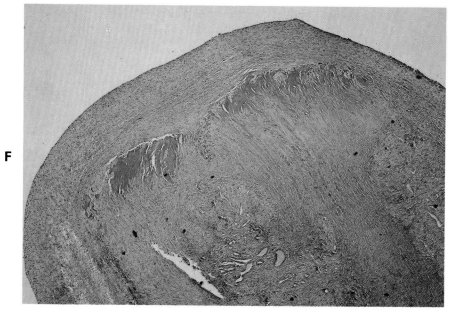

FIG. 8-20, cont'd. Vascular source.

E Arthroscopic view of smooth stump of ACL.
F Photomicrograph of same lesion with synovial vascular covering. (Trichrome stain; ×40.)

Response to injury or disease

All the tissues in and about the synovial joint respond to injury or disease. The response is unique to cell and tissue type.[61a]

Avascular normal articular cartilage responds when injured within its substance without penetration to bone. Cellular repair has not been shown in animal experiments.[42,44,45] In contrast, arthroscopic experience has shown areas of cellular response without evidence of vascular contribution (see Fig. 8-23). The avascular portion of the meniscus also shows fibrous cellular healing (see Fig. 8-54).

Restoration that is cellular in nature occurs in both synovium and bone. Repair, including scar formation, occurs in vascular connective tissue, synovial stroma, joint capsule, ligaments, and tendons. Articular cartilage repair occurs by hemorrhage, inflammatory cell formation, and fibrous repair when underlying bone is penetrated.[42,71]

Existing literature

In laboratory animal studies the effects of age and time to sacrifice as well as the size, depth, and configuration of the articular lesion have been reported.[6,7,12] The presence of compression or absence of contact with the opposing articular surface adversely affects repair.[69,81] The effects of immobilization, intermittent active motion, and continuous passive motion are different in drill holes in normal rabbit joints.[71] Cellular cultures have demonstrated further information about articular cell characteristics and metabolism.

Recent authors have held tenaciously to the concept that partial-thickness articular lesions show no cellular repair.[23,42] They further agree that if any surface response is to occur the cancellous bone must be exposed to create hemorrhage, inflammatory response, and fibrous repair. They report that the fibrous noncartilaginous repair has a limited survival time, not exceeding 1 year.[42] Postoperative application of continuous passive motion supposedly causes regeneration of hyaline cartilage in drill holes through the normal rabbit articular surface.[71]

I know of only one experimental animal study performed on the sclerotic lesions of degenerative joint disease. Richmond et al.[66] created sclerotic lesions in dogs via arthrotomy by sectioning the anterior cruciate ligament and mechanically debriding the articular cartilage off the femur. After time and development of degenerative joint disease, arthroscopic debridement of the sclerotic lesion was carried out. Postmortem examination showed that tissue type varied with the depth of the cortical bone removed. The trim cortex of dogs made it impossible to determine the depth of debridement. Those areas cut at or near the tidemark showed reparative fibrocartilage. Those areas cut into cancellous bone showed fibrous repair.

Arthroscopic observations

Arthroscopy provides a means of studying the response of human articular cartilage to injury and disease. Observations are made and can be recorded on videotape during routine diagnostic and operative arthroscopy.

Comparison studies can be made on second-look arthroscopy with the patient under local anesthesia. A biopsy can be taken of reparative areas for microscopic examination. Routine documentation and storage of information on videotape permits later study and comparison of the lesion, the surgery, and the in vivo healing.

Challenge to traditional belief

Two arthroscopic observations challenged these "established" views. The first was tissue response to partial thickness patellar debridement (see Fig. 8-23). The second concerned the intracortical bone blood supply exposure, subsequent hemorrhage, and a healing response (Figs. 8-16 and 8-33).

Arthroscopic patellar debridement was performed with a motorized rotating-cutting-suction device. The partial-thickness lesion of the patellar surface was removed. The subchondral plate was not approached or violated. No bleeding was observed. The defects were away from synovial reflection.

Immediately after surgery the debrided surface was course. Second-look arthroscopy performed between 1 month and 4 years has shown the maintenance of sealed, smooth fibrocartilaginous repair (see Figs. 8-37 to 8-40). This was not supposed to happen.

The sclerotic lesion of exposed bone in degenerative arthritis was examined by arthroscopic means and demonstrated vessels on, at, and within the cortical bone (see Figs. 8-12 and 8-13). There is profuse vascularity on the surface as well as vessels in the cancellous bone. There is no necessity to drill or decorticate into the cancellous layer to create bleeding.[39,66]

Under arthroscopic control, decortication of the sclerotic surface was performed at various depths. This showed the vascularity to be profuse and less than 1 mm from the surface. Penetration into cancellous bone also demonstrated vascularity, but this depth was not necessary to produce bleeding. The bleeding was best demonstrated by close-up viewing with the arthroscope and by the application of suction to the arthroscope-cannula system. This decompressed the joint when combined with cessation of the inflow fluid.

Clinical experience. With these observations in mind, arthroscopic intraarticular debridement was applied to full-thickness lesions. Sclerotic lesions were abraded with a motor-driven rotating burr–suction device to a depth of 1 mm. Second-look arthroscopies were combined with biopsy (see Figs. 8-37 to 8-40).

Control of size, site, and configuration of the articular lesion is not possible in humans as in animal studies. Still there were opportunities for observations by arthroscopic control for comparison to reports of animal investigations. Illustrative cases were selected that demonstrated anatomical or pathological factors to support or challenge established principles of articular cartilage healing.

The pluripotential cells of the subchondral bone have received the most attention in animal investigations.[71] The subchondral cellular contribution is emphasized, and other sources of cellular repair of human articular cartilage are ignored. Animal experiments along with the common clinical experiences with intraarticular fracture healing, drilling, or curettage of articular defects reinforce the focus on the subchondral vascular source.[32,33,60]

Six major categories of clinical experience contributed to my observation. Group I consisted of diagnostic arthroscopies that provided a look at the natural history of the following untreated lesions: torn meniscus, dislocated patella, fractures, and ligamentous injury. Group II consisted of diagnostic arthroscopies that were performed after open surgical procedures. This group included meniscectomy, drilling and curettage, open knife-blade shaving of the condyles or patella, ligamentous repairs, synovectomy, and arthroplasty, including total knee replacement. Group III consisted of second-look arthroscopies with comparison videotapes following arthroscopic intraarticular shaving of the patella or patellofemoral joint (1 month to 4 years). Group IV contained second-look arthroscopies with comparison videotapes of intraarticular arthroscopic shaving of weight-bearing condylar surfaces, but not down to bone. This procedure was often done in conjunction with arthroscopic meniscectomy, ligamentous injury repair, or repair of direct-blow trauma or done secondary to degenerative arthritis (1 month to 4 years). Group V consisted of second-look arthroscopies following arthroscopic meniscectomy. These were performed to determine the adequacy of resection early after the procedure for diagnosis, for therapeutic reasons if symptoms persisted or recurred, at the time of a second injury, or at the time of subsequent ligamentous reconstructive surgery. Group VI contained second-look arthroscopies performed following superficial scraping of exposed sclerotic lesions of degenerative articular surfaces of both patellofemoral and femorotibial joint areas. The surface was denuded to a depth of less than 1 mm to expose numerous small vessels. A subsequent routine arthroscopic inspection was performed to assess healing before weight-bearing ambulation was initiated.

When the opportunity presented, biopsy was performed of selective areas during both conventional and arthroscopic surgery. The initial biopsy site was included in the planned excision of tissue, and subsequent microbiopsies were diagnostic. In some cases the maturity of the tissue affected patient management. Cartilage maturation was determined by biopsy before increased ambulation or activities was recommended in early case experience.

ARTICULAR CARTILAGE RESPONSE TO INJURY/DISEASE
Age

In experimental studies on young animals cartilage cellular mitosis has been demonstrated.[31,79,43] The normal histological finding in young dogs is vessels in the articular cartilage halfway to the surface.[6] Partial-thickness lesions of articular cartilage in these animals healed in a vascular manner.[6]

Young people show penetration of vessels beyond the bone up to the cartilaginous tidemark.[65] These vessels disappear with maturity.[23] No vessels normally cross the bone–calcified cartilage barrier in adults (see Figs. 8-14 and 8-15).

Vascularity

Vascularity increases in degenerative arthritis.[34] The vessels penetrate the calcific layer to the tidemark (see Figs. 8-14 and 8-15). As the surface cartilage fragments the vessels penetrate deep into the degenerative areas.

It is common to observe bleeding from otherwise intact degenerative cartilage. Suction decompression performed before instrumentation demonstrates extrusion of blood from the surface. This supports the histological observations.

Debridement of deep partial-thickness degenerative lesions, though obviously not debridement to bone, demonstrates similar findings. A traumatic partial-thickness lesion shows no evidence of vessels or bleeding. An acute lesion in which articular cartilage is stripped from subchondral cortex bone shows no bleeding when the joint is distended. Decompression with suction on the arthroscope draws blood out to the surface through vascular channels in the cortex.

An acute osteochondral fracture into cancellous bone shows vascularity even with the joint distended.

Depth of lesion
Partial-thickness lesion

Experimentally, partial-thickness lesions are seen to respond differently than those that penetrate to vascular bone.[23] Light mimcroscopy shows no cellular repair,[23] and there is no reaction in the adjacent cartilage nor any cellular mitosis. The adjacent cartilage does not degenerate. Partial-thickness lesions are nonprogressive.

Electron microscopy of partial-thickness lesions in animals shows no cellular response covering the base of the defect.[23] Ghadially reports that although chondrocytes are incapable of mounting a repair reaction sufficient to fill a superficial defect, they do respond by heightened metabolic activity. A product of this activity is the creation of a layer of fine, smooth collagen fibrils that contain matrices.

There is a smoothing of the ultrastructure by "flow formations," which are caused by the pressures of weight bearing and shearing forces. This material is worn off by 2 years. The edges of the defect roll or fold in toward the defect. This response gives a smooth appearance on gross examination.

Open knife-blade shaving produces the same results in humans (Fig. 8-21).

Some experimental animal studies demonstrate cellular repair of partial-thickness lesions.[16] Callandruccio et al. reported that partial repairs showed preoperative vascularity in the area of partial-thickness defects in young animals.[6] Therefore, unlike the avascular area in mature hyaline cartilage postoperative cellular repair sections showed a vascular contribution to healing.

Ghadially writes, "one may now confidently assert that if repair tissue is seen in a so-called superficial defect, then it is not a superficial defect at all and the subchondral bone is unknowingly injured."[23]

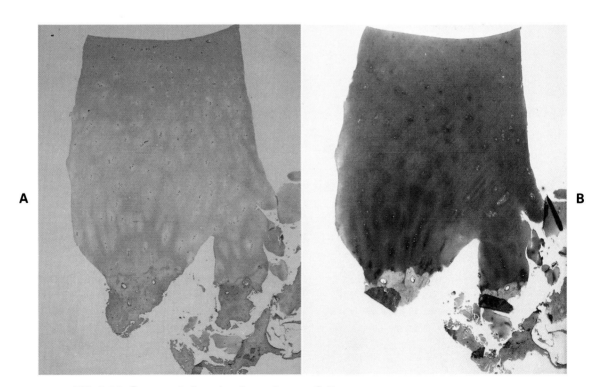

A

B

FIG. 8-21. Open patellar shaving—1-year follow-up.

A Photomicrograph of biopsy specimen. (Hematoxylin and eosin stain; ×20.)
B Low-power photomicrograph with special stain for glucosaminoglycans. Note no cellular surface repair. (Safranin O stain; ×20.)

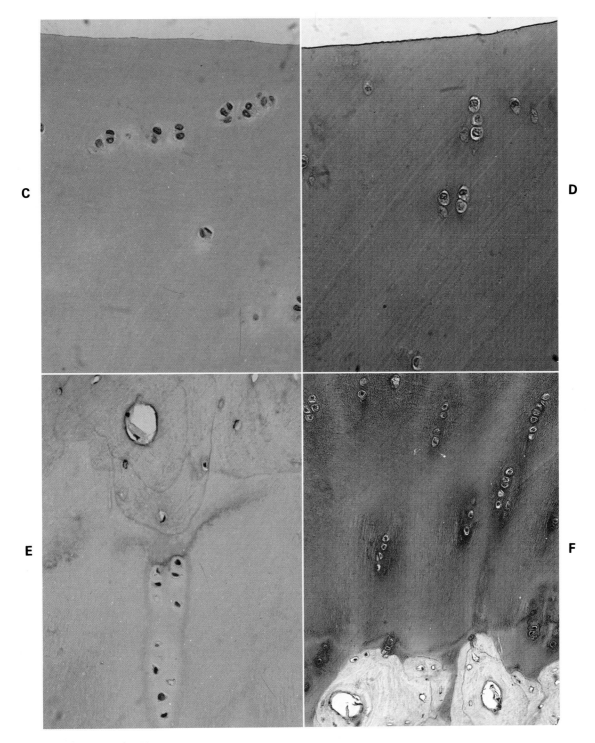

FIG. 8-21, cont'd

C High-power photomicrograph of surface shows no healing. Cellular response of clumping. (Hematoxylin and eosin stain; ×400.)

D High-power photomicrograph of surface after open knife blade shaving 1 year before. No reaction. (Safranin O stain; ×400.)

E High-power photomicrograph of tidemark showing normal vascularity. (Hematoxylin and eosin stain; ×40)

F High-power photomicrograph with safranin O shows normal cells and staining at base, 1 year after open shaving.

Arthroscopic perspective

Degenerative lesions. The fissures associated with degenerative arthritis show translucent tissue in the base of the lesion (see Fig. 8-5). The fissure is opaque and different from the adjacent edges on arthroscopic inspection. Biopsy specimens show a fibrous base in the fissure. Stellate fissures are less stable; progressive fragmentation has been observed as early as 4 months. The larger-diameter degenerative lesions show no sign of repair at repeat arthroscopy.

A lesion that appears furry on arthroscopy represents fragmentation on histological examination (see Fig. 8-9). It may appear granular or in a cobblestone-like pattern when fragmentation is accompanied by erosion of surface (see Fig. 8-10).

Progressive erosion of hyaline cartilage causes vascular penetration across the tidemark area (see Fig. 8-15). This is manifested by the appearance of bleeding from the base of the partial-thickness lesion. This vascular penetration probably is the source of repair in some partial-thickness degenerative lesions. A similar intracartilaginous vascularity contributed to healing of partial-thickness lesions in young dogs.[6]

Traumatic lesions. A smooth appearance of traumatic lesions is a common finding during diagnostic or second-look arthroscopy. The small areas (1 to 3 mm) of iatrogenic surgical scuffing are smooth within 2 months. There appears to be a translucent surface that differs from adjacent normal tissue. I have no human biopsy specimens of scuffing.

The partial-thickness traumatic hyaline cartilage lesion associated with meniscus or cruciate ligament tearing has rounded edges and a smooth or furry base. Hyaline cartilage laceration shows no sign of repair at 4 months by second-look arthroscopy.

Arthroscopic debridement. Arthroscopic observations of patellar surface repair following debridement (shaving) with motorized instrumentation reopened the controversy about the healing of partial-thickness lesions (Figs. 8-22 to 8-24).

The patellar shaving project was originally aimed at developing a motorized arthroscopic instrument for meniscectomy. I chose the pathological model of chondromalacia patella because of easy of arthroscopic access and unlikely event of worsening the patient's condition by superficial debridement (see Chapter 10).

The procedure was performed without expectation of much patient benefit, let alone consideration of tissue response or repair. I was satisfied that open patellar shaving, either as reported in the literature or in my own experience was rarely beneficial. As a result I had little clinical experience with open shaving. In severe cases I performed spongialization (Pridie procedure) or patellectomy.

I should emphasize that I performed only an average of two cases per month during a period in which I was attracting and being referred these cases. Isolated patellar shaving is an uncommonly performed surgical procedure; a case arises perhaps 5 times per year out of 600 cases, usually requiring correction of the underlying cause of patellar malposition. Therefore this initial case experience must be placed in the proper clinical perspective for present-day practice.

To my surprise the patients expressed improvement in symptoms, and physical examination showed a decrease in or the absence of crepitus. I did not expect this to be the case after such a superficial nonaggressive debridement. In fact,

Text continued on p. 549.

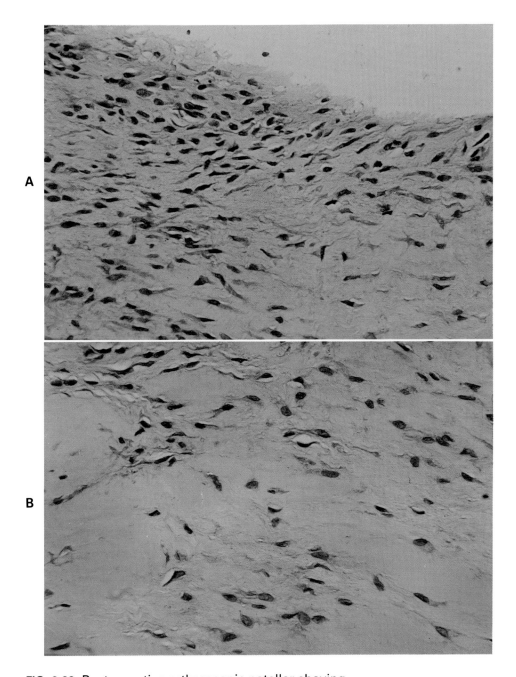

FIG. 8-22. Postoperative arthroscopic patellar shaving.

A Photomicrograph of surface biopsy 1 month postoperatively. Note fibrous repair on surface without angioblastic contribution. (Hematoxylin and eosin stain; ×400.)

B Photomicrograph of same patient with fibrous repair continuous with hyaline cartilage tissue. (Hematoxylin and eosin stain; ×400.)

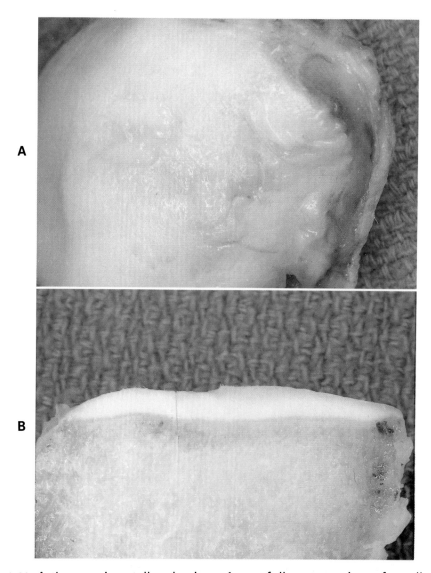

FIG. 8-23. Arthroscopic patellar shaving—1 year follow-up at time of patellectomy.

A Gross specimen shows islands of fibrous repair tissue on surface of hyaline cartilage.

B Gross specimen sectioned to show translucent tissue on surface.

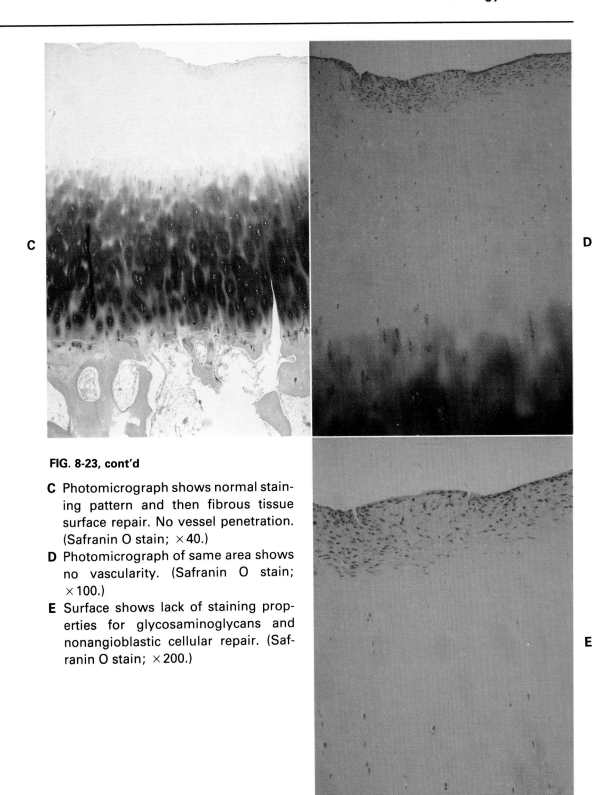

C

D

E

FIG. 8-23, cont'd

C Photomicrograph shows normal staining pattern and then fibrous tissue surface repair. No vessel penetration. (Safranin O stain; ×40.)

D Photomicrograph of same area shows no vascularity. (Safranin O stain; ×100.)

E Surface shows lack of staining properties for glycosaminoglycans and nonangioblastic cellular repair. (Safranin O stain; ×200.)

Continued.

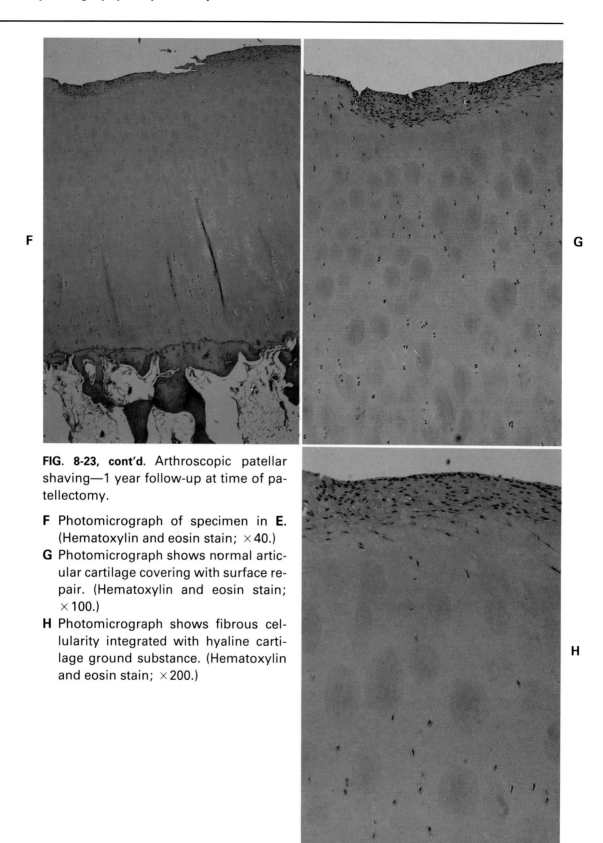

FIG. 8-23, cont'd. Arthroscopic patellar shaving—1 year follow-up at time of patellectomy.

F Photomicrograph of specimen in **E.** (Hematoxylin and eosin stain; ×40.)

G Photomicrograph shows normal articular cartilage covering with surface repair. (Hematoxylin and eosin stain; ×100.)

H Photomicrograph shows fibrous cellularity integrated with hyaline cartilage ground substance. (Hematoxylin and eosin stain; ×200.)

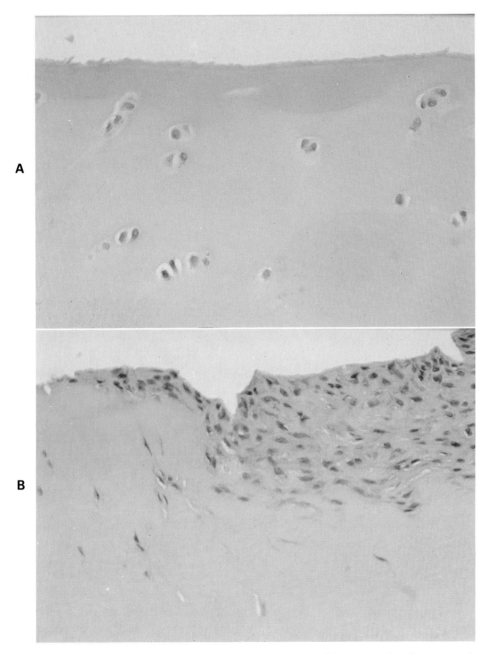

FIG. 8-24. Junction of fibrous tissue repair patch with normal adjacent articular cartilage, 1 year after arthroscopic patellar debridement. (same case as in Fig. 8-23.)

A Photomicrograph of adjacent hyaline cartilage surface. (Hematoxylin and eosin stain; ×400.)

B Junction of repair tissue and hyaline cartilage surface. (Hematoxylin and eosin stain; ×400.)

Continued.

547

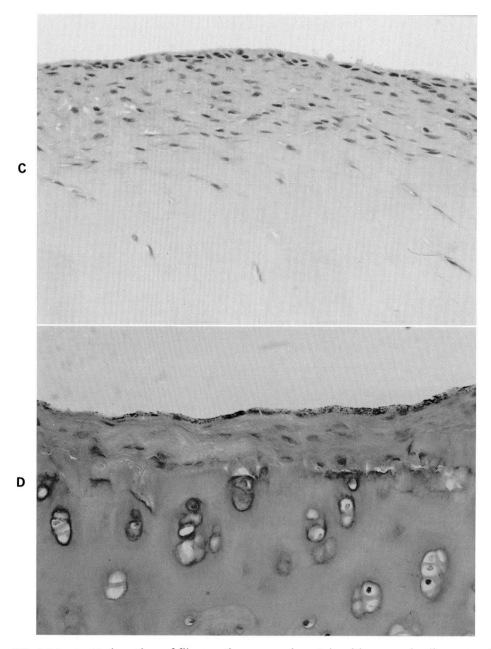

FIG. 8-24, cont'd. Junction of fibrous tissue repair patch with normal adjacent articular cartilage, 1 year after arthroscopic patellar debridement. (same case as in Fig. 8-23.)

C High-power photomicrograph of repair lesion. (Hematoxylin and eosin stain; ×400.)

D Comparison to histological fibrous tissue response in adult rabbit experiment. Repair of fibrous tissue is similar to human partial-thickness lesion created in saline environment. Particles on surface of repair are India ink placed on gross specimen for photographic purposes. (Hematoxylin and eosin stain; ×400.)

during this time, I complained that the instrument was not aggressive enough to accomplish the resection that would be possible by open methods. In some cases, I resorted to arthroscopic use of a knife blade to "complete" shaving.

I performed second-look arthroscopies out of curiosity (see Fig. 10-52). I have taken every reasonable opportunity to obtain arthroscopic second looks at previously debrided hyaline cartilage surfaces. To my surprise (and perhaps your disbelief) there was arthroscopic evidence of sealing or repair (notice I said "sealing," not "healing") of the partial-thickness lesions. The shortest interval was 1 month, performed because of a reinjury (see Fig. 8-22). The longest has been 4½ years, performed at the time of surgery on the other knee. A controlled experiment is not possible in humans, but the observations create a desire to understand the process in view of experimental evidence by open surgery.

Microbiopsies (1 mm) during subsequent arthroscopy showed fibrous repair of hyaline cartilage partial-thickness defects. Patellectomy specimens provided yet another opportunity to examine tissue response (see Fig. 8-23).

Partial-thickness lesions of the femoral and tibial condyles, both traumatic and degenerative, have been carefully debrided usually in conjunction with arthroscopic meniscectomy. These surfaces respond in the same manner as the patella as observed by arthroscopy. A few microbiopsy specimens show early fibrocartilage repair (Fig. 8-25). The repair is minimal. At 2½ to 4 years, the repair cellularity is minimal.

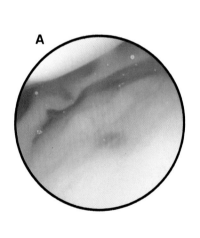

FIG. 8-25. Partial-thickness healing.

A Arthroscopic view of half-thickness tibial avulsion after debridement.

B Photomicrograph of regenerated fibrocartilage at 8 weeks without vascular contribution.

My longest second-look arthroscopy on a partial-thickness traumatic lesion is 6 years. During arthroscopic lateral meniscectomy I created an iatrogenic defect (1.0 × 0.5 cm) on the tibial condyle. Progressive degenerative arthritis in the joint resulted in repeat arthroscopy. The original videotapes were available for exact site location. The area of partial-thickness defect was filled into the surface with white, firm tissue. Posterior to the healed lesion was degeneration and a small area of exposed bone. All this occurred since the previous surgery with iatrogenic injury (Fig. 8-26, A).

A biopsy of the healed area showed mature cartilage cell histologically and diffuse histochemical staining properties for proteoglycans (Fig. 8-26). The specimen did not include underlying bone, but no area of vascularization was seen. Unfortunately, no collagen typing studies were performed.

Rationale. How do we reconcile these arthroscopic observations with experimental evidence? It seems completely inconsistent. Where could the cellular response originate?

Let us first consider the variables in arthroscopic experience that differ from reported laboratory experiments. Most laboratory experiments were performed in normal animal knees by arthrotomy in room air environment.

In arthroscopy, the species is different (*Homo sapiens*), the articular cartilage was pathologically degenerative, and the environment was normal saline irrigation medium.

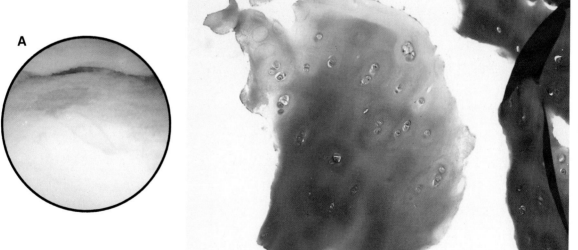

FIG. 8-26. Six years postoperatively, iatrogenic partial-thickness lesion of tibial surface. Lesion was made with cutting instrument during near-total arthroscopic meniscectomy. Progressive degenerative arthritis resulted in need for repeat arthroscopy. Original videotape was available for review and location of exact site.

A Arthroscopic view of tibial condyle with white regrown patch in area of previous iatrogenic defect.

B Photomicrograph of regrown cartilage in defect site. (Safranin O stain; ×40.)

FIG. 8-26, cont'd

C High-power view of same specimen shows cartilage cell and diffuse, positive-staining properties for proteoglycans. (Safranin O stain; ×100.)

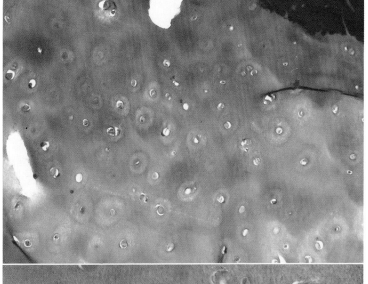

C

D High-power photomicrograph of reparative cells. (Safranin O stain; ×400.)

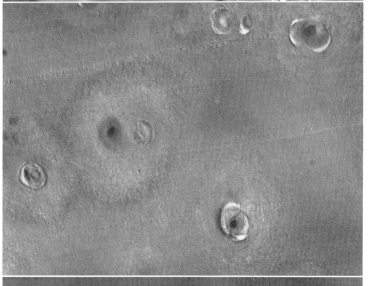

D

E High-power photomicrograph of adjacent normal hyaline cartilage. (Safranin O stain; ×400.)

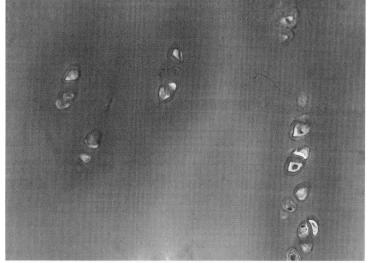

E

The only experimental report of healing of partial-thickness articular lesions was the result of decreasing proteoglycan leakage on the wound by enzymatic depression with specific dosages of papain.[62] It was concluded that proteoglycan weapage on the wound prevented blood from clotting on the surface. When proteoglycans were inhibited, clot formation attached to the lesion and fibrous tissue repair occurred.

If proteoglycans presence inhibits clot and subsequent fibrous tissue formation, let us examine proteoglycans presence in typical arthroscopic surgery.

The usual arthroscopic debridement is performed for degenerative arthritis. Degenerative arthritis has decreased proteoglycan content.[44,45] Furthermore, proteoglycans are easily extracted from degenerative hyaline cartilage.[49] They are less firmly held by diseased collagen.[49] Therefore in arthroscopic experience the proteoglycan content of the degenerative operative site was decreased to start with, and existing proteoglycan was easily removed.

Normal saline lavage used during operative arthroscopy further decreased proteoglycan presence. Reagan et al.[62] showed in vitro decreased cartilage metabolism in saline solution compared to lactated Ringer's. The in vivo experiments of Nole et al. on the toxicity of the bupivacine anesthetic agent showed that as little as 12 ml of saline injected in both young pigs and adult dogs caused profound inhibition of articular cartilage synthesis for 24 hours.[57] Return to normal synthesis took 3 days.

The arthroscopic environment starts with degenerative articular cartilage with decreased proteoglycan content that is easily extracted.[44,45,49] Subject to normal saline lavage, the already-decreased proteoglycan content is further depressed for 24 hours.[57] Therefore in the arthroscopic environment there is opportunity for blood clot formation on debrided partial-thickness lesions. This reasoning validates arthroscopic observations of fibrous tissue repair of partial-thickness lesions treated by this method and explains the discrepancy with experimental literature.

Experimental evidence. To further test this thesis, in 1985 I performed animal experiments, creating partial-thickness lesions in a closed (arthroscopic control) environment using three mediums: air, lactated Ringer's solution, and normal saline solution. The rabbits were sacrificed at 6 weeks. There was no healing of partial-thickness defects in adult rabbits subjected to the air or lactated Ringer's medium. The animals with partial-thickness defects created in the normal saline environment showed fibrous tissue healing of lesions. The experimental tissue repair was of the same character as seen in human arthroscopy using saline solution (Fig. 8-24, *D*). This will be more fully reported in the future.

Another source of cellular repair has been proposed by Barrie.[2] In his study of loose bodies the surface of hyaline cartilage sealed with cellularity, which he attributed to multiplication of mature cartilage cells. His evidence was the histological appearance of multiplication of cells in clumps, exhibiting mitosis and being continuous with reparative layer. Experimental studies of in situ hyaline cartilage do not show similar changes. I have seen this type of repair adjacent to full-thickness lesions; however, this was in the vascular area of degenerative or traumatic hyaline cartilage.

Another source of cellular repair has been attributed to perichondrium or the superficial layer of cells that covers the hyaline cartilage.[2] The synovial lining adjacent to the margins of articular cartilage will respond and fill the defect in this area, spreading over the surface. This is usually accompanied by evidence of angioblastic vascularity.

Potenza offers yet another possibility of surface cellular repair in his study of the fate of freeze-dried acellular flexor tendon grafts placed in a dog's knee joint.[59] This tissue, devoid of cells, vascularity, and viability, was coated and impregnated with layers of cells. He attributed cell origin to free synovial cells. Fibroblastic activity was observed.

The nutrition of hyaline cartilage, similar to tendon, comes from synovial diffusion.[46-48] The potential for free blood or synovial cells to participate in repair is similar in both tissues.

Full-thickness lesion

The full-thickness lesion can be an acute avulsion of cartilage off intact cortical bone, an osteochondral fracture, osteochondritis dissecans, or the sclerotic lesion of degenerative arthritis. Surgically the full-thickness lesion is created by debridement or drill holes.

Normal cortical bone and the sclerotic degenerative lesion both are vascular.[5,21,26,34] Although recognized in the pathology literature, this fact has not been fully appreciated by orthopedists. Vascular angioblastic repair is the common denominator of repair of these lesions.

Avulsion

Avulsion of articular cartilage is a common occurrence with either a direct blow, anterior cruciate ligament tear, subluxation of the joint, or meniscal tear. (Figs. 8-28 and 8-29). In addition, dislocations of the patella will frequently tear a portion of the articular cartilage off the bone, leaving a bleeding bed. The lesions are traumatic and can mimic torn meniscus by elevated chondral flap or incongruity of surface with a loose body (see Fig. 8-27).

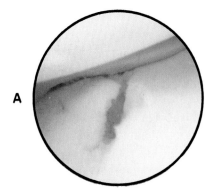
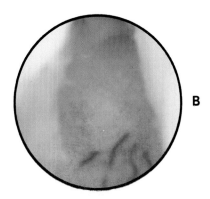

FIG. 8-27. Full-thickness traumatic fissure of lateral tibial plateau caused by trauma.

A Arthroscopic view of traumatic lesion that mimicked torn lateral meniscus.
B Depth of lesion shows vascularity after minimal debridement.

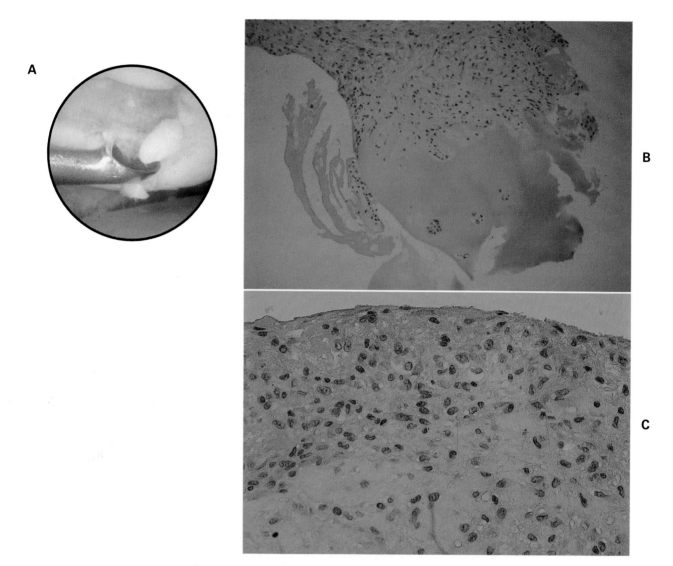

FIG. 8-28. Traumatic avulsion to exposed bone.

A Arthroscopic view of biopsy of traumatic avulsion lesion of femoral condyle.
B Photomicrograph shows junction of hyaline cartilage and fibrous repair at 8 weeks after injury.
C High-power (×400) photomicrograph of surface showing plump cells of fibrous repair. No vessels at 8 weeks after injury.

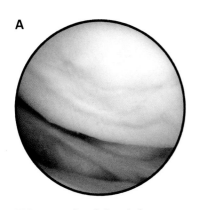

FIG. 8-29. Avulsion injury.

A Arthroscopic view at 8 weeks after surgical debridement of flap articular cartilage to exposed bone.

B Biopsy shows junction of existing cartilage and repair.

C Photomicrograph of fibrous covering of adjacent intact cartilage.

D Photomicrograph shows freeing of hyaline cartilage cells contributing to repair. This is similar to Barrie's report on loose bodies.

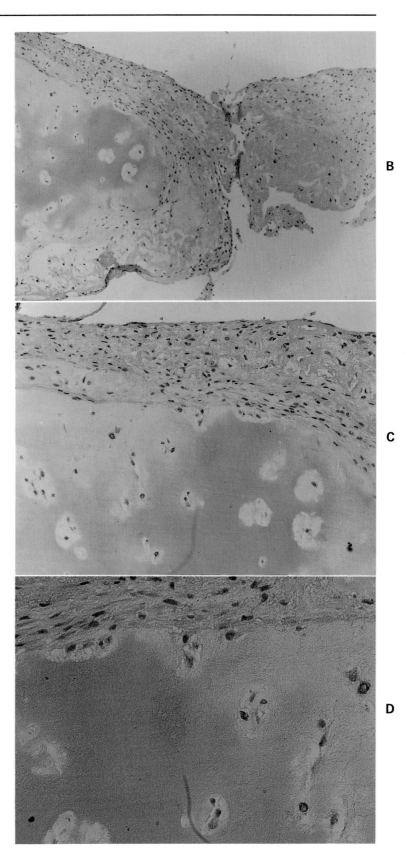

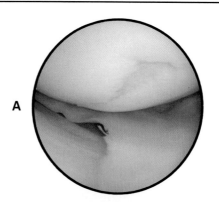

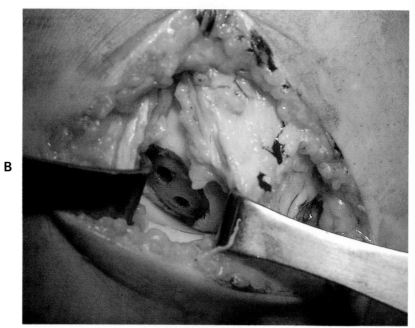

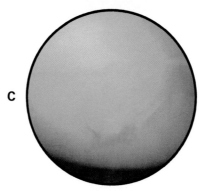

FIG. 8-30

A Natural healing of full-thickness lesion seen arthroscopically. Small loose body from defect was removed with forceps. Full-thickness avulsion treated by open surgery.

B Photograph taken through arthrotomy (circa 1972). Edges of lesion were excised perpendicularly. Base was drilled.

C Arthroscopic view of same patient, 1 year later, showing healed surface. Methylene blue was used to highlight articular surface.

The natural history of an untreated avulsion is hemorrhage, fibrous tissue proliferation, and subsequent maturation to fibrocartilage (Fig. 8-30).

Fracture

Fracture of the articular cartilage is no different histologically than a fracture elsewhere, with its attendant hemorrhage, formation of fibrocartilage, and ultimate bone[44,45] (see Fig. 9-6).

A surface fibrocartilaginous seal bridges the articular cartilage surface area. The repair even compensates for considerable offsets (2 to 3 mm) of the articular cartilage as it fills in between the two surfaces.

Experimental and open surgical debridement

Both experimental and open surgical procedures emphasize osseous debridement or drilling into cancellous bone.

Insall reported Pridie's concept of spongialization into the cancellous layer even for partial-thickness defects. The procedure included debridement of articular cartilage, cortical currettage, or placement of drill holes.

Magnuson advocated a joint debridement procedure that has come to be known as the "housecleaning."[41] The procedure, performed through an extensive arthrotomy, included meniscectomy, synovectomy, osteophyte resection, and decorticalization of bone including multiple drill holes.

The Smith-Petersen cup arthroplasty of the hip was performed using gouges and reamers to expose the cancellous bone of the femoral head and acetabulum.[75,76] Osteophytes were resected as the joint was reshaped for interposition material. Glass was used originally, but eventually Vitallium mold was introduced. Histological sections show repair cartilage covering of bone. Urist supported these observations.[84]

Similar regrowth of cartilage tissue has been reported after hip and tibial osteotomy.[5,14,15,22] Careful photographic or histological documentation of preoperative and postoperative location or tissue type was not available. The tissue was not subjected to histochemical staining, and collagen type was not known. In the photographs seen in the literature, resections appear fibrocartilaginous because of the increased cellularity diffuse throughout matrix.[75] Normal hyaline cartilage has fewer cells in clumps or rows (see Fig. 8-1, C). Both hyaline cartilage and fibrocartilage stain positively for proteoglycans; therefore the nature of tissue is not conclusive (see Fig. 8-37).

Others have advocated drilling and cutting into cancellous bone to obtain a healing response.[60,70] The bulk of experimental evidence shows full-thickness lesions repair following hemorrhage and formation of reparative fibrocartilage.[23,42] They describe the tissue response as fibrous, even "hyaline," but reported resistance to wear with breakdown after 1 year.[42,44,45] The suggestion of hyaline cartilage restoration is not supported by collagen typing.[39]

The accepted criteria for determining cartilage tissue type are light microscopic analysis of cellular pattern, histochemical staining of glycosaminoglycans and electrophoresis identification of type II collagen.

Fibrocartilage has similar characteristics of hyaline cartilage with oval cells, including eccentric nuclei surrounded by lacunae. The fibrocartilage has a diffuse cellular pattern. Reparative fibrocartilage will produce a positive diffuse histochemical stain for glycosaminoglycans[67,82,86] (Fig. 8-37).

Collagen-molecule types are differentiated by the composition of their polypeptide chains. The fibers derived from these collagen molecules are interstitial, that is, located between cellular components. Type I collagen is prevalent in all major connective tissues. Type II collagen is restricted to normal hyaline cartilage in adults. Type III collagen is found in dermis, vessels, and the uterine wall.[86]

The critical factor in establishing a tissue as hyaline cartilage is the presence of type II collagen. The cellular appearance and histochemical staining properties are similar in hyaline and reparative fibrocartilage.

Drill defects in animals

Ghadially prefers to call his full-thickness experimental drill hole lesions "core defects."[23] After placing 1.5 to 2 mm core defects through normal rabbit articular cartilage, he observed a blood clot at 4 days. The edges of the lesion showed cartilage flow and became rounded.

At 1 week there were spindle cells in loose stroma. Ghadially makes an important point concerning the repair tissue in the cartilage layer as opposed to bone: the bone defect repairs with granulation tissue, but the area of repair in cartilage consists of avascular spindle cells and not granulation tissue by definition. This factor is important in cartilage production at maturity, because vascular tissue ends up fibrous, not cartilaginous.

At 3 weeks the spindle cells showed a change to the plump configuration of chondrocytes. The tissue adheres to adjacent cartilage. Chondrocyte clusters are seen near the core defect. At 2 months the tissue appears the same but has decreased cell density. At 6 months there is decreased cell density and increased matrix formation. There is metaplastic transformation from fibrous to cartilaginous tissue. The subchondral plate reforms at 3 months.

Scanning electromicroscopic inspection of core defects show radially arranged fibroblasts at the junction with the articular cartilage. At 3 weeks the repair tissue flows over the edges of adjacent cartilage.

The appearance of core defects after 1 year is as follows:

50% had a smooth, cartilaginous-appearing "hyaline." No collagen typing evidence was presented.

25% had a fragmented fibrous plug.

25% had an absence of tissue in the defect except for a flow of tissue from normal cartilage covering the hole.

There were fissures in the adjacent hyaline cartilage. There was no migration of adjacent cartilage cells into the defect. Two-year-old core defects showed re-formed tidemark at a level higher than original.

The placement of drill holes has been the traditional surgical method for stimulating repair to articular surfaces in condylar conditions. It was believed the closest blood supply was in the cancellous bone. Furthermore this area was thought to be a source of pluripotential cells for articular surface repair. The source of repair cells is blood.[71]

Salter reported on the effects of continuous passive motion, intermittent active motion, and immobilization in healthy New Zealand white rabbits. The normal hyaline cartilage was violated experimentally with a 2 mm diameter drill hole into cancellous bone. The resultant tissue response and repair was studied with histochemical staining.

The conclusion was that those animals subjected to continuous passive motion had regenerated "hyaline" cartilage. No proof substantiates this claim. There are some deficiencies in this experiment, especially if the results are extrapolated to the response of human anatomy, pathology, and tissue type. The repair tissue in the animals was subjected *only* to histochemical staining techniques. Both human and animal fibrocartilage demonstrate pericellular staining properties for glycosaminoglycans. The specific test for hyaline cartilage is demonstration of type II collagen, but the reparative tissue was not subjected to this confirmatory examination. The 2 mm diameter specimens may have been too small for an accurate isolated biopsy to be obtained without including adjacent normal hyaline cartilage.

The concept of the pluripotential cell and its location in cancellous bone would support the necessity of drilling to cancellous bone, but tissue repair occurs from blood and inflammatory response.[23,44,45] Primitive fibrous cells result. Because of cancellous bone vascularity, pluripotential cells do not exist in any single location but rather with hemorrhagic response at any location. A vessel rupture and bleeding in cortical bone have the same potential for tissue repair.

The blood supply is within the cortical bone in both normal animals and humans. Even in the pathologically sclerotic bare lesion of degenerative arthritis the blood supply is on the surface (see Fig. 8-13). There is no need to drill to cancellous bone to expose blood vessels, because they are in abundance in the cortex.

There is a gross pathological difference between the rabbit's response to a drill hole and that seen in human tissue. The rabbit studies showed a differentiation of tissue along previous tissue layers.[71] The human drill hole does not differentiate by tissue layers but rather forms a fibrous and fibrocartilaginous plug below the level of the tidemark (Fig. 8-31).

The experimental animal model was not diseased.[70] The human model is pathological, usually degenerative arthritis, without covering articular cartilage when the drill hole is created.[41]

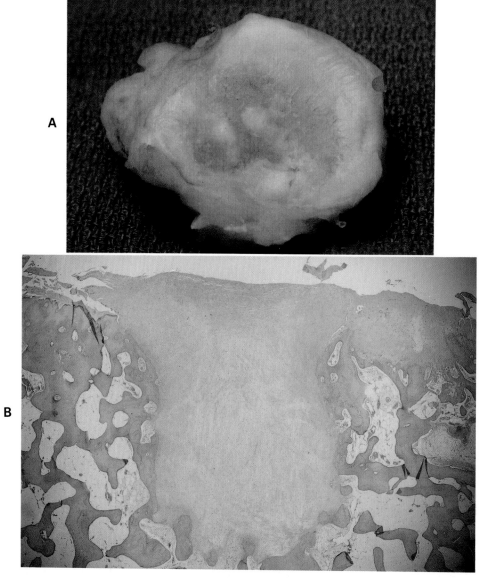

FIG. 8-31. Drill hole in human 26 months after open surgery.

A Gross photograph 26 months after open drilling of patella.
B Photomicrograph of lesion. Lesion measures 2.8 mm wide, 4.1 mm deep, and 0.7 mm high above bony platform. (Hematoxylin and eosin stain; ×40.)

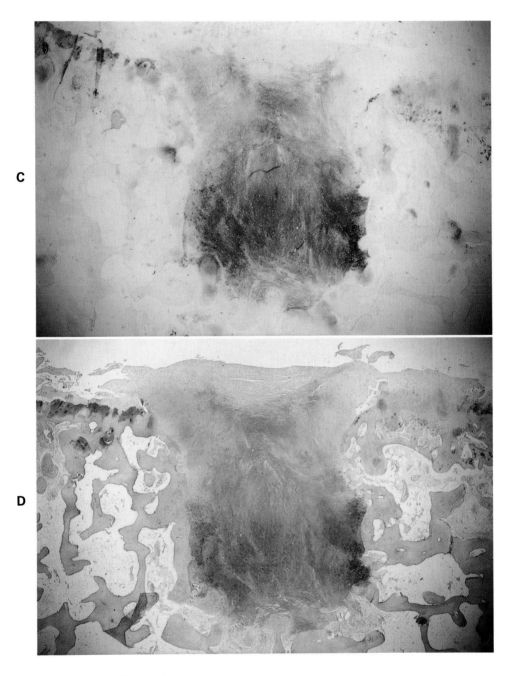

FIG. 8-31, cont'd

C Photomicrograph. (Toluidine blue stain; ×40.)
D Photomicrograph. (Safranin O stain; ×40.)

Drill holes in humans

A superficial drill hole limited to cortical bone results in hemorrhage, inflammation, fibrous tissue and fibrocartilage throughout the width and depth of the lesion (see Fig. 8-16, *A* and *B*). Spread of the fibrous repair is restricted by the surrounding surface of dead, exposed bony tissue (a bony sequestrum) (see Fig. 8-16, *C*). Multiple drill holes, superficial or deep, do not coalesce unless the surface of dead osteons is also debrided or unless drill holes are placed next to each other causing the same effect of removing dead surface tissue.

If the drill hole penetrates into the cancellous layer, the repair remains in the configuration of a plug (see Fig. 8-31, *B*). The surface is irregular and fibrous. The plug is a mixture of fibrous and fibrocartilage tissue (see Fig. 8-31, *D*). The fibrocartilage stains with safranin O, demonstrating histochemical evidence of glycosaminoglycans in the repair tissue.[67,82] The human drill hole surface remains fibrous. There is a fibrocartilaginous plug into cancellous bone or to the depth of the surgical lesion.

A surgical specimen from patellectomy taken 1 year postoperatively after open patellar drilling shows characteristic findings (see Fig. 8-31). The histochemical staining properties are positive for glycosaminoglycans. The surface is predominantly fibrous and stains weakly (Fig. 8-32, *A* and *B*). The fibrocartilage cells accompany dense histochemical staining on the edges of the drill hole near the bony vascular nutrient source (Fig. 8-32, *C*). On the other hand; the central area has fewer cells, is less densely stained, and even shows myxomatous degen-

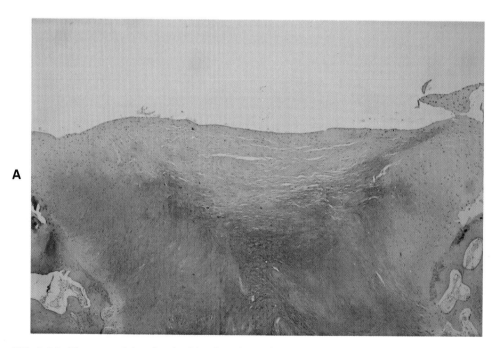

FIG. 8-32. Close-up histological look at human drill hole.

A Surface of drill hole is poorly organized fibrous tissue. (Safranin O stain; ×100.)

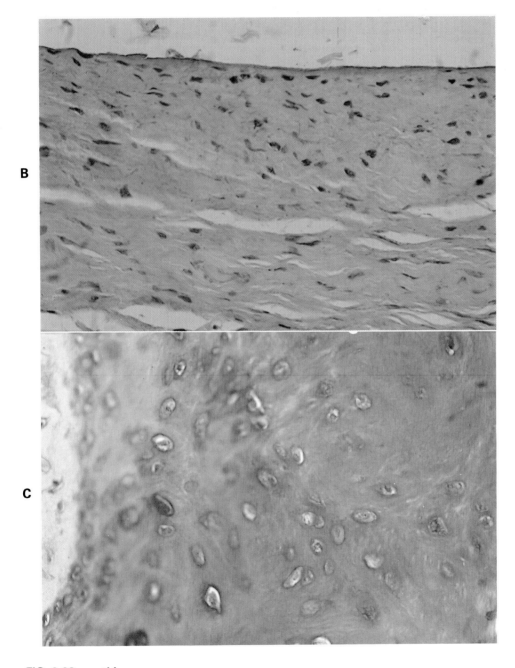

FIG. 8-32, cont'd

B Surface shows fibrous tissue. (Safranin O stain; ×400.)
C Margins of lesion show fibrocartilage near bone and blood supply of nutrition.
(Safranin O stain; ×400.)

Continued.

eration (Fig. 8-32, *D*). The size of the regenerated mass is larger than after abrasion (compare Figs. 8-31 and 8-40).

The histological and histochemical properties of the drill hole differ from those resulting from superficial debridement of a similar lesion (Fig. 8-40).

The tissue response to superficial debridement is uniformly positive histochemically and cartilaginous in nature throughout, top to bottom and side to side. The thinner mass of tissue places all cells closer to a synovial fluid source of nutrients (see Fig. 8-40). Compare the cellular appearance of fibrocartilage response to abrasion to that of a drill hole (see Fig. 8-32, *D*).

It has been suggested that a drill hole provides a better means of mechanical fixation. In practice the separation of postabrasion tissue has been clinically significant and confirmed by arthroscopy in two patients. Both cases involved rotational trauma. The abrasion technique involves creation of an irregular bony surface, providing for mechanical as well as biological fixation. Drill holes are not only unnecessary but contraindicated in the treatment of exposed bony areas on the articular surface of joints because of the failure of a uniform fibrocartilage response.

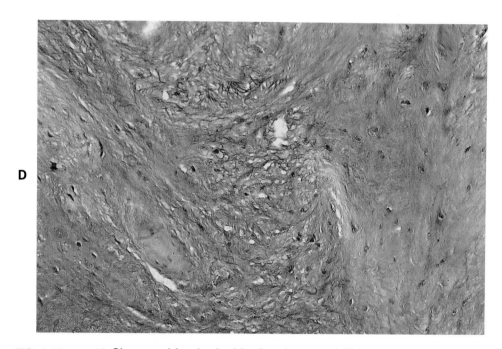

FIG. 8-32, cont'd. Close-up histological look at human drill hole.

D Center of drill hole shows irregular, acellular myxomatous tissue in area remote from source of nutrition. (Safranin O stain; ×200.)

Open conventional vs. arthroscopic surgery: effect on healing

There were no differences between healing of full-thickness lesions, whether repaired by open or arthroscopic methods. The subsequent hemorrhage and repair appeared similar on both arthroscopic and histological inspection.

Arthroscopic techniques minimize surgical exposure and allow accurate and minimal debridement. Motorized instrumentation with confined windows for resection removes only the degenerative tissue. This method preserves adjacent normal tissue, a technique not possible using knife blade by open or arthroscopic methods. The knife blade resection alters articular contours and surfaces unnecessarily, beyond the extent of the lesion.

Beyond the microresection techniques, arthroscopy includes the environmental benefit of saline effect to decrease proteoglycan weepage. This is the environmental factor that results in clot formation and repair of partial-thickness injuries.

PATHOLOGICAL TISSUE RESPONSE TO ABRASION

The debridement of the sclerotic lesion limited to the cortex results in bleeding demonstrated arthroscopically (Fig. 8-33, *A*). A blood clot forms (Fig. 8-33, *B* and *C*). Histological inspection shows the depth level to be just below the tidemark. (Fig. 8-33, *D*). A close-up of the junction shows a transition to adjacent articular cartilage (Fig. 8-33, *E*). The cortex shows hyperemia (Fig. 8-33, *D*).

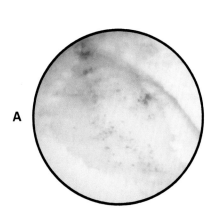

A

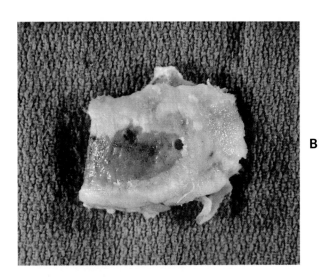

B

FIG. 8-33. Response of sclerotic lesions to intracortical abrasion.

A Arthroscopic appearance of sclerotic defect immediately after abrasion.
B Gross specimen 48 hours postoperatively, showing blood clot on surface. Specimen obtained from total knee operation by another surgeon.

Continued.

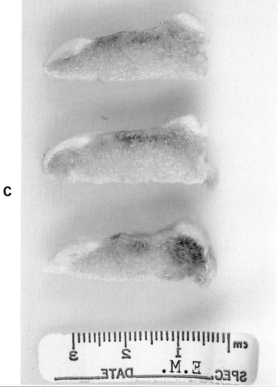

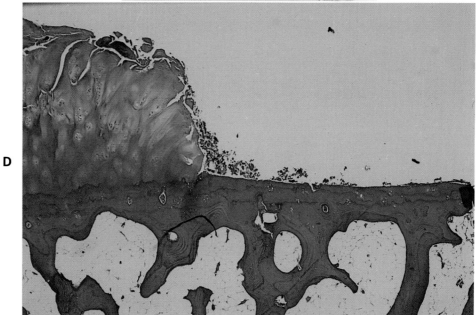

FIG. 8-33, cont'd. Response of sclerotic lesions to intracortical abrasion.

C Specimen sectioned for histopathological study. Note cortical hemorrhage (dark area) at area of abrasion.

D Photomicrograph of junction of articular cartilage and abrasion. (Hematoxylin and eosin stain; ×40.)

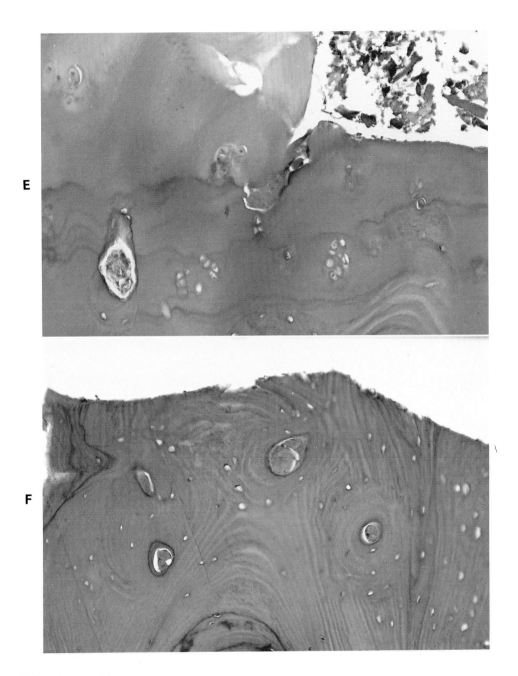

FIG. 8-33, cont'd

E Close-up of junction. (Hematoxylin and eosin stain; ×400.)

F Surface of abrasion at 48 hours shows vascular engorgement. Surface clot removed during preparation. (Hematoxylin and eosin stain; ×400.)

Arthroscopic appearance

Second-look arthroscopy shows a soft patch of fibrous tissue at 2 months (Fig. 8-34, *A*). The tissue is compressible and easily torn or elevated. There is an obvious need for continued joint protection.

The arthroscopic appearance at 3 to 4 months still may show vascular areas in otherwise avascular repair (Fig. 8-35, *A* and *B*).

Arthroscopic inspection at 6 months shows a soft, white tissue similar to a marshmallow in consistency. It is white and usually elevated above the adjacent yellow degenerative hyaline cartilage.

Arthroscopic inspection at 9 months shows firm white fibrocartilage (Fig. 8-36, *B* and *C*). It is soft to palpation and mechanically and biologically attached to cortical bone.

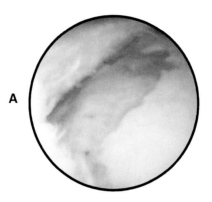

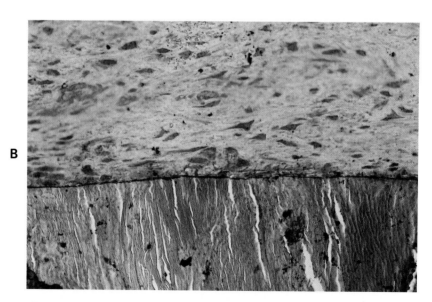

FIG. 8-34. Two months after arthroscopic abrasion arthroplasty.

A Arthroscopic view shows soft, pliable, white fibrous tissue covering defect.
B Biopsy at 2 months shows cortical bone platform and avascular spindle cell formation. (Gluteraldehyde preparation; ×400.)

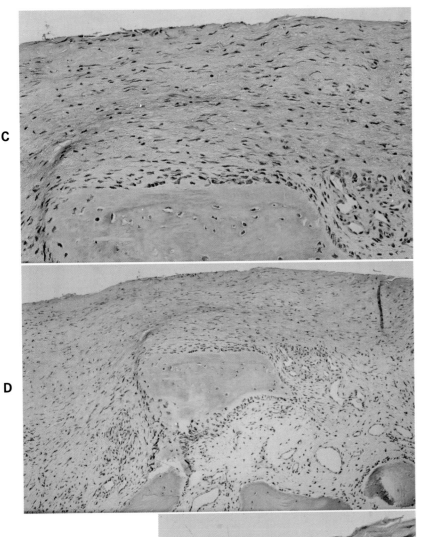

C Photomicrograph shows fibrous covering organizing on cortex. (Hematoxylin and eosin stain; ×100.)

D Photomicrograph of fibrous tissue repair at 2 months. (Hematoxylin and eosin stain; ×200.)

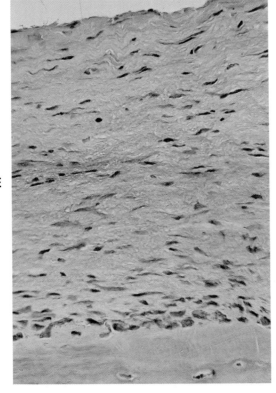

E Fibrous tissue repair on surface of live bone. Dead osteons were debrided. (Hematoxylin and eosin stain; ×400.)

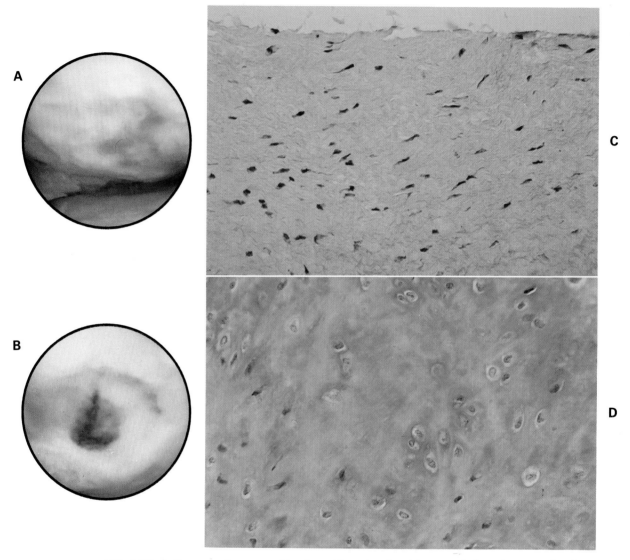

FIG. 8-35. Arthroscopic second looks with selective biopsy after arthroscopic abrasion arthroplasty.

A Arthroscopic view at 3 months after repair when cortex was excised to bleeding cancellous bone. Notice red color of vascular repair.

B Arthroscopic view at 4 months. There are still some areas of vascularity. Non-weight-bearing regimen was violated.

C Biopsy at 4 months in another patient shows healing of surface spindle cells. (Hematoxylin and eosin stain; ×400.)

D Photomicrograph of deeper area in patients shown in **C** shows fibrocartilage at 4 months. (Hematoxylin and eosin stain; ×400.)

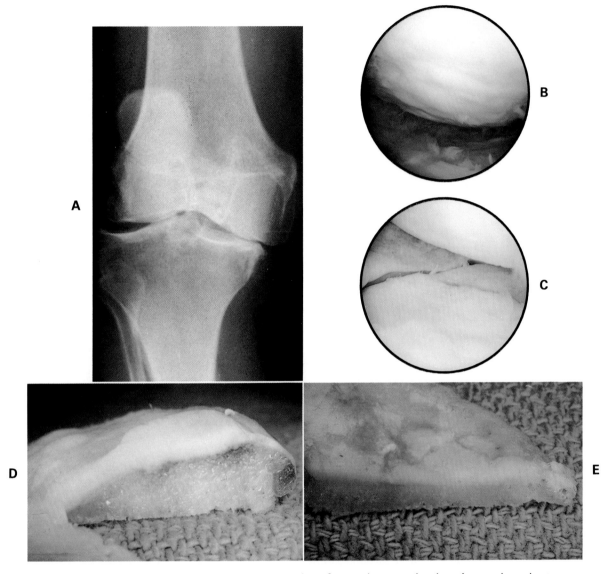

FIG. 8-36. Gross specimen—9 months after arthroscopic abrasion arthroplasty.

A Standing x-ray film shows mechanical instability, a contraindication that was unrecognized before the procedure. The following histological specimens were taken at time of subsequent total knee replacement.

B Arthroscopic view of repair tissue on femur after 9 months.

C Arthroscopic view of repair tissue on tibia after 9 months.

D Gross femoral specimen cutaway shows regrown depth of fibrocartilage at 9 months.

E Gross tibial specimen cutaway shows regrown fibrocartilage at 9 months.

Arthroscopic inspection between 1 and 3 years shows minimal surface fragmentation (see Fig. 9-58, *A*). The tissue is firmer in physically active patients, as opposed to the soft tissue seen in a sedentary person. The longest follow-up with arthroscopic inspection and biopsy is 4 years. This patient returned with degenerative change in other compartments. The reparative cartilage was smooth and firm and had a continuous seal to adjacent hyaline cartilage (see Fig. 8-40).

Gross appearance

Surgical specimens from the few patients who underwent subsequent total knee replacement afforded the best opportunity to observe the pathological process. The tissue is white and soft and often raised above adjacent cartilage (see Fig. 8-36, *D* and *E*). The compression forces of weight bearing undoubtedly level the surface. It is biologically well-secured to adjacent hyaline cartilage and cortical bone (Fig. 8-37).

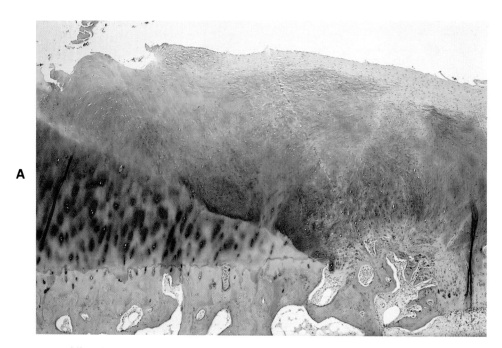

FIG. 8-37. Histological character of abrasion arthroplasty 9 months postoperatively.

A Photomicrograph shows junction of fibrocartilage and hyaline cartilage. Notice smooth biological and mechanical seal to adjacent tissue of cartilage and bone (Safranin O stain; ×40.)

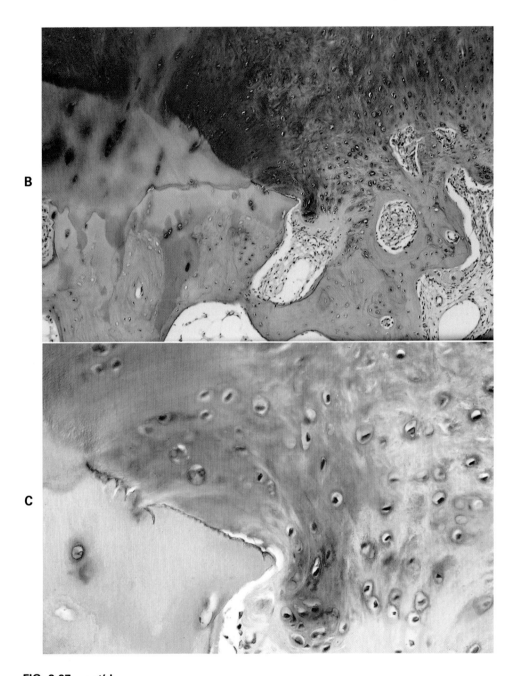

FIG. 8-37, cont'd

B Junction of fibrocartilage to bone and hyaline at tidemark. Notice vascularity in area of abrasion. (Safranin O stain; ×200.)

C High-power photomicrograph of junction at tidemark shows biological adherence. (Safranin O stain; ×400.)

Light microscopy

Hematoxylin and eosin, methylene blue, and safranin O staining methods have been applied. The special stains reflect the concentration of glycosaminoglycans in articular cartilage. The safranin O stain is thought to be a quantitative reflection of glycosaminoglycans in tissue.[67]

Histological comparison of hyaline and reparative fibrocartilage

The hyaline cartilage shows a well-defined bone-cartilage junction (Fig. 8-37) and tidemark. Vascularity is limited to the bone. The body of the cartilage shows few cells in chains or clumps (Figs. 8-38, C, and 8-39). The matrix shows increased histochemical staining for glycosaminoglycans in the pericellular zone. The surface is normally a region of flattened cells with tangentially arranged collagen (see Fig. 8-1, B).

Hyaline cartilage analysis of clinical specimens reveals degenerative change. There may be clumping of cells and fibrillation of the articular surface (see Fig. 8-38, A).

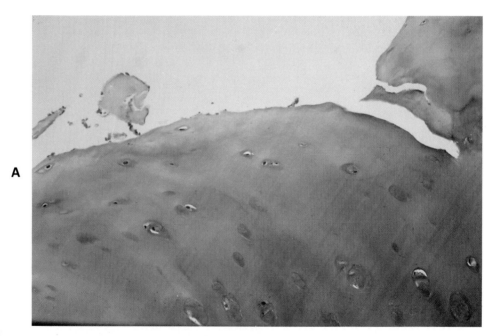

FIG. 8-38. Histological comparison of hyaline (degenerative) and adjacent reparative fibrocartilage. (Same patient as in Fig. 8-37.)

A Surface of degenerative hyaline cartilage. (Safranin O stain; ×400.)
B Surface of reparative fibrocartilage. (Safranin O ×400.)
C Central area of hyaline cartilage. (Safranin O stain ×400.)
D Central area of fibrocartilage. (Safranin O stain ×400.)

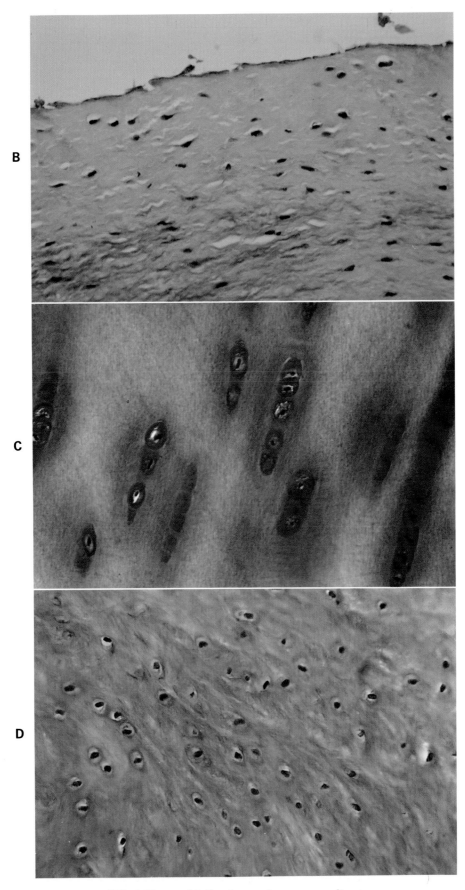

B

C

D

FIG. 8-38, cont'd. For legend see opposite page.

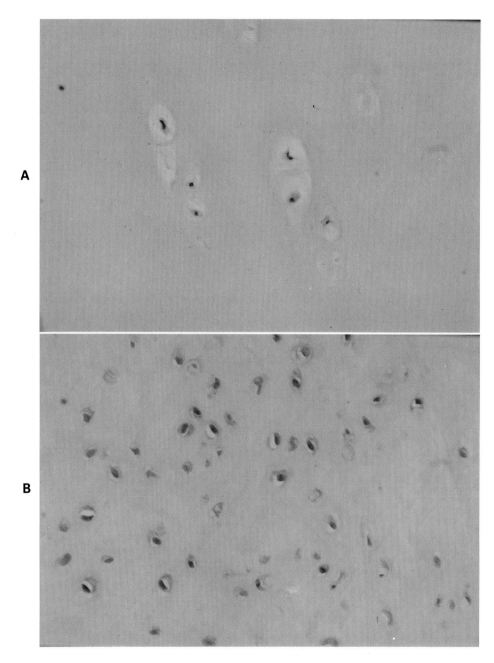

FIG. 8-39. Various staining properties of hyaline and reparative fibrocartilage. All ×400.

A Hyaline cartilage. (Hematoxylin and eosin stain; ×400.)
B Fibrocartilage. (Hematoxylin and eosin stain; ×400.)

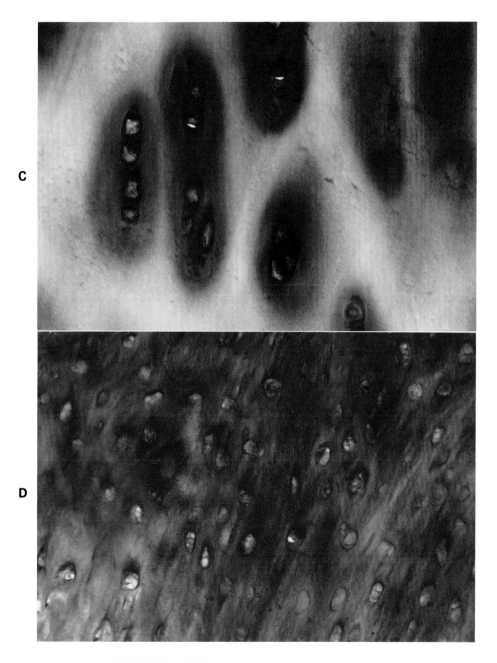

FIG. 8-39, cont'd

C Hyaline cartilage. (Toluidine blue stain; ×400.)
D Fibrocartilage. (Toluidine blue stain; ×400.)
Continued.

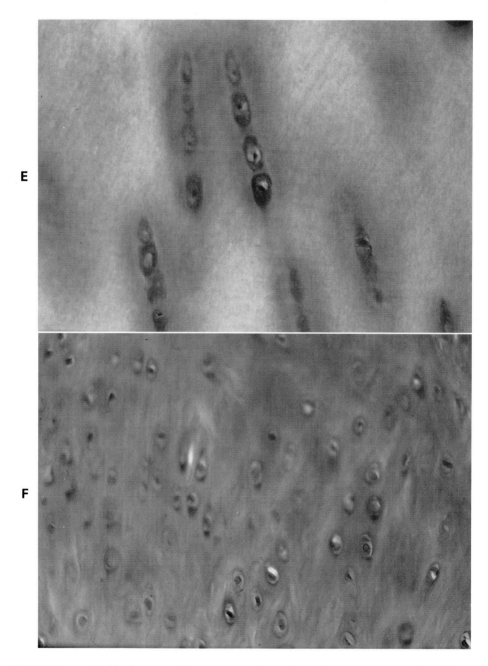

FIG. 8-39, cont'd. Various staining properties of hyaline and reparative fibrocartilage. All ×400.

E Hyaline cartilage. (Safranin O stain; ×400.)
F Fibrocartilage. (Safranin O stain; ×400.)

The reparative fibrocartilage is biologically adhered to adjacent hyaline cartilage and bone. The bone-fibrocartilage junction shows hypervascularity at 9 months (see Fig. 8-37, *C*). This is decreased at 4 years (Fig. 8-40). No tidemark is observed in biopsies through 2½ years. A specimen taken 4 years after abrasion procedures showed tissue differentiation with re-formation of the tidemark (see Fig. 8-40, *C*). The cells have a cartilaginous appearance with lacunae. The reparative fibrocartilage was very cellular, and there was no order to the pattern. There was an intense diffuse histochemical staining response for glycosaminoglycans (see Fig. 8-39, *F*).

Nearer to the surface there are fewer cells and decreased staining properties (see Fig. 8-38, *B*). Specimens taken at 9 months showed tangentially aligned fibrous tissue. The 4-year specimen showed integrity of all layers including the surface (see Fig. 8-40). This was a small area of abrasion in a physically active 40-year-old man.

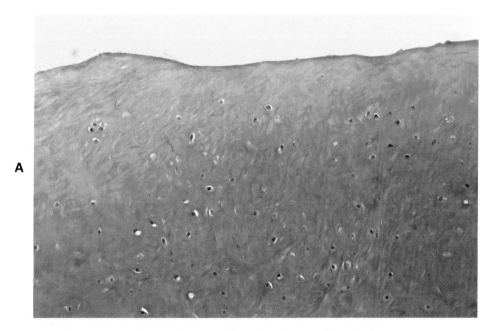

A

FIG. 8-40. Follow-up biopsy 4 years after abrasion arthroplasty.

A Photomicrograph of surface shows overview of tissue substance. Notice smooth surface. (Safranin O stain; × 100.) Tissue is 2.5 mm layer on bony platform.

Continued.

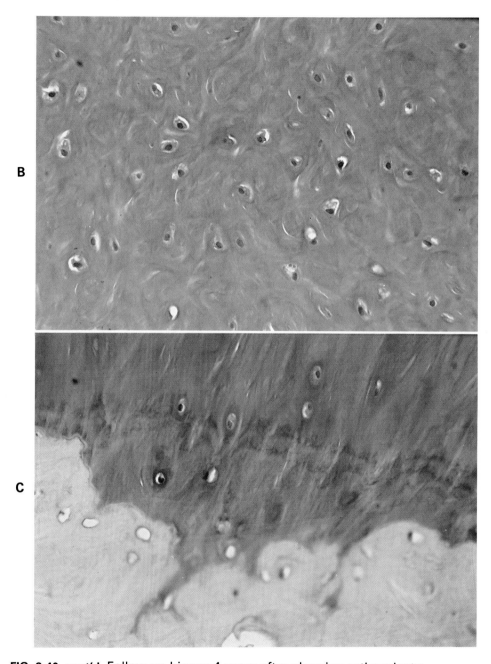

FIG. 8-40, cont'd. Follow-up biopsy 4 years after abrasion arthroplasty.

B Cellular character is cartilaginous. Staining shows positive for glycosaminoglycans. Matrix is fibrous. (Safranin O stain; ×400.)

C Regeneration of tidemark not seen in other biopsies of shorter follow-up. (Safranin O stain; ×400.)

Collagen typing of reparative fibrocartilage

I have submitted reparative fibrocartilage specimens to Dr. Fred Keeley at The Hospital for Sick Children Research Institute in Toronto for collagen typing[35] (Fig. 8-41).

There has been no evidence of type II collagen in any specimen; all of them failed the specific test to designate tissue as hyaline cartilage. The opportunity for specimens of adequate size is infrequent.

I do not know of any animal experiment or human biopsy specimen that has demonstrated regrown type II collagen. Lemperg emphatically states that articular cartilage defects in adults will not heal by formation of hyaline cartilage having mechanical and chemical properties equal to normal articular cartilage.[39] I agree. The tissue has been called "hyaline" based on cell morphological and histochemical stain findings. Any human specimen showing type II collagen must demonstrate that the exact area of biopsy correlates with the operative location. Any drilling procedure in which the surface is not completely removed leaves spaces between holes of residual hyaline cartilage islands, yielding false positive observation of type II collagen.

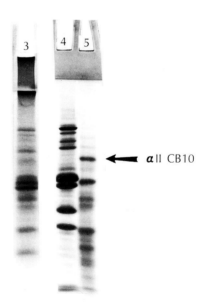

FIG. 8-41. Biochemical analysis for type II collagen shows presence in control specimen 5, none in control specimen 4 or patient specimen 3. (Courtesy of F.W. Keeley, Ph.D., Toronto, Ont.)

Cheung et al. demonstrated synthesis of type II collagen in hyaline cartilage adjacent to superficial and deep lacerations located short of the tidemark.[9] They had similar results in multiple 1 mm drill holes. Review of their article shows that the biopsies included regenerated fibrocartilage and adjacent normal hyaline cartilage. Their conclusion that the reparative tissue contained type II collagen could be incorrect, because the biopsies were not restricted to repair tissue.

Fate of regenerated tissue

Most cases demonstrate integrity of regenerated fibrocartilage for greater than 3 years following abrasion arthroplasty (see Fig. 8-40). The redevelopment of the joint space in 50% of the original series and arthroscopic second-look observations up to 4 years later support this observation (see Figs. 9-59 to 9-61).

I had two patients who had traumatic rotational injury 1 year after abrasion arthroplasty and sustained internal derangement with elevation of the fibrocartilage flap off the tibial surface (Fig. 8-42). Arthroscopic removal of the flap and repeat abrasion stabilized these conditions. In all patients with inflammatory, nonrheumatoid (seronegative) arthritis, the fibrocartilage appeared at 4 months and disappeared in 1 year. Repeat abrasion had the same result. Knee replacement was recommended.

Four patients of 102 had varus angulatory deformity exceeding 15 degrees and loss of regrown tissue. Repeat abrasion combined with osteotomy was performed (Fig. 8-43).

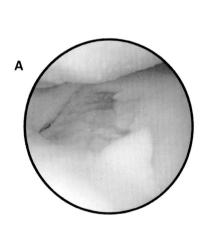
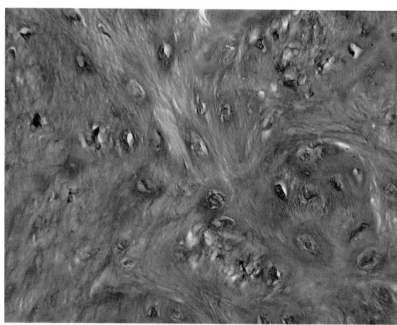

FIG. 8-42. Avulsion of regrown fibrocartilage.

A Arthroscopic view of tibial avulsion of flap of reparative fibrocartilage after rotational trauma.

B Photomicrograph shows fibrocartilage. (Safranin O stain; ×400.)

Tissue survival

How can this fibrocartilage survive when normal hyaline cartilage was unable to survive in the first place? The implication is that hyaline cartilage should be in that area, even though the joint environment has more superior properties for survival of reparative fibrocartilage. This is undoubtedly true in the normal environment of the knee joint. It must be assumed that the local environment was hostile to the hyaline cartilage, whether by pressure or biochemical wear.[19,30,69,84,86] Restoration of normal hyaline cartilage to the existing hostile joint environment may only result in the repeated demise of the cartilage. If the local environment is not altered by mechanical osteotomy or possibly some biochemical change, the regrown composite tissue or reparative fibrocartilage has proven to survive where the hyaline cartilage failed. It could then be concluded that the reparative tissue, seen to exist there in the natural historical pathological state as patches, has certain properties that allow it to maintain its integrity in an environment that is hostile to hyaline cartilage.

Why does tissue survive after abrasion arthroplasty? The bony debridement, which is minimal, creates an intact bony platform. The cortex maintains its integrity.[39] The vascular response is achieved without creating cancellous fractures. The entire area of dead osteons is resected to the margin of adequate cartilage. The resultant attachment of fibrocartilage to bone and surface is both biological and mechanical (see Fig. 8-37).

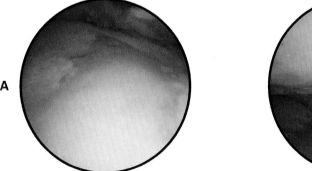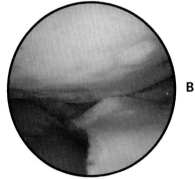

FIG. 8-43. Loss of reparative fibrocartilage in presence of severe angulatory deformity; 1 year after arthroscopic abrasion arthroplasty.

A Arthroscopic view of medial tibia.
B Arthroscopic view of medial femur shows one small patch of regrown tissue.

The minimal insult of arthroscopic abrasion permits early active motion to resist ankylosis and fibrosis. The cellular pattern of postabrasion fibrocartilage is more cartilaginous than that in human drill holes. The drill hole has more fibrous tissue (see Figs. 8-31 and 8-32). Abrasion involves a thinner layer of tissue as compared to the larger mass of deeper or wider cortical resections. Cartilage nutrition comes via diffusion from joint fluid. The thinner layer or mass of tissue places cells closer to nutrition. The deeper mass of tissue may break down from malnutrition (see Fig. 8-32, D). Tissues that depend on vascularity for nutrition become myxomatous when removed from a source of blood (see Fig. 8-32, D).

Perhaps the most important factor in success in this treatment is to cooperate with the natural healing process. The tissue is already attempting repair. The natural pathological processes of hemorrhage and islands of repair demonstrate this fact. The debridement of necrotic tissue, resultant hemorrhage, protection from loads, avascular fibrous repair, and conversion to reparative fibrocartilage are achieved.

Contrary to the ideas expressed in the literature,[42] pathological studies show reparative fibrocartilage survival, maturation, and differentiation through the first 5 years of clinical experience in properly chosen cases. I believe this finding is related to the different cellular morphological characteristics and the thin tissue mass of superficial abrasion, as opposed to that necessary in drilling or decortication.

FACTORS IN ABRASION SURGERY
Site of lesion

The tissue response was the same, independent of the location in the knee of the abraded sclerotic lesion. If the lesion was adjacent to a bone-synovial junction the synovial pannus contributed to repair in the adjacent area.

The clinical results were best in medial compartment lesions. The lateral compartment and patellar surfaces produced fair results. When the femoral trochlea was abraded, the result was poor. Multiple compartment abrasions were attempted in a few patients, all with failure. I have abandoned the use of this procedure in such cases.

Size of lesion

Experimental full-thickness lesions exceeding 3 mm up to 9 mm in horses resulted in defective repair of the femur.[12] The opposite tibial surface became degenerative when large lesions were excised into cancellous bone.

Depth was an important but unemphasized dimension of these experimental lesions. They cannot be considered the same as the pathological sclerotic lesion of degenerative joint disease. The large experimental lesions cut into cancellous bone, whereas the sclerotic lesion is confined to the cortex.

The size of the sclerotic lesion in patients is not as critical as their body weight, joint alignment, instability, or willingness to protect the joint during the postoperative period. The larger lesions (3 to 5 cm) are associated with a more severe process, even angulation, instability, or ankylosis. These factors are important to clinical success, not the pathological response.

Depth of lesion

Hjertquist and Lemperg demonstrated that cartilaginous tissue of mature appearance would not occur unless the subchondral bone plate in the base of an experimentally created defect was restored.[29] If marrow were not sealed over with bone plate (cortex), immature fibrous tissue existed. These authors theorized that the restored subchondral bone plate supports the regenerate tissue and acts as a pressure distributor, giving correct differentiation stimulus.

Richmond et al. showed that the depth of an experimental abrasion in degenerative sclerotic lesions of dogs affected the type of cellular response.[66] If debridement was limited to the cortex, cartilage cells formed. If the cortex was penetrated, only a primitive fibrous response was observed.

Both of these experimental observations support and are consistent with observations made in human abrasion arthroplasty.

Configuration of lesion

The configuration of a lesion is important only when mobile or overhanging degenerative tissue exists. Fragments are debrided. Adequate resection stabilizes the edges and promotes sealing of the lesion to adjacent tissue.

Deformity

Axial malalignment of the lower extremity may cause excessive load and wear patterns and affect the surface response[70] (see Fig. 8-43). Angulation of under 10 degrees of varus or 15 degrees of valgus is considered safe to treat the surface without osteotomy in a patient with a low activity level. All angulatory problems should be corrected in an active person unless the lesion is small (less than 2 cm).

The patella should be repositioned in young people. In older people with bony deformity and degenerative change, repositioning may accentuate symptoms because of patellofemoral incongruity. The tissue initially heals, but excessive forces cause degradation.

Range of motion

A fixed loss of motion adversely affects healing because motion is essential to surface repair. This is especially so in the shoulder joint.

The presence of a moderate decrease in range of motion has not adversely affected any articular healing following arthroscopic chondroplasty of exposed areas. I use the same criteria of motion as for osteotomy.[14,15]

Instability

Instability of the patellofemoral joint, of the knee cruciate ligament origin, or of the shoulder joint causes failure of repair caused by shearing force. Second-look arthroscopy often shows progression of the sclerotic articular condition.

The uncontrolled, unstable, anterior cruciate–deficient knee, even with the removal of offending torn meniscal fragments by arthroscopic means, sustains further articular injury. Delays in surface healing commonly occur, including production of loose bodies. Control of the instability in an abrasion patient with a brace, activity modification, muscle rehabilitation, or ligament reconstruction sustains surface healing.

A repeat subluxation or dislocation of the patella following patellar abrasion further injures or delays the articular reparative process. A patient with malalignment or lateral compression of the patella that is easily demonstrated on x-ray film and is not corrected at the time of patellar abrasion will have impaired healing of the articular surface.

The same factors affect the results of partial-thickness debridement.

Weight or force

Weight or force across a joint adversely affects the response to injury, disease, and surgical debridement. Obesity adversely affects the load on the lower extremity. Failure to repair and even loss of repair has been seen arthroscopically. The load may be in the form of excessive weight lifting during the rehabilitation process. The joint is compressed and carried through a range of motion, which adversely affects the healing tissue.

Weight-bearing pressure

Full weight bearing on either partial-thickness articular injuries or full-thickness injuries to exposed bone delayed repair and maturation to a smooth surface. Intraarticular shaving of a half-thickness lesion of a femoral condyle usually required 1 month of non-weight bearing to seal the surface. Immediate weight bearing resulted in a rough surface and even worse symptoms for the patient.

After abrasion arthroplasty or trauma to a weight-bearing bony surface, a period of 8 weeks was necessary to facilitate early tissue maturation and reduction in vascularity. Lesions as small as 4 mm were still vascular at 5 weeks when the patient walked on the extremity. In bilateral cases, unavoidable weight bearing delayed maturation and change from a vascular to a fibrocartilaginous surface beyond 6 months (Fig. 8-44). Some patients required repeat debridement and postoperative protection.

Progressive quadriceps exercises will slow the smoothing and healing that follow patellar debridement procedures. This produces synovitis, fine loose bodies, and an irregularly healed surface. Normally the patellar surface that is protected but still allowed normal daily activity will show maturation and a smooth fibrous tissue surface at 1 month.

Clinical experience with a large avulsion of the articular surface occurred from osteochondral fracture or power lawn mower avulsion injuries. There was no contact with the opposite articular surface, and there was ankylosis. These defects are usually peripheral and fill in with large masses of fibrous tissue. A non-weight-bearing activity program is instituted following condylar shaving or arthroscopic abrasion.

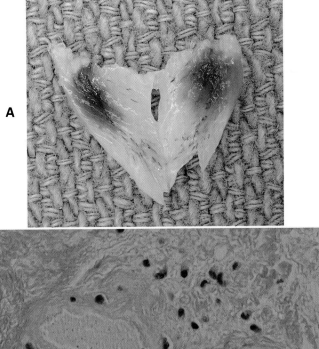

FIG. 8-44. Histological view of tissue response to weight bearing after abrasion arthroplasty.

A Gross specimen shows vascularity at 7 months of partial weight-bearing in bilateral abrasion arthroplasty.

B Photomicrograph of same patient showing fibrovascular proliferation. (Hematoxylin and eosin stain; ×400.)

Presence of meniscus

Articular cartilage loss exists both with and without a torn meniscus. Articular cartilage repair occurs both with and without a meniscal tear. The continued abnormal mobility of the tear can wear the articular surface down so that impingement no longer occurs and the surface can heal. The complete removal of a torn lateral meniscus in an adolescent has resulted in delayed articular healing and even further destruction. The same has been observed in the adult with total medial meniscus removal and tibia valgus or varus. Presence of the meniscus seems more important to the injured or deformed knee in promoting articular healing.

Mobilization

Immobilization has an adverse effect on cellular organization and results in fibrous adhesion[25,83] (Fig. 8-45). Intermittent active motion has been shown experimentally to result in better tissue formation than immobilization.[71] Continuous passive motion causes the most normal-appearing tissue, but it has not been demonstrated to produce hyaline cartilage. The evidence is histologically based and does not include collagen typing studies.[71]

Immobilization results in a greater incidence of fibrous adhesions following open or arthroscopic surgery. Arthroscopic procedures promote early motion with decreased morbidity.

Exercise

Staged activity is an important component of the healing process. Doing nothing can be as bad as doing too much. The most common cause of postoperative effusion is doing too much too soon, especially in the degenerative knee. Acceleration-deceleration exercises, including aerobic dancing, should be deferred in cases of surgical repair on the meniscus or ligaments.

In general the patient protects the joint during the healing phase, increasing the range of motion within the limits of discomfort. After healing activity may be progressively increased within tolerance.

Effect of aspirin

Simmons reported the benefit of aspirin on cartilage degeneration.[10,73] The size of the lesion was reduced. The treated rabbits showed no cellular clumping or the usual evidence of degeneration.

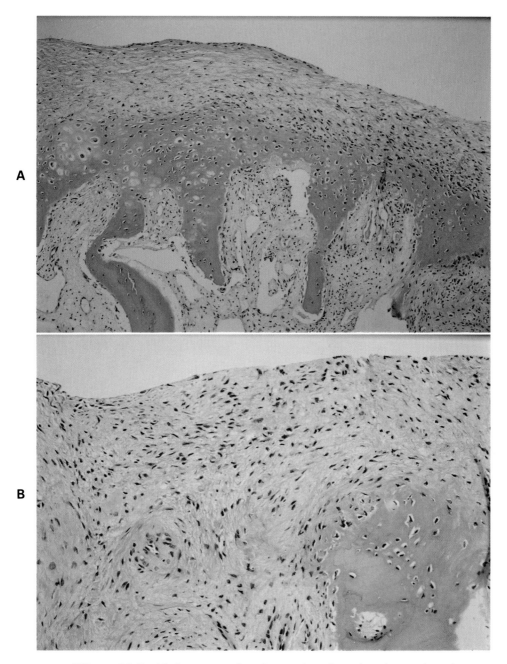

FIG. 8-45. Effect of failed joint protection 2 months after abrasion arthroplasty.

A Photomicrograph of fibrous tissue on new bone. (Hematoxylin and eosin stain; ×40.)

B Disorganized fibrous vascular tissue. (Hematoxylin and eosin stain; ×200.)

Continued.

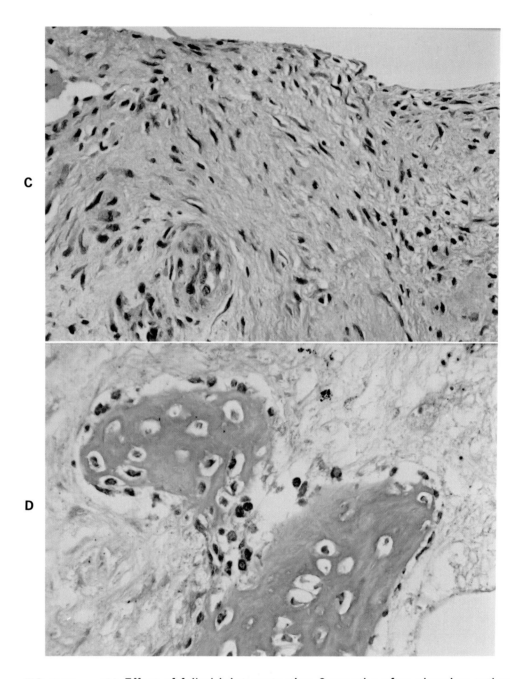

FIG. 8-45, cont'd. Effect of failed joint protection 2 months after abrasion arthroplasty.

C Spindle cell fibroblast with blood vessels at surface. Not seen with intermittent active motion (non-weight bearing). (Hematoxylin and eosin stain; ×400.)

D Osteoclastic activity not seen in protected joints. (Hematoxylin and eosin stain; ×400.)

Osteonecrosis

Osteonecrosis is a localized area of dead bone (Fig. 8-46, *A*). Although found infrequently, it is most commonly seen on the femur and less commonly on the tibia. It is usually found in a patient who has degenerative arthritis. Its onset can be sudden, although the process may be preceded by several months of pain. Osteonecrosis can be accompanied by extreme pain with weight bearing or even by fragmentation of bone or loose bodies.

In cases of longer duration, the necrotic area can be seen by x-ray film. In patients with a rather acute onset of osteonecrosis of a small area, it may only be discovered at the time of arthroscopic surgery. The area may be well localized and demonstrated only by careful probing or palpation of the femoral condyle and tibial plateau. In this case the arthroscopic surgeon becomes very much like a dentist. He or she identifies the lesion and performs debridement. Arthroscopic debridement in small, localized osteonecrosis, followed by joint protection, reduces symptoms. (less than 1 cm) A corrective osteotomy may be performed.

In areas where there is gross loss of the articular surface on the femur, a hemiarthroplasty or total knee replacement is indicated (see Fig. 8-46, *A*).

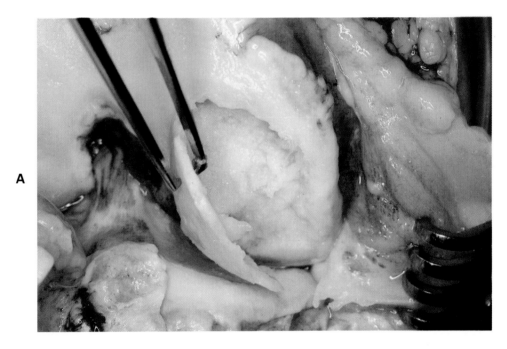

A

FIG. 8-46. Osteonecrosis.

A Operative photograph of large osteonecrotic area held with forceps off of medial condyle.

Continued.

It is interesting to note that the surface bone of a sclerotic lesion is osteonecrotic (Fig. 8-46, *B* to *D*). Most cases that I have seen of so-called clinical osteonecrosis with a well-circumscribed cavity have featured a degenerative joint, loss of articular surface, necrosis over a wide surface area, and a well-localized area of necrosis deeper on the femoral condyle. The exact etiological relationship is not known at this time.

B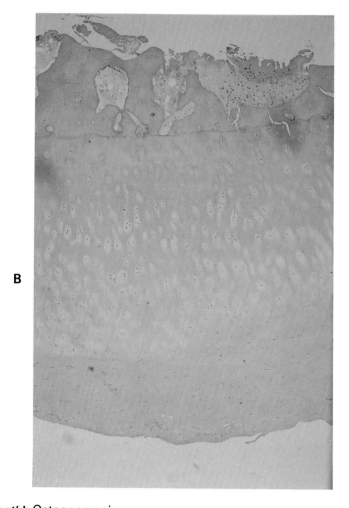

FIG. 8-46, cont'd. Osteonecrosis.

B Photomicrograph of loose articular fragment of bone at base. (Hematoxylin and eosin stain; ×20.)

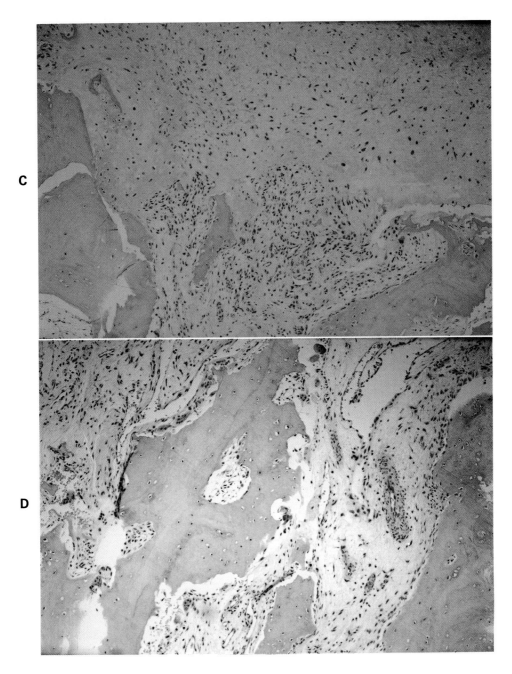

FIG. 8-46, cont'd

C Photomicrograph of fibrovascular invasion in base of lesion. (Hematoxylin and eosin stain; ×100.)

D Photomicrograph shows osteoclasts and fibrovascular invasion at base of lesion. (Hematoxylin and eosin stain; ×100.)

Osteochondritis dissecans

Osteochondritis dissecans, although not common in the general population, is common in an orthopedic surgeon's practice. It occurs in a young person with the onset of pain in the knee joint. It occurs in the elbow as Panner's disease. It may manifest itself by the presence of loose bodies in the initial stages and has a high incidence of being bilateral.

The pathological lesion is separation of a portion of bone, usually on the medial femoral condyle in the knee, although it occasionally can occur laterally (Fig. 8-47, A). The base of the defect is covered with a fibrocartilaginous tissue, very much as if the patient has had a fracture or an avulsion (Fig. 8-47, B and C). The piece will be alive if it is still attached to vascularity or by a pedicle to synovium. If it is separated from the bone, it becomes a loose body. As Barrie has described, bone necrosis occurs in the absence of blood supply in the free loose body.

The bone surface is covered with an fibrocartilaginous or fibrous tissue. On pathological analysis neither the base nor the piece is considered normal where there is already fragmentation.

In the early stages where there is no separation of articular cartilage on the surface, it is possible that the bone could be reconstituted if the lesion were drilled. My experience has not been uniformly satisfactory. At this time, I combine debridement of the base of the fragment and defect with compression screws to create immobilization (see Fig. 9-19).

In the case of loose (yet attached) fragments, the pathological findings dictate taking the lesion apart. The base of the fragment is debrided to vascularity, but not so deep that the fragment cannot be set back in. The joint is decompressed so that bleeding can be seen. If there is not enough bone or there is a

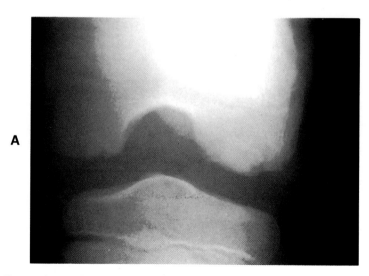

A

FIG. 8-47. Osteochondritis dissecans.

A Anteroposterior x-ray film of knee shows osteochondritis dessicans lesion of medial femoral condyle and nonpathological growth variation on lateral femoral condyle.

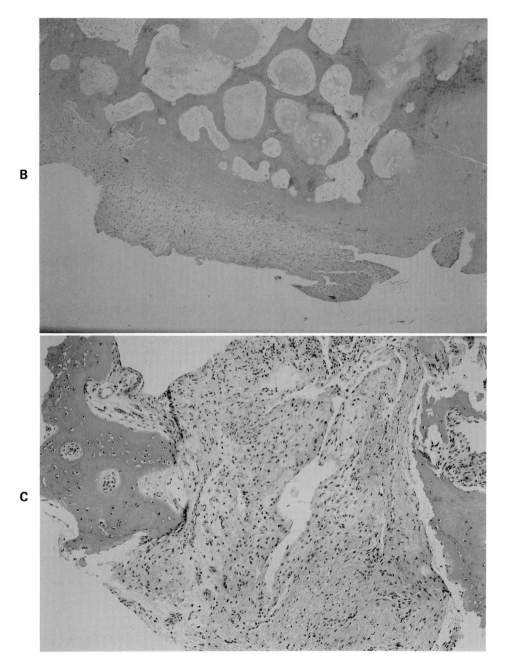

FIG. 8-47, cont'd

B Photomicrograph of biopsy specimen of base shows fibrous tissue covering deep side of fragment. (Hematoxylin and eosin stain; ×40.)
C Biopsy of femoral defect base shows fibrovascular proliferation. (Hematoxylin and eosin stain; ×100.)

lack of integrity or vascularity the chances of success are reduced. After the fibrous tissue is debrided to ensure vascularity on both sides, adequate fixation and protection are required until there is an osseous union.

If the fragment is partially dislodged, arthroscopic debridement and repair with internal fixation result in union by 8 weeks. If the piece has dislodged or fragmented, the crater is covered with fibrous tissue. The loose bodies are removed. Superficial debridement results in repair bleeding into surgically smoothed adjacent cartilage. Repair is fibrous and often with depression of the surface. Second-look arthroscopic follow-up 5 years later shows intact fibrocartilage with surface degeneration.

Replacement of long-standing loose bodies has had mixed results in my experience.

Loose bodies

Loose bodies can be of meniscus or articular cartilage. This is determined by histological identification.

The presence of loose bodies results in effusion that adversely affects the chemical and enzymatic joint environment (see Fig. 8-7). A large loose body may cause giving-out of the knee joint or repeat injury with locking. The natural history of small loose bodies is eventual absorption or engulfment by synovium (see Fig. 8-8). Before that, they rest in gravity-dependent recesses, especially around popliteus tendon.

The most common and smallest loose bodies are wear particles of the articular cartilage.[53] These can be seen in people who have developed overuse syndrome from considerable running, weight lifting, or other forms of exercise that involve carrying the knee through a range of motion with excessive loads.

These loose bodies appear arthroscopically within the joint like small, fine, floating "bacon strips." These are easily vacuumed out at the time of the diagnostic arthroscopy with suction on the arthroscope.

As the fragments become a little larger and gain some depth, breadth, and width, they can be more easily visualized. They appear as multiple, fine loose bodies in and about the joint. These loose bodies are engulfed by the synovium and then absorbed (see Fig. 8-7).

It is diagnostic and therapeutic to vacuum the loose bodies. They can be seen on microscopy if the cell block is carried out on the joint aspirate. The debris is visualized in the cell block. It is possible to make a diagnosis of its origin, whether it be articular, meniscal, or synovial.

Histological studies on the loose bodies show fibrous tissue over the area with live cartilaginous tissue and nonviable bony tissue (see Fig. 8-19).

An excellent article by Barrie[2] gives a very clear description of the pathological process of loose bodies.

Preoperatively, care must be taken to ascertain whether a loose body is present within the joint. Care must be taken to ensure that its presence does not involve a mimicking avulsion fracture or an ossicle within the meniscus, one in the juxtaarticular position in the fat pad, or even one outside the synovium.

Chondrocalcinosis

Chondrocalcinosis may be seen by x-ray examination in the intraarticular cartilage and menisci[58,68,90] (Fig. 8-48, *A*). Arthroscopic inspection clearly shows chondrocalcinosis accompanying degenerative changes in the articular surfaces (Fig. 8-48, *B* and *C*). These are differentiated by polarized light from deposition of gouty crystals, pseudogout, and previous injections of hydrocortisone acetate (Fig. 8-48, *D* and *E*). In some areas of bare bone, patches of white cartilage must be differentiated.

Histologically the crystalline lesions usually occur near the surface. They are often surrounded by a myxomatous, acellular change and include the crystalline material. There is no reaction by synovium, cellular proliferation, or vascularization.

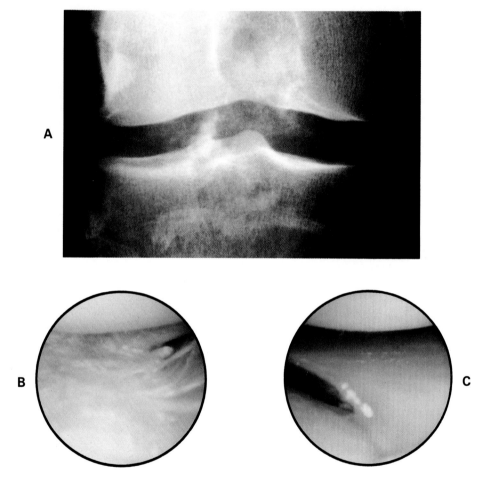

FIG. 8-48. Chondrocalcinosis.

A Anteroposterior x-ray film shows calcific deposits in articular cartilage and meniscus.

B Arthroscopic view of degenerative meniscus with fragmentation and calcific deposits.

C Arthroscopic view of calcium deposits on inner margin of meniscus.

Continued.

597

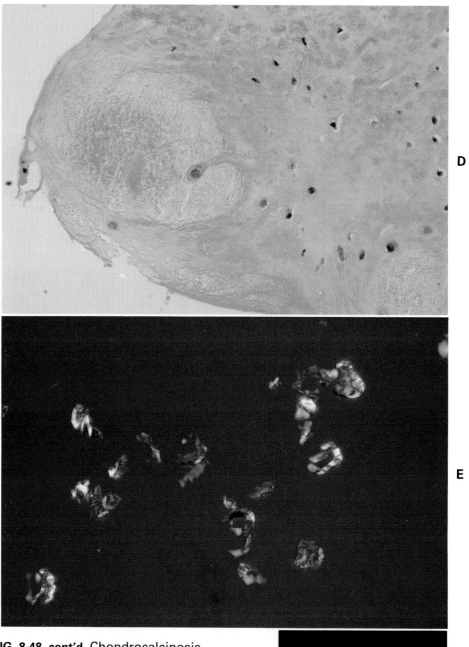

FIG. 8-48, cont'd. Chondrocalcinosis.

D Photomicrograph shows calcium deposit in tip of meniscus (Hematoxylin and eosin stain; ×200.)

E Polarized light shows berefringement crystals (Hematoxylin and eosin stain; ×400.)

F Cross-section of meniscus in pseudogout.

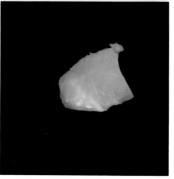

MENISCAL DISEASE

The meniscus is altered by trauma and/or degeneration. To differentiate the exact role of each process is difficult. Repeated trauma in young athletes shows premature degeneration. An acute, minimal tear in a previously asymptomatic knee will often show signs of degeneration in a meniscal specimen.

Trauma

Clear, traumatic, etiological factors are present in younger patients (Fig. 8-49). These are usually longitudinal, transverse, or bucket-handle tears (Fig. 8-50).

The natural history of an untreated traumatic tear is to shrink in size, to become rounded on the edge, and to seek a position away from weight-bearing surfaces. On histological analysis this tear, which was created by trauma, subsequently shows degeneration in tissue (see Fig. 8-53).

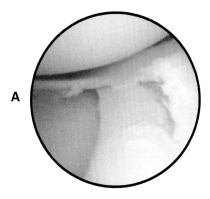

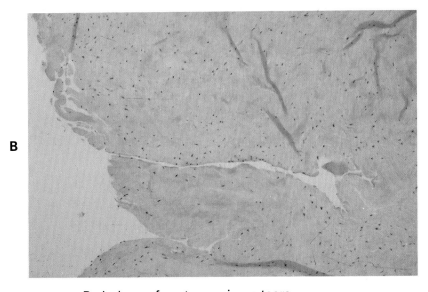

FIG. 8-49. Pathology of acute meniscus tears.

A Arthroscopic view of longitudinal tear of medial meniscus.
B Photomicrograph of tear. (Hematoxylin and eosin stain; ×40.)

Continued.

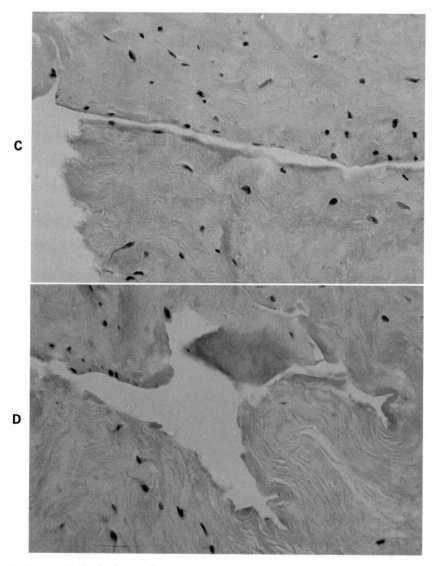

FIG. 8-49, cont'd. Pathology of acute meniscus tears.

C Photomicrograph of tear shows absence of cellular or vascular repair. (Hematoxylin and eosin stain; ×200.)

D Base of cleft shows myxomatous change of acellularity. (Hematoxylin and eosin stain; ×400.)

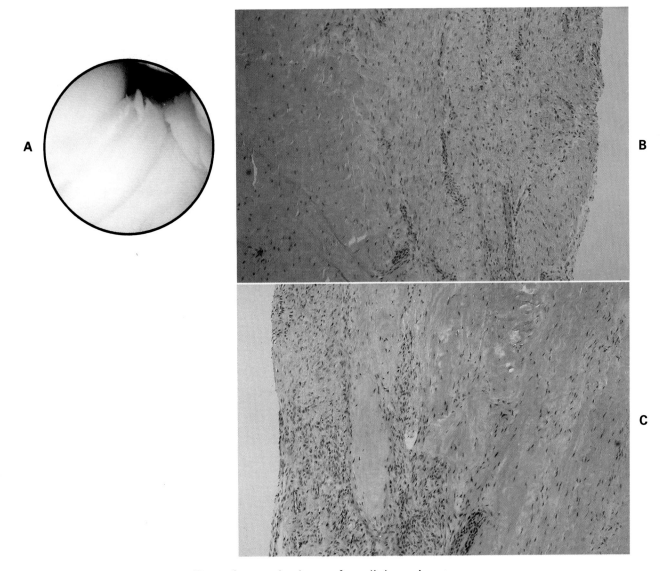

FIG. 8-50. Tear of posterior horn of medial meniscus.

A Arthroscopic view of posterior horn longitudinal tear from posteromedial approach.

B Photomicrograph of thin fibrovascular covering of meniscus. (Hematoxylin and eosin stain; ×40.)

C Photomicrograph of section of edge of capsular margin tears. Notice fibrous cellular and vascular proliferation over capsular tissue. (Hematoxylin and eosin stain; ×40.)

Trauma can cause deformation of the meniscus shape without rupture. Interstitial tissue separation can exist without rupture through the meniscus, which prevents visual identification. Often surface alterations show separation of the surface with an interstitial lesion but no penetration.

Degeneration

The degenerative process occurs on the surface and within the substance of the meniscus[50] (Figs. 8-51 and 8-52). Degenerative changes are seen on the inner rim of the meniscus. These are readily identified by arthroscopy. The first sign of degeneration is the loss of the normal opaque appearance of the inner rim. It becomes translucent like glass.

A separation of the translucent rim becomes a tag (see Fig. 8-51). These usually separate, become free in the joint, and eventually become absorbed by synovium. They are usually asymptomatic and found incidentally. A larger separation becomes a fringe tear. This size of tear may produce symptoms in an otherwise normal meniscus. When such a lesion is identified arthroscopically, superficial debridement is performed.

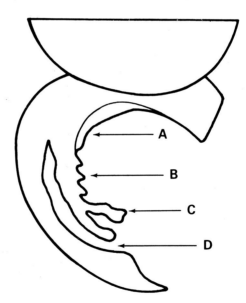

FIG. 8-51. *A,* Translucent inner border is first sign of degeneration of meniscus. *B,* Fringe tags occur when some translucent area sloughs off. *C,* Fringe tags of or elevations of translucent inner degeneration may catch in joint and mimic positive McMurray sign. *D,* Cleft tears or complete tears within meniscus can occur when collagen bundles completely separate.

A greater separation of the inner margin develops a tear with a sharp margin, often referred to as a parrot-beak type. A transverse tear may occur (see Fig. 8-51). This is most often at the posterior horn of the medial meniscus or the midportion of the lateral meniscus.

Degeneration within the meniscal substance causes loss of mobility, flexibility, and consistency of substance as well as increased tissue hardness.

The surface of the meniscus changes from opaque white to yellow. Deposits of crystalline material often separate collagen bundles. These are visualized arthroscopically.

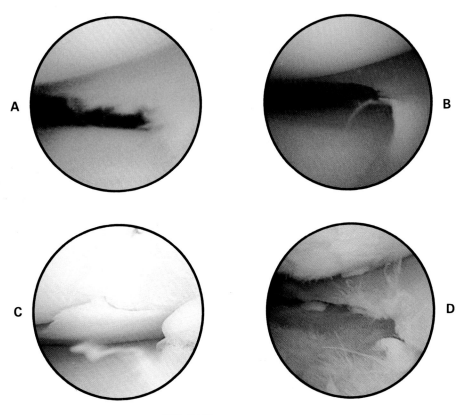

FIG. 8-52

A Fringe tags.
B Fringe tear.
C Cleft tear.
D Diffuse degeneration.

Interstitial degeneration may produce pain, especially with myxomatous or cystic change but no arthroscopically identifiable lesion (see Fig. 8-53). Resection should be deferred in the absence of a tear or deformation.

Longitudinal and horizontal cleft tears are the first manifestations of degenerative meniscal separation (Fig. 8-53). The combination of tears in both planes appears as complex tear. The complex tear has a high association with articular degeneration.

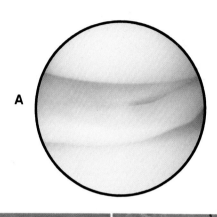

A

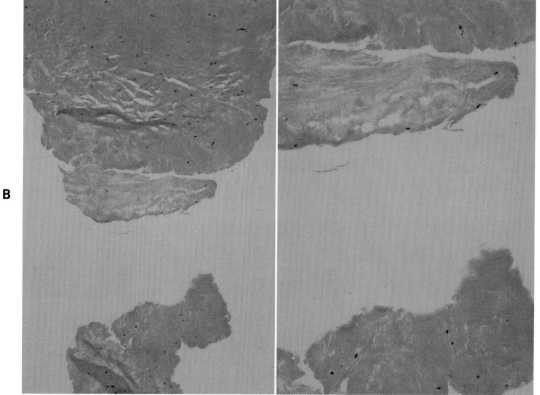

B

C

FIG. 8-53. Traumatic tear by history that is degenerative in nature.

A Arthroscopic view of posteromedial longitudinal tear

B Photomicrograph shows cleft and necrotic edges at tear. (Hematoxylin and eosin stain; ×100.)

C Close-up shows acellular myxomatous changes on margin tear. (Hematoxylin and eosin stain; ×200.)

In evaluating a degenerative meniscus in a degenerative compartment, etiological factors are important to treatment and prognosis. The degenerative meniscal tear causing articular changes is weighed against a diffuse degenerative process involving both meniscus and articular cartilage. The question is, Will meniscectomy reduce the patient's symptoms and interrupt the process of mechanical origin? If the condition is diffuse degeneration, osteotomy or even joint replacement should be the treatment choice. Most often this etiological determination is not possible because of the late stage of both meniscal and cartilage degeneration.

Total removal of a meniscus that is in an already degenerative compartment will lead to progressive symptoms and further degeneration. The disease process involves more of the joint than just the meniscus.

Diagnostic and treatment implications

The meniscus should be visualized and probed for the most subtle surface and interstitial changes. Sometimes flap tears are hidden under meniscus that has reshaped to the joint contour.

Interstitial tears may be incomplete, not breaking through the surface. Some normal diagnostic examinations have been followed by persistent symptoms. Later arthroscopy, even as early as 2 months, has shown obvious tearing. This was assumed to have existed within the substance, but not seen until exposed to the surface.

Histological observations of torn meniscus

The traumatic tear shows separation of tissue without adjacent tissue degeneration (see Fig. 8-49). If the tear is in the outer one third of the meniscus, biopsies show vascular response and fibrous tissue proliferation on both sides (see Fig. 8-50). The capsular side of a tear has abundant vascularity in its depths and on its surface (see Fig. 8-50, C).

The meniscal side shows very minimal surface vascularity without substance penetration (see Fig. 8-50, B). A fibrous tissue response covers the surface. The tear matures to a fine synovial or fibrous tissue covering with decreased surface vascularity.

Histological characteristics of the degenerative meniscus include loss of cells, decreased staining intensity, and subsequent myxomatous and cystic degeneration (see Fig. 8-53, B and C). Crystalline deposits are evident in some cases.

Classification

Meniscal tears are classified by their etiological nature, age, site, and configuration. The various description choices are listed in the computer-assisted operative report (see Chapter 5) and are illustrated in Chapter 11. The classification assists the surgeon in appreciating the cause, treatment choices, and prognosis.

Response to injury
Natural history

The joint responds to the torn meniscus in a self-protective manner. Pain is produced, which signals the need for protection. If mechanical impingement occurs the joint motion is automatically restricted. If the patient decides to force activity or motion, the meniscus can be displaced to a noncontact area. This occurs with a bucket-handle tear in the notch. A flap tear often rolls under the intact meniscus rim. The meniscus will shrink in size and become rounded on the edges (Fig. 8-54, *A* to *C*). A large fragment that is subjected to repeated intercondylar impingement often separates from a bucket-handle tear into two flap tears, thereby reducing articular impingement.

Small, stable peripheral tears heal spontaneously.

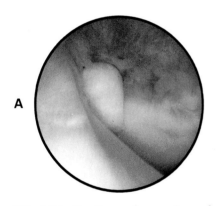

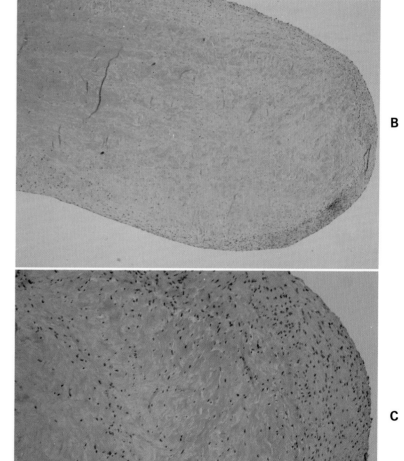

FIG. 8-54. Healing of margins of flap tear.

A Arthroscopic view of flap tear—smooth.

B Photomicrograph of tear shows fibrous avascular covering of surface (Hematoxylin and eosin stain; ×40.)

C Section shows avascular normal meniscus covered with fibrous coating. (Hematoxylin and eosin stain; ×100.)

Meniscal healing

The cellular response to meniscal tear comes from four potential sources: the adjacent synovium, capsule vascularity, intraarticular hemorrhage, and free synovial cells.[1,37,59]

The adjacent synovium contributes angioblastic and cellular tissue for peripheral meniscal tears (Fig. 8-55). The synovium proliferates in the area and "flows" over the meniscus in a way similar to the pannus seen on articular cartilage defects.

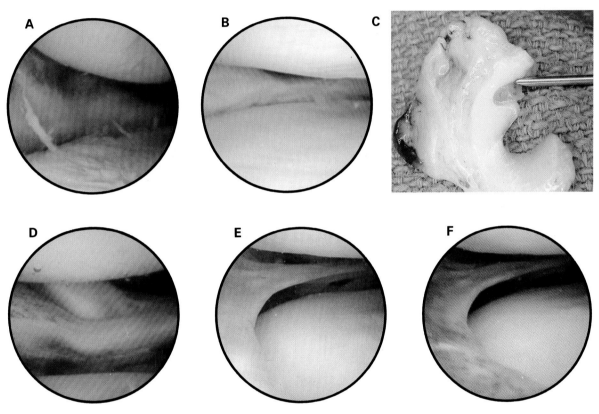

FIG. 8-55.

A Arthroscopic view of arthroscopic total meniscectomy 3 months after surgery. Notice synovial contribution to small regenerated meniscus and mild degenerative arthritis in tibial plateau.

B Ten years after open total meniscectomy. Notice smooth articular cartilage and small regenerated rim from capsular and synovial contribution.

C Experimental lesion produced in dog meniscus showing synovial contribution filling defect at 2 weeks.

D Arthroscopic view of lateral compartment and popliteus tendon shows a regenerated meniscus 2½ months after virtually complete arthroscopic meniscectomy.

E Arthroscopic view taken of regenerated meniscal rim 3 months following total meniscal removal. Tourniquet is elevated.

F Arthroscopic view of patient in **E** but with tourniquet released. At 3 months there is still considerable vascular contribution of regrown fibrous tissue.

Tears within the outer one third of the meniscus have abundant vascularity for hemorrhage and angioblastic proliferation. From the joint capsule (Fig. 8-56, A and B). The potential for peripheral repair is greater for these reasons. The avascular area of the meniscus shows a fibrous tissue healing response 4 to 6 weeks postoperatively (Fig. 8-56, C).

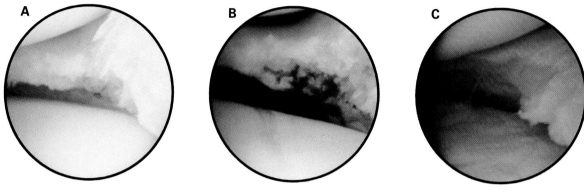

FIG. 8-56

A Arthroscopic view taken at the completion of subtotal or selective arthroscopic meniscectomy. Tourniquet just released.

B After tourniquet release. Notice vascularity coming into meniscus in area heretofore not recognized.

C Arthroscopic view taken 2 months following subtotal or selective arthroscopic meniscectomy. Notice bridge of regrown tissue added to medial meniscus.

Arthroscopic observations have shown an affinity of blood for the resected margin of meniscus (see Fig. 8-56, B). This is observed when a partial meniscal resection accompanies anterior cruciate ligament reconstruction. The joint is decompressed for a time, during the harvest of semitendosus graft. Even under tourniquet control, the joint fills with some blood from the drill holes in the intercondylar notch. After redistention of the joint and cleaning of blood for exposure, inspection of the meniscal margin shows adherence of blood. This occurs within 5 to 10 minutes. The adherence is such that mechanical means are necessary to strip it away. The organized clot on the meniscus is transformed into a translucent inner-margin avascular reshaping of the meniscus. This fibrous tissue also covers irregularly shaped retained posterior horns in cases of free meniscal grafts. My in vitro studies show blood and not synovial fluid contributes to this healing.

Regeneration

Smillie proposed that complete meniscal resection resulted in a better regenerated replica of the meniscus.[74] Complete meniscectomy also removed all of the diseased tissue. This concept prevailed until recent years. I was instructed in this method and probably was one of its last advocates.

A meniscus resected to the periphery will form a triangular replica (Fig. 8-57). It is smaller in all dimensions, softer in consistency, and has no normal meniscal tissue. There is no regeneration of normal meniscal tissue regardless of the extent of resection.

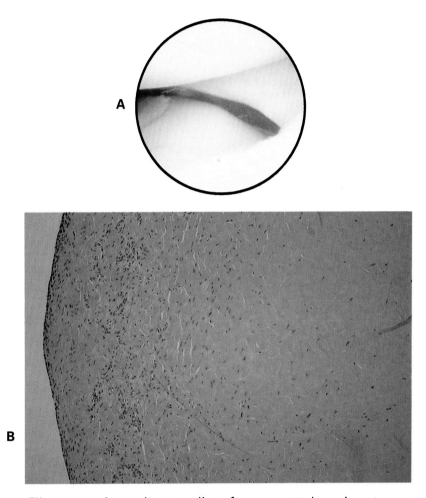

FIG. 8-57. Fibrous repair meniscus replica after open total meniscectomy.

A Arthroscopic view of regrown rim of medial meniscus.
B Photomicrograph of biopsy specimen of inner edges of medial meniscus replica. (Hematoxylin and eosin stain; × 100.) *Continued.*

FIG. 8-57, cont'd. Fibrous repair meniscus replica after open total meniscectomy.

C Higher power shows fibrous and vascular regeneration when resection is near synovial reflection. (Hematoxylin and eosin stain; ×200.)

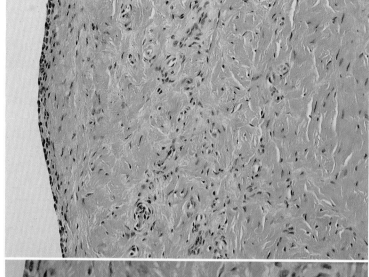

C

D High-power photomicrograph shows synovial margin of fibrovascular body of meniscus replica. This differs from avascular tissue that grows from partial resection. (Hematoxylin and eosin stain; ×400.)

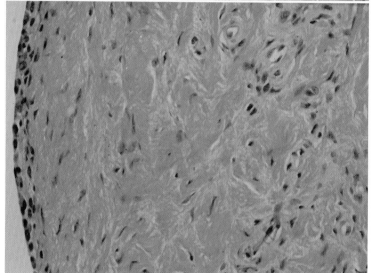

D

E Another patient showed fibrovascular synovial covering of rim of meniscus when all but thin remnant was resected. (Hematoxylin and eosin stain; ×400.)

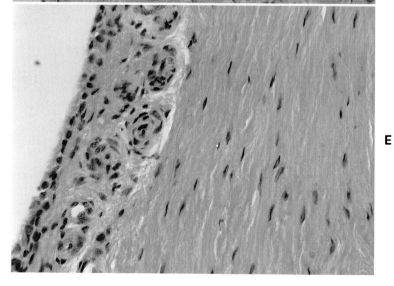

E

Present treatment of meniscus tears includes minimal debridement and maximal preservation of tissue, even resuturing. A total lateral meniscectomy will often redevelop a fibrous bridge in front of the popliteus sheath (see Fig. 8-55, *D*).

Every second-look arthroscopy after total meniscectomy has shown some degree of degenerative arthritis.

Meniscectomy tissue study

Tissues resected by open or arthroscopic surgery provide an opportunity to study the meniscal response to injury and repair.

The bucket-handle tear shows no evidence of vascularity. Serial sections show cellularly inactive tissue with some degeneration (Fig. 8-58). After the gross specimen is resected, representative sections are taken for histological study (Fig. 8-58, *B*). There is no evidence of synovial covering except near the attachment to the joint wall. There is no vascularity; therefore a resutured bucket-handle tear is histologically the same as the free meniscal graft.

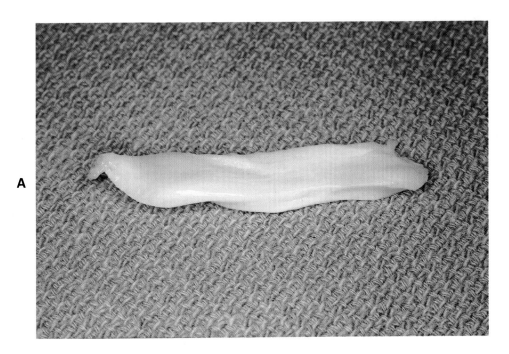

FIG. 8-58. Bucket-handle tear of medial meniscus

A Gross specimen.

Continued.

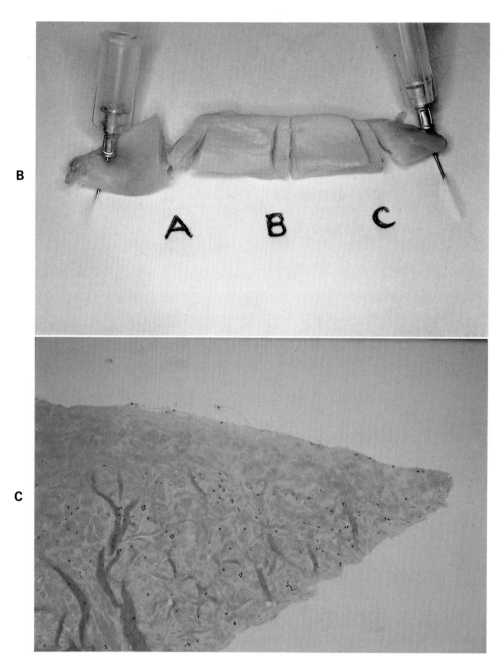

FIG. 8-58, cont'd. Bucket-handle tear of medial meniscus

B Serial sectioning shows no vessels in bucket-handle tear.
C Photomicrograph of lead edge of bucket handle tear. (Hematoxylin and eosin stain; × 100.)

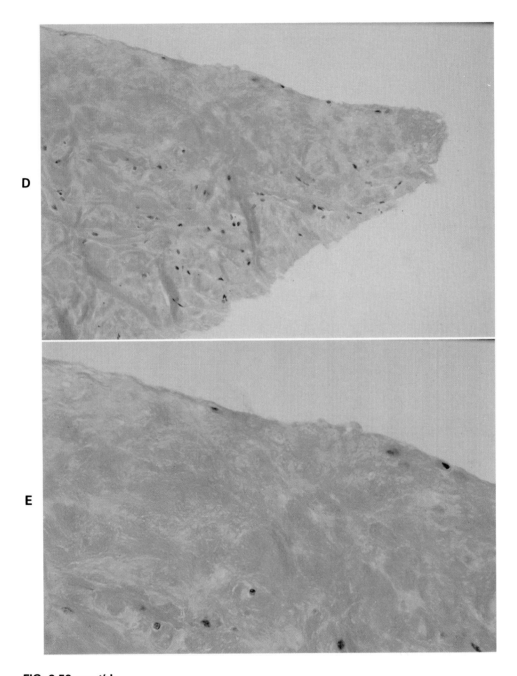

FIG. 8-58, cont'd

D Same specimen without vessels. (Hematoxylin and eosin stain; ×200.)
E High-power photomicrograph of edge of meniscus. (Hematoxylin and eosin stain; ×400.)

Continued.

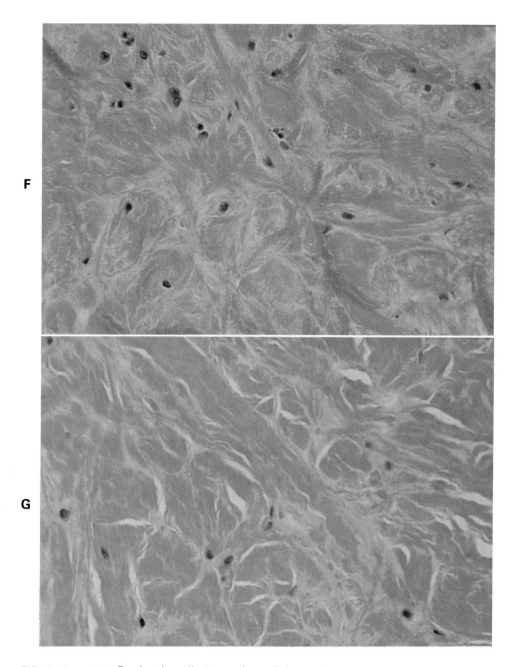

FIG. 8-58, cont'd. Bucket-handle tear of medial meniscus

F High-power photomicrograph of substance of bucket handle tear. (Hematoxylin and eosin stain; ×400.) Notice fibrocartilage without vessels.

G Another section in body of tear shows fewer cells and fibrous tissue separation. (Hematoxylin and eosin stain; ×400.)

Inspection of resected retained posterior horn left behind from open surgery shows vascular proliferation adjacent to the synovial margins (Fig. 8-59) and accellular encasement in other cases (Fig. 8-60).

The inner rim of meniscal healing shows similar tissue attached to the inner margin of the meniscus (Fig. 8-61).

Text continued on p. 620.

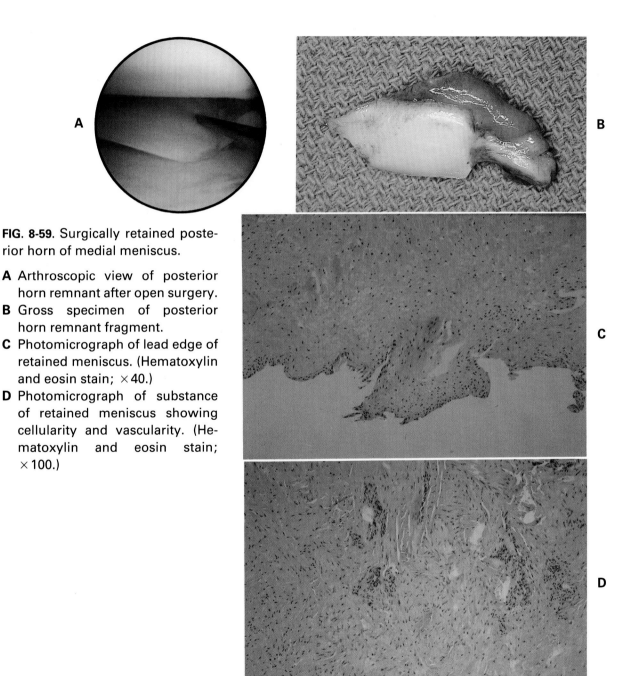

FIG. 8-59. Surgically retained posterior horn of medial meniscus.

A Arthroscopic view of posterior horn remnant after open surgery.

B Gross specimen of posterior horn remnant fragment.

C Photomicrograph of lead edge of retained meniscus. (Hematoxylin and eosin stain; ×40.)

D Photomicrograph of substance of retained meniscus showing cellularity and vascularity. (Hematoxylin and eosin stain; ×100.)

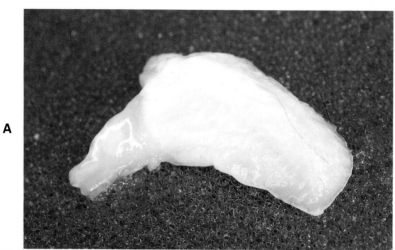

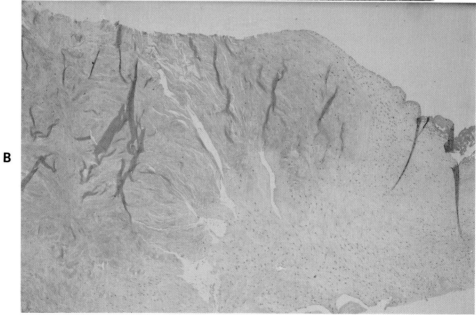

FIG. 8-60. Avascular cellular healing potential of meniscal tissue.

A Gross specimen of surgically retained posterior horn shows encasement with clear fibrous tissue at 2 years after incomplete open meniscectomy.

B Photomicrograph shows meniscus at junction with pale fibrous repair (Hematoxylin and eosin stain; ×200.)

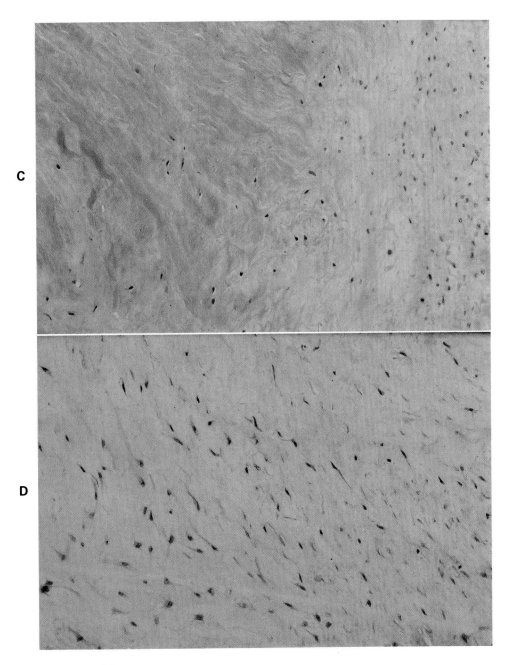

FIG. 8-60, cont'd

C Junction of meniscus and loose avascular cellular repair. (Hematoxylin and eosin stain; ×200.)

D High-power photomicrograph shows loose spindle cells. No increased density within 2 years. (Hematoxylin and eosin stain; ×200.)

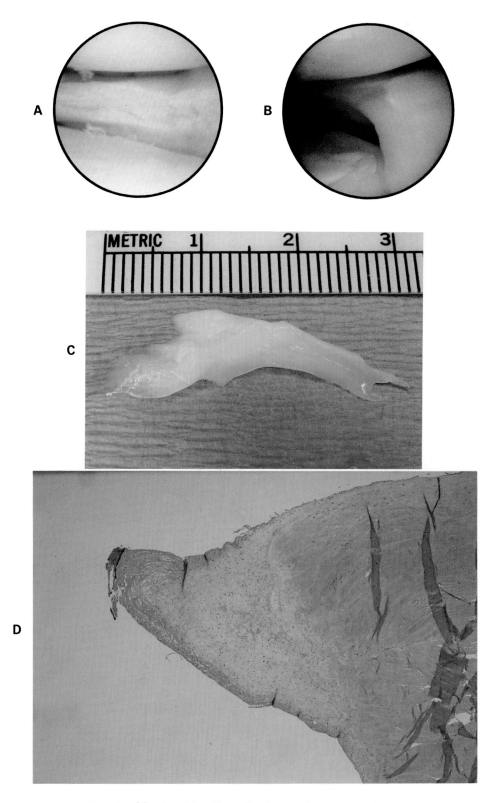

FIG. 8-61. Meniscal healing. For legend see opposite page.

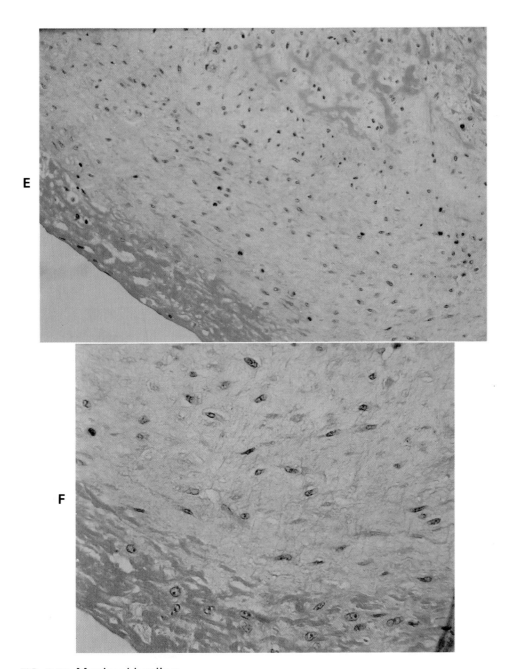

FIG. 8-61. Meniscal healing.

A Arthroscopic view immediately after resection of medial meniscus in avascular area in young person.

B Arthroscopic view of avascular repair of inner margin of medial meniscus.

C Gross specimen of different patient with same avascular regenerated rim attached to avascular area of meniscus.

D Photomicrograph of avascular regrown tissue tip of inner rim of meniscus. Notice meniscal tissue at base. (Hematoxylin and eosin stain; ×40.)

E Photomicrograph shows loose avascular covering of meniscus. (Hematoxylin and eosin stain; ×200.)

F High-power photomicrograph of margin of meniscus edge repair, partial resection. It is loose fibrocartilage with minimal fibrous repair. (Hematoxylin and eosin stain; ×400.)

Factors adversely affecting repair of meniscus

Torn meniscal tissue evokes little cellular response. Cross-sectional histological sections of bucket-handle tears show minimal surface vascular and cellular response at areas of attachment (see Fig. 8-58). The substance attachments and the remainder of the meniscal mass have no vascular ingrowth or cellular response.

As much as 70% of the inner portion of the meniscus is avascular[1] (see Fig. 8-63, *A* and *B*). A tear in this area does not hemorrhage and thus is eliminated a source of inflammatory cells for repair or blood vessels for the possibility of vascular budding. The inner area is also removed from the synovium. Free blood in the joint could attach to the area.

The torn meniscus becomes mobile within the joint. This motion prevents adhesion to adjacent tissue because of repeated mechanical disruption of the vascular and cellular response.

Degenerative changes are common in the area of meniscal tears (Fig. 8-62). The adjacent tissue has decreased cellularity, poor histological staining properties, and even necrotic areas. There are no areas of vascular penetration even in peripheral degenerative tears. Arthroscopic second-looks show no growth of fibrous tissue over exposed areas of resection in degenerative meniscus. This is in

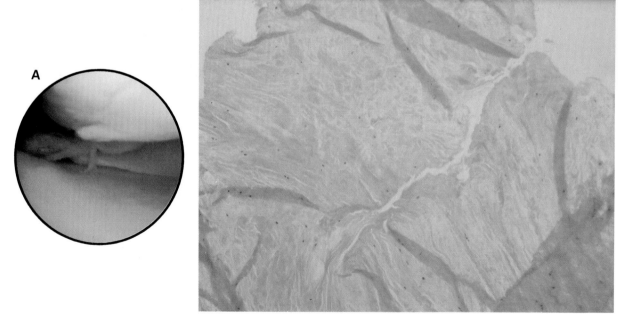

Fig. 8-62. Degenerative tear of meniscus.

A Arthroscopic view of meniscal degenerative posterior horn tear and femoral condyle.

B Photomicrograph degeneration tear shows cleft, decreased cells, no vessels, and no repair. (Hematoxylin and eosin stain; × 100.)

contrast to nondegenerative resected margins that hold blood clots and remodel to achieve a fibrous tissue repair.

Synovitis and effusion produce a hostile environment for collagen synthesis.[44,45] In cases of degenerative arthritis or persistent loose articular debris, no meniscal margin healing is seen on second-look arthroscopy.

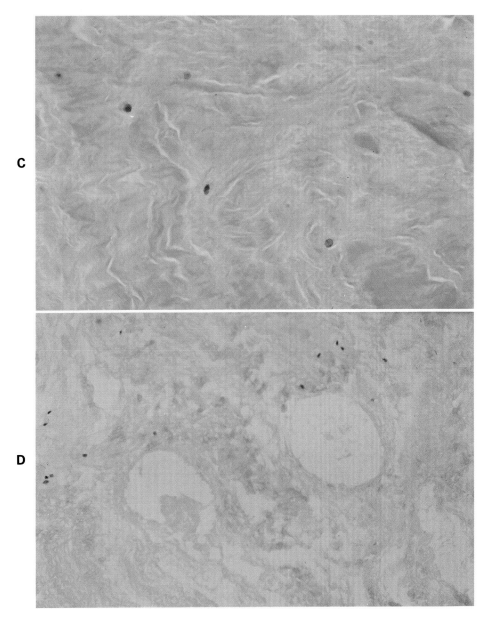

FIG. 8-62, cont'd

C High-power photomicrograph shows decreased cells, fiber separation, and pale staining. (Hematoxylin and eosin stain; ×400.)

D Myxomatous and cystic changes deep in degenerative meniscus (Hematoxylin and eosin stain; ×400.)

MENISCUS REPAIR

Second-look arthroscopy provides the opportunity to compare meniscus lesions and their repair and results. I have performed repairs in the avascular area. If a lesion is well secured to capsule with nonabsorbable suture material in an otherwise stable knee, retear is unlikely. Henning reports repairs in this area with combined open methods and permanent suture material. He has shown fibrous coalition of the surface on arthrography and second-look arthroscopy. His highest failure rate was in the avascular area (43%).

Repairs in the outer one-third of the meniscus result in a fibrous tissue seal of the surfaces as seen arthroscopically (Fig. 8-63, C to E). Core biopsy shows minimal tissue reaction at the area of repair (Fig. 8-64). There is fibrous cell repair with few small vessels. There is minimal collagen formation at the repair state and no vascular or collagen penetration into the substance of the repaired meniscus (see Fig. 8-63, D and E).

The punctures produced by the needles were filled in and smooth with the meniscus surface 12 weeks after the procedure. Exposed nonabsorbable sutures have been covered with translucent fibrous tissue.

On one occasion I had a second look at a vascular access channel of 2 mm diameter. It too was sealed over smoothly with the meniscus surface at the twelfth week. (The tissue in the suture and vascular access channel appeared as

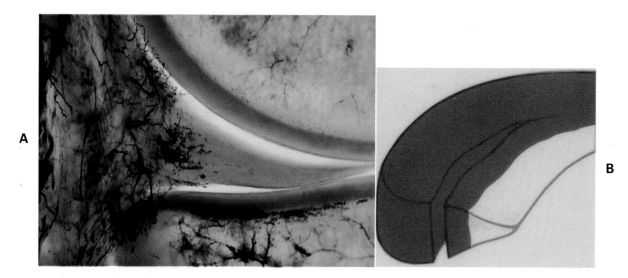

FIG. 8-63. Meniscal vascularity.

A Cross-section of meniscus with India ink vascular injection. Notice extent of vascularity into peripheral margin of meniscus. Notice dye in tibial cortical vascular network. (Courtesy of S.P. Arnoczky, D.V.M., New York, New York.)

B Graphic of torn meniscus in vascular area. Mulholan's concept of red-red tear.

translucent fibrous tissue.) I did not obtain a biopsy specimen. This same patient subsequently suffered a torn meniscus in the area of the vascular access channel.

It will be interesting to learn how far the human vascular access channel brings regrown vessels into the meniscal substance. As to whether vascular access channels are necessary or contraindicated, I am inclined to believe they are both. In both such procedures I performed, the channel was the source of a stress riser and a tear. The meniscus is basically avascular tissue, not requiring or needing vascular penetration.

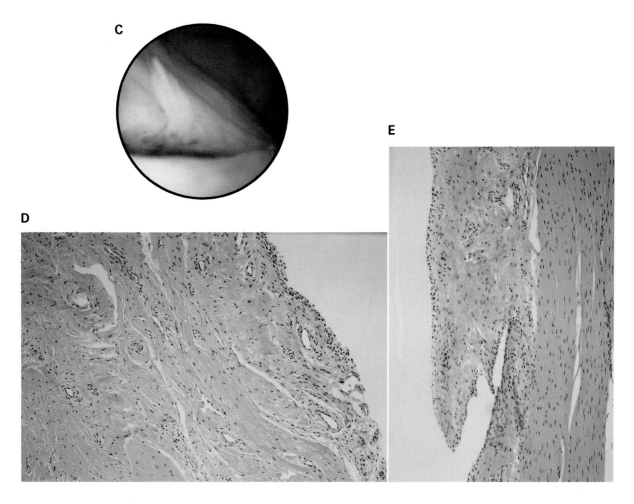

FIG. 8-63, cont'd

C Arthroscopic view of peripheral red-red tear. Posteromedial compartment.

D Photomicrograph of capsular side. Notice vessels. (Hematoxylin and eosin stain; ×100.)

E Photomicrograph of meniscus side showing thin surface layer of regrown vessels and synovium. Notice avascular meniscus fibrous tissue below.

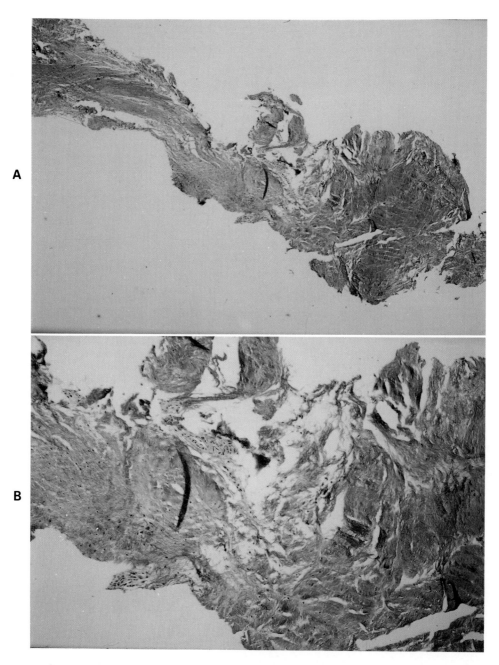

FIG. 8-64. Histological studies of meniscal repair 3 months postoperatively. Biopsy performed at time of anterior cruciate staple removal.

A Photomicrograph of core biopsy meniscus to right, capsule to left. (Trichrome stain; ×40.)

B High-power photomicrograph of repair site. Meniscus to right, vascular capsule to left. (Trichrome stain; ×100.)

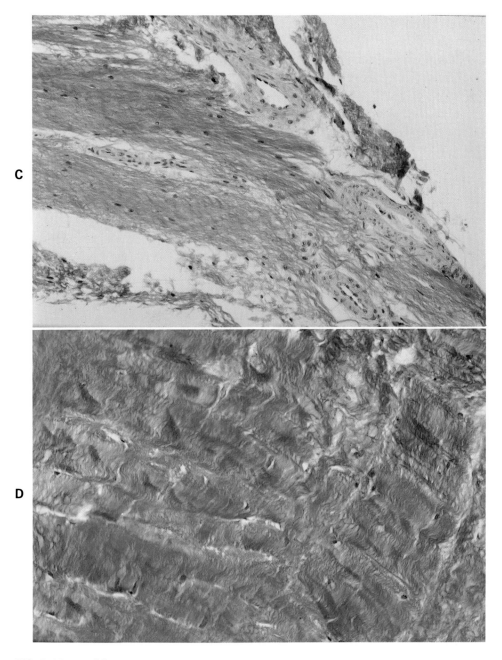

FIG. 8-64, cont'd

C Vascular capsular area. (Trichrome stain; ×200.)
D Avascular, low-cellular, normal dense meniscal tissue. (Trichrome stain, ×200.)

The outer one third of the meniscus heals with vascular and fibrous repair (Fig. 8-65, *A* and *B*). Lesions in the inner two thirds repair with a superficial cellular covering, probably from blood clot (see Fig. 8-56, *C*).

Rotational meniscus grafts were performed to fill meniscal defects. After healing, biopsies showed hypervascularization of grafted tissue. The normal appearing meniscal tissue was invaded by vascularization. They were lacking in firm fibrocartilage mass. It was like a sponge (Fig. 8-66).

The free meniscal grafts show fibrous covering over margins with normal-appearing avascular meniscus at 12 weeks (Fig. 8-67).

Biopsy specimens of free meniscal grafts taken 6 months postoperatively show integrity of meniscal tissue and no vascular penetration. There is synovial covering with vessels at the attachment area (Fig. 8-68). The inner margin is covered with avascular fibrous tissue similar to the repair tissue seen with partial meniscectomy.

Combined clinical and experimental evidence shows that the meniscus tissue is predominantly avascular except at the outer rim in the capsular attachment area. The repair of peripheral meniscus is achieved both by vascular budding and avascular cellular repair.

The area of the repair has neither cellular nor vascular penetration of the reattached meniscal tissue. Histological inspection shows an encapsulation of meniscus with a synovial vascular response at the capsular margin and an avascular cellular covering of the remaining meniscus (see Fig. 11-70). Recent laboratory experiments confirmed that avascular cellular repair contribution is from blood products (see Fig. 11-52).

Avascular meniscus receives its nutrition by diffusion. Attempts at vascularization, as in rotational pedicle graft, change the histological characteristics of the meniscus to hypervascular tissue with loss of fibrocartilage integrity.

It would therefore seem that repairs should not include attempts to vascularize except in the outer margin. Complete vascular access channels have been the sites of two subsequent tears.

Knowing the nonpenetrating nature of encapsulated repair suggests that using permanent suture material in minimal repairs and grafts would be of benefit. This permanent suture would act as internal fixation for repair that does not result in integration of the collagen material of the adjacent tissues. Further observations are necessry to determine the best suture material.

Text continued on p. 632.

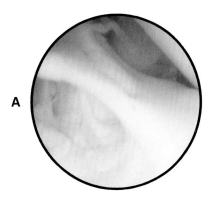

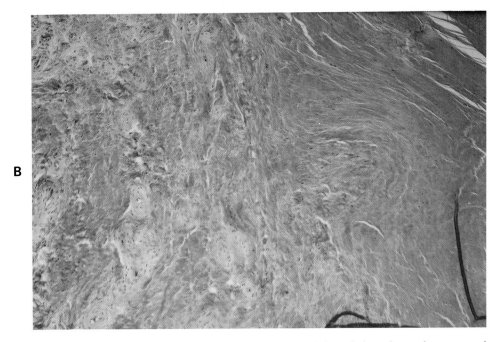

FIG. 8-65. Second-look arthroscopy of posteromedial peripheral meniscus repair.

A Arthroscopic posteromedial view through notch shows repair and transverse fibrous adhesion to posterior wall after 1 year.

B Core biopsy shows meniscus to right (avascular) and vascular (red) repair to capsule. Meniscus is secure without penetration of vascularity into normal meniscus. (Trichrome stain; × 100.)

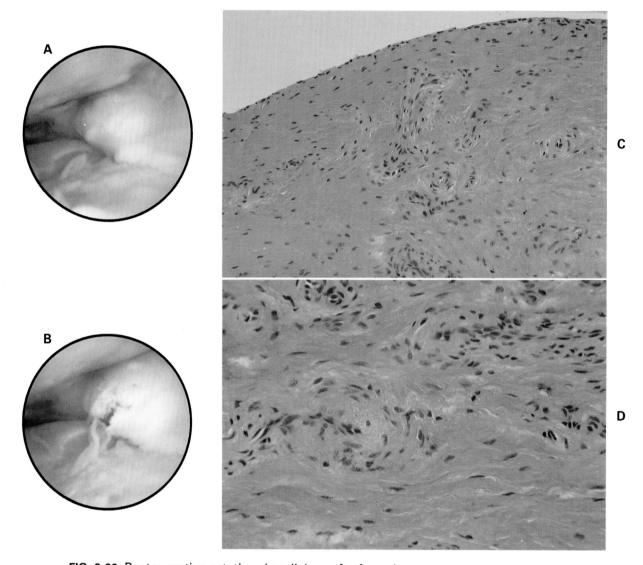

FIG. 8-66. Postoperative rotational pedicle graft of meniscus.

A Arthroscopic view of graft in center within cellular envelope.

B Biopsy site shows bleeding in previously avascular meniscus tissue.

C Photomicrograph of hypervascular meniscus pedicle graft. (Hematoxylin and eosin stain; ×100.)

D High-power photomicrograph shows loss of normal meniscal architecture with invasion of angioblasts. (Hematoxylin and eosin stain; ×400.)

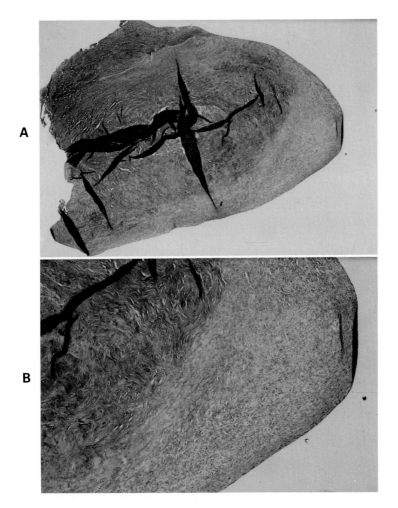

FIG. 8-67. Histological studies of free meniscal graft, 12 weeks postoperatively.

A Biopsy of inner margin shows same acellular repair as posterior horn, meniscal repair in avascular area or bucket handle. (Trichrome stain; ×40.)
B Junction of meniscus graft and repair tissue. No vessels are seen. (Trichrome stain; ×100.)

Continued.

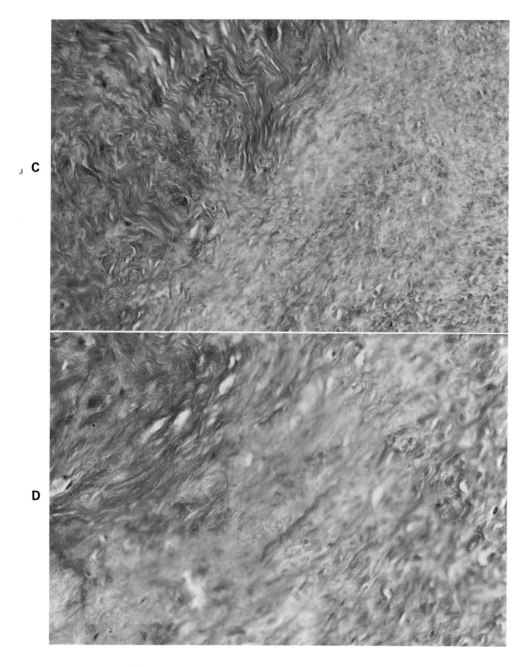

FIG. 8-67, cont'd. Histological studies of free meniscal graft, 12 weeks postoperatively.

C Junction shows avascularity of both areas. Repair tissue is less dense. (Trichrome stain; ×200.)

D High-power photomicrograph of junction shows biological adherence. Note absence of angioblastic contribution to repair. (Trichrome stain; ×400.)

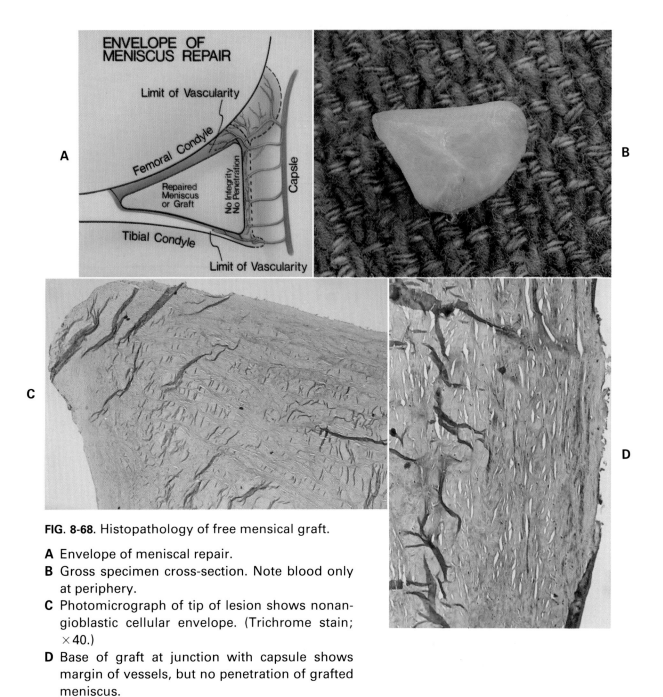

FIG. 8-68. Histopathology of free mensical graft.

A Envelope of meniscal repair.

B Gross specimen cross-section. Note blood only at periphery.

C Photomicrograph of tip of lesion shows nonangioblastic cellular envelope. (Trichrome stain; ×40.)

D Base of graft at junction with capsule shows margin of vessels, but no penetration of grafted meniscus.

Cystic meniscus

A cystic meniscus is most commonly seen on the lateral side (see Fig. 11-46). Rarely, one involves the medial meniscus (Fig. 8-69, *A*). The cyst has both myxomatous and gelatinous cavities (Fig. 8-69, *A*).

Diskoid meniscus

The diskoid meniscus is usually located on the lateral side. It is a broad lesion in the substance in which cleavage tears that look like "pita bread" can be seen. The tears are not seen from the outside and often not discovered until pathologic specimen inspection. Histological sections show fibrous bundle separation (Fig. 8-70, *A* and *B*).

When resected or reshaped, the inner margin heals over with avascular fibrous tissue (Fig. 8-70, *C* and *D*).

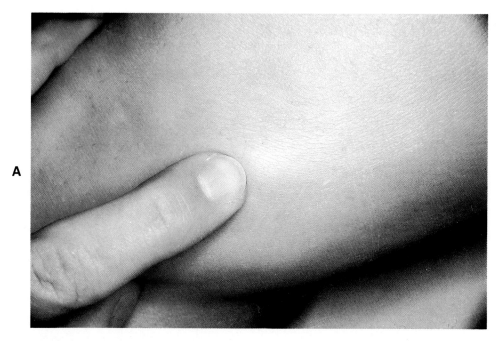

FIG. 8-69. Cystic medial meniscus.

A Clinical photograph of cystic medial meniscus. This site is less common than lateral.

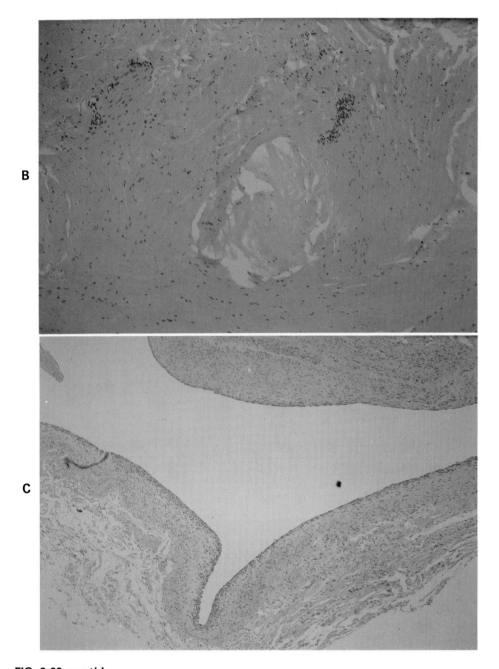

FIG. 8-69, cont'd

B Photomicrograph of cystic changes deep in meniscus—first sign of degeneration. (Hematoxylin and eosin stain; ×100.)

C Low-power photomicrograph of cystic wall. Notice clear, defined synovial lining. Center is filled with ganglion gelatinous material. (Hematoxylin and eosin stain; ×40.)

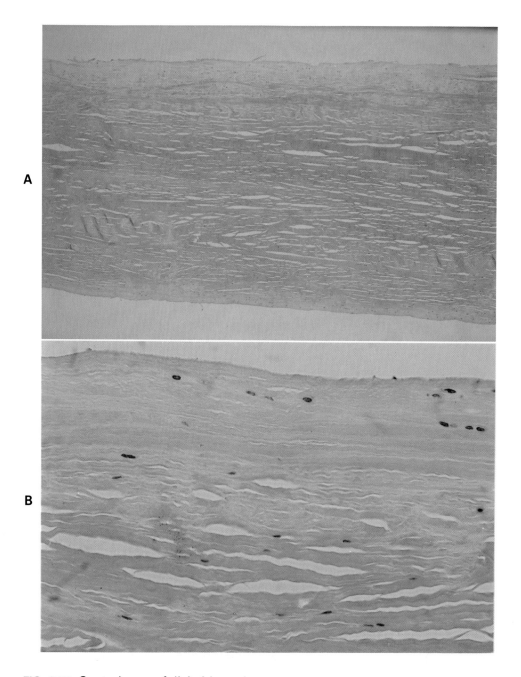

FIG. 8-70. Central area of diskoid meniscus.

A Photomicrograph of resected central area of diskoid meniscus. Notice longitudinal separation of fibrous bundles. (Hematoxylin and eosin stain; ×40.)

B High-power photomicrograph of surface of diskoid meniscus showing fibrous separations. (Hematoxylin and eosin stain; ×200.)

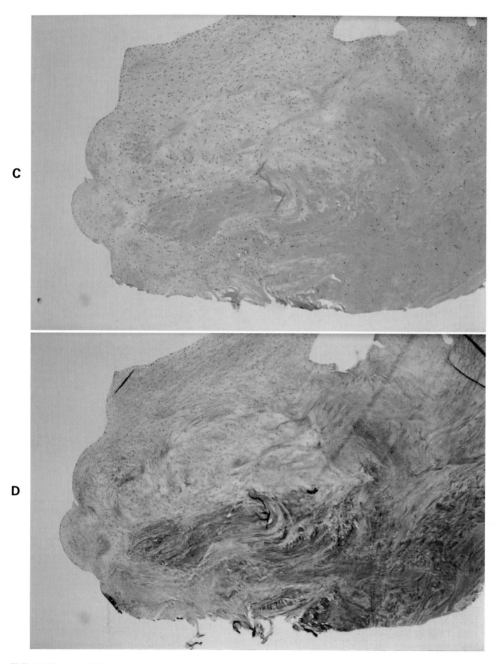

FIG. 8-70, cont'd

C Biopsy of regrown edge of diskoid meniscus done 6 months after resection Notice avascular spindle cell over edge. (Hematoxylin and eosin stain; ×40.)

D Trichrome stain of specimen in **C** shows darker meniscal tissue and nonangioblastic cellular repair.

LIGAMENTS AND TENDONS

The normal anterior cruciate ligament has a synovial and a prominent vascular covering. It receives the majority of its nutrition from diffusion.[63,88] No blood supply enters from either bony attachment.[72] Its histological characteristics are that of wavy collagen bundles with sparse cellularity and minimal vascularity (Fig. 8-71).

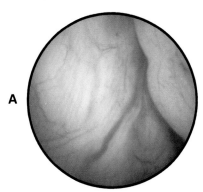

FIG. 8-71. Normal anterior cruciate ligament.

A Arthroscopic view showing vein on surface.

Ligamentous healing is both vascular and cellular in origin. Torn, exposed anterior cruciate ligament evokes a pathological vascular and fibrous response to injury.

The emphasis on replacing vascularity for ligamentous repair has been overemphasized. The nutrition of the anterior cruciate ligament has been shown to be supplied primarily through synovial diffusion.

The hand surgery literature on tendon healing is of interest in a discussion of anterior cruciate ligament grafting procedures with tendon substitutes. The hand flexor tendon, like the anterior cruciate ligament, receives its nutrition by diffusion from the synovial environment.[46-48] Although small vessels exist within and on the surface, little nutrition comes from this source.

Experimentally, a free avascular flexor tendon segment in the synovial sheath or free in the knee joint maintains its viability through 160 days (the length of the experiment).[40,59] There is no necrosis or evidence of this segment acting as a scaffolding for vascular or collagen repair.

The source of cellular repair of flexor tendon grafts is from the tendon itself and from the free synovial cells.[40,47] The original vascularity or subsequent vessels of adhesions contribute little to the nutrition of flexor tendons.[48]

Of further interest is the healing process of implanted tendon to bone.[13,20] A tendon placed in a bone drill hole repairs with hemorrhage and marrow contribution to fibrosis. It is continuous with adjacent bone within 3 months. The histological picture is that of a normal tendon-bone interface: tendon to fibrocartilage to bone.

The anterior cruciate ligament is most available for pathological study and is arthroscopically accessible for biopsy. Injury to this ligament is common. The anatomical and functional complexity of this ligament far exceed its arthroscopic profile.

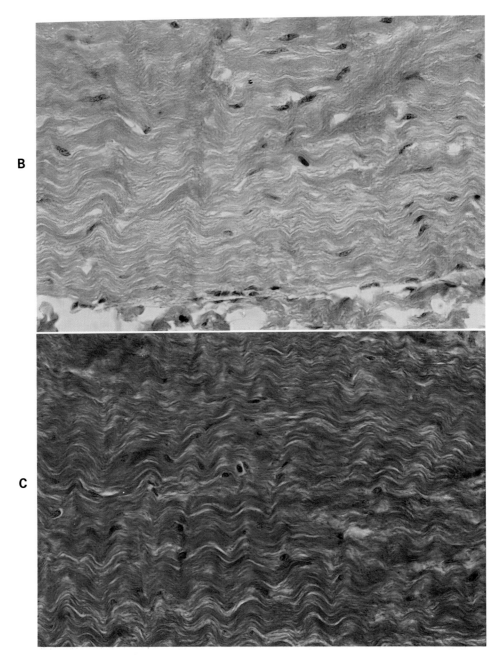

FIG. 8-71, cont'd

B Photomicrograph. Note wave pattern of collagen. (Hematoxylin and eosin stain; ×400.)

C Photomicrograph shows no vessels with special stain. (Trichrome stain; ×400.)

The structure of importance is the anatomical attachment of the anterior cruciate ligament around the posterior cruciate ligament to the inner wall of the medial femur (see Fig. 7-16). This structure along with the common synovial covering of both cruciate ligaments results in the torn anterior cruciate ligament being healed to the posterior cruciate. I have called this "pedicle of the anterior cruciate ligament," because it resembles the surgically created pedicles of skin in plastic surgery. The pedicle has synovial covering, vascularity, and remnants of the original cruciate collagen (see Fig. 8-73).

Acute tear

The tear of the anterior cruciate ligament starts with interstitial disruption. If the tear is interrupted at this stage, the synovium may remain intact. Further stress results in elongation followed by disruption (Fig. 8-72, *A*).

My arthroscopic experience has led me to believe that most tears are interstitial. Elongation occurs, and the tear is near the femoral side. In the past 3 years I have only seen a few tears that did not have arthroscopic evidence to support this process.

These observations were confirmed by a hole drilled through the lateral femoral condyle to the intercondylar notch at the attachment of the anterior cruciate ligament. If a cannula is placed in this transosseous approach and the obturator is removed, the flow of the saline carries the ligament out at its point of attachment. It travels beyond the point that could be anticipated from a midsubstance tear. The fact that elongation occurs before the tear does give a longer fragment. However, if it had been a true midsubstance tear, even with elongation, tissue would be seen going out from both proximal and distal attachments. In fact, this rarely happens. Most of the tissue that is carried out the drill hole with the flow of fluid is secured to the tibial side and flows out through the femoral drill hole. This technique facilitates mechanical repair of the anterior cruciate ligament.

The midsubstance tear has been observed to be the most common area for separation. Torn fragments observed at open surgery appear this way. The femoral-end intraligamentous tear is next in frequency. Occasionally the anterior cruciate ligament tears off the tibia and avulses bone (see Fig. 12-32). This occurs in younger age groups. A femoral avulsion with bone is least common (see Fig. 12-33).

An isolated tear of the posterolateral bundle is common (see Fig. 12-19). I have not seen an isolated tear of anteromedial bundle.

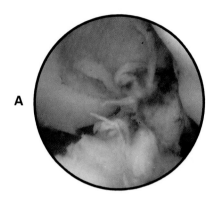

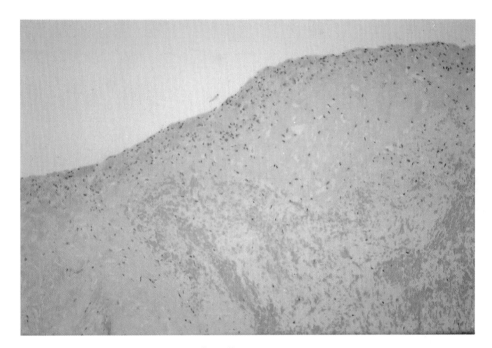

FIG. 8-72. Acute tear anterior cruciate ligament.

A Arthroscopic view of recent tear. Notice hemorrhage.
B Photomicrograph of recent tear with hemorrhage. (Hematoxylin and eosin stain; ×100.)

Continued.

On histological inspection the acute tear shows ligamentous disruption with hemorrhage (see Fig. 8-72, *B*). Contraction and smoothing of the torn ligament occurs in the first week. The end of the ligament may appear as a contracted ball of hemorrhagic tissue (see Fig. 12-19). This is more common with a posterolateral bundle that is anatomically separate from the posterior cruciate ligament connection.

The cellular and vascular response is abundant. Biopsy shows a massive synovial, vascular, and fibrocellular reaction (see Fig. 8-72, *C* to *E*).

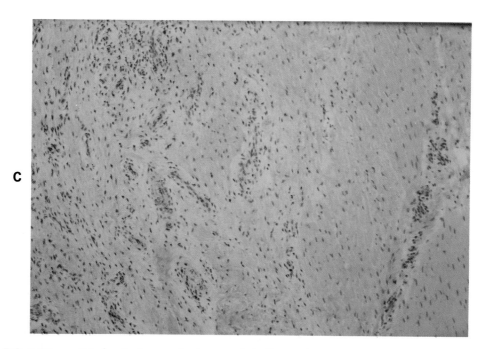

FIG. 8-72, cont'd. Acute tear anterior cruciate ligament.

C Only 1 week after injury, angioblastic activity is visible. (Hematoxylin and eosin stain; ×100.)

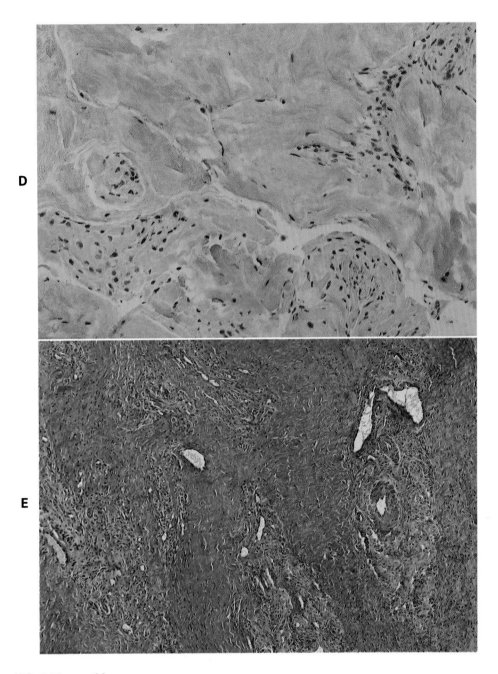

FIG. 8-72, cont'd

D Photomicrograph of 3-week-old tear with vascular penetration between bundles of ligament.
E Trichrome stain shows vascularity (red) between ligament bundles (blue).

Anterior cruciate pedicle

The anatomical juxtaposition of the cruciate ligaments results in femoral attachment tears attaching to the posterior cruciate ligament (Fig. 8-73). The attachment of synovium and anterior cruciate ligament extension restricts distal displacement and contraction. The natural history of most anterior cruciate ligament tears is healing to the posterior cruciate ligament.

Some patients with complete loss of the anterior cruciate ligament attachment to the lateral femoral condyle have a normal physical examination, even while under anesthesia. When the anterior cruciate ligament is attached to the posterior cruciate ligament and to the medial femoral condyle above and posterior, the ligamentous integrity of the knee is maintained.

Arthroscopic inspection from a distance shows a normal-appearing anterior cruciate ligament with a broad-based tibial insertion and normal girth as it crosses the posterior cruciate. Only scope penetration, combined with anterior tibial displacement, identifies the femoral detachment (see Fig. 12-22).

The histological picture is synovium-covered ligamentous tissue showing mature collagenization. The vascularity is diminished, but not to normal levels. There is greater cellularity than normal (see Fig. 8-73).

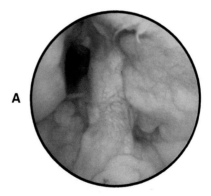

A

FIG. 8-73. Anterior cruciate pedicle attached to posterior cruciate ligament.

A Arthroscopic photograph of pedicle.

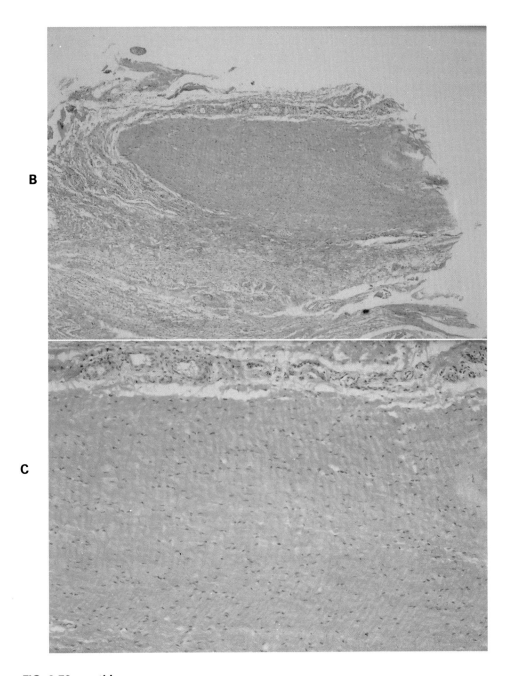

FIG. 8-73, cont'd

B Biopsy pedicle shows anterior cruciate ligament with surrounding synovial vascular envelope. (Hematoxylin and eosin stain; ×40.)

C Photomicrograph of same lesion showing anterior cruciate ligament without vascular invasion. (Hematoxylin and eosin stain; ×200.)

Chronic anterior cruciate ligament tears

Chronic anterior cruciate ligament tears with gross capsular ligamentous disruption become very fragmented (Fig. 8-74, *A*). There is often an accompanying torn meniscus and degenerative changes. The histological picture is gross disruption, fragmentation, disorganization, and decrease in both collagen bundles and cellularity (Fig. 8-74, *B* and *C*).

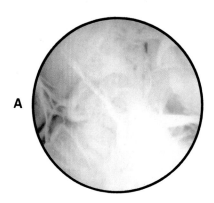

FIG. 8-74. Old anterior cruciate ligament tear.

A Arthroscopic photograph of old tear with degeneration. There is no synovial or vascular response on frayed ends.

B Photomicrograph of old, fragmented anterior cruciate ligament tear. (Hematoxylin and eosin stain; ×100.)

C Disorganization of ligament bundles with necrotic areas and minimal cellular response. (Hematoxylin and eosin stain; ×200.)

Absent anterior cruciate ligament

The most common cause of absent anterior cruciate ligament is its previous surgical resection. I mention this only to condemn resection and to recommend preservation of anterior cruciate ligament tissue. The principles of harvesting remnants of anterior cruciate ligament preserve unique properties for repair. Congenital absence of anterior cruciate ligament is rare (see Fig. 12-30), and other abnormalities accompany the condition.

Histological response to repair

Arthroscopic techniques have provided a means of anterior cruciate ligament repair. Second-look arthroscopy with biopsy has provided insight into the healing process.

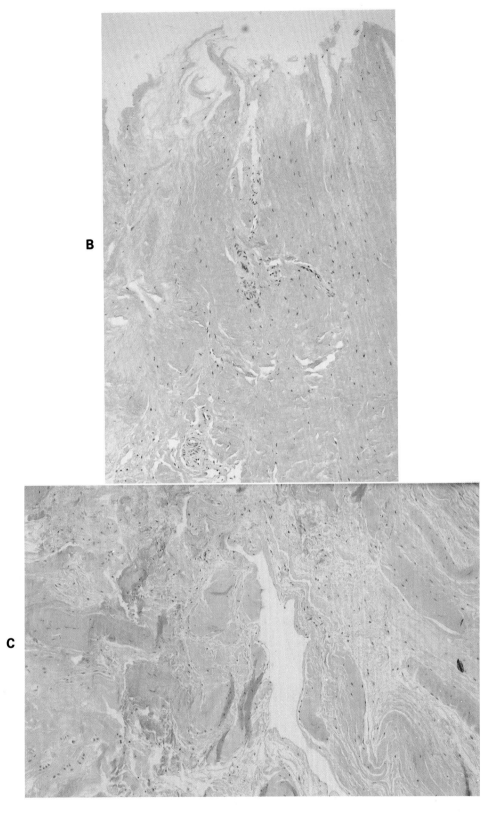

FIG. 8-74, cont'd. For legend see opposite page.

Acute tears

The arthroscopic repair of acute anterior cruciate ligament tears shows an abundance of soft tissue response (see Fig. 8-72, *B* to *E*). A blood clot immediately covers and adheres to the repaired ligament. A synovial covering with fibrous tissue surrounds the repair by the sixth week. Routine staple implant removal in early cases provided the opportunity for biopsy. This was because proliferation of tissue was so abundant that incision in repair tissue was necessary to expose the staple (Fig. 8-75). In some cases the ligament-bone junction was so adherent that resection was necessary to gain increased motion. This occurred at 6 weeks (Fig. 8-76). In three cases strong intraarticular adhesions necessitated lysis and resection to see the repair and provide joint motion.

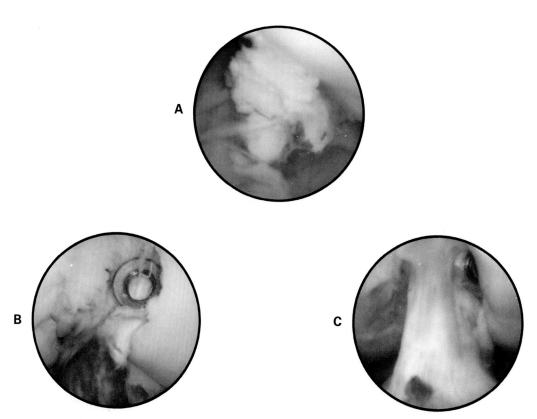

FIG. 8-75. Healing of acute anterior cruciate ligament tear 12 weeks postoperatively.

A Arthroscopic photograph of acute tear.
B Immediate postoperative appearance of tear with staple implant reattachment.
C Postoperative view same patient 12 weeks later.

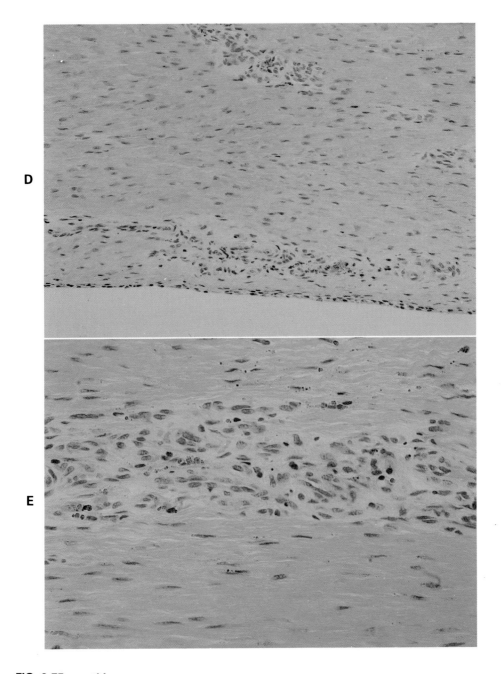

FIG. 8-75, cont'd

D Photomicrograph of biopsy specimen of repair at 12 weeks. Notice blood product and collagen pattern (Hematoxylin and eosin stain; ×100.)

E Higher-power photomicrograph of same patient with collagen bundles and oriented vascular pattern. No synovial invasion. (Hematoxylin and eosin stain; ×400.)

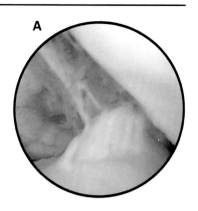

FIG. 8-76. Bone ligament junction 3 months after acute repair.

A Arthroscopic view of repaired ligament.
B Biopsy of junction bone and ligament. (Trichrome stain; ×200.)
C High-power photomicrograph of bone-ligament junction. (Trichrome stain; ×400.)

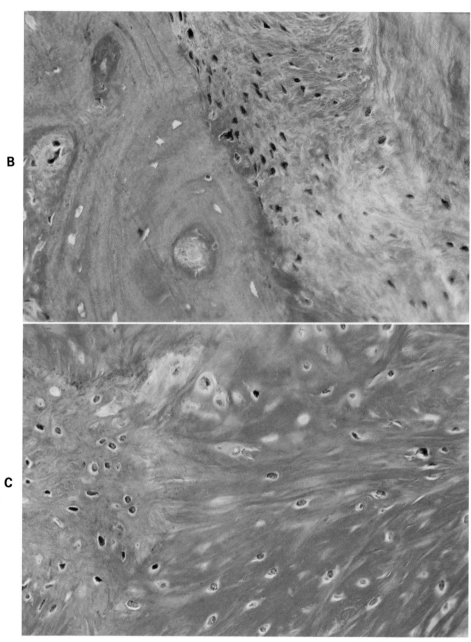

Pedicle graft repair

In patients with low activity expectations, reattachment of the loose pedicle to the lateral femoral wall reduced instability. Second-look arthroscopies and staple removal provided opportunities for biopsy (Fig. 8-77). The acute reaction of osseous debridement provided immediate blood clot covering. A well-defined synovial encasement was seen by 10 weeks.

FIG. 8-77. Postoperative repair of anterior cruciate pedicle.

A Arthroscopic photograph of 10-week-old repair of anterior cruciate pedicle.

B Low-power photomicrograph of biopsy specimen of repair. (Hematoxylin and eosin stain; ×20.)

C Trichrome stain of same specimen as in **B**.

Continued.

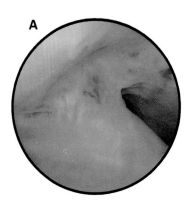

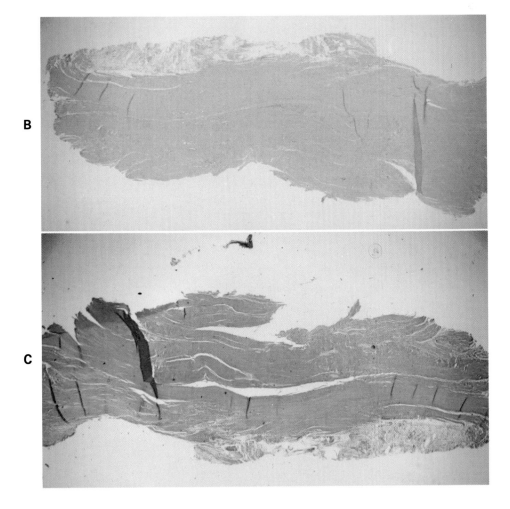

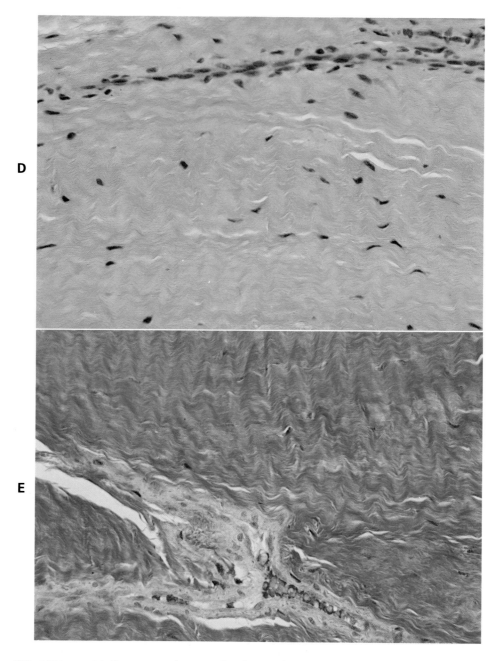

FIG. 8-77, cont'd. Postoperative repair of anterior cruciate pedicle.

D High-power pedicle repair with vessels aligned with collagen. (Hematoxylin and eosin stain; ×400.)

E Special stain shows dense, normal-appearing anterior cruciate ligament *(blue)* with linear vessels along repaired area. (Trichrome stain; ×400.)

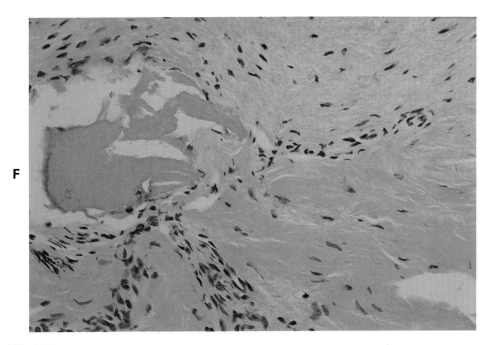

FIG. 8-77, cont'd

F Anterior cructiate pedicle-bone junction 6 months after pedicle repair was done for second injury and tear. (Hematoxylin and eosin stain; ×400.)

The surface adherence to bone was biologically sound but mechanically vulnerable to retear. Retears of pedicle repair occurred with active patients with reinjury, usually in sports. These retorn pedicles were seen to expose bone at the site of detachment. Biopsy during subsequent reconstruction showed mature collagenization with vascularization and recent hemorrhage. The mechanical fault was not in the ligamentous pedicle but in the superficial interface to bone. Deeper attachment into bone was not possible because of lack of pedicle length, unlike tendon grafts.

Semitendinosus augmentation reconstruction

It has been assumed that a free tendon graft would die and serve as scaffolding for revascularization, cellular repair, and collagenization.

Arthroscopic inspection of previously implanted, large-diameter tendon grafts of patellar tendon or iliotibial tract has shown them to be bulky, pale, and loose. Knee joint extension was blocked by the bulk of the graft, and resection was necessary to provide improved motion. The tissue showed large, cystic areas and fibrosis (Figs. 8-78 and 8-79).

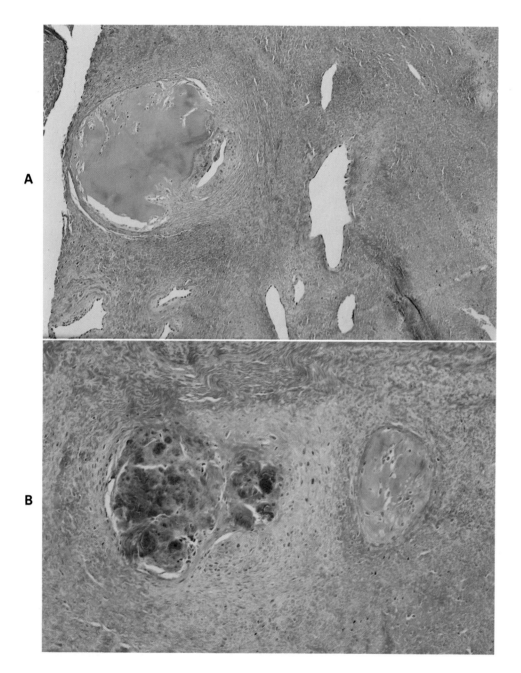

FIG. 8-78. Histopathologic studies of large-diameter tendon grafts after open surgical placement.

A Photomicrograph of vascularized patellar tendon graft. Notice cystic and necrotic areas and absence of linearity. (Trichrome stain; ×40.)
B Closer look at cystic, necrotic areas. (Trichrome stain; ×100.)

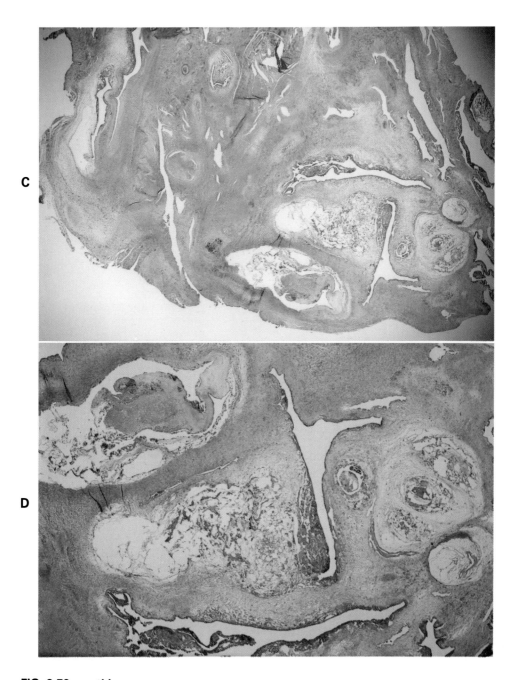

FIG. 8-78, cont'd

C Solid areas of repair still showed degeneration. (Trichrome stain; ×200.)
D Calcific deposits in ligament repair after open reconstruction. (Trichrome stain; ×100.)

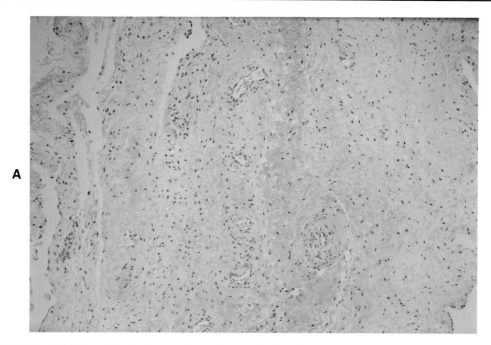

FIG. 8-79. Histopathologic studies of vascularized patellar tendon graft.

A Biopsy of patellar tendon graft shows hypervascularity, disorganization, and minimized collagen linearity. (Hematoxylin and eosin stain; ×100.)

Puddo and Ippolito reported histological inspection of 16-month-old semitendinosus graft to the anterior cruciate ligament.[61] The patient had a satisfactory result until he injured the ligament. Biopsy demonstrated a fibrovascular repair. In light of my observations I doubt if the exact area of semitendinosus graft was examined.

Biopsy specimens taken by Zaricznyj do not show evidence of revascularization or recollagenization.[89]

I have had two cases of semitendinosus double-loop grafts with second-look arthroscopy and biopsy 1 year postoperatively. A review of the operation on videotape showed the exact placement of the grafts. This provided direction for identification of the grafts at the second arthroscopy.

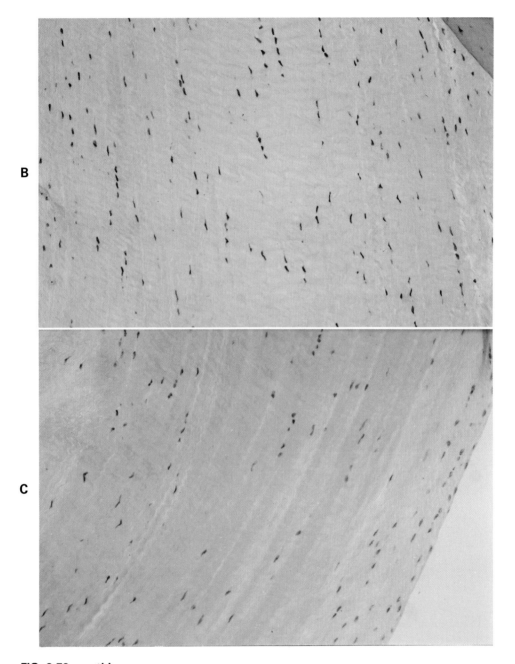

FIG. 8-79, cont'd

B Biopsy of area that looked to be the best ACL graft tissue. Notice linearity and cellular alignment. (Hematoxylin and eosin stain; ×20.)

C Same patient. Biopsy of adhesion for comparison to ACL graft. More densely staining collagen, but similar pattern. (Hematoxylin and eosin stain; ×200.)

On gross examination the notch was seen to have re-formed fibrous membranous ligament (Fig. 8-80, A). Debridement of adhesions above the notch and suprapatellar pouch was performed. Removal of the loose fibrous tissue of the regrown membranous ligament was necessary to see graft (Fig. 8-80, B). In both cases, the cruciate ligament remnants had been sandwiched between the two limbs of the graft (see Fig. 8-80, B).

A 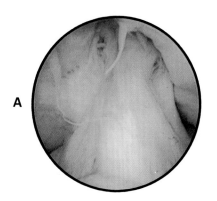 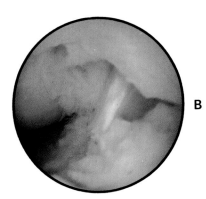 B

FIG. 8-80. Semitendinosus graft of anterior cruciate ligament 1 year postoperatively.

A Arthroscopic view of ligament mass with synovial covering.
B Arthroscopic view with loose synovial tissue removed, exposing graft.

The tendon grafts were relaxed at 90 degrees of flexion. They became tight with anterior displacement of the tibia. There was no restriction of motion in extension. There was a 10-degree loss of flexion. The ligaments lent some support, but not as much as the cruciate tissue that healed in between the grafts. This gave the most integrity to the knee. The grafts were covered with loose areolar tissue and had a yellow-pinkish color.

Biopsy of the medial band in the first patient and lateral band on the second were studied under light microscopy (Figs. 8-80, C and D, and 8-81). Both hematoxylin and eosin plus trichrome stains were used. There was no evidence of necrosis, revascularization, or cellularization. The tendons maintained their viability. Comparison to preoperative semitendinosus remnants showed similar architecture cellularity and paratenon with sparse vascularity. The lateral tendon specimen was taken near the bone attachment and showed more vascularity than the medial midportion biopsy. This should not be surprising in light of the literature on free tendon graft implantation.[13,20]

To summarize, experimental evidence shows that hand flexor tendons, like the anterior cruciate ligament, receive their nutrition by diffusion through synovial pathways.

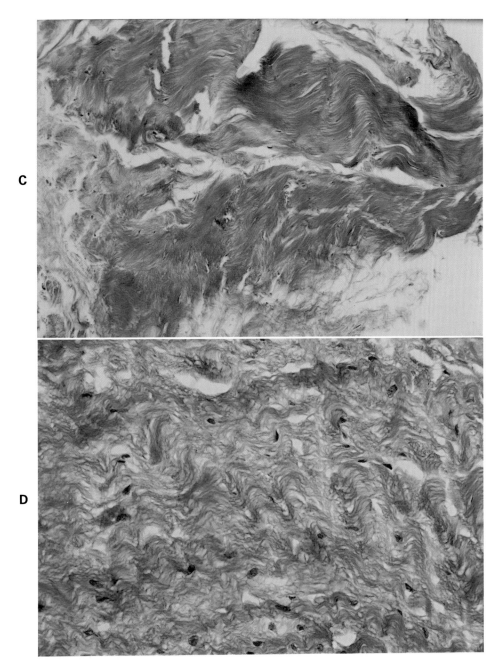

FIG. 8-80, cont'd

C Photomicrograph of biopsy of edge of graft. (Trichrome stain; ×40.)
D High-power photograph shows avascular, viable graft without evidence of re-organization (Trichrome stain; ×400.)

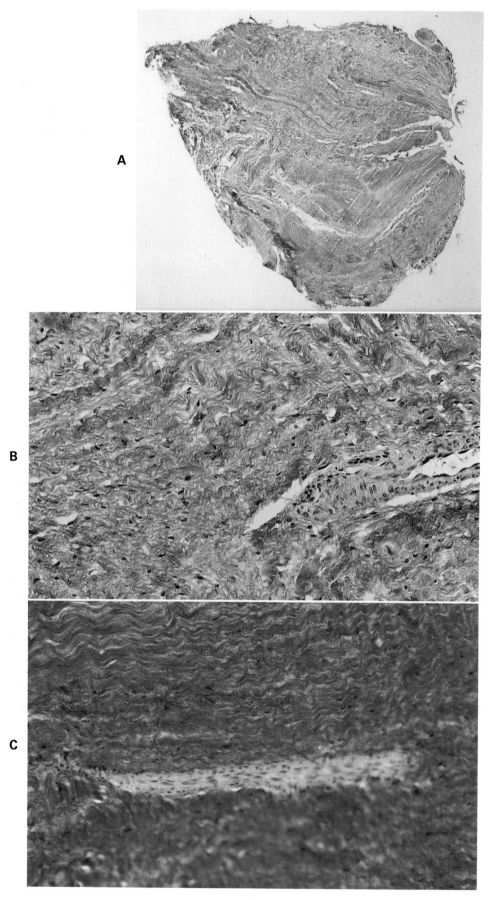

FIG. 8-81. For legend see opposite page.

A free tendon graft does not become necrotic in the synovial cavity.[40,59] Free tendon grafts in fingers remained viable in the absence of blood supply. The profundus tendon segments placed as loose bodies in the dog's knee joint showed smoothing of the uninterrupted surface and cut surfaces.[40] The cellular origin was proposed to be from the tendon (as some segments were enclosed in dialysis bags). Potenza, using 14½-year-old freeze-dried profundus tendon as free bodies in the dog knee joint, showed synovial origin of cellularization.[59] The sheets of synovial cells penetrated into spaces within the previously acellular collagen mass. Free synovial cells contribute to cellularization of these loose bodies. This has implications for other loose bodies as well as cut surfaces of meniscus and articular cartilage.

Lundborg and Rauk,[40] Manske, and Becker have shown that free tendon graft tissue contributes to repair. Becker et al. showed free tendon graft in tissue culture growing into a circular defect in the tendon substance.

There are three sources of free tendon healing: the adjacent adhesions to lacerated ends, the free synovial cells, and the tendon itself.

I theorize that the reason for survival may be related to the smaller cross-sectional diameter of the semitendinosus graft and to its paratenon integrity. The larger mass of tendon from the patella or iliotibial tract has a greater mass for diffusion of nutrients. This may explain the evidence of necrosis and vascular repair with larger grafts.

FIG. 8-81. Semitendinosus graft of anterior cruciate ligament 1 year postoperatively in another patient.

A Photomicrograph of biopsy specimen taken near lateral tibial attachment. (Trichrome stain; × 200.)
B Minimal vascularity appears red. (Trichrome stain; × 400.)
C Dense collagen without evidence of reorganization. Vessels seen near margins and near bone.

Normal tendon-bone junction

The normal tendon-ligament attachment is a transition from tendon via fibrocartilage to bone. A surgically implanted tendon to bone is transformed to the same histological appearance in 3 months.[13,20,87]

The tendon graft into bone forms a blood clot. By 8 days there is a marked cellular reaction. This is followed by osteoclastic activity. By 3 weeks the tunnel is filled with fibroblasts. Bone callus is formed at the same time. At 5 weeks the adjacent fibrous tissue blends into tendon, and at 3 months there is a mature tendon-cartilage-bone interface.

The blood supply of flexon tendor is on the paratenon surface and within the substance coming from bony and fibrous attachments. The terminal input serves only one-third of the tendon. Most tendon nutrition comes from the synovium by diffusion.

Another explanation is that previous biopsies did not isolate the graft areas. In a recent case of massive ankylosis, I resected all tissue except the graft. I found it interesting that all adjacent tissues were very vascular, but the graft itself underneath was not (Fig. 8-82). This further supports the notion that vascularity is lacking in even previously vascularized tendon grafts.

My question is, why perform vascularized tendon graft? Tendon does not normally have vessels. It does not need them for nutrition and does not require them for survival. Furthermore, if a tendon graft is transplanted with vessels, it does not appear to maintain them.

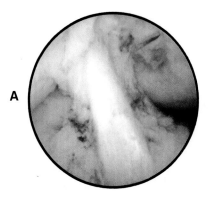

A

FIG. 8-82. Vascularized patellar tendon graft 9 months postoperatively.

A Arthroscopic view of graft after resection of massive scar. Note vascularity of adjacent tissue.

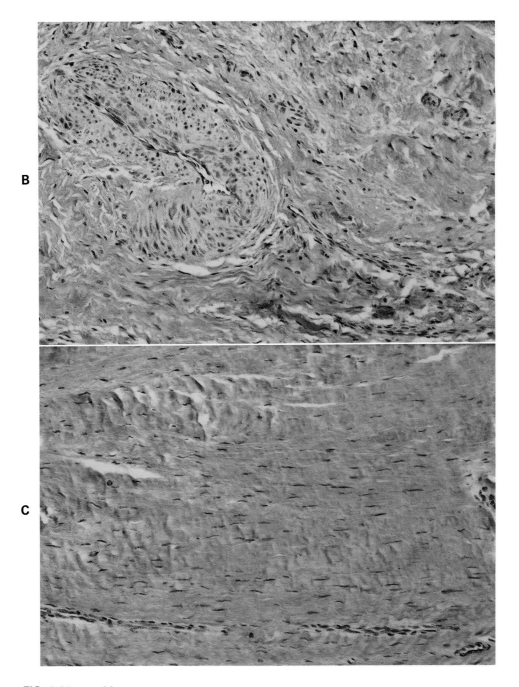

FIG. 8-82, cont'd

B Photomicrograph of paratendinous fibrovascular repair. (Trichrome stain; ×200.)

C Photomicrograph of vascular tendon graft with minimal vessels and no evidence of necrosis or repair. (Trichrome stain; ×200.)

Vascularization

The normal anterior cruciate ligament has no vessels from bone to ligament. The interstitial vascularity is minimal. There are surface vessels in synovium. Much attention has been given to the need for vascular supply to the area of anterior cruciate ligament grafts.

Surgical techniques have been devised to cause synovial covering, even transplantation, of vascularized tendon grafts. I do not understand the rationale for these. Although the normal anterior cruciate ligament has a minimal number of vessels, a torn cruciate evokes an enormous vascular response from adjacent synovium. It seems the issue should be controlling vascularity rather than supplying more. It is acknowledged that anterior cruciate nutrition is nonvascular in origin.

The issue in anterior cruciate ligament substitution should be viability. With maintenance of graft viability, the issues of strength, shear, stress, creep, stretch, and breakage become of less concern. Preservation of existing anterior cruciate tissue provides the source of collagenization.

Augmentation with meniscal tissue

The meniscus has been reported as a substitute for both the anterior and posterior cruciate ligaments.[11,80,85] Clinically, the best use has been with the posterior cruciate ligament in a recent injury with an already irreparably torn medial meniscus.

The advantages of meniscal tissue are its juxtaposition in the joint, its maintenance of viability by diffusion, and its strength. The disadvantages are that the tissue evokes little reaction beyond its synovial covering. Tissue that will provoke a vascular response or collagen tissue is minimal. Sacrifice of the meniscus has its own disadvantages to the knee (see Chapter 11).

I have used meniscus for augmentation only if an irreparable tear existed. I use only tissue that would be excised during the normal course of meniscectomy. This has limited my experience to 2 to 3 mm wide strips of the inner border of the meniscus. I have left the anterior attachment intact. The free end is included with the ligament repair; I consider this a temporary mechanical backup to healing of the ligament. Second-look arthroscopy shows incorporation into the cruciate repair mass and the synovial covering (see Fig. 12-43). I have taken no biopsy specimen.

Mobilization

Patients who are immobilized in casts or inactive because of pain demonstrated fibrous bands from the synovium to the articular surface (Fig. 8-83). Occasionally, transchondylar fibrous bands were seen in the early postoperative repair phase. These were most commonly seen after major open reconstructive surgery and arthroscopic lateral release with extensive disruption of the capsular tissues. Open curettage of femoral lesions demonstrated transchondylar bands from 4 to 8 weeks during any immobilization period.

No patient was on a continuous passive motion program. The patient with minimal injury or morbidity, such as is common with arthroscopic surgery, was able to initiate early active motion and usually to avoid any fibrous articular adhesions.

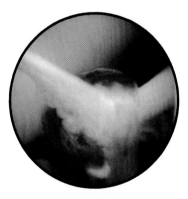

FIG. 8-83. Early fibrous adhesion approximately 6 weeks after arthrotomy. Maturation appears at approximately 3 to 6 months, with fibrosis replacing vascularity.

REFERENCES

1. Arnoczky, S.P., and Warren, R.F.: Microvasculature of the human meniscus, Am. J. Sports Med. **10**:90, 1982.
2. Barrie, H.J.: Intra-articular loose bodies regarded as organ cultures *in vivo*, J. Pathol. **125**:163, 1978.
3. Becker, H., et al.: Intrinsic tender cell proliferation in tissue culture, J. Hand Surg., **6**:616, 1981.
4. Bentley, G., Chondromalacia patellae, J. Bone Joint Surg. **52A**:221, 1970.
5. Byers, P.D.: The effect of high tibial osteotomy on osteoarthritis of the hip, J. Bone Joint Surg. **56B**:279, 1974.
6. Calandruccio, R.A., and Gilmer, W.S.: Proliferation, regeneration and repair of articular cartilage of immature animals, J. Bone Joint Surg. **44A**:431, 1962.
7. Campbell, C.J.: The healing of cartilage defects, Clin. Orthop. **64**:45, 1969.
8. Carlson, H.: Reactions of rabbit patellar cartilage following operative defects, Acta Orthop. Scand. suppl. 28, 1957.
9. Cheung, H.S., et al. In vitro synthesis of tissue specific type II collagen by healing cartilage. I. Short-term repair of cartilage by mature rabbits, Arthritis Rheum. **23**:211, 1980.
10. Chrisman, O.D., Snook, G.A., and Wilson, T.C.: The protective effect of aspirin against degeneration of human articular cartilage, Clin. Orthop. **84**:193, 1972.
11. Collins, H.R., et al.: The meniscus as a cruciate ligament substitute, Am. J. Sports Med. **2**:11, 1974.
12. Convery, F.R., Akeson, W.H., and Keown, G.H.: The repair of large osteochondral defects, Clin. Orthop. **82**:253, 1972.
13. Cooper, R.R., and Misol, S.: Tendon and ligament insertion J. Bone Joint Surg. **52A**:1, 1970.
14. Coventry, M.B.: Osteotomy about the knee for degenerative and rheumatoid arthritis, J. Bone Joint Surg. **55A**:23, 1978.
15. Coventry, M.B.: Upper tibial osteotomy for gonarthrosis: the evolution of the operation in the last 18 years and long term results, Orthop. Clin. North Am. 191, 1979.
16. DePalma, A.F., McKeever, C.D., and Subin, D.K.: Process of repair of articular cartilage demonstrated by histology and autoradiography with tritiated thymidine, Clin. Orthop. **48**:229, 1966.
17. Evans, C.H., Mears, D.C., and Stanitski, C.L.: Ferrographic analysis of wear in human joints (Evolution by comparison with arthroscopic examination of symptomatic knees), J. Bone Joint Surg. **64B**:572, 1982.
18. Farkas, T., et al.: Papain induced healing of superficial lacerations in articular cartilage of adult rabbits, Presented at 23rd annual meeting of the Orthopaedic Research Society, Las Vegas, Feb. 1-3, 1977.
19. Ficat, C.: Les confusions du cartilage articulaire, etude experimetale, Rev. Chir. Orthop. **62**:493, 1976.
20. Forward, A.D., and Cowan, R.J.: Tendon suture to bone, J. Bone Joint Surg. **45A**:807, 1963.
21. Freeman, M.A.R.: Adult articular cartilage, ed. 2, Pitman Medical Publishing, 1979.
22. Fujisawa, Y., Masuhara, K., and Shiomi, S.: The effect of high tibial osteotomy on osteoarthritis of the knee: an arthroscopic study of 54 knee joints, Orthop. Clin. North Am. **10**:585, 1979.
23. Ghadially, F.N.: Fine structure of synovial joints, Butterworths, 1983.
24. Gideon P., Mazeeves, B., and Ficat, P.: La confussion du cartilage articulaire etude experimental et deductions cliniques, J. Chir. (Paris) **1**:115, 1978.
25. Hall, M.C.: Cartilage changes after experimental immobilization of the knee joint of the young rat, J. Bone Joint Surg, **45A**:36, 1963.
26. Harrison, M.H.M., Schajowicz F., and Toueta, J.: Osteoarthritis of the hip: a study of the nature and evolution of the disease, J. Bone Joint Surg. **35B**:598, 1953.
27. Heatley, F.W.: The meniscus—can it be repaired? An experimental investigation in rabbits, J. Bone Joint Surg, **62B**:397, 1980.
28. Henning, C.E., Jolly, B.L., and Scott, G.A.: Arthroscopic intra-articular meniscus repair—healing parameters, Presented at the annual meeting of the American Academy of Orthopaedic Surgeons, Las Vegas, 1985.

29. Hjertquist, S.O., and Lemperg, R.: Histological, autoradiographic and microchemical studies of spontaneously healing osteochondral articular defects in adult rabbits, Calc. Tiss. Res. **8**:54, 1971.

30. Hotchkiss, R.N., Tew, W.P., and Hungerford, D.S.: Cartilaginous debris in the injured human knee (correlation with arthroscopic findings) Clin. Orthop. **168**:144, 1982.

31. Hulth, A., Lindberg, L., and Techag, H.: Mitosis in human osteoarthritic cartilage, Clin. Orthop. **84**:197, 1972.

32. Insall, J.N.: Intra-articular surgery for degenerative arthritis of the knee: a report of the work of the late K.H. Pridie, J. Bone Joint Surg. **49B**:211, 1967.

33. Insall, J.N.: The Pridie debridement operation of osteoarthritis of the knee, Clin. Orthop. **101**:61, 1974.

34. Jaffe, H.L.: Metabolic degenerative and inflammatory disease of bones and joints, Philadelphia, 1972, Lea & Febiger, 735.

35. Kelley, F.W.: Personal communication, 1982–85.

36. Kewpson, G.E., et al.: Correlations between stiffness and chemical constituents of the human femoral head, Biochem. Biophys. Acta **215**:70, 1970.

37. King, D.: The healing of semilunar cartilage, J. Bone Joint Surg. **18B**:333, 1936.

38. Landells, J.W.: The reaction of injured human articular cartilage, J. Bone Joint Surg. **45B**:150, 1957.

39. Lemperg, R.: Can articular cartilage heal? In Peckett, J.C., and Radin, E.L.: Chondromalacia of the patella, Baltimore, 1983, Williams & Wilkins.

40. Lundborg, G. and Rank, F.: Experimental studies on cellular mechanisms involved in healing of animal and human flexor tendon in synovial environment, The Hand, **12**:3, 1980.

41. Magnusson, P.B.: Technique of debridement of the knee joint for arthritis, Surg. Clin. North Am. **26**:249, 1976.

42. Mankin, H.J.: The response of articular cartilage to mechanical injury, J. Bone Joint Surg. **64A**:460, 1982.

43. Mankin, H.J.: Localization of tritiated thymidine in articular cartilage of rabbits. I. Growth in immature cartilage, J. Bone Joint Surg. **44A**:682, 1962.

44. Mankin, H.J.: The reaction of articular cartilage to injury and osteoarthritis (first of two parts), N. Engl. J. Med. **291**:1285, 1974.

45. Mankin, H.J.: The reaction of articular cartilage to injury and osteoarthritis (second of two parts), N. Engl. J. Med. **291**:1335, 1974.

46. Manske, P.R., and Lesker, P.A.: Nutrient pathways of flexor tendons in primates, J. Hand Surg. **7**:436, 1982.

47. Manske, P.R., Lesker, P.A., and Bondwell, K.: Experimental studies in chickens on the initial nutrition of tendon grafts J. Hand Surg. **4**:565, 1979.

48. Manske, P.R., Whiteside, L., and Lesher, P.A.: Nutrient pathways to flexor tendons using hydrogen washout technique, J. Hand Surg. **3**:32, 1978.

49. McDersitt, C.A., and Muir, H.: Biochemical changes in the cartilage of the knee in experimental and natural osteoarthritis in the dog, J. Bone Joint Surg. **58B**:94, 1976.

50. Meachim, G.: The state of knee meniscal fibrocartilage in Liverpool necropsics, J. Pathol. **119**:167, 1976.

51. Meachim, G., and Osborn, G.V.: Repair of the femoral articular cartilage surface in osteoarthritis of the hip, J. Pathol. **102**:1, 1970.

52. Meachim, G., and Roberts, C.: Repair of the joint surface from subarticular tissue in the rabbit knee, J. Anat. **109**:317, 1971.

53. Milgram, J.W., The classification of loose bodies in human joints, Clin. Orthop. **124**:282, 1977.

54. Mindell, E.R.: Personal communication, 1982.

55. Mitchell, N., and Shepard, N.: The resurfacing of adult rabbit articular cartilage by multiple perforations through subchondral bone, J. Bone Joint Surg. **58A**:230, 1976.

56. Mori, Y.: Debris observed by arthroscopy of the knee, Orthop. Clin. North Am. **10**:559, 1979.

57. Nole, R., Munson, N.M.L., and Fulherson, J.P.: Bupivacaine and saline effects on articular cartilage, Arthroscopy **1**:123, 1985.

58. O'Connor, R.L.: The arthroscope in management of crystalline induced synovitis of the knee, J. Bone Joint Surg. **55A:**1443, 1973.

59. Potenza, A.D., and Herte, M.C.: The synovial cavity as a "tissue culture in situ:" science or nonsense, J. Hand Surg. **7:**196, 1982.

60. Pridie, K.W.: A method of resurfacing osteoarthritic knee joints, J. Bone Joint Surg. **41B:**618, 1959.

61. Puddu, G., and Ippolito, E.: Reconstruction of the anterior cruciate ligament using the semitendonosis tendon: histological study of a case, Am. J. Sports Med. **11:**14, 1983.

61a. Radin, E.L., and Burr, D.B.: Hypothesis: joints can heal, Sem. Arthritis Rheum. **13**(3), 1984.

62. Reagan, B.F., et al.: Irregating solutions for arthroscopy, J. Bone Joint Surg. **65A:**629, 1983.

63. Renzoni, S.A., et al.: Synovial nutrition of knee ligaments, Orthop. Trans. Orthop. Res. Soc., **8:**(2), 1984.

64. Repo, R.U., and Finlay, J.B.: Survival of articular cartilage after controlled impact., J. Bone Joint Surg. **59A:**1068, 1977.

65. Repo, R.U., and Mitchel, N.: Collagen synthesis in mature cartilage of the rabbit, J. Bone Joint Surg. **53B:**541, 1971.

66. Richmond, J.C., et al.: A canine model of osteoarthritis with histologic study of repair tissue following abrasion arthroplasty, Presented at the annual meeting of the Arthroscopy Association of North America, Boston, April 1985.

67. Rosenberg, L.: Chemical basis for the histological use of safranin-O in the study of articular cartilage, J. Bone Joint Surg. **53A:**69, 1971.

68. Ryan, L.M., and McCarty, D.J.: Calcium pyrophosphate crystal deposition disease; pseudogout: articular chondrocalcinosis. In McCarty, D.J., ed.: Arthritis and allied conditions, Philadelphia, 1985, Lea and Febiger.

69. Salter, R.B., and Field, P.: The effects of continuous compression on living articular cartilage: an experimental investigation, J. Bone Joint Surg. **42A:**31, 1960.

70. Salter, R.B., McNeill, O.R., and Carbin, R.: Pathological changes in articular cartilage associated with persistent joint deformity, an experimental investigation. In Studies of rheumatoid disease: proceedings of the Third Canadian Conference on the Rheumatic Diseases, Toronto, Canada, 1965.

71. Salter, R.B., et al.: The biological effect of continuous passive motion on the healing of full thickness defects in articular cartilage: an experimental investigation in the rabbit, J. Bone Joint Surg. **62A:**1232, 1980.

72. Scapinelli, R.: Studies of the vasculature of the human knee joint, Acta Anat. (Basel) **70:**305, 1968.

73. Simmons, D.P., and Chrisman, O.D.: Salicylate inhibition of cartilage degeneration, Arthritis Rheum. **8:**960, 1965.

74. Smillie, I.S.: Injuries of the knee joint, ed. 4, London, 1975, Churchill Livingstone.

75. Smith-Petersen, M.N.: Arthroplasty of the hip: a new method, J. Bone Joint Surg. **21:**269, 1939.

76. Smith-Petersen, M.N.: Evolution of mould arthroplasty of the hip joint, J. Bone Joint Surg. **30B:**59, 1948.

77. Sokaloff, L.: The joints and synovial fluid, 2 vols., New York, 1980, Academic Press.

78. Tanaka, H.: Proceedings: an experimental study on the influence of immobilization on the knee joint after removal of articular cartilage, Calcif. Tissue Res. **15:**165, 1974.

79. Telhag, H.: Mitosis of chondrocytes in experimental "osteoarthritis" in rabbits, Clin. Orthop. **86:**224, 1972.

80. Tillburg, B.: The late repair of torn cruciate ligaments using meniscus, J. Bone Joint Surg. **59B:**15, 1977.

81. Trias, A.: Effect of persistant pressure on articular cartilage: an experimental study, J. Bone Joint Surg. **43B:**376, 1961.

82. Troyer, H.: A microspectophotometric study of metachromasia, J. Histochem. Cytochem. **22:**1118, 1974.

83. Troyer, H.: The effect of short-term immobilization on the rabbit knee joint cartilage: a histochemical study, Clin. Orthop. **107:**249, 1975.

84. Urist, M.R.: The repair of articular surfaces following arthroplasty of the hip, Clin. Orthop. **12:**209-229, 1958.

85. Walsh, J.J.: Meniscal reconstruction of the ACL, Clin. Orthop. **89:**171, 1972.

86. Weiss, C.: Normal and osteoarthritic articular cartilage, Orthop. Clin. North Am. 1979, **10:**175, 1979.

87. Whiston, T.B., and Walmsley, R.: Some observations on the reaction of bone and tendon after tunnelling of bone and insertion of tendon, J. Bone Joint Surg. **42B:**377, 1960.

88. Whiteside, L.A., and Sweeny, R.E., Jr.: Nutrient pathways of the cruciate ligaments, J. Bone Joint Surg. **62A:**1176, 1980.

89. Zaricznyj, B.: Reconstruction of anterior cruciate ligament using free tendon graft, Am. J. Sports Med. **11:**164, 1983.

90. Zarins, B., and McInerney, V.K.: Calcium pyrophosphate and pseudogout, Arthroscopy **1:**8, 1985.

Index